AF412491

# BIOMEDICAL SENSORS

# BIOMEDICAL SENSORS

EDITED BY
**DERIC P. JONES**

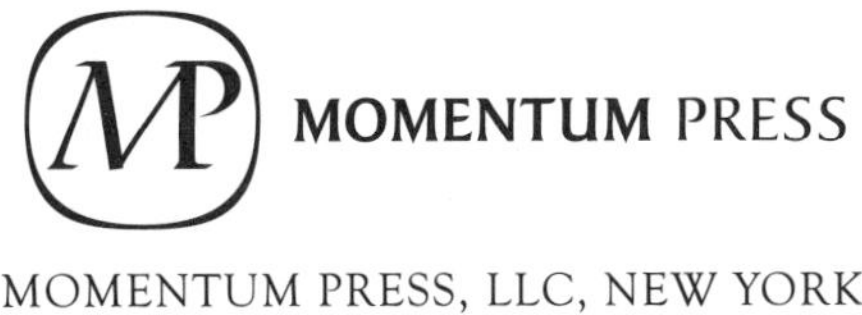

MOMENTUM PRESS, LLC, NEW YORK

Biomedical Sensors
Copyright © Momentum Press®, LLC, 2009

All rights reserved. No part of this publication may be reproduced, stored in a retrieval system, or transmitted in any form or by any means—electronic, mechanical, photocopy, recording or any other except for brief quotations, not to exceed 400 words, without the prior permission of the publisher

First published in 2010 by
Momentum Press®, LLC
222 East 46th Street, New York, N.Y. 10017
www.momentumpress.net

ISBN-13: 978-1-60650-056-9 (hard back, case bound)
ISBN-10: 1-60650-056-2 (hard back, case bound)

ISBN-13: 978-1-60650-058-3 (e-book)
ISBN-10: 1-60650-058-9 (e-book)

DOI forthcoming

A publication in the Sensors Technology series, edited by Joe Watson, PhD, published by Momentum Press®, LLC

Cover Design by Jonathan Pennell
Interior Design by Scribe, Inc. (www.scribenet.com)

First Edition: October 2010

10 9 8 7 6 5 4 3 2 1

Printed in Taiwan

# CONTENTS

# SENSORS TECHNOLOGY SERIES
# EDITOR-IN-CHIEF'S PREFACE

In recent years the interface between the life sciences and the physical sciences has become inhabited by researchers and practitioners with knowledge and expertise in both areas. This is a very welcome trend because traditionally it has been difficult for the physical scientist to appreciate the needs of the life scientist or medical practitioner, and equally difficult for the biomedical community to ascertain what might be possible in physical terms. Happily, this gulf is rapidly being filled. In particular, the development of instruments based on physical, chemical, and biological principles has burgeoned. Inevitably, as with all things, there are downsides, the predominant one in the medical context being related to cost, which for some installations can represent several millions of dollars.

However, rather more modest analytical instruments require sensors of various types as well, and this volume presents a selection of these, complete with detailed background material on the scientific and technical principles relevant to each. Such multifaceted work represents a major ongoing international endeavor and, as such, merits more comprehensive bibliographical material than do some of the more mature topics in other volumes of the series. The descriptive material and relevant bibliographies in the present compilation have been provided by an author list of leading scientists in their various specialties assembled by the volume editor, Deric Jones, who has drawn upon his experience as Head of Medical Electronics & Physics at the Medical School of St. Bartholomew's Hospital in the University of London. These authors have in turn drawn upon their own experiences to present authoritative reviews of sensors ranging from basic devices for measuring temperature and flow, through both ionizing and nonionizing radiation, to transducers for ultrasound, chemical, and biological sensing.

J. Watson
Editor-in-Chief
July 2010

## ABOUT THE EDITOR-IN-CHIEF

**Joseph Watson** is an electrical engineering graduate of the University of Nottingham, England, and the Massachusetts Institute of Technology. He has published books and papers in various areas including electronic circuit design, nucleonics, biomedical electronics, and gas sensors and has been a visiting professor at the University of Calgary, Canada, and the University of California, Davis and Santa Barbara. Dr. Watson has held various consultancies with firms in the United States, Canada, and Japan and since retirement from the University of Wales, Swansea, has continued as chairman of the UK-based Gas Analysis and Sensing Group and as editor-in-chief for the Sensors Technology Series for Momentum Press.

# PREFACE

## BACKGROUND

In 400 B.C. the Greek physician Hippocrates placed his hand on a patient's forehead and used the sense of touch to estimate body temperature. The five human senses were effectively the only sensors available to the "father of medicine" and his descendents until the seventeenth century when the first objective biomedical sensor in the form of a crude thermometer was devised. However, it was only toward the end of the nineteenth century that developments in science made possible significant advances in biomedical sensor technology. The twentieth century and the modern era of biomedical technology may have been ushered in when, in November 1895, Wilhelm Röntgen astonished the medical profession and the world with an X-ray image of his wife's hand that he obtained using photographic film as a sensor. Twenty-four centuries after Hippocrates, sensors now extend the range of human senses to make possible diagnostic and therapeutic techniques that the ancient Greeks could never have envisioned. Almost all modern biomedical measurement and imaging systems depend upon sensors of one kind or another, although in many cases they are not immediately evident, often being hidden deep within the medical instrument. Today it is quite common for there to be a number of sensors embedded within the same medical device; for example, the ubiquitous hospital blood gas analyzer will routinely incorporate more than half a dozen sensors, one for each gas and substance to be analyzed.

## WHAT IS A SENSOR?

The broadest and simplest definition of a *sensor* is "anything that responds to an input of interest." However, a general-purpose dictionary definition is "a device that detects or measures some condition or property and records, indicates, or otherwise responds to the information received." Although this is an excellent everyday definition, for biomedical engineering and medical physics purposes it is too imprecise. A device that merely "detects some condition or property," presumably by registering the presence or absence of a physical quantity with a simple yes-or-no response, would be called a "detector," not a sensor. Although detectors have important uses in medicine, especially as the basis of alarms, they are not generally regarded as sensors. For practical biomedical applications a *sensor* is better defined as "*a device that responds to a physical input of interest with a recordable functionally related output that is usually electrical or optical.*" In a biomedical context, of course, the term *physical input* is taken to include chemical and biochemical quantities and concentrations. A device with an electrical output satisfies the "records or indicates" criterion in the general dictionary definition because electrical signals can be amplified and processed readily to give a display on a monitor, an output on a chart recorder, or an input to a digital data storage system. Sometimes a sensor's optical output signals *are* the required output—in imaging, for example—but any optical output signal can usually be converted fairly easily into an electrical signal by means of a photosensor.

It is the requirement that the output be *functionally related* to the physical quantity of the input that distinguishes a sensor from a yes–no detector. The most desirable functional relationship is a simple linear one, whereby a doubling of the input physical quantity results in a doubling of the electrical or optical output. Such a relationship usually leads to a relatively simple calibration procedure. Unfortunately, many common and widely utilized sensors do not exhibit such linear behavior— a thermistor for temperature measurement, for example—but nevertheless they can still be made into useful practical devices by using suitable, if more elaborate, calibration methods (see Chapter 1).

The terms *sensor* and *transducer* are often used synonymously, although there are times when this may not be appropriate. It seems to be generally accepted in science and technology that a working definition of a *transducer* is "a device that converts one form of energy into another, the latter often being electrical." A sensor usually meets this criterion and can therefore also be described as a transducer. Even sensors of biochemical quantities or concentrations are somehow converting chemical energy into electrical or optical energy. However, a transducer, unlike a sensor, does not necessarily have an electrical or optical output that is intended to be recordable and also functionally related to its input. An example of this is in ultrasonic imaging (see Chapter 6), where the same probe has two quite separate functions: (1) to generate the ultrasonic waves that enter the human body and (2) to respond to, or sense, the ultrasonic echoes from tissue interfaces within the body. In the first case the probe is acting as a *transducer*, converting a short pulse of electrical energy into ultrasonic mechanical energy; in the second case the probe acts as a *sensor*, converting the incident ultrasonic mechanical energy in the echo into an electrical signal that is processed to give the recorded image. On the basis of this distinction, transducers can sometimes be regarded as components of sensors. For example, a diaphragm in a microphone or a pressure sensor converts sound or pressure energy into strain energy in the diaphragm; a second transducer stage is required to convert this strain energy into recordable electrical energy in order to make a complete sound or pressure sensor. The use of the word *sensor* allows a distinction to be made between a device that gives a measurable recordable output that is functionally related to changes in a physical quantity at its input, and a device for converting one form of energy into another—a *transducer*, which may not necessarily have the properties of a sensor.

## SCOPE OF THIS VOLUME

This volume includes a wide range of topics in biomedical engineering and medical physics. However, the subject of biomedical sensors has grown very rapidly in the last three decades and now encompasses such a huge field that even a "comprehensive" treatment of this sensor technology must, of necessity, be selective. The choice of topics was influenced principally by their clinical relevance and also to some extent by the contents of a long-established graduate-taught master's course at the Medical School of St. Bartholomew's Hospital, London, UK, that the editor organized. It was decided to include sensors associated with the measurement of temperature, fluid flow, radiation (including ionizing radiation, non-ionizing radiation, and ultrasound), and also chemical and biochemical sensors, including biosensors. Those sensors associated with purely mechanical physical quantities have not been treated as primary subjects in this volume. Hence, sensors for the measurement of position, force, pressure, and acceleration, which are all of particular importance in the field of biomechanics, have been left for the present.

The aim here is to emphasize the technological principles and the practical applications of bio-medical sensors rather than the theoretical concepts. The treatments in the chapters usually include details of the technical principles of the sensor together with those of any associated peripheral devices essential for registering the response of the sensor. Examples of the practical applications of the systems associated with the sensors have been included, but detailed discussions of the operations of complete systems have been avoided. Generally the volume concentrates on sensors that are currently used in practice or are likely to be used in the near future. Research laboratory techniques that are speculative or a long way from being practically viable in a clinical context have not been included. Some chapters, where appropriate, contain critical comparisons of manufacturers' sensor data.

## READERSHIP

This volume is intended to provide a good initial introduction and reference source for biomedical engineers and medical physicists who need to become acquainted with new fields and topics. It should act as a reliable guide to the bewildering array of more specialized literature and texts on the subject. The contents should be accessible to a broad range of professionals in biomedicine, including practic-ing experienced biomedical engineers, medical physicists, clinical technologists, and clinicians working in a hospital or other health care environment.

Academics in higher education institutions will find the book an invaluable resource to further their scholarship and advance research projects on sensors and other medical devices. In addition, students should benefit from a well-written, advanced textbook suitable for those final-year undergraduate, postgraduate, and research students aiming to pursue a career in the field of medical physics or biomedical engineering.

Engineers and applied physicists working for health care providers or for the pharmaceutical and medical instrumentation industries will find in this volume a rich source of relevant information. It also contains essential tools to help solve practical problems encountered in both routine applications and the challenges of advanced development work.

## THE CONTENTS

The majority of the distinguished authors who have contributed to *Biomedical Sensors* have had decades of practical experience in biomedical engineering and medical physics. Moreover, the authors have well-established international reputations and many are world-renowned experts in their fields.

The chapters are organized according to the measurand being considered, that is, the physical quantity being sensed and measured (e.g., temperature, ionizing radiation, or chemical concentration).

The first chapter deals with the measurement of the temperature of the human body. Temperature has been used by physicians since the earliest times for the diagnosis and monitoring of disease. Given its fundamental importance, it is surprising that there have been so few comprehensive reviews of the subject. It is almost as if it is taken for granted that anyone can measure body temperature accurately if required. This chapter shows that this is not necessarily true, particularly as there are now so many possible techniques, some intended for specific applications, that the choice of an appropriate method to give accurate reliable results is often not easy. Chapter 1 provides a timely overview of modern clinical thermometry and gives a critical assessment of the accuracy and applicability of the various methods available to the physician, surgeon, parents, and others for whom assessing the temperature of the human body is of vital importance.

Chapter 2 is primarily concerned with the most important liquid in the body, which is, of course, blood. The measurement of blood velocity and blood flow in arteries and veins is a major activity for large numbers of biomedical engineers and medical physicists. The quantitative estimation of blood flow in the limbs and in various organs is of great value in many diagnostic investigations, and advances in the subject have made significant contributions to cardiology. The chapter provides a comprehensive review of the traditional flow measurement techniques, such as indicator dilution methods, plethysmography, and ultrasound for arteries and veins. It also covers more modern techniques such as ultrasonic Doppler methods in cardiology and functional magnetic resonance imaging (MRI) in the brain. More advanced topics, such as the use of contrast agents in ultrasonic imaging and MRI in the quantitative analysis of dynamic processes are also discussed. The chapter ends with a brief overview of the measurement of flow in other fluids, including urine, saliva, tears, and gastric acids.

Chapter 3, on respiratory flow sensors, considers another fluid, namely, the gas that flows out of and into the human lung. It requires the use of quite specialized techniques that are different from those outlined in Chapter 2 for liquids. Every large hospital has a pulmonary function laboratory, because respiratory disease is one of the most significant public health burdens in developed countries. Indeed, respiratory diseases account for about one-third of all deaths in the United States. It might be thought that the measurement of airflow is relatively simple, but there are many technical challenges associated with the application of flow sensors in pulmonary medicine. These are dealt with in an exemplary manner in this chapter.

Chapter 4 deals comprehensively with ionizing radiation sensors in medicine, a field that is primarily the preserve of medical physicists, but also engages numerous engineers in the design, development, and maintenance of medical X-ray equipment. The importance of ionizing radiation can be judged from the fact that it is likely that two-thirds or more of all the clinical engineers and scientists working in hospital environments are employed in X-ray or other ionizing radiation–related activities in diagnostic imaging, radiotherapy, nuclear medicine, and radiation protection. The chapter gives an overview of the basic requirements for sensing ionizing radiation, the interactions with materials, and the criteria for assessing the performance of the sensors. It goes on to treat sensors for dosimetry ranging from semiconductors and radiographic film to diamond and outlines their advantages and disadvantages. Next, sensors for imaging are reviewed, including radiographic film and flat-panel detectors, while the characteristics of various scintillator materials for sensors are also outlined. Specific applications and advances in imaging in computed tomography (CT), mammography, single photon emission computed tomography (SPECT), and positron emission tomography (PET) are also covered. The final part deals with sensors for ionizing radiation spectroscopy and concludes with examples of detector selection in a series of case studies.

Chapter 5 deals with nonionizing electromagnetic radiation and radiometric and photometric measurements. Lasers have played an important role in biomedicine for more than three decades, finding significant applications in ophthalmology, surgery, and photodynamic therapy for cancer treatment. In Europe, recent directives on the use of artificial optical radiation in the workplace are being implemented, while in the United States, the Food and Drug Administration (FDA) Center for Devices and Radiological Health produces similar guidance notes. There is also an increasing use of ultraviolet (UV) light therapy for the treatment of eczema and hyperbilirubinemia in newborn babies, up to 60% of whom may suffer from this condition. This authoritative chapter is timely, as there is a growing need to understand the challenges faced in obtaining accurate dosimetry measurements with nonionizing radiation, particularly when it is required to make comparisons with other treatment centers. There is an explanation of radiometric and photometric terms and a review of measurement sensors. Radiometric sensors for the measurement of UV irradiance in phototherapy treatment and their application are discussed. The chapter ends with a section on the objective measurement of solar radiation at the earth's surface and, in particular, the measurement of sun-burning UV radiation, a topic of some importance with the increasing incidence of skin cancer worldwide.

Ultrasonic imaging was originally developed in the 1960s to replace potentially damaging X-rays in fetal imaging. It now finds applications not only in obstetrics, but in a wide range of disciplines from cardiology to ophthalmology and gastroenterology. Chapter 6 reviews in depth the probes that generate and sense the ultrasonic signals that enter the human body in ultrasonic imaging. It complements the sections on ultrasonic flow measurements in Chapter 2. The principles of operation of the probes are outlined and various practical electrical and acoustical models of the sensors are developed. The construction of single-element probes and multielement arrays is considered and the characteristics of various modern piezoelectric materials used to make the probes are compared. Focusing principles and performance criteria are established, followed by some examples of the clinical applications of phased and linear arrays. Finally, advanced topics such as multimode operation and the construction of two-dimensional arrays are considered.

The measurement of the concentrations of the various chemical components of blood is of great importance in the diagnosis and treatment of disease. Blood gas analyzers are among the most significant of medical instruments and operate 24 hours a day, every day, in all major hospitals. Gas sensors also perform a vital role in anesthesia, measuring accurately the concentrations of the anesthetic agents. Chapter 7 is a comprehensive overview of the principles of the sensors used to measure these and other chemical compounds. Electrochemical sensors for the measurement of pH, $pO_2$ (the partial pressure of oxygen), and $pCO_2$ (the partial pressure of carbon dioxide) in blood both noninvasively and invasively are described. Advanced miniature microelectromechanical systems (MEMS) for sensing blood $pO_2$ and $pCO_2$ and similar ion-selective field effect transistors (ISFETs) for pH are covered. Optical fiber chemical sensors for pH, $pCO_2$, and invasive and noninvasive blood oximetry are reviewed. The principles of gas phase sensors for the real-time measurement of the concentrations of oxygen, carbon dioxide, and anesthetic gases in respiratory medicine and anesthesia are outlined. There is also a review of a variety of methods for blood glucose sensing from optical and electrochemical sensors to biosensors. Some of the latter part of this section complements the following chapter on biosensors. Finally, a highly sensitive acoustic chemical sensor is described that makes use of a quartz crystal microbalance coated with zeolite to detect acetone in the breath for the diagnosis of diabetes and for other clinical analyses.

Biosensors have evolved from the marriage of two disciplines: optoelectronics technology, exemplified by microcircuits and optical fibers, and molecular biology. They are among the most exciting and challenging developments in analytical devices and have the potential to make continuous measurements of blood chemistry at the bedside or, by means of a chip on a catheter, in a patient's vein. They incorporate a biological recognition element that interacts with a target molecule to provide a highly selective sensor. Drugs, metabolites, proteins, and nucleic acids are all targets for biosensors. Chapter 8 introduces and reviews enzyme-based biosensors—in particular, those based on glucose oxidase, used to estimate blood glucose, and urease for the estimation of blood urea. Enzyme immobilization techniques are described, from physical entrapment and chemical immobilization to surface adsorption. Optical biosensors, including optical fibers, surface plasmon resonance, and attenuated total reflection types are covered. Modified electrochemical biosensors that can be used for home glucose monitoring are also described. Microfabricated enzyme-linked field effect transistors (ENFETs), whole cell biosensors, and nanobiosensors are discussed. Biosensors have enormous potential, but there are also formidable challenges for practical utilization, which are outlined clearly in this chapter. The problems include robustness and lifetime and operational stability, but these are being resolved using a variety of sensors, formatting techniques, and MEMS.

Medical thermography is the ultimate noninvasive investigative technique in which clinically relevant information is obtained without any contact with the patient and without the use of penetrating radiation. It is the subject of the final chapter and uses infrared (IR) radiation that is passively emitted by the human body. Medical thermography is a fine example of "swords into plowshares" technology transfer, because most of the significant advances in the challenging field of IR imaging have been made for military purposes. Thermography is unique in providing quantitative information on inflammatory processes (e.g., in rheumatic diseases), and modern cameras are even capable of detecting infection in passengers at airport gates. In addition, skin diseases, nerve injuries, industrial and sports injuries, and disruptions to the peripheral circulation have all been investigated using IR imaging. This chapter complements Chapter 5, in that it describes a practical application of IR radiometry. It begins with an historical overview of IR detection and imaging and the development of early thermographic cameras. The IR spectrum and its subdivisions and the laws governing the emission of IR radiation are then described. Next, IR camera characteristics and the measurement of IR radiation using IR thermometers and thermal imagers are reviewed, followed by an outline of the development of modern focal-plane imaging arrays. Finally, the characteristics of a variety of sensors, from miniature bolometers to photon detectors, are described and figures of merit for assessing thermal camera performance are discussed.

The design, manufacture, distribution, and maintenance of sensors and the biomedical systems that depend on them are of immense and growing commercial significance. Multimillion-dollar companies, such as the biomedical divisions of General Electric, Philips, and Siemens, together with scores of other smaller enterprises, all base their prosperity on sensors, since virtually all their biomedical products depend critically on the reliable functioning of sensors of one kind or another.

Advanced biomedical sensors represent a commendable application of cutting-edge technology for the benefit of humanity. The practice of modern medicine would be impossible without them. The authors of this volume have communicated not only their consummate expertise, but also their enthusiasm for the subject. Readers will find here a rich source of practical knowledge and, it is hoped, the inspiration to make their own contributions to this rapidly expanding and important field.

## ACKNOWLEDGMENTS

It is a pleasure to acknowledge the encouragement of Stuart J. Meldrum of the Norfolk and Norwich University Hospital, United Kingdom, and Michael R. Neuman of Michigan Technological University in the initial stages of this project. I am grateful to Stuart Meldrum for reading and providing invaluable comments on the manuscript of Chapter 3. I should also like to express my gratitude to all the distinguished authors who have interrupted their busy schedules to contribute to this volume. Without them it would not exist. The original concept for the "Comprehensive Sensor Technology" series came from Joe Watson, the series editor. His steadfast enthusiasm, determination, and tenacity have overcome many obstacles to ensure that the series is being published. I am deeply indebted to him for his sound advice, for his unfailing support, and for much more. Finally, I would like to thank my wife, Jennifer, for her forbearance and patience.

Deric P. Jones
Editor
Biomedical Engineering
School of Engineering & Mathematical Sciences
City University
Northampton Square, London
July 14, 2010

## ABOUT THE EDITOR

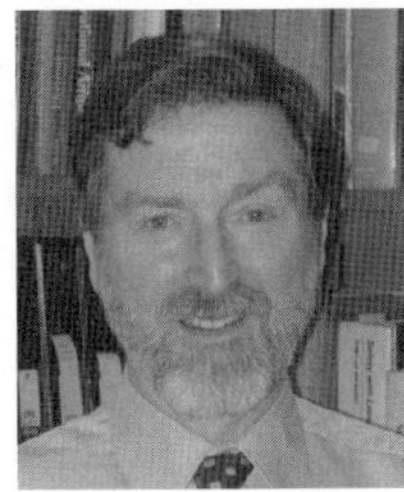

**Professor Deric Powell Jones** BSc DIC PhD was born in Monmouthshire, South Wales, and received the degrees of BSc in physics and PhD in the superconductivity of alloys from Imperial College, London. He worked as a medical physicist at St. Bartholomew's Hospital and then as a lecturer at the Medical School. During more than twenty-five years spent at St. Bartholomew's he became a reader in the University of London and head of Medical Electronics and Physics in the Medical School. His research interests include the application of opto-electronic techniques in anesthesia and surgery and also the development of new techniques for physiological measurements in respiration and ophthalmology. He is a fellow of the UK Institute of Physics and of the UK Institute of Physics and Engineering in Medicine and a chartered engineer and a senior member of the Institute of Electrical and Electronics Engineers. Professor Jones is currently affiliated to the Biomedical Engineering Department at City University, London.

# CHAPTER 1

# BIOMEDICAL SENSORS

## TEMPERATURE SENSOR TECHNOLOGY

P. A. Kyriacou

*School of Engineering and Mathematical Sciences*
*City University, London, UK*

> The clinical thermometer ranks in importance with the stethoscope. A doctor without his thermometer is like a sailor without his compass.
>
> —*Family Physician*, 1882

## 1.1. INTRODUCTION

Human body temperature is of vital importance to the well-being of the person and therefore it is routinely monitored to indicate the state of the person's health. Despite the fact that temperature

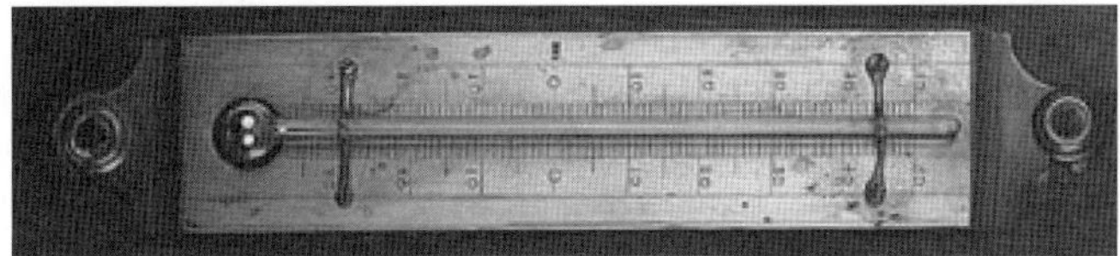

Celsius thermometer (attached to a barometer) made by J. G. Hasselström, Stockholm, late eighteenth century.

measurement in humans seems so simple, a wide variety of devices are available to record a temperature from skin, oral or rectal mucosa, or the tympanic membrane. The choice of clinical thermometers for health professionals and parents has never been so complicated.

This chapter attempts to provide an overview of temperature-sensing technologies in medicine. The introductory sections give a brief and general description of temperature and its effect on the human body. A synoptic historical review on the evolution of the thermometer, including the clinical thermometer, is given in section 1.3. Section 1.4 describes the main sensors and transducers used in the development of clinical thermometers, such as thermocouples, thermistors, resistance temperature detectors (RTDs), semiconductor temperature sensors, liquid crystal temperature sensors, and infrared (IR) radiation sensors. These thermometers have been designed and developed for application in various parts of the body such as the rectum, mouth, axilla, esophagus, bladder, ear, temporal artery, and skin, and are discussed in section 1.5. It is impossible for this chapter to cover every possible application and evaluation study relating to different thermometers, however, an effort is made in section 1.6 to provide an integrative review of studies comparing selected invasive and noninvasive temperature measurement methods.

## 1.2. TEMPERATURE

In the literature one can find many definitions of temperature, including the following:

1.  Temperature is the degree of "hotness" of a body: more precisely it is the potential for heat transfer. In our everyday lives, we are aware of different temperatures through the sensation of touch, but how hot or cold something feels is subjective. We can say that the kettle is hotter than the ice cream, but not by how much. Measurement, on the other hand, must be objective and a thermometer is used.

2.  Temperature can be defined in macroscopic terms, using concepts of thermodynamics, as an intrinsic property of matter that quantifies the ability of one body to transfer thermal energy (heat) to another body. Temperature can also be defined on a microscopic scale as proportional to the random kinetic energy of an assemblage of molecules or atoms (Kerlin & Shepard 1982).

3.  Temperature is a measure of how fast the atoms and molecules of a substance are moving. In a qualitative manner, we can describe the temperature of an object as that which determines the sensation of warmth or coldness felt from contact with it. It is easy to demonstrate that when two objects of the same material are in thermal contact, the object with the higher temperature cools while the cooler object becomes warmer until a point is reached after which no more change occurs, and to our senses, they feel the same. When the thermal changes have stopped, we say that the two objects or systems are in *thermal equilibrium*. We can then define the temperature of the system by saying that the temperature is the quantity that is the same for both systems when they are in thermal equilibrium. If we experiment further with more than two systems, we find that many systems can be brought into thermal equilibrium with each other; thermal equilibrium does not depend on the kind of object used. Put more precisely, *if two systems are separately in thermal equilibrium with a third, then they must also be in thermal equilibrium with each other*, and they all have the same temperature regardless of the kind of systems they are. The statement in italics, called the *zeroth law of thermodynamics* may be restated as follows:

- If three or more systems are in thermal contact with each other and all in equilibrium together, then any two taken separately are in equilibrium with one another (Quinn 1990).
- Now one of the three systems could be an instrument calibrated to measure the temperature—that is, a thermometer. When a calibrated thermometer is put in thermal contact with a system and reaches thermal equilibrium, we then have a quantitative measure of the temperature of the system. For example, a mercury-in-glass clinical thermometer is put under the tongue of a patient and allowed to reach thermal equilibrium in the patient's mouth—we then see by how much the silvery mercury has expanded in the stem and read the scale of the thermometer to find the patient's temperature (Quinn 1990).

### 1.2.1. BODY TEMPERATURE

The human body regulates temperature by keeping a tight balance between heat production and heat loss. For example, when the body is too hot, the blood vessels in the skin expand (dilate) to carry the excess heat to the skin's surface. When the body is too cold, the blood vessels narrow (contract or vasoconstrict) so that blood flow to the skin is reduced to conserve body heat. In both cases the body employs various mechanisms to regulate the body temperature (e.g., the body sweats, and as the sweat evaporates it helps cool the body). Also, shivering causes the muscles to contract involuntary, which helps to generate more heat. Under normal conditions, these mechanisms keep the body temperature within a narrow, safe range.

Humans regulate heat generation and preservation to maintain their internal body temperature or core temperature. Temperature regulation is controlled by the hypothalamus (in the brain), which is often called the body's thermostat. Normal core temperature varies between 97.7°F and 99.5°F (36.5°C and 37.5°C). For adults, fever occurs when the oral temperature is above 100°F (37.8°C) or the rectal or ear temperature is above 101°F (38.3°C). For children, fever occurs when the rectal temperature is 100.4°F (38°C) or higher (Herzog & Coyne 1993; Mackowiak, Wasserman, & Levine 1992).

An abnormally low (hypothermia) or high (hyperthermia) body temperature can be serious and even life threatening. Low body temperature may occur from cold exposure, shock, alcohol or drug use, or certain metabolic disorders such as diabetes or hypothyroidism. A low body temperature may also be present with an infection, particularly in newborns, older adults, or people who are frail. At high body temperatures, heatstroke occurs and the body fails to regulate its own temperature (body temperature continues to rise). Symptoms of heatstroke include mental changes (such as confusion, delirium, or unconsciousness) and skin that is red, hot, and dry, even under the armpits (Marieb, 1992).

Body temperature can be measured in many locations on the body, including the mouth, ear, armpit, rectum, forehead, bladder, skin, and esophagus. Such temperature measuring techniques will be discussed in more detail in the following sections.

## 1.3. WHAT IS A THERMOMETER?

The word thermometer is derived from two smaller word fragments: *thermo* from the Greek for heat and *meter* from the Greek meaning to measure. Thermometers measure temperature. This is possible by using materials that change in some way when they are either heated or cooled. For example, in a mercury or alcohol thermometer the liquid expands when it is heated and contracts when it is cooled, therefore the length of the liquid column is longer or shorter depending on the temperature (http://en.wikipedia.org/wiki/Thermometer).

A thermometer is a device that provides a measure of the temperature of a system in a quantitative manner. The easiest way to do this is to find a material that has a property that changes in a regular way with its temperature. The most direct "regular" way is a linear one:

$$t(x) = ax + b, \tag{1.1}$$

where $t$ is the temperature of the substance that changes as the property $x$ of the substance changes. The constants $a$ and $b$ in equation 1.1 depend on the substance used and may be evaluated by specifying two temperature points on the scale, such as 32°F for the freezing point of water and 212°F for its boiling point.

For example, the element mercury is liquid in the temperature range of −38.9°C to 356.7°C (the Celsius scale will be discussed later). As a liquid, mercury expands as it gets warmer; its expansion is linear and can be accurately calibrated.

The mercury-in-glass thermometer illustrated in Figure 1.1 contains a bulb filled with mercury that expands into a capillary. The mercury's expansion is then calibrated on a scale imprinted on the glass tube. Modern thermometers are calibrated in standard temperature units such as Fahrenheit or Celsius.

## 1.3.1. THE DEVELOPMENT OF THERMOMETERS AND TEMPERATURE SCALES

In this section a general historical review of the development of the thermometer is presented, with special references to the evolution of the clinical thermometer. The historical highlights in the development of thermometers and their scales given in this section are mostly based on *Temperature* by T. J. Quinn (1990) and *Heat* by J. M. Cork (1942) and a recent historical review of clinical thermometers by J. M. S. Pearce (2002).

Of the many tools and instruments regarded as essential to the clinical examination, none has had such widespread application as the clinical thermometer. In the time of Hippocrates, only the hand was used to detect the heat or cold of the human body, although fever and chills were known as signs of morbid processes. In Alexandrine medicine, the pulse was observed as an index of disease, superseding the crude assessment of temperature. In the Middle Ages, the four humors were assigned the qualities of hot, cold, dry, and moist, and thus fever again acquired importance (Pearce, 2002).

The first attempt at standardization of temperature scales took place in approximately 170 A.D. when Galen, in his medical reports, suggested a standard "neutral" temperature made up of equal quantities of boiling water and ice. Four degrees of heat and four degrees of cold were on either side of this temperature (http://www.eo.ucar.edu/skymath/tmp2.html).

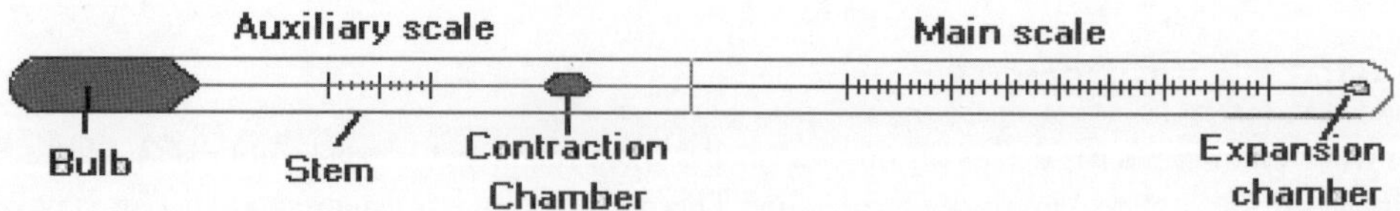


**Figure 1.1.** Mercury-in-glass thermometer.

Some of the earliest devices that were used to measure temperature were called thermoscopes. In 1592 Galileo developed a rudimentary temperature-measuring instrument that had no scale and therefore no numerical readings. This temperature-measuring device comprised a glass bulb having a long tube extending downward into a container of colored water (some say Galileo, in 1610, is supposed to have used wine; see Fig. 1.2). Some of the air in the bulb was expelled before placing it in the liquid, causing the liquid to rise into the tube. As the remaining air in the bulb was heated or cooled, the level of the liquid in the tube varied, reflecting the change in air temperature. An engraved scale on the tube allowed for a quantitative measure of the fluctuations. The air in the bulb is referred to as the *thermometric medium,* that is, the medium whose property changes with temperature (Cork, 1942; Quinn, 1990).

A large step forward was achieved by Santorio, who invented a mouth thermometer. Santorio (1561–1636) was an Italian physiologist and a professor at Padua. He made quantitative experiments in temperature, as well as other physiological measurements such as respiration and weight. He produced several thermometer designs, but all were cumbersome and required a long time to measure the oral temperature. In 1641 the first sealed thermometer that used liquid rather than air as the thermometric medium was developed for Ferdinand II, Grand Duke of Tuscany. This thermometer used a sealed alcohol-in-glass device, with fifty "degree" marks on its stem, but no "fixed point" was used to zero the scale. These were referred to as "spirit" thermometers. In 1664 Robert Hook, curator of the Royal Society, used a red dye in the alcohol. His scale, for which every degree represented an equal increment of volume equivalent to about 1/500 of the volume of the thermometer liquid, needed only one fixed point. He selected the freezing point of water. Hook showed that a standard scale could be established for thermometers in a variety of sizes. Hook's original thermometer became known as the standard of Gresham College and was used by the Royal Society until 1709 (http://www.brannan .co.uk/thermometers/invention.html).

In 1665 Christiaan Huygens added a scale extending from the freezing point to the boiling point of water, the original centigrade system. In 1702 the astronomer Ole Roemer of Copenhagen based his scale on two fixed points: snow (or crushed ice) and the boiling point of water, and he recorded the daily temperatures at Copenhagen in 1708 and 1709 with this thermometer. In 1709 the alcohol thermometer was invented by Daniel Gabriel Fahrenheit (1686–1736). Fahrenheit based his new scale on

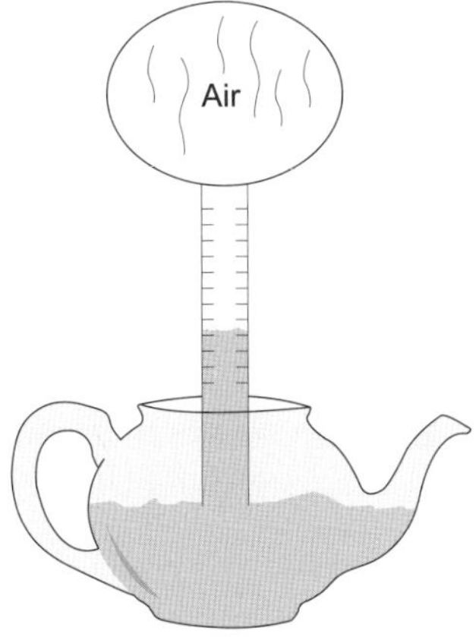



**Figure 1.2.** Florentine wine thermoscope.

a mixture of ice and ammonium chloride as the lower point. In 1724 Fahrenheit used mercury as the thermometric liquid; he found mercury more useful than water, as it expanded and contracted more rapidly. Mercury's thermal expansion is large and fairly uniform, it does not adhere to the glass, and it remains a liquid over a wide range of temperatures. Also, its silvery appearance makes it easy to read. On this scale, Fahrenheit measured the boiling point of water to be 212°F. Later he adjusted the freezing point of water to 32°F so that the interval between the boiling and freezing points of water could be represented by the more rational number 180. Temperatures measured on this scale are designated as degrees Fahrenheit (°F; Pearce, 2002).

The thermometer was not generally used for medical applications until Hermann Boerhaave (1668–1738), with his students Gerard L. B. Van Swieten (1700–1772) and Anton De Haen (1704–1776), and George Martine started to use the thermometer at the bedside. De Haen studied diurnal changes in normal subjects and observed changes in temperature with shivering or fever. He also observed the acceleration of the pulse when the temperature was raised and thus found that temperature was a valuable indication of the progress of an illness. However, his colleagues were not impressed, and therefore the thermometer was not widely used (Pearce, 2002).

Technological development of the thermometer continued, and in 1742 the Swedish astronomer Anders Celsius (1701–1744) reintroduced the centigrade scale. Centigrade means "consisting of or divided into 100 degrees." The Celsius scale has 100 degrees between the freezing point (0°C) and boiling point (100°C) of pure water at sea level air pressure. The term "Celsius" was adopted in 1948 by an international conference on weights and measures. In 1745 Carolus Linnaeus of Uppsala, Sweden, described a scale in which the freezing point of water was 0 and the boiling point 100, making it a *centigrade* (one hundred steps) scale (http://www.eo.ucar.edu/skymath/tmp2.html).

The Celsius scale is defined by the following two items, which will be discussed later in this section:

1.    The triple point of water is defined as 0.01°C.
2.    A degree Celsius equals the same temperature change as a degree on the ideal-gas scale.

When using the Celsius scale, the boiling point of water at standard atmospheric pressure is 99.975°C, in contrast to the 100°C defined by the centigrade scale. To convert from Celsius to Fahrenheit, multiply degrees Celsius by 1.8 and add 32:

$$°F = 1.8 \times °C + 32. \tag{1.2}$$

In 1780 J. A. C. Charles (a French physician) demonstrated that for the same increase in temperature, all gases exhibit the same increase in volume. Because the expansion coefficient of gases is almost the same, it is possible to create a temperature scale based on a single fixed point rather than two fixed points, such as the Fahrenheit and Celsius scales. This brings us back to a thermometer that uses a gas as the thermometric medium (http://www.eo.ucar.edu/skymath/tmp2.html).

In a constant volume gas thermometer, a large bulb B of gas (hydrogen, for example) under a set pressure connects with a mercury-filled "manometer" by means of a tube of very small volume, as shown in Figure 1.3. The level of mercury at C may be adjusted by raising or lowering the mercury reservoir R. The pressure of the hydrogen gas, which is the $x$ variable in the linear relation with temperature in equation 1.1, is the difference between the levels D and C plus the pressure above D (Cork, 1942; Quinn, 1990).

Despite improvements in the thermometer, its use in the medical setting remained largely neglected until the late nineteenth century, when, in 1868, Carl Wunderlich published temperature recordings from more than 1 million readings in more than 25,000 patients made with a foot-long thermometer

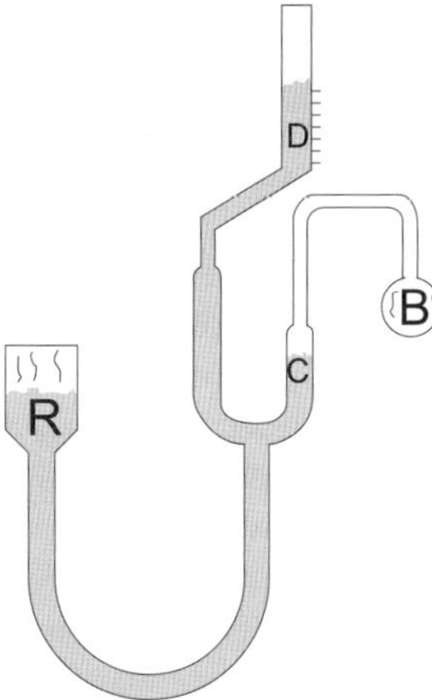

**Figure 1.3.** Constant volume gas thermometer.

used in the axilla. He established a range of normal temperatures from 36.3°C to 37.5°C. Temperatures outside this range suggested disease. In 1852 William Aitkin made a mercury instrument with a narrower tube sited above a bulb reservoir. This ensured that the mercury did not drop back after the reading had been taken. The size of this thermometer (used by Wunderlich and Aitkin) was a major disadvantage until 1866, when Thomas Clifford Allbutt (1836–1925) designed a conveniently portable 6-inch clinical thermometer, able to record a temperature in 5 minutes. This new thermometer replaced the foot-long model, which required 20 minutes to determine a patient's temperature. The measurement of temperature soon became an inescapable routine (Pearce, 2002).

At about the same time, William Thomson, Lord Kelvin (1824–1907), among his other achievements, took the whole process one step further with his invention of the Kelvin scale in 1848. The Kelvin scale measures the ultimate extremes of hot and cold. Kelvin developed the idea of absolute temperature, what is called the "Second Law of Thermodynamics," and developed the dynamic theory of heat. In 1887 P. Chappuis conducted extensive studies of gas thermometers with constant pressure or with constant volume using hydrogen, nitrogen, and carbon dioxide as the thermometric medium. Based on his results, the *Comité International des Poids et Mesures* (International Committee of Weights and Measures) adopted the constant volume hydrogen scale, based on fixed points at the ice point (0°C) and the steam point (100°C), as the practical scale for international meteorology.

Experiments with gas thermometers have shown that there is very little difference in the temperature scale for different gases. Thus it is possible to set up a temperature scale that is independent of the thermometric medium if it is a gas at low pressure. In this case, all gases behave like an "ideal gas" and have a very simple relation between their pressure ($p$), volume ($V$), and temperature ($T$):

$$pV = (\text{constant})\,T. \tag{1.3}$$

This temperature is called the *thermodynamic temperature* and is now accepted as the fundamental measure of temperature. There is a naturally defined zero on this scale: it is the point at which the pressure of an ideal gas is zero, making the temperature also zero. With this as one point on the scale, only one other fixed point need be defined.

In 1933 the International Committee of Weights and Measures adopted this fixed point as the triple point of water (the temperature at which water, ice, and water vapor coexist in equilibrium); its value is set as 273.16. The unit of temperature on this scale is called the kelvin, after Lord Kelvin, and its symbol is K (no degree symbol is used). To convert from Celsius to kelvin, add 273:

$$K = {}^\circ C + 273. \tag{1.4}$$

In 1871 Sir William Siemens proposed a thermometer that uses a metallic conductor whose resistance changes with temperature. The element platinum does not oxidize at high temperatures and has a relatively uniform change in resistance with temperature over a large range. The platinum resistance thermometer is now widely used as a thermoelectric thermometer, covering a temperature range from about –260°C to 1235°C.

Returning to the clinical thermometer, during World War II a pioneering biodynamicist and flight surgeon with the Luftwaffe, Theodore Hannes Benzinger, invented the ear thermometer, and much later, in 1984, David Phillips invented the IR ear thermometer. Dr. Jacob Fraden, chief executive officer (CEO) of Advanced Monitors Corporation, invented the world's best-selling ear thermometer, the Thermoscan human ear thermometer.

Many different kinds of temperature sensors are currently used by themselves or installed in different types of probes (surface, indwelling), catheters, or needles making contact with or introduced to the object site of the body. A description of such sensors is the subject of the next section.

## 1.4. TEMPERATURE SENSORS, TRANSDUCERS, AND THERMOMETERS

Both the words *sensor* and *transducer* are used in the description of measurement systems. The word *sensor* is most popular in the United States, whereas the word *transducer* is more frequently used in Europe. A dictionary definition of *sensor* is a device that detects a change in a physical stimulus and turns it into a signal that can be measured or recorded. A corresponding definition of *transducer* is a device that transfers power from one system to another in the same or in a different form. A sensible distinction is to use *sensor* for the sensing element itself and *transducer* for the sensing element plus any associated circuitry. All transducers would thus contain a sensor and most (though not all) sensors would also be transducers. In the context of this chapter, both words will be used interchangeably (Cromwell, Weibell, & Pfeiffer, 1980).

The past decade has seen the introduction of many new clinical thermometers to replace the traditional mercury-in-glass thermometer. These include contact and noncontact temperature sensors. Some of the most common temperature sensors used in the development of the majority of clinical thermometers, including thermocouples, thermistors, RTDs, semiconductor temperature sensors, liquid crystal temperature sensors, and IR radiation sensors, will be discussed in this section (Crawford, Hicks, & Thompson, 2006; Michalski, Eckersdorf, & McGhee, 1991).

### 1.4.1. CONTACT TEMPERATURE SENSORS

Contact temperature sensors measure their own temperature. One infers the temperature of the object by assuming or knowing that the two objects are in thermal equilibrium, that is, there is no heat flow between them.

### 1.4.1.1. Thermocouples

Thermocouples are one of the most popular contact temperature sensors. They can measure a wide range of temperatures, are interchangeable, and have standard connectors. Around 1821 the German-Estonian physicist Thomas Johann Seebeck discovered that the junction between two metals generates a voltage that is a function of temperature (http://www.picotech.com/applications/thermocouple .html). Such an effect is known as the thermoelectric or Seebeck effect (Michalski et al., 1991; Togawa, Tamura, & Oberg, 1997). Although almost any two metals can be used to make a thermocouple, a number of standard metals are used because they give predictable output voltages and tolerate large temperature gradients. A photograph and a diagrammatic representation of one of the most popular thermocouples, the K-type thermocouple, are shown in Figure 1.4. Standard tables show the voltage produced by thermocouples at any given temperature; for example, in Figure 1.4, the K-type thermocouple at 300°C will produce 12.2 mV.

It is not possible to simply connect up a voltmeter to the thermocouple, as shown in Figure 1.4, to measure voltage because the connection of the voltmeter leads makes a second, undesired thermocouple junction. To make accurate measurements, this must be compensated for by using a technique known as cold junction compensation (CJC). Connecting a voltmeter to a thermocouple makes several additional thermocouple junctions (leads connecting to the thermocouple, leads to the meter, inside the meter, etc.). The law of intermediate metals states that a third metal inserted between the two dissimilar metals of a thermocouple junction will have no effect, provided that the two junctions are at the same temperature. This law is important in the construction of thermocouple junctions. Thermocouple junctions are made by welding the two metals together, not soldering them, as this ensures that the performance is not limited by the melting point of solder. Thermocouple standard tables allow for a second cold thermocouple junction on the assumption that it is kept at exactly 0°C. This is done with a constructed ice bath, thus the term *cold* junction compensation. Maintaining an ice bath is not practical for most measurement applications, so instead the actual temperature at the point of connection of the thermocouple wires to the measuring instrument is recorded (Togawa et al., 1997).

Typically cold junction temperature is sensed by a precision thermistor or a semiconductor temperature sensor that is in good thermal contact with the input connectors of the measuring instrument. This second temperature reading, along with the reading from the thermocouple itself, is used by the measuring instrument to calculate the true temperature at the thermocouple tip. Understanding CJC

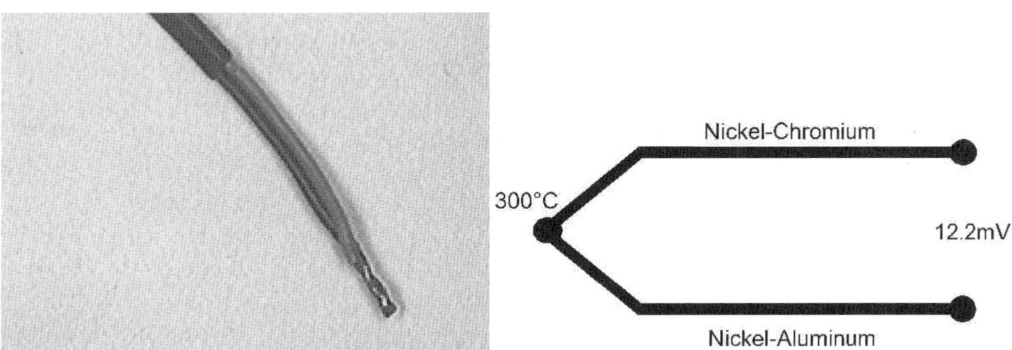


**Figure 1.4.** K-type thermocouple.

is important because any error in the measurement of cold junction temperature will lead to the same error in the measured temperature from the thermocouple tip.

As well as dealing with CJC, the measuring instrument must also allow for the fact that the thermocouple output is nonlinear. The relationship between temperature and output voltage is a complex polynomial equation (fifth to ninth order depending on the thermocouple type). The integrated circuit (IC) amplifier in Figure 1.5 has a compensation circuit for the reference temperature assembled in the same package (AD594/595; Analog Devices, Norwood, MA). The AD594/595 is a complete instrumentation amplifier and thermocouple cold junction compensator on a monolithic chip. It combines an ice-point reference with a precalibrated amplifier to produce a high-level, low-impedance, 10 mV/°C linear voltage output directly from the thermocouple signal. The nominal absolute accuracy at 25°C is ±1°C, and the effect of package temperature is less than ±0.025°C per 1°C. Thus a stability of ±0.25°C will be attained by limiting the package temperature in a range of ±10°C (Togawa et al., 1997).

Thermocouples are available as either bare wire "bead" thermocouples (Fig. 1.4), which offer low cost and fast response times, or they are built into probes. A wide variety of thermocouple probes are available, including needle, insulated, catheter, capsule, direct immersion, surface mount, and micro-thermocouple, suitable for different measuring applications (industrial, scientific, food temperature, clinical thermometry, etc.). Each type of thermocouple is made using different techniques. Details of such techniques can be found in the literature. When selecting probes, care must be taken to ensure they have the correct type of connector. The two common types of connector are "standard" with round pins and "miniature" with flat pins.

### 1.4.1.1.1. Thermocouple Types

As mentioned previously, when selecting a thermocouple consideration should be given to the thermocouple type, insulation, and probe construction. Such considerations will have an effect on the measurable temperature range, accuracy, and reliability of the readings. The following is a guide to thermocouple types (http://www.picotech.com/applications/thermocouple.html):

- **Type K (chromel [Ni-Cr alloy]/alumel [Ni-Al alloy])**: The "general purpose" thermocouple. It is low cost and, owing to its popularity, it is available in a wide variety of probes. They are available in the –200°C to 1200°C range. Sensitivity is approximately 41 µV/°C.

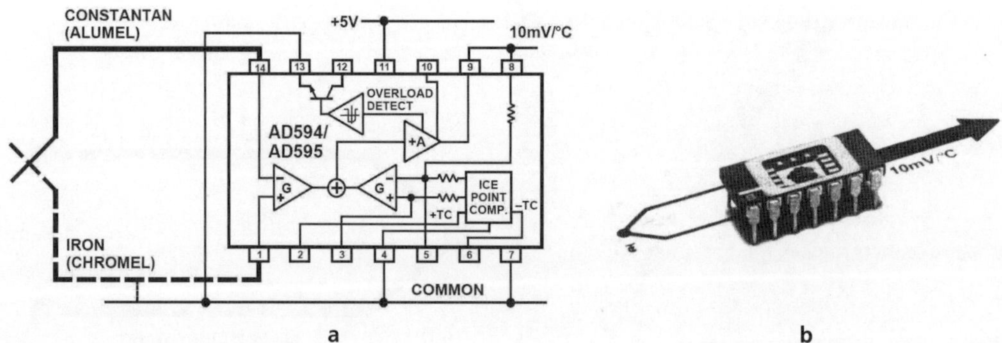


**Figure 1.5.** (a) Thermocouple amplifier having a compensation circuit for the reference temperature; (b) diagrammatic functionality of the IC (Analog Devices AD594/595).

- **Type E (chromel/constantan [Cu-Ni alloy])**: Has a high output (68 μV/°C) that makes it well suited to low-temperature (cryogenic) use.
- **Type J (iron/constantan)**: Limited range (–40°C to 750°C) makes type J thermocouples less popular than type K. The main application is with old equipment that cannot accept modern thermocouples. Type Js have a sensitivity of ~52 μV/°C.
- **Type N (nicrosil [Ni-Cr-Si alloy]/nisil [Ni-Si alloy])**: High stability and resistance to high temperature oxidation makes type N thermocouples suitable for high-temperature measurements without the cost of platinum (B, R, S) types. They can withstand temperatures above 1200°C. Sensitivity is about 39 μV/°C at 900°C.

Thermocouple types B, R, and S are all noble metal thermocouples and exhibit similar characteristics. They are the most stable of all thermocouples, but due to their low sensitivity (approximately 10 μV/°C) they are usually only used for high-temperature measurements (>300°C).

## 1.4.1.1.2. Considerations for Using Thermocouples

Most measurement problems and errors with thermocouples are caused by a lack of understanding of how thermocouples work. The following are some of the more common thermocouple problems:

- **Connection problems**. Many measurement errors are caused by unintentional thermocouple junctions. In the event that longer length thermocouple leads are needed, the correct type of thermocouple extension wire should be used.
- **Lead resistance**. Thermocouples are made from thin wire. This can cause the thermocouple to have a high resistance, which can make it sensitive to noise and can also cause errors due to the input impedance of the measuring instrument. It is recommended that thermocouple leads be kept short. If longer leads are needed, thermocouple extension wire (which is much thicker and thus has a lower resistance) should be used.
- **Decalibration**. This is the process of unintentionally altering the makeup of thermocouple wire. The usual cause is the diffusion of atmospheric particles into the metal at the extremes of operating temperature. If operating at high temperatures, check the specifications of the probe insulation.
- **Noise**. The output from a thermocouple is a small signal that is prone to electrical interference. Most measuring instruments reject any common mode interference, and interference can be minimized by twisting the cables together to help ensure both wires pick up the same interference signal.
- **Common mode voltage**. Although the thermocouple signal is very small, much larger voltages often exist at the input to the measuring instrument. These voltages can be caused by either inductive pickup or by "earthed" junctions. Common mode voltages can be minimized by using the same cabling precautions outlined for noise and by using insulated thermocouples.
- **Thermal shunting**. All thermocouples have some mass. Heating this mass takes energy and thus will affect the temperature you are trying to measure. If thermocouples with thin wires are used, lead resistance must be considered. The use of a thermocouple with thin wires connected to much thicker thermocouple extension wire often offers the best compromise.

## 1.4.1.1.3. Advantages and Disadvantages of Thermocouples

Thermocouples are wonderful sensors to experiment with because of their robustness, wide temperature ranges, and other unique properties (immune to shock and vibration, simple to manufacture, require no excitation power, no self-heating, and can be made very small). Because of their physical characteristics, thermocouples are the preferred method of temperature measurement in many applications, including clinical applications. No other temperature sensor provides this degree of versatility. On the downside, thermocouples produce a relatively low output signal that is nonlinear. These characteristics require a sensitive and stable measuring device that is able to provide reference junction compensation and linearization. Also, the low signal level requires that a higher level of care be taken when installing thermocouples to minimize potential noise sources (Michalski et al., 1991; Togawa et al., 1997).

### 1.4.1.2. Thermistors

The thermistor was invented by Samuel Ruben in 1930. The semiconductor thermistor is usually made up of small beads of complex materials such as cobalt, nickel, iron, zinc, and glass, the resistance of which is very temperature dependent. Thermistors were named by Bell Telephone Laboratories and the name is short for thermal resistors (http://www.kele.com/tech/monitor/Temperature/TRefTem4.html).

Thermistors are used inside many devices as temperature-sensing and correction devices as well as in specialty temperature-sensing probes for commerce, science, and industry, including the new digital thermometers used in medicine. Also, thermistors are used on pulmonary artery catheters for thermal dilution measurements of cardiac output. Thermistors typically work over a relatively small temperature range compared to other temperature sensors such as thermocouples, but are highly sensitive within this range, as resistance falls exponentially with temperature (Fig. 1.6). The main disadvantage of thermistors is their nonlinear resistance versus temperature characteristic. However, thermistors remain highly popular because of their low cost, miniature size, and convenience (Michalski et al., 1991; Togawa et al., 1997).

There are basically two types of thermistors, the *negative temperature coefficient (NTC)* type, used mostly in temperature sensing, and the *positive temperature coefficient (PTC)* type, used mostly in electric current control. The resistance of a thermistor has a negative temperature coefficient of about –0.04/K and its sensitivity is about ten times that of a platinum wire temperature probe. Such sensitivity makes a thermistor a suitable temperature-sensing element for use in physiological temperature measurement where relatively higher resolution is required in a narrow temperature range (Togawa et al., 1997). In a thermistor, the relationship between its resistance and the temperature is highly

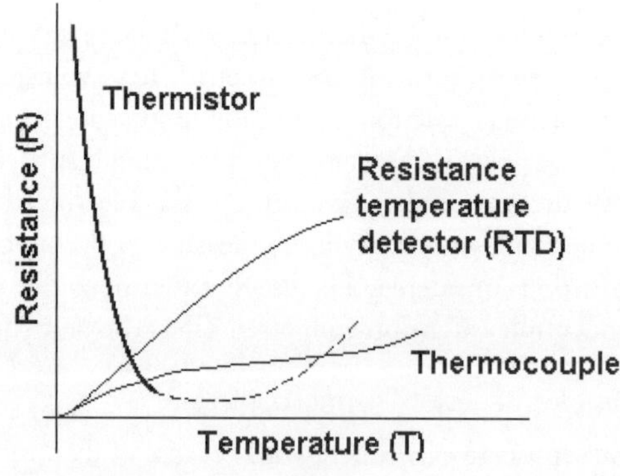


**Figure 1.6.** Thermistor characteristic curve of resistance versus temperature.

nonlinear. The resistance of a thermistor changes negatively and sharply with a positive change in temperature, as shown in Figure 1.6.

The thermistor resistance–temperature relationship can be approximated by

$$R = R_{Ref} \times e^{\beta\left(\frac{1}{T} - \frac{1}{T_{Ref}}\right)} \tag{1.5}$$

where $T$ is temperature (in kelvin); $T_{Ref}$ is the reference temperature, usually room temperature; $R$ is the resistance of the thermistor (in ohms), $R_{Ref}$ is the resistance at $T_{Ref}$; and $\beta$ is a calibration constant depending on the thermistor material, usually between 3000 K and 5000 K.

The thermistor resistance can easily be measured, but the temperature is buried inside an exponential. To solve for temperature ($T$), a natural logarithm is applied to both sides of equation 1.5:

$$\frac{1}{T} = \frac{1}{T_{Ref}} + \frac{1}{\beta}\left[\ln(R) - \ln(R_{Ref})\right]$$

$$\Rightarrow T = \frac{T_{Ref} \times \beta}{\beta + T_{Ref}\left[\ln(R) - \ln(R_{Ref})\right]}. \tag{1.6}$$

Alternatively, some references use the NTC $\alpha$ to describe the sensitivity of a thermistor:

$$\alpha = \frac{1}{R}\frac{dR}{dT}$$

$$\Rightarrow \alpha = -\frac{\beta}{T^2}. \tag{1.7}$$

Typically the value of $\alpha$ falls between –2% and –8%. Using the previous equations, the temperature can be directly obtained from the measured resistance.

Various types of thermistor probes for general use or medical use are commercially available. Figure 1.7 shows examples of thermistor probes.

From the characteristic curve (see Fig. 1.6), it can be seen that not only is the thermistor nonlinear, but it also has a negative temperature coefficient (i.e., its resistance decreases with increasing temperature). A typical circuit, shown in Figure 1.8, is used to convert thermistor ohms to a direct current (DC) voltage.

The output of the circuit is found using the formula

$$V_{out} = -V_{Ref} \times \frac{R_f}{R_i} \tag{1.8}$$

where $V_{Ref}$ is a fixed reference voltage and $R_i$ is the sum of the thermistor's resistance, $R_T$, plus 10 k$\Omega$. Using specific values of $R_T$ found in the manufacturer's data manual, a table can be created that shows $V_{out}$ as a function of temperature. For the development of a digital thermometer, the output voltage, $V_{out}$, can then be fed into a microcontroller that determines the temperature of the thermistor by converting the analog input, either voltage or current, to a temperature value. This is accomplished using

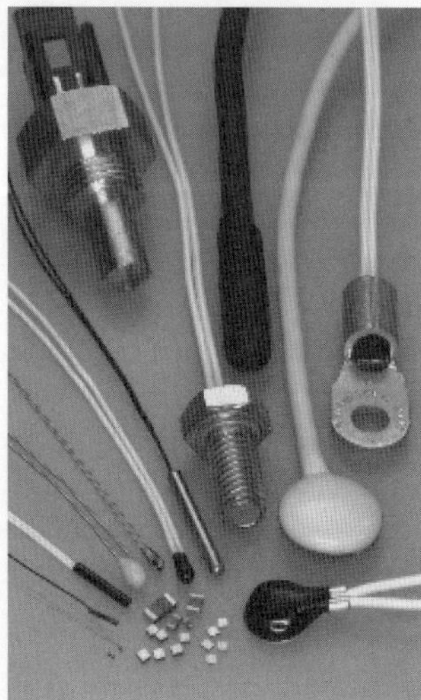

**Figure 1.7.** Thermistor probes.

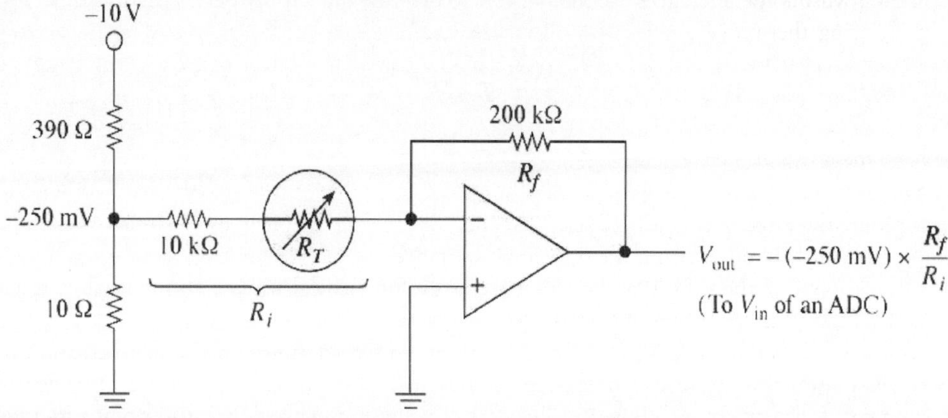


**Figure 1.8.** Circuit used to convert thermistor ohms to a DC voltage.

either a "look-up" table or by programming into the software the equations that relate resistance to temperature.

Another familiar method of utilizing a thermistor to measure temperature is to use a Wheatstone bridge with the thermistor as one leg of the bridge. The circuit in Figure 1.9 is one example of a circuit that utilizes a thermistor to sense temperature. As temperature increases, the voltage output increases. The selection of $R_1$, $R_2$, and $R_3$ will determine the sensitivity of the circuit as well as the temperature range for which the circuit is best suited.

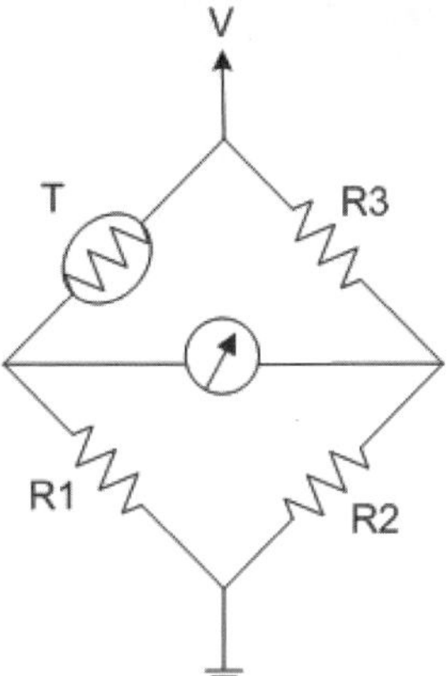


**Figure 1.9.** Wheatstone bridge—Voltage mode.

### 1.4.1.3. Resistance Temperature Detectors

Resistance thermometers or resistance temperature detectors (RTDs) are wire-wound and thin-film temperature sensors that change in resistance with varying temperature. Resistance thermometers are slowly replacing thermocouples in many industrial applications because they have greater stability, accuracy, and repeatability. The resistance tends to be almost linear with temperature, and platinum is usually used because of its linear resistance–temperature characteristic, chemical inertness, and stability with temperature. Resistance thermometers require a small current be passed through in order to determine the resistance, which can lead to self-heating. Their main advantages include a wide operating range, high accuracy, and a high suitability for precision applications. Compared to thermistors, resistance thermometers are less sensitive to small temperature changes and have a slower response time (http://www.temperatures.com).

### 1.4.1.4. Semiconductor Thermometer Devices

Semiconductor thermometers are produced in many types and shapes in the form of ICs. Most are very small and their fundamental design results from the fact that semiconductor diodes have voltage–current characteristics that are temperature sensitive. That means that semiconductor triodes or transistors are also temperature sensitive. These devices have temperature measurement ranges that are small compared to thermocouples and RTDs, but they can be quite accurate and inexpensive and very easy to interface with other electronics for display and control. The major uses are where the temperature range is limited to about –25°C to 200°C.

A typical example is the LM35 series (National Semiconductor, Santa Clara, CA) precision IC temperature sensors, whose output voltage is linearly proportional to the Celsius (centigrade) temperature (see Fig. 1.10). The LM35 thus has an advantage over linear temperature sensors calibrated in kelvin, as the user is not required to subtract a large constant voltage from its output to obtain convenient centigrade measurements. The LM35 does not require any external calibration or trimming to provide typical accuracies of ±¼°C at room temperature and ±¾°C over a full –55°C to 150°C temperature range.

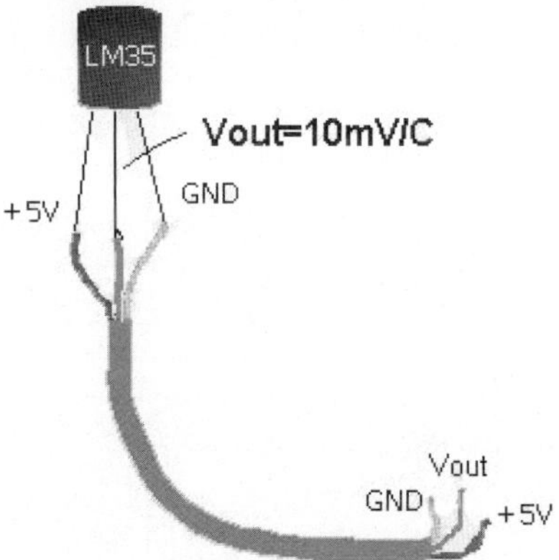


**Figure 1.10.** LM35 IC linear temperature sensor.

### 1.4.1.5. Liquid Crystal Temperature Sensors

Friedrich Reinitzer, an Austrian scientist, and Otto Lehman discovered and coined the term "liquid crystal" (a substance that can be between a liquid and a solid state). Today liquid crystals can be found in most state-of-the-art technologies, including liquid crystal displays (LCDs) in watches, computer screens, televisions, and clinical thermometers (http://kicp-yerkes.uchicago.edu/2003-winter/pdf/ywi2003-liquid_crystals.pdf).

Liquid crystal temperature sensors are thin, flat pieces of plastic with heat-activated chemical dots (heat-sensitive liquid crystals) on the surface that are designed to change color in accordance with the temperature sensed. They are used for disposable clinical liquid crystal thermometers or plastic strip thermometers. Disposable liquid crystal thermometers are mainly used on the skin, such as the forehead, but they can also be used in the mouth or rectum. When a plastic strip thermometer is placed on the skin it initially looks black in color; the color then changes depending on the temperature to red, yellow, green, or blue. Liquid crystal thermometers are made with cholesteric liquid crystals.

Under the microscope, liquid crystals look like small rodlike structures. In their solid state, the liquid crystal rodlike structures form layers parallel to each other. In their liquid state the structures are shifted at various angles in relationship to each other. In their liquid crystal state the rods form layers, but adjacent layers run in slightly different directions from those above or below them. This is shown in Figure 1.11.

The distance over which the liquid crystals twist is called the pitch (Fig. 1.12), and it determines the color of the light that is reflected.

Liquid crystals, when exposed to different temperatures change state from solid to liquid to gas, which has an effect on the pitch distance (decreases with heat) and the angle of twisting between the rods (increases with heat). These changes determine the color of light that is reflected. For example, when the distance equals half of the wavelength of red light the liquid crystal will reflect red light. If the distance is shortened to half the wavelength of blue light it will reflect blue light.

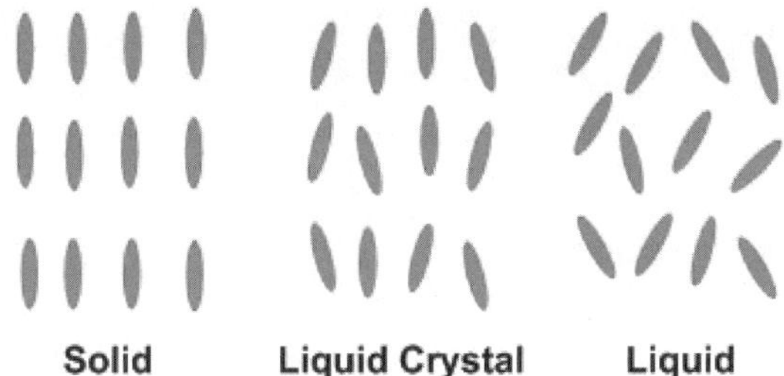



**Figure 1.11.** Cholesteric liquid crystals in their solid, liquid crystal, and liquid states.

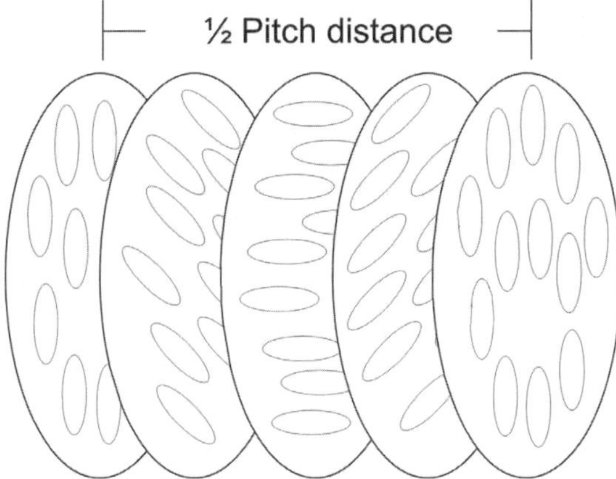



**Figure 1.12.** Distance over which the liquid crystals twist.

## 1.4.2. NONCONTACT TEMPERATURE SENSORS

Noncontact temperature measurement can be realized using radiation heat transfer (Togawa et al., 1997). Noncontact temperature measurement is the preferred technique for small, moving, or inaccessible objects. The uses of noncontact temperature sensors are many, but the understanding of their use is, in general, relatively poor. Part of this misunderstanding comes with the need to deal with emissivity, or more precisely, with spectral emissivity. This quality defines the fraction of radiation emitted by an object as compared to that emitted by a perfect radiator (blackbody) at the same temperature. Emissivity is determined in part by the type of material and its surface condition, and may vary from close to 0 (for a highly reflective mirror) to almost 1 (for a blackbody simulator). Emissivity is used to calculate the true temperature of an object from the measured brightness or spectral radiance. Because an object's emissivity may also vary with wavelength, a radiation thermometer with spectral response matching regions of high emissivity should be selected for a specific application. Emissivity values are listed in the literature for a variety of materials and spectral bands, or these values can be determined empirically (http://www.omega.com/temperature/Z/NoncontactTM.html).

In many industrial plants, noncontact sensors have not yet been standardized to the extent that thermocouples and RTDs are. More recently the medical world has adopted the IR noncontact ear thermometer (discussed in the next section), which is basically a single waveband radiation thermometer (http://www.temperatures.com).

### 1.4.2.1. Infrared-Sensing Thermometers

Infrared thermometers are useful because they do not need physical contact with the thermal source. IR sensors absorb and detect IR emissions given off by a heated surface (Fig. 1.13). The incoming radiation is converted to an electric signal that corresponds to a particular temperature. Near the human body temperature, the peak of the thermal radiation is in the far-IR region (Togawa et al., 1997).

A typical IR clinical thermometer is the ear or tympanic thermometer. The sensor can be introduced intermittently into a speculum in the external auditory meatus. The sensor is in sight of the eardrum and gathers information from the tympanic membrane over a period of 1 second. The data are then processed to produce a temperature reading. Such a device has been found to correlate well with the pulmonary artery temperature during rewarming in cardiopulmonary bypass surgery. However, both research and practice have shown that user technique is very important for an accurate temperature reading. An IR ear thermometer will display the temperature of whatever it is directed at, therefore correct placement in the ear canal is critical. If the probe tip is not well into the ear canal, the chances are the coolest portions of the ear canal will be measured. If, on the other hand, the probe tip is inserted well into the canal the reading is much more likely to include the warmest part of the ear—the tympanic membrane—and give a true reading of core body temperature. A major advantage of this technique is that readings can be made quickly and the site of measurement is generally easily accessible (http://www.graduateresearch.com/thermometry).

## 1.5. CLINICAL THERMOMETERS

Since the mercury-in-glass thermometer was introduced at the start of the twentieth century, the measurement of body temperature has become easy and accurate (Togawa, 1985; Togawa et al., 1997).

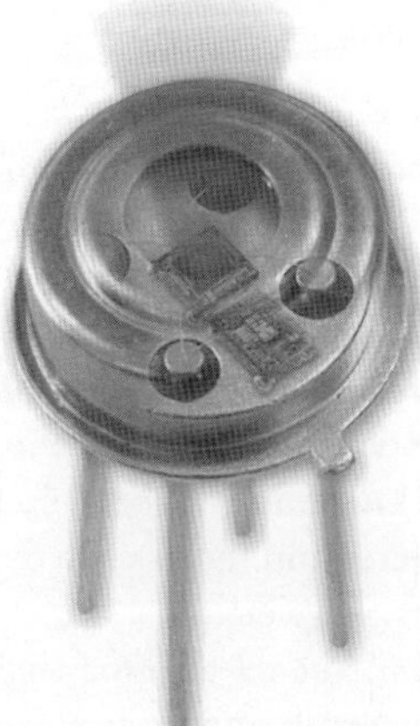

**Figure 1.13.** Infrared thermometer sensor for noncontact temperature measurements. *Image credit: http://www.melexis.com*

This thermometer has proven for many years to be a reliable, easy-to-use, and low-cost device. However, there are many occasions when the use of a glass thermometer might not be the best choice, especially when fast response and continuous temperature monitoring is required. The traditional mercury thermometer has gradually been replaced by the more "user friendly" digital thermometer. Since the accuracy is comparable with both instruments and mercury contamination is also a serious issue in hospitals, the use of mercury thermometers is no longer recommended (Press & Quinn, 1997).

Over the last several years many different kinds of clinical thermometers have been introduced that use the various temperature sensors and transducers described in section 1.4. These thermometers have been designed and developed for application in various parts of the body, including the rectum, mouth, axilla, esophagus, bladder, ear, temporal artery, and skin. This section discusses the most widely used clinical thermometers.

## 1.5.1. RECTAL THERMOMETRY

A typical rectal temperature probe is a flexible catheter with a thermistor (see section 1.4.1.2) at the tip. Rectal temperature provides accurate measurements of core temperature and rectal thermometry has traditionally been considered the gold standard for temperature measurement (Brown, Christmas, & Ford, 1992; Cereda & Maccioli, 2004; McCarthy, 1998). Rectal thermometers could be either the traditional glass thermometer or an electronic digital thermometer, as shown in Figure 1.14. Despite its wide acceptance, rectal thermometry also presents some limitations (Cereda & Maccioli, 2004; Robinson et al., 1998). Rectal temperatures are slow to change in relation to changing core temperature, and they have been shown to stay more elevated (0.2°C to 0.3°C) than those obtained in other parts of the body (Cranston, Gerbrandy, & Snell, 1954; Eichina et al., 1951; Isley, Rutten, & Runciman, 1983). Rectal readings are also affected by the depth of the measurement (usually 8 to 15 cm from the anal sphincter), conditions affecting local blood flow, and the presence of stool (Togawa et al., 1997). Rectal perforation is another major limitation, especially in infants and small children (Blainey, 1974; Kenney et al., 1990). Rectal thermometry has the capacity to spread contaminants that are commonly found in stool, therefore proper sterilization techniques are necessary. Despite these limitations, rectal thermometry can be a reasonable choice to monitor temperature (Cereda & Maccioli, 2004).

## 1.5.2. ORAL THERMOMETRY

Oral thermometry is the most common method of taking a temperature. Traditionally the mercury-in-glass thermometer was used for measuring temperature where the temperature sensor was positioned

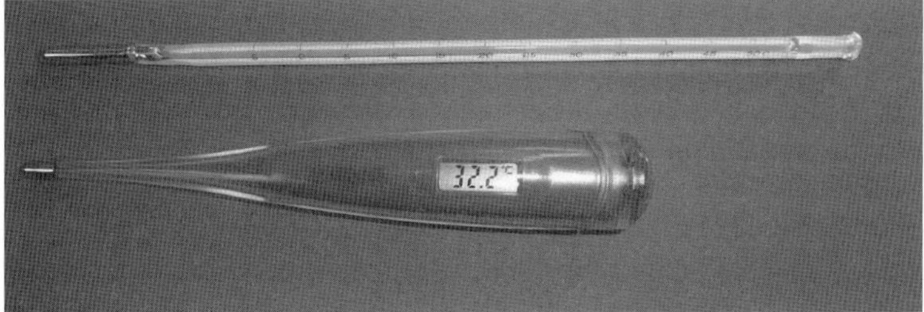

**Figure 1.14.** Typical oral and rectal thermometers.

under the tongue (sublingual). Today the mercury-in-glass thermometer has been replaced by mercury-free glass thermometers (manufacturers use galinstan, a liquid alloy of gallium, indium, and tin, as a replacement for mercury) or digital thermometers, which with the press of a button, provide an easy-to-read temperature in about 60 seconds (Fig. 1.14). The sublingual site is easily accessible and reflects the temperature of the lingual arteries. Oral temperature measurement is easily accessible, less prone to operator error, and quickly reflects changes in core body temperature. However, oral temperature is easily influenced by the ingestion of food or drink and by mouth breathing (Jaffe, 1995). Also, for the correct measurement of temperature when using a sublingual probe the mouth should remain sealed, with the tongue depressed for 3 to 4 minutes (for glass thermometers), which can be a difficult task, especially with children or unconscious or uncooperative patients. Also, safety is an issue, as patients may accidentally bite or break the thermometer. Safety is increased by using nonbreakable probes instead of glass probes. The main advantages of this method are easy accessibility and that it is noninvasive. Oral thermometers are not recommended for infants or very young children because of the previously mentioned limitations. The accuracy of the oral thermometer is somewhere between that of rectal and axillary thermometers, however, its accuracy increases when it is properly applied.

## 1.5.3. AXILLARY THERMOMETRY

Axillary (armpit) thermometry relies on traditional temperature measurement using a mercury-in-glass temperature sensor (or mercury-free glass temperature sensor) or digital thermometer, such as the ones shown in Figure 1.14, placed over the axillary artery (Seguin & Terry, 1999). Such a technique can be influenced by environmental conditions and also by vasoconstriction and vasodilation of the underlying vasculature. Axillary thermometry is an easy and very practical method to use (compared with oral or rectal measurements). The thermometer should be kept clamped under the arm against the chest for 3 to 4 minutes. The time needed to record the temperature using this technique is one of its limitations, however, axillary thermometry allows for repeatable temperature measurements without any significant discomfort. Unfortunately this technique has been found to be the worst estimate of core temperature in children (Jaffe, 1995; McCarthy, 1998) and shows low sensitivity and specificity in detecting fever. Despite these limitations, axillary thermometry has been recommended by the American Academy of Pediatrics as a screening test for fever in neonates because of the risk (very low) of rectal perforation when using a rectal thermometer (Kresch, 1994).

## 1.5.4. ESOPHAGEAL THERMOMETRY

Esophageal temperature is mainly monitored during anesthesia (Hooper & Andrews, 2006). Usually after induction of general anesthesia, a flexible esophageal thermistor-type probe (76 cm in length) is inserted through the mouth or the nose into the lower one-third of the esophagus. The length of the probe is covered with a white polyvinyl chloride (PVC) sleeve that prevents exposure of the lead wire and acts as a barrier to moisture. The tip of the thermistor is insulated, reducing the risk of electrical shocks or burns. The top of the probe is round and smooth for nontraumatic insertion (Fig. 1.15). Esophageal temperature is considered an accurate and precise estimate of core temperature in almost all conditions. However, misplacement of the esophageal temperature probe close to the trachea, where there is a flow of cooler gases (more proximal positioning), can lead to falsely lowered temperature values (Whitby & Dunkin, 1971).

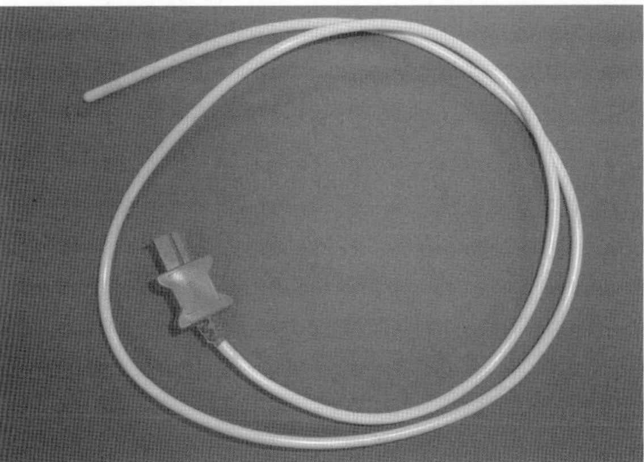

**Figure 1.15.** Esophageal thermometer.

Also, there is evidence that esophageal temperature can artifactually decrease during thoracotomy and rapid infusion of cold fluids and can also be affected by the temperature of inspired gases (Bissonnette, Sessler, & LaFlamme, 1989). Another reported limitation is patient discomfort and trauma, especially postoperatively when the patient is not fully anesthetized and the probe has been inserted into the esophagus through the mouth (it is more tolerable when the probe is inserted through the nose; Whitby & Dunkin, 1968). Also, in rare cases, complications such as esophageal perforations and burns have been reported.

## *1.5.5. PULMONARY ARTERY CATHETER THERMOMETRY*

Temperature measured invasively in the pulmonary artery is considered the gold standard in temperature monitoring, but it is highly unsuitable for a majority of patients because of its invasiveness (Bock et al., 2005). A pulmonary artery catheter (PAC), frequently referred to as a Swan-Ganz catheter, in honor of its inventors Jeremy Swan and William Ganz, is inserted through a major vein (often the internal jugular, subclavian, or femoral vein) and a thermistor is embedded in the tip (about 3 cm behind the tip) of the PAC lying in the pulmonary artery. This method is often used as a reference for other monitoring devices (Bock et al., 2005; Milewski, Ferguson, & Terndrup, 1991). The use of this measurement site is restricted to critically ill patients in whom a pulmonary artery catheter is required for hemodynamic monitoring.

## *1.5.6. BLADDER THERMOMETRY*

Bladder temperature is monitored using a thermistor-tipped Foley bladder catheter (Togawa et al., 1997). The Foley catheter with temperature sensor is used for urinary drainage and simultaneous monitoring of bladder temperature. Bladder temperature is determined primarily by urine flow, and high flow rates are necessary for the bladder temperature to reflect core temperature. Low urinary flow makes bladder temperature difficult to interpret in relation to true core temperature. Based on several studies, bladder temperature is reliable, accurate, and safe for core temperature monitoring. During hypothermia, this method is less reliable. The temperature in the bladder is close to the core temperature (Cork, Vaughan, & Humphrey, 1983) and has been found to correlate highly with rectal, esophageal, and pulmonary arterial temperatures. However, the accuracy of this measurement site decreases with low urinary output and during surgery in the lower abdomen.

### 1.5.7. TYMPANIC THERMOMETRY

Because the eardrum is in the vicinity of the carotid artery, the brain, and the hypothalamus, tympanic temperature is often considered a gold standard of core temperature measurement and is used as a reference for other sites. To measure this temperature, a transducer is placed in contact with the tympanic membrane (Fig. 1.16). The first devices used to measure tympanic membrane temperature did so by being in direct contact with the tympanic membrane.

Small thermocouples and thermistor probes have been used for tympanic temperature measurements since 1963, when Benzinger and Taylor described tympanic temperature sensors in which copper-constantan wires were connected side by side at the tip and drawn into fine polyethylene tubing (Togawa et al., 1997). In 1969 it was shown that such a device measured core temperature better than a rectal thermometer (Benzinger & Benzinger, 1972). However, thermistors in direct contact with the tympanic membrane are not practical for everyday use. Direct visualization with an otoscope is required for correct positioning of the probe, as malpositioning can cause inaccurate measurements (Webb, 1973). In addition, bleeding and perforation of the eardrum from contact tympanic probes have been reported (Tabor, Blaho, & Schriver, 1981; Wallace et al., 1974). For these reasons, tympanic temperature is measured mainly for research purposes and for those conditions in which knowledge of brain temperature is particularly desired, such as during hypothermic cardiopulmonary bypass (Webb, 1973).

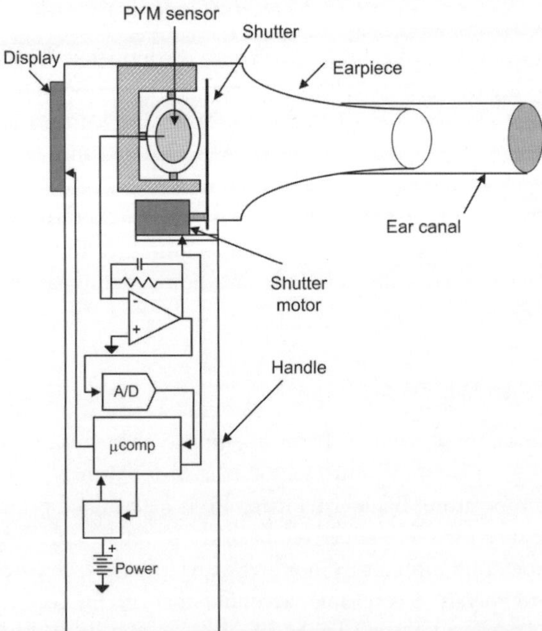


**Figure 1.16.** A diagram of a typical tympanic thermometer.

Instead of being in direct contact with the tympanic membrane, today's tympanic thermometers measure the thermal radiation emitted from the tympanic membrane and the ear canal, and are thus called IR emission detectors (IREDs). Tympanic IR thermometry (noncontact) has received a great deal of the attention over the last few years in the clinical setting, and a large number (more than one hundred since the early 1990s) of peer reviewed articles have been published demonstrating its applicability in the clinical setting and comparing its accuracy and sensitivity with other more traditional temperature measuring techniques, some of them described in this review. Some of these comparison studies will be reported in the following sections.

The thermal radiation emitted is in proportion to the tympanic membrane's temperature, therefore the IRED accurately estimates tympanic membrane temperature (Chamberlain et al., 1995). The blood supply of the tympanic membrane is similar in temperature and location to the blood bathing the hypothalamus, the site of the body's thermoregulatory center, and therefore it is an ideal location for core temperature estimation (Childs, Harrison, & Hodkinson, 1999; Terndrup et al., 1997). Crying, otitis media, or earwax have not been shown to change tympanic readings significantly.

Tympanic thermometers became available commercially in the early 1990s. The First-Temp ear thermometer, manufactured by Intelligent Medical Systems, Carlsbad, CA, was the first ear thermometer on the market and sold for a list price of $695. Today a state-of-the-art tympanic thermometer, such as the Braun Thermoscan Pro 4000 ear thermometer, manufactured by Welch Allyn, Inc., Skaneateles Falls, NY, can be purchased for about $200. Tympanic membrane thermometers at prices ranging from $20 to $40 are also available.

A tympanic thermometer can measure the IR radiation of the tympanic membrane in two ways. A thermopile sensor (composed of thermocouples connected in either series or parallel) with a light pipe installed at the tip of the probe detects the level of heat in the area directly proximal to the tympanic membrane by taking multiple readings very quickly. Also, measurements can be taken by employing a pyrosensor (PYM sensor), which is a heat flow detector that measures the speed at which the thermal energy flows through a sensor. The pyrosensor takes a "snapshot" of the heat that it records from the tympanic membrane, just like photographic film (Fig. 1.16). In both methods the tip of the tympanic membrane probe is inserted into the external auditory canal (Fig. 1.17; Betta, Cascetta, & Sepe, 1997; O'Hara & Phillips, 1986, 1988).

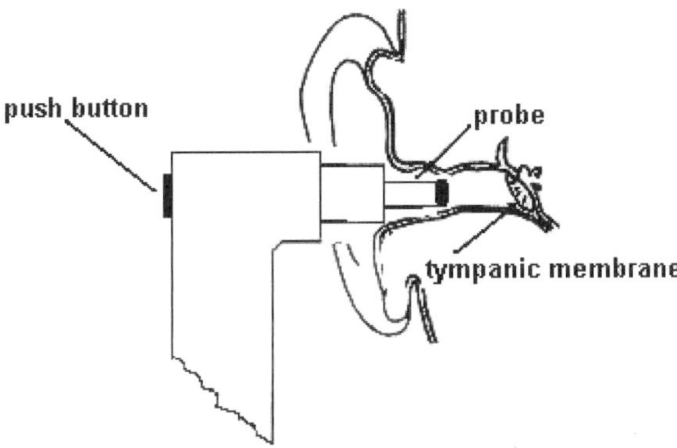


**Figure 1.17.** Tympanic IR temperature measurement with a probe placed into the external auditory canal.

In conclusion, ear temperature measurement with an IR tympanic thermometer offers a reasonable estimate of core temperature within 1 to 2 seconds and can be tolerated by awake patients, allowing its use in those situations in which esophageal temperature is difficult to obtain, such as during regional anesthesia. Although ear temperature measurement is common in the recovery room, intensive care unit, and in general on many hospital floors, its intraoperative use is probably still relatively rare.

## 1.5.8. TEMPORAL ARTERY THERMOMETRY

Exergen Corporation, Watertown, MA, recently (late 1990s) developed the TemporalScanner temporal artery noninvasive IR thermometer (Pompei, 1999). The temporal artery and surrounding tissue was investigated as a new and potentially more suitable temperature measurement site (Sandlin, 2003). The temporal artery area is a site with a long history of temperature measurement, actually dating back to the early centuries B.C. and the first recorded references to palpation of the head for assessment of fever (Pompei, 1999). As a temperature measurement site, the temporal artery is easily accessible and usually quite visible, poses no risk of injury for the patient, and contains no mucous membranes (eliminating the risk of contaminates; Ikeda et al., 1997). Also, perfusion of the temporal artery remains relatively constant, thus ensuring the stability of blood flow required for the measurement method. Exergen Corporation developed and validated three IR devices: one a professional model for clinical use, one for home use, and the other a professional model for use in neonatal intensive care (Pompei, 1999).

Because the temporal artery thermometer measures temperature at the outer surface of the head, the absolute temperature will not be the same as the arterial temperature of interest (core temperature). A technique known as the arterial heat balance (AHB) method, which accounts for temperature losses due to ambient temperature, is employed (Pompei, 1999). The difference between normal ambient temperature and arterial temperature is about 17°C. If the cooling effect at the skin surface from the radiated heat loss to the environment is taken into consideration, measurement errors of more than 3°C could be present (Pompei, 2006). The AHB method incorporated into the IR thermometer accounts for the radiated heat loss by measuring ambient temperature at the same time it is measuring the absolute temperature of the skin surface (2000 times per second) over the temporal artery. It then computes arterial temperature by restoring the measured heat loss to the absolute peak surface temperature measurement. The AHB method solves the heat balance equation multiple times per second, selects the highest of the readings, and discards all the others. The final temperature displayed is the solution to the algorithm, which gives the maximum reading during a particular measurement (Pompei, 1999).

## 1.5.9. SKIN THERMOMETRY

The temperature of the skin is often measured using thermocouples or liquid crystals enclosed in adhesive pads (Cereda & Maccioli, 2004). A thermocouple skin temperature sensor and a liquid crystal temperature sensor are shown in Figure 1.18(a) and Figure 1.18(b), respectively. These sensors can be applied on various regions of the body, usually the shoulder, toe, or forehead. Interpretation of skin temperature values can be difficult and must be done with caution, as they cannot be considered to reflect the core temperature. As discussed previously for temporal artery temperature measurements, even when the skin temperature reading is adjusted, the resulting value might not accurately estimate core temperature (Cork et al., 1983). The differences in temperature between periphery and core continuously change during

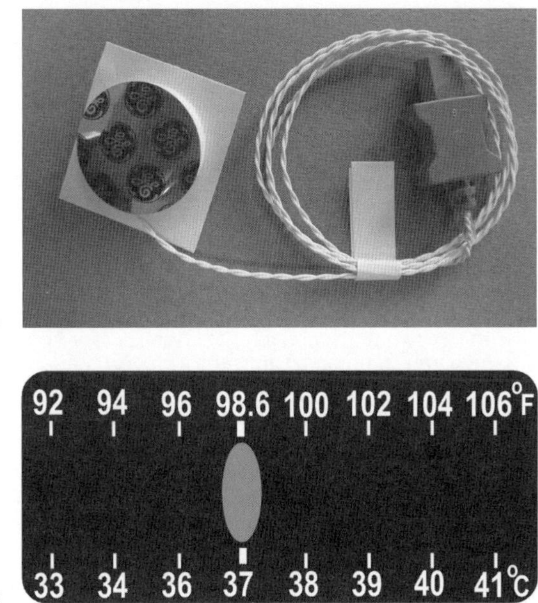



**Figure 1.18.** (a) A thermocouple skin temperature sensor; (b) a liquid crystal temperature sensor.

anesthesia; such changes can be caused by the duration of anesthesia, use of body warmers such as blankets, environmental temperature, and vasomotor status (Bissonnette et al., 1989).

However, skin temperature sensors are used quite extensively, especially in cases when esophageal or other invasive temperature probes would be impractical, such as during regional anesthesia. In fact, most anesthesiologists who monitor temperature during regional anesthesia use skin temperature sensors (Frank et al., 1999). Also, skin thermometers such as liquid crystal strip thermometers are safe to use, as they do not contain glass, latex, or mercury, and they are accurate to within ±0.2°F (±0.1°C; Vaughan, Cork, & Vaughan, 1982). Such temperature sensors have been reported to work well for screening in older children (Reisinger, Kao, & Grant, 1979).

## 1.5.10. PACIFIER THERMOMETRY

The pacifier is a digital baby thermometer intended for oral measurement of body temperature in babies and toddlers up to 3 years of age. The pacifier digital baby thermometer allows parents to take their baby's temperature accurately and conveniently, without causing distress. The thermometer consists of two parts. The first part includes a silicone orthodontic comfort nipple to place in the baby's mouth, a base element, and a washer. The second part includes a thermometer housing and thermometer electronics that fit into the washer for attachment to the base. The thermometer includes a flexible thermocouple that extends into the hollow nipple and an end that rests on the interior of the nipple. The nipple is made of silicone and is heat conductive, thus the temperature of the baby's tongue is effectively transmitted to the thermocouple. The temperature is then displayed by the thermometer (Braun, 2006; Press & Quinn, 1997).

### 1.5.11. INGESTIBLE THERMOMETRY

Ingestible temperature sensors used for monitoring core temperature (in humans and animals) were described as early as the 1960s, but they have never received widespread clinical application. HQ Inc., Palmetto, FL, designed and now manufactures an ingestible (pill form) temperature sensor (CorTemp). The sensor was developed with the goal of monitoring the core temperature of football players during games, wirelessly transmitting core body temperatures to trainers on the sidelines. The pill was originally developed in the mid-1980s by NASA so the space agency could monitor the body temperatures of astronauts on the space shuttle. There is little published technical information regarding this sensor, but in brief, the biocompatible ingestible sensor contains a temperature-sensitive quartz crystal oscillator. Once inside the gastrointestinal tract, the crystal sensor vibrates at a frequency related to the temperature of the substance (body) surrounding it, producing a magnetic flux and transmitting the signal harmlessly through the body. The CorTemp Ambulatory Data Recorder picks up, displays, and stores the data in a solid-state memory until the data are downloaded into a computer. The sensor is covered with a protective silicone coating, is approximately 10 mm in diameter and 20 mm long, and is energized by an internal silver-oxide battery. The technology is expensive and works for only 1 to 2 days (Byrne and Lim, 2007).

## 1.6. APPLICATION, EVALUATION, AND COMPARISON OF THERMOMETRY AND MEASUREMENT ROUTES

### 1.6.1. INTRODUCTION

Probably the most common reason to monitor body temperature is to examine the patient's thermal balance. The body can counterbalance for small increases or decreases in temperature by activating the thermoregulatory system. Extremes in temperature can affect hypothalamic functions, disrupt thermoregulation, and lead to death, thus it is important to continuously monitor temperature. Since it is not easy to measure directly the temperature of the hypothalamus, proximal sites such as the tympanic membrane, the pulmonary artery, and esophagus are better suited for these measurements (Miller, 2000).

A response to an increase in body temperature is to remove excess moisture from body tissues by way of perspiration. A response to a decrease in body temperature is for the body to generate heat by shivering. Shivering is an involuntary contraction and expansion of muscle tissue. Heat is also conserved by vasoconstriction of poorly perfused tissues. Temperature in the pulmonary artery remains unchanged and hence is not ideal for monitoring these responses. Unless the hypothalamic functions fail or heat cannot be appropriately conserved or generated, the pulmonary artery shows only a gradual decrease in temperature. Both fever and hyperthermia can cause disruption to the central nervous system due to a rapid increase in temperature.

It is important to monitor temperature during regional and general anesthesia. When general anesthetic is given, the core temperature of patients is a vital measurement. Anesthesia can greatly alter the thermoregulatory system, causing a decrease in cold-response limit and an increase in warm-response limit. This results in the blocking of thermoregulatory defenses. Hyperthermia is an acute condition wherein the amount of heat produced or absorbed by the body is much more than it can dissipate. This can result in the failure of hypothalamic functions, that is, the hypothalamus fails to trigger necessary cooling mechanisms. The mechanisms of the body that regulate heat are unable to deal with this heat efficiently, and hence there is an uncontrollable increase in body temperature. Unless necessary steps are taken to cool the body, irreversible brain damage and death will occur.

Therefore accurate temperature measurement is critical to the assessment and management of temperature fluctuations in acutely ill patients. Temperature monitoring, using the previously described noninvasive and invasive technologies, is now widely practiced in many fields of medicine, including anesthesia, surgery, and intensive care, for all types of patients (neonates, children, and adults; Busic & Das-Gupta, 2004; Cattaneo et al., 2000; Frank et al., 1999; Gilbert, Barton, & Counsell, 2002; Hooper & Andrews, 2006; Kaukuntla et al., 2004; Krenzischek, Frank, & Kelly, 1995; Nussmeier, 2005; Tabbutt et al., 2006; Van Dam, Nduka, & Carver, 2003; Young & Sladen, 1996). There are numerous reports in the literature describing the use of such techniques in different clinical applications, and the majority of such reports not only discuss the application of a particular clinical thermometer but also compare different thermometers. It is impossible for this section to cover every possible application and evaluation study relating to different thermometers, however, an effort has been made to provide a review of studies comparing selected invasive and noninvasive temperature measurement methods discussed previously in this chapter.

## *1.6.2. COMPARISON OF MULTIPLE CLINICAL THERMOMETERS*

A study that compares skin core temperature-corrected liquid crystal thermography, axillary electronic, and oral electronic thermistor readings with temperatures obtained by IR tympanic membrane thermometry from 215 postanesthesia care unit (PACU) patients was conducted by Darm, Hecker, and Rubal (1994). The measurement of patient body temperature in the PACU is an important parameter in patient management and failure to achieve minimal acceptable body temperature standards has been associated with physiological derangement, the application of additional therapy, and prolonged PACU stays. Regression analysis results from this study suggested that when compared with tympanic temperature, the oral method is more accurate and has greater precision than either the liquid crystal or axillary methods, concluding that the incidence of hypothermia depends on the method chosen to assess body temperature, with significant nursing implications.

Patel et al. (1996) compared esophageal, tympanic membrane, and forehead skin temperatures in forty patients undergoing elective surgeries. They concluded that there was a lack of agreement between the clinically accepted measurements (lower esophageal and tympanic membranes) and the skin temperature measurement. The data suggested that forehead skin temperature is not interchangeable with standard core temperature measurements, and that sole reliance on forehead skin measurement in the perioperative setting could adversely affect patient care. Also, a study by Jensen et al. (2000) attempted to compare a number of electronic tympanic, oral, axillary, and rectal measurements with those taken with a standard rectal mercury thermometer in a group of two hundred patients in a county hospital in Denmark. They found that the rectal electronic measurements were closest to the rectal mercury readings, with a mean of –0.05°C (standard deviation [SD] 0.12°C), whereas the other measurements gave unacceptable SDs of temperature differences ranging from 0.41°C to 0.53°C. They concluded that the electronic rectal temperature measurements are the most accurate and they did not recommend electronic tympanic, oral, or axillary measurements.

A comparative study on the accuracy of liquid crystal forehead, digital electronic axillary, IR tympanic, and mercury-in-glass rectal thermometers in 200 infants and young children ages 0 to 48 months (Kongpanichkul & Bunjongpak, 2000) showed that tympanic thermometry had the best performance while forehead thermometry had the poorest. The authors concluded that the three clinical thermometers are not suitable as a substitute for a mercury-in-glass rectal thermometer in assessment of fever in infants and young children. More recently Lefrant et al. (2003) conducted a temperature study in forty-two intensive care patients, comparing bladder, esophageal, rectal, axillary, and inguinal temperatures versus pulmonary artery temperature. Temperature was simultaneously monitored with PAC, bladder, esophageal, and rectal electronic thermometers and with axillary and inguinal gallium-in-glass thermometers. A total of 529 temperature measurement comparisons were carried out. They concluded that in critically ill patients, bladder and esophageal electronic thermometers are more reliable than the electronic rectal thermometer, which is better than inguinal and axillary gallium-in-glass thermometers for measuring core temperature.

Monitoring temperature in critically ill children is an important component of care, yet the accuracy of methods is often questioned. Temperature measured in the pulmonary artery is considered the gold standard, but this route is unsuitable for the majority of patients. However, an accurate, reliable, and less invasive method has yet to be established in pediatric intensive care work. To determine which site most closely reflects core temperature in babies and children following cardiac surgery, Maxton, Justin, and Gillies (2004) compared pulmonary artery temperature to the temperature measured at rectal, bladder, nasopharyngeal, axillary, and tympanic sites. In this study, bladder temperature was shown to be the best estimate of pulmonary artery temperature, closely followed by the temperature measured by the nasopharyngeal probe. The results support the use of bladder or nasopharyngeal catheters to monitor temperature in critically ill children after cardiac surgery.

Farnell et al. (2005) conducted a study to assess the accuracy and reliability of two noninvasive methods, a chemical (Tempa.DOT) and tympanic thermometer (Genius First Temp M3000A), against the gold standard PAC, and to determine the clinical significance of any temperature discrepancy using an expert panel. A total of 160 temperature sets were obtained from twenty-five adult intensive care patients over a 6-month period. Their findings showed that the chemical thermometer was more accurate and reliable and was associated with fewer clinically significant temperature differences compared with the tympanic thermometer.

### 1.6.3. EVALUATION OF TEMPORAL THERMOMETRY

As described in section 1.5.8, IR arterial temperature can be measured with a device that is positioned in the temporal area. Greenes and Fleisher (2001) assessed the accuracy of the noninvasive temporal artery thermometer in infants and compared its accuracy with that of a tympanic thermometer, using rectal thermometry as the criterion standard. A sample of 304 infants younger than 1 year was included in the study. They found that the temporal artery thermometer has limited sensitivity for detecting cases of fever in infants. However, they pointed out that the temporal artery thermometer is more accurate than the tympanic thermometer in infants, and it is better tolerated by infants than rectal thermometry.

Roy, Powell, and Gerson (2003) have also compared a noninvasive temporal artery thermometer with rectal and ear thermometry. In this case, temperatures were measured in healthy patients 0 to 18 years of age. This study provided information about temporal artery temperatures in healthy infants and children that can serve as a basis for interpreting temperature measurements in ill children when the same instrument is used. In a recent trial (Schuh et al., 2004) in a busy pediatric emergency department, the temporal artery device was shown to have a sensitivity of about 80% in identifying fever (as determined by rectal measurements). It was concluded that temporal artery thermometry may be a promising tool for screening children at low risk in the emergency department but cannot yet be recommended for home use or hospital use when definitive measurements are required. Also, Schuh et al. (2004) compared the temporal artery thermometer with the rectal thermometer in 327 children less than 24 months of age. The conclusion was that the temporal thermometer cannot replace the rectal thermometer and it was found to be inadequate for the detection of fever.

A study by Myny et al. (2005) was conducted to evaluate the accuracy and variability of the temporal artery thermometer (TAT) in intensive care unit (ICU) patients. Fifty-seven adult patients with indwelling PACs were studied. Body temperature was measured simultaneously with the TAT and the axillary thermometer and was compared with the temperature recording of the PAC. The authors concluded that the temporal scanner has a relatively good reliability, with acceptable accuracy and variability in patients with normothermia. The results were comparable to those of the axillary thermometer, but they did not seem to give any substantial benefit compared to rectal, oral, or bladder thermometry. In the same year, Hebbar et al. (2005) compared seventy-five temperature pairs that were obtained from forty-four pediatric ICU patients. They found that temporal artery and axillary temperature measurements showed variability compared to rectal temperatures, with marked variability in febrile children. Neither was sufficiently accurate to recommend replacing rectal or other invasive methods. In conclusion, since temporal artery and axillary methods provide similar accuracy, TATs may serve as a suitable alternative for patients in whom invasive thermometry is contraindicated.

Studies by Kistemaker, Den Hartog, and Daanen (2006) and Suleman et al. (2002) evaluated the reliability of an IR forehead skin thermometer (SensorTouch) for core temperature measurements. Kistemaker et al. (2006) conducted two experiments in which the body temperature was measured with a rectal sensor, with an esophageal sensor, and with the SensorTouch. They concluded that the SensorTouch did not provide reliable readings of body temperature during periods of increasing body temperature, but the SensorTouch might work under stable conditions. Suleman et al. (2002) studied fifteen adults and sixteen children who developed mild fever—a core temperature of at least 37.8°C—after cardiopulmonary bypass. Temperature was recorded with the SensorTouch thermometer and from the pulmonary artery (adults) or bladder (children). They found that the SensorTouch accuracy was poor in the adults and suboptimal in the infants and children.

## 1.6.4. EVALUATION OF TYMPANIC THERMOMETRY

Ear temperature measurement using an IR tympanic thermometer is widely used today, especially in neonatal and pediatric temperature monitoring, and offers a reasonable estimate of core temperature (Dew, 2006; Shinozaki, Deane, & Perkins, 1988). However, despite its popularity, its intraoperative use is probably still relatively rare. Androkites, Werger, and Young (1998) conducted a study to determine whether IR tympanic membrane thermometry can replace mercury-in-glass temperatures as an assessment tool for detecting fevers earlier and more reliably in a pediatric oncology outpatient setting. A total of 313 patient visits had IR tympanic temperatures and axillary temperatures taken simultaneously (obtained by using mercury-in-glass thermometers). The tympanic thermometry resulted in a significantly higher temperature reading than the axillary method. They concluded that to prevent unnecessary medical intervention, it is recommended that mercury-in-glass thermometers verify elevated tympanic temperatures.

In 1999 Childs et al. investigated tympanic membrane temperature as a measure of core temperature with a goal of determining the variability of a single user's tympanic membrane (ear) temperature measurements. They studied forty-two afebrile, healthy children and twenty febrile children with acute burns. In the afebrile children, measurements made in both ears (and within just a few minutes of each other) differed by as much as 0.6°C. In the group of febrile, burned children, core temperature was measured hourly at a number of sites (ear, rectum, axilla, and bladder). They found that the measurement error from one recording to the next is probably acceptable, at about 0.1°C to 0.2°C. They recommended that to limit the variations in temperature between one ear and the other, the same ear should be used throughout the temperature monitoring period. They also suggested that nurses and parents take more than one temperature reading from the same ear whenever possible.

In a direct comparison between tympanic and rectal temperature in febrile patients Sehgal et al. (2002) studied sixty febrile children. Two readings of ear temperature were taken in each child with an IR thermometer. Rectal temperature was recorded by a digital electronic thermometer. Both techniques were compared and it was observed that mean ear temperature was 38.9°C ± 0.90°C and for rectal temperature it was 38.8°C ± 0.80°C. The difference between readings taken from two ears was not significant. They concluded that the tympanic thermometer, which is a noninvasive and nonmucous device, is accurate over a wide range of temperatures and could be very useful.

Infrared ear thermometry was also evaluated in fifty critically ill patients (León et al., 2005) in order to determine its accuracy compared to axillary temperature. A total of 429 simultaneous measurements of axillary temperature and tympanic temperature were made. The authors concluded that the IR tympanic thermometer produced highly reliable measurements when compared to axillary temperature measured using a conventional mercury-in-glass thermometer. In a more recent study by Woodrow et al. (2006), the tympanic thermometer was compared with the no-touch temporal thermometer. This research compared 178 simultaneous measurements from five clinical areas. The two thermometers were found not to be equivalent, with a rather ambiguous final conclusion that this research could not identify which thermometer was more accurate.

Other comparative studies of the IR tympanic thermometer in children have been conducted in the past few years. Nimah et al. (2006) conducted a study to determine whether IR tympanic thermometry (ITT) measurements more accurately reflect core body temperatures than axillary, forehead, or rectal measurements during fever cycles in children. Thirty-six critically ill children less than 7 years of age with indwelling bladder catheters were recruited. The authors found that ITT measurements more accurately reflected core temperatures than any of the other measurement sites during febrile and afebrile periods in children. They concluded that ITT measurements are a reproducible and relatively noninvasive substitute for bladder or rectal measurements in febrile children.

Dodd et al. (2006) investigated the sensitivity and specificity of IR ear thermometry compared to rectal thermometry in detecting fever in children. Their results suggested that IR ear thermometry would fail to diagnose fever in three or four out of every ten febrile children (with fever defined as a rectal temperature of 38°C or higher).

In a pediatric study, El-Radhi and Patel (2006) investigated 106 infants whose body temperature was measured in the daytime with an IR tympanic thermometer, at the axilla with an electronic thermometer, and at the rectum. They found that there was greater agreement between the tympanic measurement and the rectal measurement than the axillary with the rectal in both febrile and afebrile infants, concluding that tympanic thermometry is more accurate than measurements of temperature with an electronic axillary thermometer, and thus they recommended its use in the pediatric emergency setting.

In 2007 Moran et al. undertook a prospective trial to compare the accuracy of tympanic, urinary, and axillary temperatures with pulmonary artery core temperature measurements. A total of 110 adult patients were enrolled in a prospective observational cohort study. The accuracy of tympanic (averaged over both ears), axillary (averaged over both sides), and urinary temperatures was referenced (as mean difference, $\Delta°C$) to pulmonary artery temperatures as standard in 6703 recordings. Their results showed that agreement of tympanic with pulmonary artery temperature was inferior to that of urinary temperature, which, on overall assessment, seemed more likely to reflect pulmonary artery core temperature.

Devrim et al. (2007) conducted a study comparing tympanic IR thermometers with the conventional temperature option, a mercury-in-glass thermometer. They recruited a total of 102 randomly selected pediatric patients and simultaneous temperature measurements were performed via the axilla and external auditory canal with three different techniques. For external auditory recordings, the IR tympanic First Temp Genius for clinical use and Microlife IR 1DA1 for home use were used. Classic mercury-in-glass thermometers were used for axillary recordings. For each method, 886 measurements were performed. The results showed that there was a significant difference between the recordings with different thermometers, and this variance was present in both higher and lower readings. They concluded by recommending that the home-use IR tympanic thermometer could be used for screening but it must not be considered as a tool for determining patient follow-up treatment.

## 1.6.5. EVALUATION OF LIQUID CRYSTAL THERMOMETRY

Forehead skin temperature measured by a strip of liquid crystal material was compared to esophageal, rectal, and axillary temperatures measured by thermistor probes in patients having general anesthesia for coronary artery bypass grafting (Burgess et al., 1978). They found that during rapid warming, forehead skin temperature rose concurrently with the other temperatures measured, but remained significantly different. They concluded that liquid crystal strip may be useful as a safe, convenient method for routine monitoring of temperature trends during general anesthesia in patients whose exact core temperature need not be continuously monitored. However, they noted that infant patients undergoing extracorporeal circulation, major abdominal, vascular, or neurosurgical procedures, or patients with a history of temperature regulatory problem are probably best monitored by a method that more exactly reflects core temperature.

Vaughan et al. (1982) studied seventy-one adult postsurgical patients by comparing simultaneous measurement of core (tympanic membrane) and shell (liquid crystal adhesive temperature strip) cutaneous temperatures. Their results suggested that shell temperature (temperature strip) is not a reliable or valid indicator of core temperature (tympanic membrane) in postanesthetic adults. Also, Allen, Horrow, and Rosenberg (1990) evaluated the ability of forehead liquid crystal thermometry (LCT), rectal temperature, and axillary skin temperature to reflect distal esophageal temperature during rapid warming on cardiopulmonary bypass. In twenty-four patients undergoing open heart surgery, temperatures were measured during the rapid warming phase on bypass (12–35 minutes). Polynomial regression analysis revealed that LCT, but not axillary or rectal temperatures, correlated with esophageal temperature. They concluded that forehead LCT may be useful in monitoring temperature trends and detecting rapid elevations in body temperature when more invasive temperature monitoring is inappropriate or unavailable.

A two-part study by Brull et al. (1993) compared liquid crystal skin temperature with other temperature monitors that are used routinely during surgery in order to assess whether liquid crystal skin thermometry accurately reflects core temperature. The first part compared liquid crystal with esophageal temperature during general inhalational anesthesia. The second part compared liquid crystal with esophageal, pulmonary artery, and bladder temperatures during the periods of rapid temperature change associated with cardiopulmonary bypass. This study suggested that liquid crystal, an inexpensive and noninvasive means of temperature monitoring, reflects trends in temperature changes in the clinical setting.

## 1.6.6. EVALUATION OF BRAIN AND INTRACRANIAL THERMOMETRY

The introduction of brain temperature monitoring technology has made it possible to examine the difference between core and brain temperatures. Intracranial temperature measurement may play a pivotal role in the prognosis and treatment of neurological and neurosurgical patients (Alessandri et al., 2004; Childs et al., 2005, 2006). A review by Mcilvoy (2004) examined the published literature comparing core temperatures (blood, rectal, bladder, and esophageal) with brain temperatures (measured by direct contact with the brain or measured in any of the spaces surrounding the brain, excluding intraoperative measurements). Fifteen studies (between 1990 and 2002) found that the brain temperature was higher than all measures of core temperature, with mean differences of 0.39°C to 2.5°C. Three of the studies found statistical significance after a $t$ test. Temperatures greater than 38°C were found in eleven studies. This review demonstrates that brain temperatures have been found to be higher than core temperatures. However, Mcilvoy (2004) found that existing studies are limited by low sample sizes, limited statistical analysis, and inconsistent measurements of brain and core temperatures.

## 1.6.7. EVALUATION OF SKIN THERMOMETRY

There are many studies comparing the accuracy, reliability, validity, and responsiveness of skin temperature thermometers. This section will cover some recent studies.

Burnham, McKinley, and Vincent (2006) conducted a study to compare a thermistor thermometer (thermistor) and two different IR thermometers (one designed to measure tympanic temperature and one for skin temperature). Reliability and validity were evaluated by making two separate measurements from the skin at identical spots on each hand, forearm, shoulder, thigh, shin, and foot in seventeen healthy subjects. Intramuscular temperature was recorded at the hand and shin sites. They found that the performance of the IR thermometers was equal to or superior to that of the traditionally used thermistor. All three devices were highly reliable and valid, whereas the IR skin device was slightly more responsive.

Buono et al. (2007) conducted a study to determine the validity of noncontact IR thermometry measuring mean skin temperature in resting and exercising subjects in cold, thermoneutral, and hot environments. The subjects for the study were six healthy volunteers. Skin temperature was measured at three sites—the forearm, chest, and calf—on each subject using both contact thermistors and a noncontact IR thermometer. The results of the study strongly suggested that IR thermometry is a valid measure of skin temperature during rest and exercise in both hot and cold environments.

## 1.6.8. EVALUATION OF PACIFIER THERMOMETRY

Rectal temperature measurement is considered the most accurate way of assessing temperature in infants, but sometimes it may be difficult to obtain correctly. On the other hand, axillary temperature is easily obtained but is often inaccurate. Tympanic temperature devices are commonly used, but some studies have indicated their accuracy may be questionable, especially in infants and young children. This section focuses on some of the studies evaluating the pacifier thermometer.

Banco, Jayashekaramurthy, and Graffam (1988) assessed the utility and accuracy of a temperature-sensitive pacifier in screening for fever in ill children less than 2 years of age. Of 189 candidates for study, 83 (42%) did not use pacifiers, and of the 106 who did, 25 (24%) could not sustain a suck for 5 minutes of direct observation. Among those eighty-one children who could sustain 5 minutes of sucking, only two of twenty children with rectal temperatures above 100°F (37.8°C) were correctly identified as febrile. They concluded that the temperature-sensitive pacifier did not accurately identify fevers in most infants who are shown to have fevers by rectal temperature determination, suggesting that the use of this pacifier for screening fever in ill infants cannot be recommended. About a decade later Press and Quinn (1997) conducted a study to determine the correlation between supralingual temperatures obtained with a new electronic pacifier thermometer (Steridyne) and rectal temperatures obtained with a digital electronic thermometer. They studied one hundred patients, ages 7 days to 24 months. They concluded that the pacifier thermometer was an accurate means of temperature measurement when recorded temperatures were adjusted upward by 0.5°F. The approximate 3 minutes required for a final temperature determination makes the pacifier thermometer most appropriate for use in low-volume ambulatory care settings and in the home. However, they recommended further investigation of the device.

In 2003 Callahan conducted a study on the reliability of perceived, pacifier, rectal, and temporal artery temperatures in infants. A sample of 200 babies younger than 3 months of age presenting to an emergency department was evaluated for parental perception of fever and with temporal artery, pacifier, and rectal temperatures. He found that the sensitivity and specificity of perceived and temporal artery detection of fever were similar, at 91% and 79% and 83% and 86%, respectively. Febrile pacifier readings had a sensitivity of 99%, but a specificity of only 46%. He concluded that rectal thermometry must remain the standard for infants younger than 3 months of age. More recently Braun (2006) conducted a study to determine the validity and reliability of one type of pacifier thermometer in approximating core body temperature using a prospective, within-subjects design, comparing pacifier and rectal temperatures in children ($n$ = 25) ages 7 days to 24 months in one pediatric hospital-based setting. The correlations between the rectal and adjusted pacifier temperature was 0.772 and between the 3- and 6-minute pacifier temperatures it was 0.913. These data provide support to previous assertions that pacifier thermometry is an acceptable method of temperature approximation in young children.

## 1.6.9. EVALUATION OF INGESTIBLE TELEMETRIC THERMOMETRY

Sparling, Snow, and Millard-Stafford (1993) monitored core temperature during exercise using an ingestible sensor and a rectal thermistor in six trained subjects (three cyclists, three runners) during 30 to 90 minutes of progressive cycling or treadmill exercise. Testing was conducted 3 to 9 hours after ingestion of the capsule. The telemetric temperature was lower than the rectal temperature both at rest and during exercise in every subject. The mean temperature difference increased by 58% from rest (0.59°C) to peak exercise (0.93°C). These preliminary results demonstrated a consistently lower temperature from the capsule sensor located within the gastrointestinal tract compared to rectal thermistors.

More recently Byrne and Lim (2007) studied the agreement between intestinal sensor temperature, esophageal temperature, and rectal temperature across numerous previously published validation studies. Also, they reviewed the application of this technology in field-based exercise studies. They found that the intestinal temperature responds less rapidly than the esophageal temperature at the start or cessation of exercise or to a change in exercise intensity, but more rapidly than rectal temperature. The intestinal thermometer has been used in many applications, including sport and occupational applications, continuous measurement of core temperature in deep-sea saturation divers, in distance runners, and in soldiers undertaking sustained military training exercises. They concluded that the ingestible telemetric temperature sensor represents a valid index of core temperature and shows excellent utility for ambulatory field-based applications.

## REFERENCES


Alessandri, B., Hoelper B. M., Behr, R, & Kempski, O. (2004). Accuracy and stability of temperature probes for intracranial application. *Journal of Neuroscience Methods, 139*(2), 161–165.

Allen, G. C., Horrow, J. C., & Rosenberg, H. (1990). Does forehead liquid crystal temperature accurately reflect "core" temperature? *Canadian Journal of Anaesthesia, 37*(6), 659–662.

Androkites, A. L., Werger, A. M., & Young, M. L. (1998). Comparison of axillary and infrared tympanic membrane thermometry in a pediatric oncology outpatient setting. *Journal of Pediatric Oncology Nursing, 15*(4), 216–222.

Banco, L., Jayashekaramurthy, S., & Graffam, J. (1988). The inability of a temperature-sensitive pacifier to identify fevers in ill infants. *American Journal of Diseases of Children, 142*(2), 171–172.

Benzinger, M., & Benzinger, T. (1972). Tympanic clinical temperature. In H. P. Thomas, T. P. Murray, & R. L. Shepard (Eds.). *Fifth Symposium on Temperature* (pp. 2089–2102). Washington, DC: American Institute of Physics, Instrument Society of America, National Bureau of Standards.

Betta, V., Cascetta, F., & Sepe, D. (1997). An assessment of infrared tympanic thermometers for body temperature measurement. *Physiological Measurement, 18*, 215–225.

Bissonnette, B., Sessler, D. I., & LaFlamme, P. (1989) Intraoperative temperature monitoring sites in infants and children and the effect of inspired gas warming on esophageal temperature. *Anesthesia and Analgesia, 69*, 192–196.

Blainey, C. G. (1974). Site selection in taking body temperature. *American Journal of Nursing, 74*, 1859–1861.

Bock, M., Hohlfeld, U., Von Enfeln, K., Meier, P. A., Motsch, J., & Tasman, A. J. (2005). The accuracy of a new infrared ear thermometer in patients undergoing cardiac surgery. *Canadian Journal of Anaesthesia, 52*(10), 1083–1087.

Braun, C. A. (2006). Accuracy of pacifier thermometers in young children. *Pediatric Nursing, 32*(5), 413–418.

Brown, P. J., Christmas, B. F., & Ford, R. P. (1992). Taking an infant's temperature: Axillary or rectal thermometer? *New Zealand Medical Journal, 105*, 309–311.

Brull, S. J., Cunningham, A. J., Connelly, N. R., O'Connor, T. Z., & Silverman, D. G. (1993). Liquid crystal skin thermometry: An accurate reflection of core temperature? *Canadian Journal of Anaesthesia, 40*(4), 375–381.

Buono, M. J., Jechort, A., Marques, R., Smith, C., & Welch, J. (2007). Comparison of infrared versus contact thermometry for measuring skin temperature during exercise in the heat. *Physiological Measurement, 28*(8), 855–859.

Burgess, G. E., III, Cooper, J. R., Marino, R. J., & Peuler, M. J. (1978). Continuous monitoring of skin temperature using a liquid-crystal thermometer during anesthesia. *Southern Medical Journal, 71*(5), 516–518.

Burnham, R. S., McKinley, R. S., & Vincent, D. D. (2006). Three types of skin-surface thermometers: A comparison of reliability, validity, and responsiveness. *American Journal of Physical Medicine and Rehabilitation, 85*(7), 553–558.

Busic, V., & Das-Gupta, R. (2004). Temperature monitoring in free flap surgery. *British Journal of Plastic Surgery, 57*(6), 588.

Byrne, C., & Lim, C. L. (2007). The ingestible telemetric body core temperature sensor: A review of validity and exercise applications. *British Journal of Sports Medicine, 41*(3), 126–133.

Callahan, D. (2003). Detecting fever in young infants: reliability of perceived, pacifier, and temporal artery temperatures in infants younger than 3 months of age. *Pediatric Emergency Care, 19*(4), 240–243.

Cattaneo, C. G., Frank, S. M., Hesel, T. W., El-Rahmany, H. K., Kim, L. J., & Tran, K. M. (2000). The accuracy and precision of body temperature monitoring methods during regional and general anesthesia. *Anesthesia and Analgesia, 90*(4), 938–945.

Cereda, M., & Maccioli, G. (2004). Intraoperative temperature monitoring. *International Anesthesiology Clinics, 42*(1), 41–54.

Chamberlain, J. M., Terndrup, T. E., Alexander, D. T., Silverstone, F. A., Wolf-Klein, G., O'Donnell, R., & Grandner, J. (1995). Determination of normal ear temperature with an infrared emission detection thermometer. *Annals of Emergency Medicine, 25*(1), 15–20.

Childs, C., Harrison, R., & Hodkinson, C. (1999). Tympanic membrane temperature as a measure of core temperature. *Archives of Disease in Childhood, 80*, 262–266.

Childs, C., Vail, A., Leach, P., Rainey, T., Protheroe, R., & King, A. (2006). Brain temperature and outcome after severe traumatic brain injury. *Neurocritical Care, 5*(1), 10–14.

Childs, C., Vail, A., Protheroe, R., King, A., & Dark, P. (2005). Differences between brain and rectal temperatures during routine critical care of patients with severe traumatic brain injury. *Anaesthesia, 60*(8), 759–765.

Cork, J. M. (1942). *Heat.* New York, NY: John Wiley & Sons.

Cork, R. C., Vaughan, R. W., & Humphrey, L. S. (1983). Precision and accuracy of intraoperative temperature monitoring. *Anesthesia and Analgesia, 62*(2), 211–214.

Cranston, W. I., Gerbrandy, J., & Snell, E. S. (1954). Oral, rectal and esophageal temperatures and some factors affecting them in man. *Journal of Physiology, 126*(2), 347.

Crawford, D. C., Hicks, B., & Thompson, M. J. (2006). Which thermometer? Factors influencing best choice for intermittent clinical temperature assessment. *Journal of Medical Engineering and Technology, 40*(4), 199–211.

Cromwell, L., Weibell, F., & Pfeiffer, E. (1980). *Biomedical instrumentation and measurements* (2nd ed.). Upper Saddle River, NJ: Prentice-Hall.

Darm, R. M., Hecker, R. B., & Rubal, B. J. (1994). A comparison of noninvasive body temperature monitoring devices in the PACU. *Journal of Post-Anesthesia Nursing, 9*(3), 144–149.

Devrim, I., Kara, A., Ceyhan, M., Tezer, H., Uludağ, A. K., Cengiz, A. B., . . . & Seçmeer, G. (2007). Measurement accuracy of fever by tympanic and axillary thermometry. *Pediatric Emergency Care, 23*(1), 16–19.

Dew, P. L. (2006). Is tympanic membrane thermometry the best method for recording temperature in children? *Journal of Child Health Care, 10*(2), 96–110.

Dodd, S. R., Lancaster, G. A., Craig, J. V., Smyth, R. L., & Williamson, P. R. (2006). In a systematic review, infrared ear thermometry for fever diagnosis in children finds poor sensitivity. *Journal of Clinical Epidemiology, 59*(4), 354–357.

Eichina, L. W., Berger, A. R., Rader, B., & Becker, W. H. (1951). Comparison of intracardiac and intravascular temperatures with rectal temperatures in man. *Journal of Clinical Investigation, 30*, 353.

El-Radhi, A. S., & Patel, S. (2006). An evaluation of tympanic thermometry in a paediatric emergency department. *Emergency Medicine Journal, 23*(1), 40–41.

Farnell, S., Maxwell, L., Tan, S., Rhodes, A., & Philips, B. (2005). Temperature measurement: Comparison of noninvasive methods used in adult critical care. *Journal of Clinical Nursing, 14*(5), 632–639.

Frank, S. M., Nguyen, J. M., Garcia, C. M., & Barnes, R. A. (1999). Temperature monitoring practices during regional anesthesia. *Anesthesia and Analgesia, 88*(2), 373–377.

Gilbert, M., Barton, A., & Counsell, C. (2002). Comparison of oral and tympanic temperatures in adult surgical patients. *Applied Nursing Research, 15*(1), 42–47.

Greenes, D. S., & Fleisher, G. R. (2001). Accuracy of a noninvasive temporal artery thermometer for use in infants. *Archives of Pediatrics and Adolescent Medicine, 155*(3), 376–381.

Hebbar, K., Fortenberry, J. D., Rogers, K., Merritt, R., & Easley, K. (2005). Comparison of temporal artery thermometer to standard temperature measurements in pediatric intensive care unit patients. *Pediatric Critical Care Medicine, 6*(5), 557–561.

Herzog, L. W., & Coyne, L. J. (1993). What is fever? Normal temperature in infants less than 3 months old. *Clinical Pediatrics, 32*(3), 142–146.

Hooper, V. D., & Andrews, J. O. (2006). Accuracy of noninvasive core temperature measurement in acutely ill adults: the state of the science. *Biological Research for Nursing, 8*(1), 24–34.

Ikeda, T., Sessler, D. I., Marder, D., & Xiong, J. (1997). Influence of thermoregulatory vasomotion and ambient temperature variation on the accuracy of core-temperature estimates by cutaneous liquid crystal thermometers. *Anesthesiology, 86*(3), 603–612.

Isley, A. H., Rutten, A. J., & Runciman, W. B. (1983). An evaluation of body temperature measurement. *Anaesthesia and Intensive Care, 11*(1), 31–39.

Jaffe, D. M. (1995). What's hot and what's not: The gold standard for thermometry in emergency medicine. *Annals of Emergency Medicine, 25*(1), 97–99.

Jensen, B. N., Jensen, F. S., Madsen, S. N., & Løssl, K. (2000). Accuracy of digital tympanic, oral, axillary, and rectal thermometers compared with standard rectal mercury thermometers. *European Journal of Surgery, 166*(11), 848–851.

Kaukuntla, H., Harrington, D., Bilkoo, I., Clutton-Brock, T., Jones, T., & Bonser, R. S. (2004). Temperature monitoring during cardiopulmonary bypass—do we undercool or overheat the brain? *European Journal of Cardio-Thoracic Surgery, 26*(3), 580–585.

Kenney, R. D., Fortenberry, J. D., Surratt, S. S., Ribbeck, B. M., & Thomas, W. J. (1990). Evaluation of an infrared tympanic membrane thermometer in pediatric patients. *Pediatrics, 85*(5), 854–858.

Kerlin, T. W., & Shepard, R. L. *(1982). Industrial temperature measurement.* Research Triangle Park, NC: Instrument Society of America.

Kistemaker, J. A., Den Hartog, E. A., & Daanen, H. A. (2006). Reliability of an infrared forehead skin thermometer for core temperature measurements. *Journal of Medical Engineering and Technology, 30*(4), 252–261.

Kongpanichkul, A., & Bunjongpak, S. (2000). A comparative study on accuracy of liquid crystal forehead, digital electronic axillary, infrared tympanic with glass-mercury rectal thermometer in infants and young children. *Journal of The Medical Association of Thailand, 83*(9), 1068–1076.

Krenzischek, D., Frank, S., & Kelly, S. (1995). Forced air warming versus routine thermal care and core temperature measurement sites. *Journal of Post-Anesthesia Nursing, 10*(2), 69–78.

Kresch, M. J. (1994). Axillary temperature as a screening test for fever in children. *Journal of Paediatric Child Health, 104*(4), 596–599.

Lefrant, J. Y., Muller, L., de la Coussaye, J. E., Benbabaali, M., Lebris, C., Zeitoun, N., Mari, C., Saïssi, G., Ripart, J., & Eledjam, J. J. (2003). Temperature measurement in intensive care patients: comparison of urinary bladder, oesophageal, rectal, axillary, and inguinal methods versus pulmonary artery core method. *Journal of Intensive Care Medicine, 29*(3), 414–418.

León, C., Rodríguez, A., Fernández, A., & Flores, L. (2005). Infrared ear thermometry in the critically ill patient. *Journal of Critical Care, 20*(1), 106–110.

Mackowiak, P. A., Wasserman, S. S., & Levine, M. M. (1992). A critical appraisal of 98.6°F, the upper limit of the normal body temperature, and other legacies of Carl Reinhold August Wunderlich. *Journal of the American Medical Association, 268*(12), 1578–1580.

Marieb, E. N. (1992). *Human anatomy and physiology* (2nd ed.). San Francisco, CA: Benjamin Cummings.

Maxton, F. J., Justin, L., & Gillies, D. (2004). Estimating core temperature in infants and children after cardiac surgery: a comparison of six methods. *Journal of Advanced Nursing, 45*(2), 214–222.

McCarthy, P. L. (1998). Fever. *Pediatrics in Review, 19*(12), 401–407.

Mcilvoy, L. (2004). Comparison of brain temperature to core temperature: A review of the literature. *Journal of Neuroscience Nursing, 36*(1), 23–31.

Michalski, L., Eckersdorf, K., & McGhee, J. (1991). *Temperature measurement.* New York, NY: John Wiley & Sons.

Milewski, A., Ferguson, K. L., & Terndrup, T. E. (1991). Comparison of pulmonary artery, rectal, and tympanic membrane temperatures in adult intensive care unit patients. *Clinical Pediatrics (Philadelphia), 30*(4 suppl.), 13–16.

Miller, R. (2000). *Anesthesia* (5th ed., Vol. 2). New York, NY: Churchill Livingstone.

Moran, J. L., Peter, J. V., Solomon, P. J., Grealy, B., Smith, T., Ashforth, W., . . . & Peisach, A. R. (2007). Tympanic temperature measurements: Are they reliable in the critically ill? A clinical study of measures of agreement. *Critical Care Medicine, 35*(1), 155–164.

Myny, D., De Waele, J., Defloor, T., Blot, S., & Colardyn, F. (2005). Temporal scanner thermometry: A new method of core temperature estimation in ICU patients. *Scottish Medical Journal, 50*(1), 15–18.

Nimah, M. M., Bshesh, K., Callahan, J. D., & Jacobs, B. R. (2006). Infrared tympanic thermometry in comparison with other temperature measurement techniques in febrile children. *Pediatric Critical Care Medicine, 7*(1), 48–55.

Nussmeier, N. A. (2005). Management of temperature during and after cardiac surgery. *Texas Heart Institute Journal, 32*(4), 472–476.

O'Hara, G. J., & Phillips, D. B. (1986). Method and apparatus for measuring internal body temperature utilizing infrared emissions. U.S. Patent 4602642. Retrieved from U.S. Patent Office Web site: http://patft.uspto.gov

O'Hara, G. J., & Phillips, D. B. (1988). Method and apparatus for measuring internal body temperature utilizing infrared emissions. U.S. Patent 4790324. Retrieved from U.S. Patent Office Web site: http://patft.uspto.gov

Patel, N., Smith, C. E., Pinchak, A. C., & Hagen, J. F. (1996). Comparison of esophageal, tympanic, and forehead skin temperatures in adult patients. *Journal of Clinical Anesthesia, 8*(6), 462–468.

Pearce, J. M. S. (2002). A brief history of the clinical thermometer. *Quarterly Journal of Medicine, 95*(4), 251–252.

Pompei, F. (2006). A brief report on the normal range of forehead temperature as determined by noncontact, handheld, infrared thermometer. *American Journal of Infection Control, 34*(4), 248–249.

Pompei, M. (1999). Temperature assessment via the temporal artery: Validation of a new method. Boston, MA: Exergen Corp.

Press, S., & Quinn, B. (1997). The pacifier thermometer: Comparison of supralingual with rectal temperatures in infants and young children. *Archives of Pediatrics and Adolescent Medicine, 151*(6), 551–554.

Quinn, T. J. (1990). *Temperature.* New York, NY: Academic Press.

Reisinger, K. S., Kao, J., & Grant, D. M. (1979). Inaccuracy of the Clinitemp skin thermometer. *Pediatrics, 64*(1), 4–6.

Robinson, J. L., Seal, R. F., Spady, D. W., & Joffres, M. R. (1998). Comparison of esophageal, rectal, axillary, bladder, tympanic, and pulmonary artery temperatures in children. *Journal of Pediatrics, 133*(4), 553–556.

Roy, S., Powell, K., & Gerson, L. W. (2003). Temporal artery temperature measurements in healthy infants, children, and adolescents. *Clinical Pediatrics (Philadelphia), 42*(5), 433–437.

Sandlin, D. (2003). New product review: Temporal artery thermometry. *Journal of Perianesthesia Nursing, 18*(6), 419–421.

Schuh, S., Komar, L., Stephens, D., Chu, L., Read, S., & Allen, U. (2004). Comparison of the temporal artery and rectal thermometry in children in the emergency department. *Pediatric Emergency Care, 20*(11), 736–741.

Seguin, J., & Terry, K. (1999). Neonatal infrared axillary thermometry. *Clinical Pediatrics (Philadelphia), 38*(1), 35–40.

Sehgal, A., Dubey, N. K., Jyothi, M. C., & Jain, S. (2002). Comparison of tympanic and rectal temperature in febrile patients. *Indian Journal of Pediatrics, 69*(4), 305–308.

Shinozaki, T., Deane, R., Perkins, F. M. (1988). Infrared tympanic thermometer: Evaluation of a new clinical thermometer. *Critical Care Medicine, 16*(2), 148–150.

Sparling, P. B., Snow, T. K., & Millard-Stafford, M. L. (1993). Monitoring core temperature during exercise: ingestible sensor vs. rectal thermistor. *Aviation, Space, and Environmental Medicine, 64*(8), 760–763.

Suleman, M. I., Doufas, A. G., Akça, O., Ducharme, M., & Sessler, D. I. (2002). Insufficiency in a new temporal-artery thermometer for adult and pediatric patients. *Anesthesia and Analgesia, 95*(1), 67–71.

Tabbutt, S., Ittenbach, R. F., Nicolson, S. C., Burnham, N., Hittle, S., Spray, T. L., Gaynor, J. W. (2006). Intracardiac temperature monitoring in infants after cardiac surgery. *Journal of Thoracic and Cardiovascular Surgery, 131*(3), 614–620.

Tabor, M., Blaho, D. M., & Schriver, W. R. (1981). Tympanic membrane perforation: Complication of tympanic thermometry during general anesthesia. *Oral Surgery, Oral Medicine, Oral Pathology, Oral Radiology, and Endodontology, 51*(6), 581–583.

Terndrup, T., Crofton, D., Mortelliti, A., Kelley, R., & Rajk, J. (1997). Estimation of contact tympanic membrane temperature with a noncontact infrared thermometer. *Annals of Emergency Medicine, 30*(2), 171–175.

Togawa, T. (1985). Body temperature measurement. *Clinical Physics and Physiological Measurement, 6*(2), 83–108.

Togawa, T., Tamura, T., & Oberg, P. A. (1997). *Biomedical transducers and instruments.* Boca Raton, FL: CRC Press.

Van Dam, H., Nduka, C., & Carver, N. (2003). No touch free-flap temperature monitoring. *British Journal of Plastic Surgery, 56*(8), 835.

Vaughan, M. S., Cork, R. C., & Vaughan, R. (1982). Inaccuracy of liquid crystal thermometry to identify core temperature trends in postoperative adults. *Anesthesia and Analgesia, 61*, 284–287.

Wallace, C. T., Marks, W. E., Adkins, W. Y., & Mahaffey, J. E. (1974). Perforation of the tympanic membrane, a complication of tympanic thermometry during anesthesia. *Anesthesiology, 41*(3), 290–291.

Webb, G. E. (1973). Comparison of esophageal and tympanic temperature monitoring during cardiopulmonary bypass. *Anesthesia and Analgesia, 52*(5), 729–733.

Whitby, J. D., & Dunkin, L. J. (1968). Temperature differences in the oesophagus. *British Journal of Anaesthesia, 40*(12), 991–995.

Whitby, J. D., & Dunkin, L. J. (1971). Cerebral, oesophageal, and nasopharyngeal temperatures. *British Journal of Anesthesia, 43*(7), 673–676.

Woodrow, P., May, V., Buras-Rees, S., Higgs, D., Hendrick, J., Lewis, T., . . . & McHenry, M. (2006). Comparing no-touch and tympanic thermometer temperature recordings. *British Journal of Nursing, 15*(18), 1012–1016.

Young, C. C., & Sladen, R. N. (1996). Temperature monitoring. *International Anesthesiology Clinics, 34*(3), 149–174.

## WEB SITES

http://en.wikipedia.org/wiki/Thermometer
http://kicp-yerkes.uchicago.edu/2003-winter/pdf/ywi2003-liquid_crystals.pdf
http://www.brannan.co.uk/thermometers/invention.html
http://www.eo.ucar.edu/skymath/tmp2.html
http://www.graduateresearch.com/thermometry
http://www.kele.com/tech/monitor/Temperature/TRefTem4.html
http://www.melexis.com
http://www.omega.com/temperature/Z/NoncontactTM.html
http://www.picotech.com/applications/thermocouple.html
http://www.temperatures.com

## ABOUT THE AUTHOR

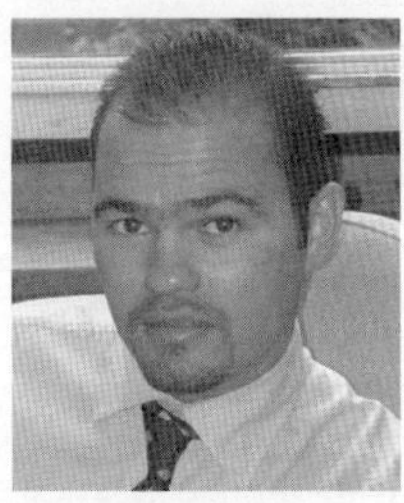

**Professor P. A. Kyriacou** BESc, MSc, PhD, CEng, CPhys, CSci, FIET, FIPEM, SMIEEE, MInstP received a BESc degree in electrical engineering from the University of Western Ontario, Canada and MSc and PhD degrees in medical electronics and physics from St. Bartholomew's Medical College, University of London. His PhD research was in the field of medical optics and biomedical instrumentation. He is currently a professor of biomedical engineering at City University in London. He is also the associate dean for postgraduate studies in the School of Engineering and Mathematical Sciences and the director of the Biomedical Engineering Research Group. His research activities are primarily focused upon the understanding, development, and applications of instrumentation, sensors, and physiological measurement for the facilitation of the diagnosis and treatment of disease and the rehabilitation of patients.

# CHAPTER 2

# FLOW SENSORS FOR LIQUIDS

M. Mischi and J. A. Blom

*Department of Electrical Engineering*
*Eindhoven University of Technology, Eindhoven, The Netherlands*

## 2.1. INTRODUCTION

Flow is a general word addressing a variety of realities. This is particularly true for the flow of liquids in a biomedical context. In the human body, blood flow is of major importance for the characterization of the cardiovascular system, but the flow of other fluids, such as urine, must also be considered.

In physics, the flow of something denotes the rate at which that something (e.g., blood) passes a given cross section (e.g., in a blood vessel). If a cross section perpendicular to the flow is chosen, the value of the flow is determined by the product of the cross section and the velocity of the flow. Blood vessel cross sections differ greatly, from 10 cm$^2$ in the ascending aorta to less than 10$^{-6}$ cm$^2$ for small capillaries. Blood velocities can vary from an average of 33 cm s$^{-1}$ in the aorta to less than 1 mm s$^{-1}$ in the microcirculation. In arteries, the flow is strongly nonstationary (pulsatile), whereas it is more stationary (nonpulsatile) in veins.

The blood velocity inside a vessel may change greatly depending on where it is measured. Remarkably, the errors that result from assuming a uniform velocity across the vessel ("plug flow") are often acceptable. Another often-encountered assumption is that of a parabolic flow profile ("Poiseuille flow"), where the highest velocity occurs in the vessel's center and the velocity is zero at the vessel walls. This idealization is valid only under strict conditions (e.g., a constant flow through rigid, straight tubes without branches) that do not occur in the circulatory system, where vessels are compliant and tortuous, flow is pulsatile, and branches are ubiquitous.

Different assumptions and simplifications lead to different measurement strategies and computational approaches. These various characterizations of flow in the human body are reflected in the several different techniques that are employed for its measurement. These techniques are based on different principles and they typically show a low correlation with each other. Therefore, once a decision for one technique has been made, it is better to monitor the flow variations in one subject by employing the same technique. This improves the significance of the measured variations.

In this chapter the available sensors and sensing techniques are first divided on the basis of the object of measurement. Therefore, sensors for flows in arteries and veins (section 2.2) are separated from sensors for flows in tissues and microcirculation (section 2.3) and sensors for flows of substances other than blood (section 2.4).

Some techniques depend on the injection of indicators (sections 2.2.1 and 2.2.2). When such indicators are used, sometimes contact between the indicator and sensors is required, resulting in invasive techniques. The specific technique employed depends on the indicator utilized. Other techniques make direct use of properties of the flowing mass: echo-Doppler ultrasound makes use of the fact that the blood contains moving particles (mainly red blood cells); magnetic resonance techniques image flowing hydrogen nuclei (spins); and the electrical conductivity of blood can be used, as well as volume variations due to vessel elasticity. These techniques are discussed in sections 2.2.3 through 2.2.6.

Sensors for flow in tissues and the microcirculation are typically based on perfusion imaging. An indicator, which in this context is typically referred to as a "contrast agent," is injected and detected noninvasively by an imaging technique of the location of interest. The imaging techniques that are usually adopted for quantitative analysis are positron emission tomography (PET) or single photon emission computerized tomography (SPECT), contrast echography, and contrast magnetic resonance imaging (MRI), which use radionuclides, microbubbles, and paramagnetic agents, respectively, as contrast agents. These techniques, which are mostly semiquantitative because of the complexity of the perfusion hemodynamics and the small size of the microvasculature, are discussed in sections 2.3.1 through 2.3.3. A special case is the assessment of blood perfusion in the brain. Because of the increased flow produced by the activation of specific areas of the cortex, the quantity of deoxyhemoglobin decreases. Since deoxyhemoglobin is a paramagnetic substance, variations in concentration can be detected by MRI and related to flow and perfusion. This technique, referred to as functional MRI (fMRI), is discussed in section 2.3.4.

Sensors for flows of other fluids are mainly used to analyze the clearance of substances such as glucose from the blood pool, as in hemodialysis. Other fluids that do not circulate with blood and whose flow is measured for diagnostic purposes include urine, saliva, tears, and gastric acid. All these measurements are briefly reported in section 2.4.

## 2.2. SENSORS FOR FLOW IN ARTERIES AND VEINS

Several techniques are available for the measurement of flow in arteries and veins. Here, a clear distinction is made between those techniques and sensors that make use of an indicator to be detected and those that do not need the dilution of indicators. The first type are typically aimed at the measurement of cardiac output (CO), which is defined as the flow produced by the left ventricle (LV) into the aorta in liters per minute. In section 2.2.1 the basic principles are explained; in section 2.2.2 the different techniques and sensors, depending on the type of indicator, are discussed. The techniques that do not need the injection of indicators can be used for different vessels, including those in the arms and legs.

The most common of these techniques are based on ultrasound flowmeters (section 2.2.3), magnetic resonance angiography (MRA; section 2.2.4), electromagnetic flowmeters (section 2.2.5), and plethysmography (section 2.2.6).

## 2.2.1. INDICATOR DILUTION PRINCIPLES

### 2.2.1.1. Flow Measurement by Indicator Dilution

Indicator dilution theory is based on the following basic concept: if the concentration of an indicator that is uniformly dispersed in an unknown volume $V$ is determined and the volume of the indicator (dose) is known, then the unknown volume can also be determined. Let $\Phi(t)$ and $V(t)$ be, respectively, the instantaneous flow and volume of the carrier fluid, and $m$ and $C(t)$ be, respectively, the indicator mass and its concentration at time $t$. Since $\Phi(t) = dV(t)/dt$ and $C(t) = dm/dV$, the following differential equation can be derived:

$$\Phi(t) = \frac{dV(t)}{dt} = \frac{1}{C(t)} \cdot \frac{dm}{dt} \, .$$

(2.1)

A typical approach for flow measurements makes use of the rapid injection of an indicator dose. This permits relaxing the constraints about the nature of the indicator, as only a small bolus of indicator is injected. However, methods based on continuous indicator infusion are commonly used as well.

In rapid injection methods, $C(t)$ in equation 2.1 is not constant. In practice, as shown in Figure 2.1, the indicator is rapidly injected into a fluid dynamic system where a carrier fluid (in this case, blood) is flowing, and the indicator concentration $C(t)$ is measured, as a function of time, downstream from the injection. This measurement permits the registration of a curve that is referred to as an indicator dilution curve (IDC). The IDC contains the necessary information to estimate the flow. Its value is derived from equation 2.1 by integration over time, as shown in equation 2.2. The flow $\Phi$ is assumed to be constant, so that it can be moved out of the integration. The resulting equation is the Stewart–Hamilton equation, which provides an estimate of the mean flow $\Phi$ (Hamilton et al., 1928; Stewart, 1897). Thus the injection and subsequent detection of an indicator allows the measurement of mean flow.

$$\int_0^\infty \Phi C(t)\, dt = \Phi \int_0^\infty C(t)\, dt = \int_0^\infty \frac{dm}{dt}\, dt = m$$

$$\Downarrow$$

$$\Phi = \frac{m}{\displaystyle\int_0^\infty C(t)\, dt}$$

(2.2)

The calculation of the integral in equation 2.2 is not trivial. Since the circulatory system is a closed system, the recirculation of the indicator produces increases in the concentration that mask the tail (downslope) of the first pass IDC (see Fig. 2.2). However, equation 2.2 is based only on the first-pass IDC: the time integral of the indicator mass is equal to the injected dose $m$. In addition, the IDC is often very noisy. Therefore the estimation of the integral of the first-pass IDC in equation 2.2 requires

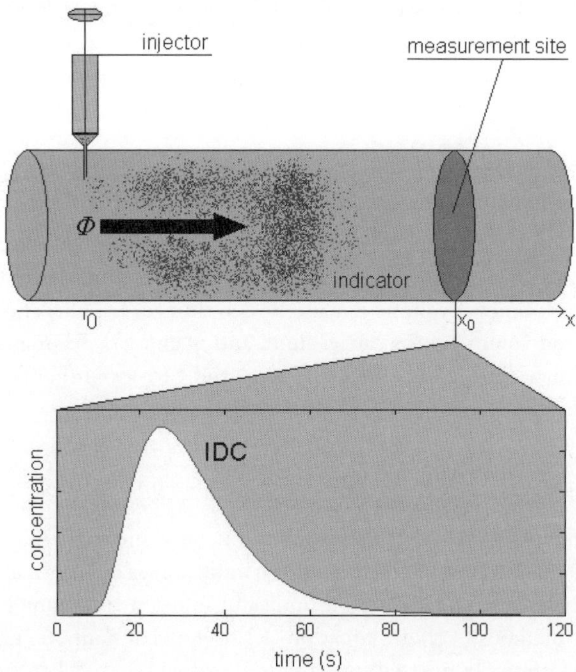


**Figure 2.1.** Simplified indicator dilution curve (IDC) measurement model. An indicator bolus is injected upstream, and its concentration is subsequently measured downstream for the derivation of an IDC.

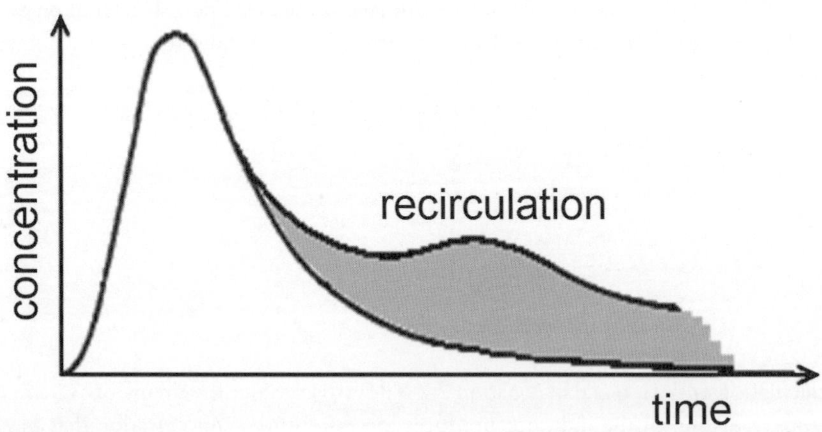


**Figure 2.2.** Effect of the recirculation of the indicator on the shape of the IDC. The tail of the IDC is masked by the recirculation rise.

the use of an appropriate model that interpolates the first part of the IDC and estimates the tail, which is masked by recirculation.

In the next section, the models that are most commonly used are briefly discussed. It is important to highlight the assumptions on which the indicator dilution theory is based:

- The average blood flow is constant during the measurement (typically longer than 30 s).
- The indicator has an instantaneous and uniform mixing.
- The injection is sufficiently fast to be modeled by a Dirac impulse.
- The loss of indicator is either absent or known.

These assumptions are also the major cause of inaccuracy in these methods (Gefen et al., 1999; Jansen, 1995).

### 2.2.1.2. Indicator Dilution Curve Modeling

The first IDC model was developed by Hamilton (Hamilton et al., 1928; Stewart, 1897; Zierler, 2000), who noticed that the IDC is characterized by a sharp rise followed by a smoother descent that resembles an exponential function. He modeled this descent by an exponential decay with time-constant $\tau$ as

$$C(t) = C(t_0)e^{-\frac{t-t_0}{\tau}}, \tag{2.3}$$

where $C(t)$ is the IDC (i.e., the concentration-time curve) and $t_0$ is the injection time. As a first step, the model interpretation of an IDC requires the fitting of the model to the measured IDC data. In the case of an exponential model, the IDC is interpolated along a short segment in the downslope of the curve before the rise given by the contrast recirculation. The fitting, based on the exponential model, can also be made by a linear regression in the log-transformed IDC data.

The IDC in equation 2.3 can also be viewed as the impulse response of a monocompartment model, which corresponds to the washout curve after the rapid injection of an indicator bolus in the compartment. Consider a chamber (compartment) of volume $V$ with one input and one output where a fluid (blood) is flowing. If the chamber is not elastic and the fluid incompressible, the input and output flows $\Phi$ are equal. From the mass conservation principle, the variation of indicator mass in the chamber ($VdC(t)$) equals the mass of the indicator that leaves the chamber ($C(t)dV$). Therefore, since $C(t)dV = C(t)\Phi dt$, the system can be described by the differential equation

$$VdC(t) = -C(t)\Phi dt. \tag{2.4}$$

If an indicator bolus is rapidly injected into the chamber at time $t_0$ and the mixing is perfect, then $C_0 = C(t_0) = mV^{-1}$ (with $m$ equal to the injected mass of the indicator). The solution of equation 2.4 is then given as in equation 2.3, with $\tau = V\Phi^{-1}$. In fact, all the compartmental models assume implicitly an instantaneous and complete mixing of the indicator in the compartments.

Another model that is often adopted in the IDC theory is the two-compartment model, which is obtained by adding a second equation (representing the second compartment) to equation 2.4. This model is clearly related to cardiac functionality, where the heart can be seen as two pumps with two compartments each. The resulting differential equations are given in equation 2.5, where $C_1(t)$ and $C_2(t)$ are the contrast concentrations in the two chambers of volume $V_1$ and $V_2$, respectively (see Fig. 2.3):

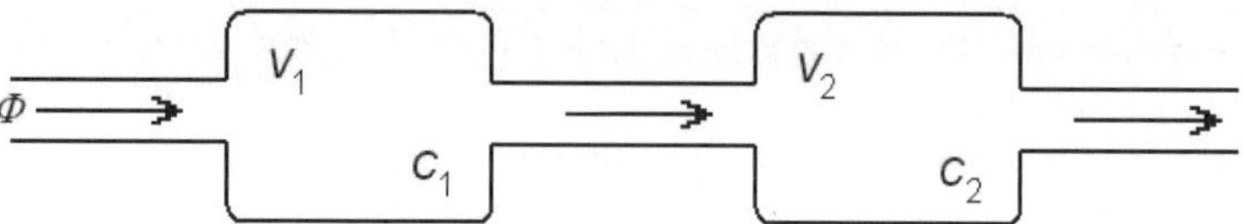

**Figure 2.3.** Two-compartment model made of two mixing chambers of volume $V_1$ and $V_2$, respectively. Because of the hypothesis of complete instantaneous mixing, the concentrations $C_1$ and $C_2$, respectively, in the first and second compartment, are homogeneous. $\Phi$ represents the flow.

$$\frac{V_1}{\Phi}\frac{dC_1(t)}{dt} + C_1(t) = 0$$

$$\frac{V_2}{\Phi}\frac{dC_2(t)}{dt} + C_2(t) - C_1(t) = 0 .$$

$$(2.5)$$

A solution of equation 2.5 for $V_1 \neq V_2$ gives $C_1(t)$ and $C_2(t)$ as

$$C_1(t) = \frac{m}{V_1} e^{-\frac{t}{\tau_1}}$$

$$C_2(t) = \frac{m}{V_1 - V_2}\left(e^{-\frac{t}{\tau_1}} - e^{-\frac{t}{\tau_2}}\right),$$

$$(2.6)$$

where $\tau_1 = V_1\Phi^{-1}$ and $\tau_2 = V_2\Phi^{-1}$. The injection time $t_0$, without any loss of generality, is assumed to be zero.

The IDC in a cascade of $n$ equal chambers is an interesting model as well (Chen et al., 1998; Norwich, 1977; Sheppard, 1962). The $n$th equation of the system is given as

$$\frac{V}{\Phi}\frac{dC_n(t)}{dt} + C_n(t) - C_{n-1}(t) = 0 .$$

$$(2.7)$$

For each chamber the initial condition is $C(0) = 0$. If the input to the first chamber ($n = 1$) is an impulse (Dirac function) at time $t_0 = 0$ of area $m\Phi^{-1}$, then, for $n \geq 1$, $C_n(t)$ can be expressed as (Linton, Linton, & Band, 1995)

$$C_n(t) = \frac{mt^{n-1}e^{-\frac{t}{\tau}}}{\Phi\tau^n(n-1)!} .$$

$$(2.8)$$

Since the injected mass $m$ is known, $C_n(t)$ in equation 2.8 is a distribution with three parameters that are related to the flow and the number and volume of the compartments. If the volumes of the chambers are different, then a multiexponential model is obtained and the number of degrees of freedom of the model increases.

The impulse response of the compartment could also be chosen according to different criteria. Often the IDC is interpreted by means of distributed models, which are usually chosen as some statistical distribution. Distributions that are commonly adopted to fit the IDC are the lognormal and the gamma variate (Chen et al., 1998; Linton, Linton, & Band, 1995; Lopatatzidis & Millard, 2001; Thompson et al., 1964). Even without a hemodynamic interpretation, these models provide accurate IDC interpolations. The formulation of the lognormal and the gamma model (for $t > 0$) that is typically used for the IDC fitting is provided in equations 2.9 and 2.10, respectively:

$$C(t) = \frac{K}{\sqrt{2\pi a_2 t}} e^{\frac{(\ln(t)-a_1)^2}{2a_2^2}}, \tag{2.9}$$

$$C(t) = Kt^{b_1} e^{-tb_2}. \tag{2.10}$$

The parameter $K$ scales the model amplitude, while $a_1$, $a_2$, $b_1$, and $b_2$ are the model shape parameters. The integrals of equations 2.9 and 2.10, which are used for flow estimates according to equation 2.2, equal $K$ and $K \cdot [b_2^{-(b_1+1)} \cdot \Gamma(b_1+1)]$, respectively.[1]

In practice, the first statistical moments of the distributions in equations 2.9 and 2.10 are also important. The first statistical moment is defined as

$$\mu^1 = \int_0^\infty tC(t)\,dt \left( \int_0^\infty C(t)\,dt \right)^{-1} \tag{2.11}$$

and is equal to $e^{a_1 + \frac{a_2^2}{2}}$ and $(1 + b_1)b_2^{-1}$ for the lognormal and the gamma model, respectively. The first moment resembles the time constant $\tau$ of the monocompartment model and defines the mean transit time (MTT), that is, the time that the contrast takes to cover the distance between the injection and the detection sites. This parameter is important in several applications that evaluate the level of perfusion and the blood volume in regions such as the myocardium or the brain.

Beyond the models of equations 2.9 and 2.10, other distributed models that provide an interesting interpretation of the indicator dispersion process are the local density random walk (LDRW) and the first passage time (FPT) models (Bogaard et al., 1986; Norwich, 1977; Sheppard, 1962; Wise, 1966). These models are based on the assumption of Brownian motion, and therefore the random walk of the indicator particles. The interest in these models is because of their relationship with the physical description of the dilution process. The dilution process of a contrast bolus dispersed in a carrier fluid that moves in one direction ($x$) is usually described by the "diffusion with drift" equation, which is given as

$$\frac{\partial C(x,t)}{\partial t} = D\frac{\partial^2 C(x,t)}{\partial x^2} - v\frac{\partial C(x,t)}{\partial x}, \tag{2.12}$$

where $C(x,t)$ is the contrast concentration at time $t$ and position $x$, $D$ is the diffusion constant of the dilution system, and $v$ is the velocity of the carrier fluid. As a result, a tight link can be found between the LDRW and FPT model parameters and the coefficients $v$ and $D$ in equation 2.12 (Bogaard et al., 1984).

---

1   $\Gamma$ represents the Gamma function $\Gamma(z) = \int_0^\infty x^{z-1}e^{-x}\,dx,\ \mathrm{Re}[z] > 0$, whose fundamental property is that

$\Gamma(z+1) = z\Gamma(z)$. If $z$ is a positive integer, $\Gamma(z) = (z-1)!$.

## 2.2.2. INDICATOR DILUTION TECHNIQUES

The field of indicator dilution applications for flow measurement in vessels is vast and the methods and sensors used vary depending on the adopted indicator. A major distinction has to be made between those methods that are based on a continuous infusion of the indicator and those that are based on the injection of a single bolus. Although the former methods are suitable for the continuous monitoring of flow, because of the large amount of injected indicator, this must be totally harmless to the body. The latter methods allow a relaxation of these requirements for the indicator, but such methods are not suitable for continuous flow monitoring. In this section the most common methods for flow measurement in large vessels (e.g., the measurement of CO) are discussed, starting with continuous methods (the Fick method and warm thermodilution) and moving on to the single bolus methods (cold thermodilution, dye dilution, and lithium dilution).

### 2.2.2.1. The Fick Method

The Fick method, proposed by Adolf Eugen Fick in 1870, uses a continuous indicator infusion. Because a large amount of indicator is injected, the indicator must be absolutely inert, harmless, and nontoxic. An indicator that fulfills these requirements is oxygen ($O_2$), which is used in the Fick method.

In the Fick method the indicator concentration is measured at two sites (see Fig. 2.4): the first site, $a$, is located before the injection point, while the second site, $b$, is located downstream. Assuming constant indicator concentrations $C_a$ and $C_b$ at the measurement locations $a$ and $b$, steady flow $\Phi = dV_a/dt = dV_b/dt$, and using equation 2.1, equation 2.13 can be derived:

$$C_b - C_a = \frac{\dfrac{dm_b}{dt}}{\dfrac{dV_b}{dt}} - \frac{\dfrac{dm_a}{dt}}{\dfrac{dV_a}{dt}} = \frac{1}{\Phi} \cdot \frac{d(m_b - m_a)}{dt}. \tag{2.13}$$

Since $d(m_b - m_a)/dt$ represents the tracer injection $dm/dt$ between the sampling points, equation 2.13 can be expressed as equation 2.14, which is the basic equation of the Fick method:

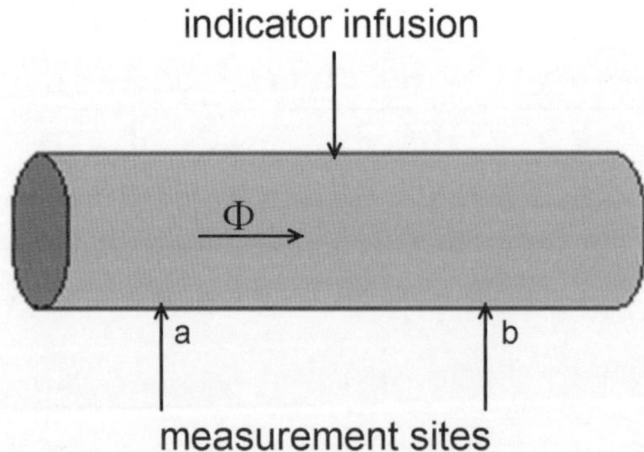


**Figure 2.4.** The Fick method model. Two measurements are continuously performed (a) upstream and (b) downstream with respect to the indicator infusion site.

$$\Phi = \frac{\dfrac{dm}{dt}}{C_b - C_a}.$$  (2.14)

An interesting characteristic of this method is that the injection is naturally performed by the lungs, and $C_a$ and $C_b$ are, respectively, the venous and the arterial concentration of $O_2$. Since the concentration of $O_2$ is different in the different venous returns, the sampling point $a$ is placed in the pulmonary artery, after the venous blood has been mixed by the right ventricle (RV). The blood samples of the so-called mixed venous blood are drawn by a catheter inserted through the jugular vein (or the subclavian vein) across the right atrium (RA) and RV up to the pulmonary artery. Then the blood samples are analyzed by a gas analyzer to determine the concentration of $O_2$. The choice of the arterial sampling site is not critical, since the blood from the lung capillaries is well mixed and little or no $O_2$ is lost in the blood's traversal through the arteries. An arm or a leg artery is normally used.

Measurement of the injected tracer (i.e., the inhaled $O_2$) is performed by making the patient breath pure $O_2$ from a spirometer (Webster, 1999). Typically an optical spirometer is used, which counts the light interruptions due to the rotation of a flow-driven fan. The exhaled carbon dioxide ($CO_2$) is absorbed by a soda-lime absorber, so that the $O_2$ injection rate $dm/dt$ (or $O_2$ consumption) can be directly measured by the net gas flow. However, attention must be paid to the different temperature of the gas during inspiration and expiration, which, at a fixed pressure (Boyle's law, $PVT^{-1}$ is constant), results in different volumes (Blom, 2003). Since during expiration the gas is saturated with water vapor, another important aspect that should be considered when measuring airflow is the presence of water vapor, which does not obey Boyle's law. A compensation for the effects due to temperature variation and the presence of water vapor on the measured volumes can be implemented, as given in equation 2.15),

$$V_i = V_e \cdot \left[ \frac{P_e - P_{H_2O}(T_e)}{P_i - P_{H_2O}(T_i)} \right] \cdot \frac{T_i}{T_e},$$  (2.15)

where $V_i$, $P_i$, and $T_i$ are, respectively, the gas volume, pressure, and temperature during inspiration; $V_e$, $P_e$, and $T_e$ are, respectively, the gas volume, pressure, and temperature during expiration; and $P_{H_2O}$ is the water vapor pressure.

As an alternative to the soda-lime absorber, the concentration of $CO_2$ can be measured by a capnograph, which measures the absorption of infrared (IR) light (4.3 μm wavelength). This light absorption is related to the concentration of $CO_2$ (Blom, 2003).

Fick's method was regarded as the standard technique for flow and CO measurements until thermodilution replaced it.

### 2.2.2.2. Thermodilution

Another indicator that fulfills the strict requirement for continuous infusion is heat, which is used in the thermodilution technique. Like $O_2$, heat is nontoxic and naturally cleared, therefore it is a perfect indicator for use in a continuous infusion technique. Thermodilution, first introduced by Fegler (1954), can be based either on a continuous infusion of the indicator or on a single bolus injection. In the first case, the indicator consists of the heat generated by a resistor, and the resulting technique is referred to as warm thermodilution. In the second case, the indicator consists of a cold saline bolus, and the resulting technique is referred to as cold thermodilution.

In both cases a Swan-Ganz catheter (see Fig. 2.5) is inserted via a central vein (usually the internal jugular or subclavian) through the RA and RV, so that its tip lies in the pulmonary artery (Swan et al., 1971). This catheter is carried to the correct position by the dragging force of the flowing blood thanks to a doughnut-shaped, air-filled balloon on the tip of the catheter.

### 2.2.2.2.1. Warm Thermodilution

In warm thermodilution (Yelderman, 1990), the catheter (described in Fig. 2.5[a]) includes circuitry for a thermistor that measures the temperature in the pulmonary artery and wires for the heating coil (resistor) that lies in the RA. A thermistor is a semiconductor thermometer that uses the relation between temperature and material resistivity for temperature measurement (Webster, 1999).

Heat is an extravascular indicator, as it can also be dissipated through the walls of the blood vessels. Therefore the distance between the injection and the sampling site should be as short as possible to limit the indicator loss. Unfortunately, in order to have adequate mixing, this distance should be long, so a compromise becomes necessary. The compromise that is usually adopted consists of infusing the indicator in the RA and sampling it in the pulmonary artery.

Warm thermodilution is also based on equation 2.14. The term $dm/dt$ is given by the heat derivative $Q'$ (expressed in watts), and the term $C_b - C_a$ is given by the temperature difference $T_b - T_a$ (expressed in kelvin) times the specific heat of blood $c_b$ (about 3700 J kg$^{-1}$ K$^{-1}$) times the blood density $\rho_b$ (about 1060 kg m$^{-3}$). Thus the reformulation of equation 2.14 for the thermodilution becomes

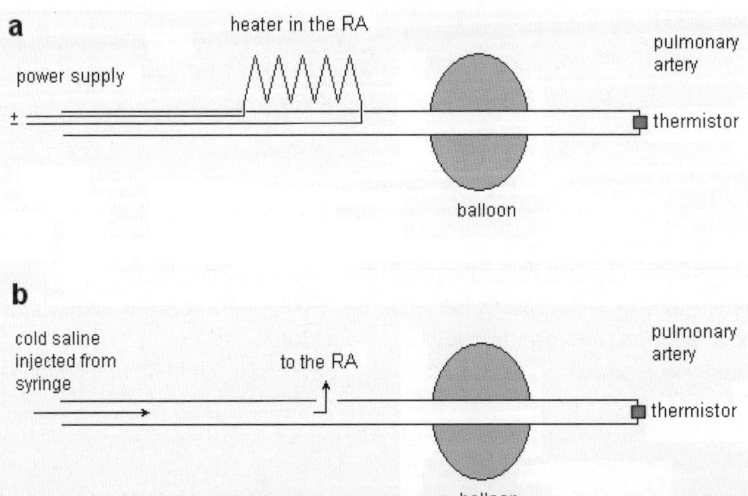


**Figure 2.5.** Scheme of a Swan-Ganz catheter for (a) warm and (b) cold thermodilution. In (a), heat is produced by a resistor, while in (b), a bolus of cold saline is injected through a dedicated line in the catheter. In both cases the temperature is measured by a thermistor on the tip of the catheter. The balloon is used to drag the catheter to the right position.

$$\Phi = \frac{Q'}{c_b\rho_b(T_b - T_a)}. \tag{2.16}$$

The mass of the tracer is now represented by the amount of supplied energy $Q$ (in joules) and its concentration is given in joules per cubic meter (J m$^{-3}$) by the term $c_b\rho_b T$. The thermistors are usually placed in a Wheatstone configuration (Webster, 1999). This technique has become very common in clinical practice and everything is integrated in a single catheter. The advantage of these methods is that they provide continuous monitoring of flow, which is of particular interest for CO.

### 2.2.2.2.2. Cold Thermodilution

Cold thermodilution is a different application of equation 2.1 that makes use of an injection of a cold indicator bolus, which can be either cold dextrose or saline (NaCl blood-isotonic solution). In this case, the resistor is replaced by a port for the bolus injection, as shown in Figure 2.5(b), which is performed by a syringe. The cold solution mixes with blood in the RA and RV before passing into the pulmonary artery, where the temperature decrease is sensed by a thermistor on the side of the catheter. The CO is then calculated from the time–temperature curve (see Fig. 2.6). Using the same interpretation of heat and temperature as in equation 2.16, equation 2.2 can be rewritten as

$$\Phi = \frac{Q}{c_b\rho_b\displaystyle\int_{t_0}^{\infty} -\Delta T(t)\,dt}, \tag{2.17}$$

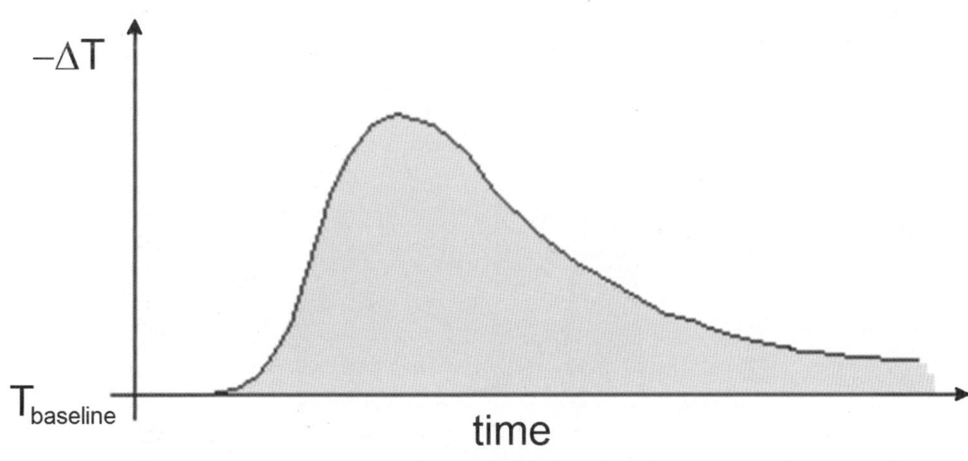


**Figure 2.6.** Example of time–temperature curve. Notice that the curve is flipped around the time axis since the IDC is given by the temperature decrease −ΔT.

where $Q$ is the total injected heat, $\Delta T$ is the temperature decrease, and $c_b$ and $\rho_b$ are the same as in equation 2.16. Since this method requires the injection of a bolus followed by its downstream detection, it is not suitable for continuous CO monitoring.

A pulmonary artery catheterization is not always possible or indicated. In these cases, a transpulmonary (also referred to as aortic) thermodilution is performed, which has been shown to provide high agreement with pulmonary artery thermodilution flow assessments (Sakka, Reinhart, & Meier-Hellmann, 1999). A bolus can be injected into the RA and detected in the aorta by a second catheter, which is usually inserted through the femoral artery. Transpulmonary thermodilution between the RA and aorta can be performed in children to assess the CO when cardiac catheterization is complicated by the small size of the heart.

Cold thermodilution can also be combined with pressure and heart rate measurements in order to provide continuous flow measurement (Gödje et al., 1996). The thermodilution measurement can be used for calibration purposes. The arterial pressure curve is linearly scaled so that its integral during systole (until the dicrotic notch; see Fig. 2.7) is equal to the stroke volume, that is, the CO divided by the heart rate. After calibration the CO can be derived continuously (beat by beat) by analysis of the measured arterial pressure curve. This approach has been reported to correlate well with continuous thermodilution, even when the pressure is measured noninvasively by finger-cuff photoplethysmography (see the end of section 2.2.6; Lieshout & Jansen, 2007; Lu & Mukkamala, 2006).

### 2.2.2.3. Dye Dilution

A colored dye such as indocyanine green, usually referred to as cardiogreen, can be used as an indicator since it is inert, nontoxic, measurable, and inexpensive. Using the principle of absorption photometry, the concentration of cardiogreen, which is usually injected into the pulmonary artery, can be detected by the light absorption peak at a wavelength of 805 nm.

In the past, blood samples had to be drawn by a catheter placed in the femoral or brachial artery and analyzed by an external photometry device. Today, the use of optical fibers allows for in situ measurements.

The kidneys clear about 50% of the dye in the first 10 minutes, so that repeated measurements are also possible. Once the system is calibrated, that is, the peak absorption is related to the concentration $C(t)$ of the dye, the flow is directly given by equation 2.2.

Other dye indicators, such as Evans blue (absorption peak at 640 nm and 50% clearance in 5 days) and Coomassie blue (absorption peak around 590 nm and 50% clearance in 15–20 minutes) are also suitable indicators that are used in clinical practice.

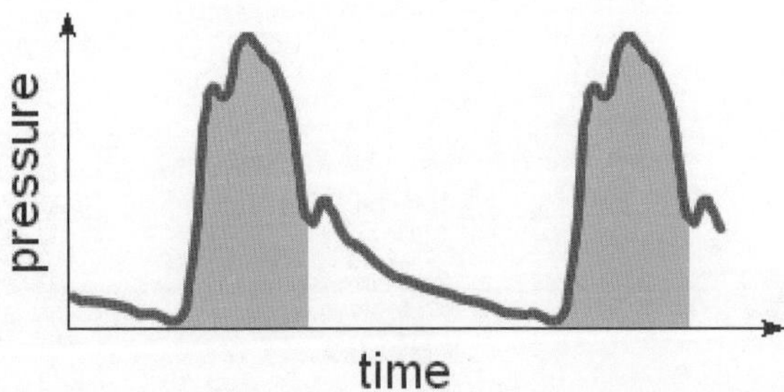


**Figure 2.7.** Arterial pressure waveform. The integral during systole until the dicrotic notch is indicated in gray.

### 2.2.2.4. Lithium Dilution

Linton et al. (1993) first proposed lithium as a possible indicator for clinical measurements (Jonas, Hett, & Morgan, 2002; Kurita et al., 1999). Lithium is a fluid that can be injected and detected by a lithium-selective electrode in a flow-through cell. Two silver–silver chloride (Ag-AgCl) electrodes measure the potential across a lithium-selective membrane. According to the Nernst equation (Webster, 1999), the electric potential $E$ across a membrane is given as

$$ E = \frac{RT}{nF} \ln\left( \frac{C_{ext}}{C_{int}} \right), \tag{2.18} $$

where $C_{ext}$ and $C_{int}$ are the external and the internal (with respect to the membrane) lithium activities, which correspond to the lithium ionic concentrations, $R$ is the gas constant ($8.314$ J mol$^{-1}$ K$^{-1}$), $T$ is the absolute temperature (kelvin), $F$ is the Faraday constant ($96485$ C mol$^{-1}$), and $n$ is the valence of the ions, which for lithium ions (Li$^+$) is 1. As a result, the transducer measures a voltage that is logarithmically related to the lithium concentration. The sensor is connected to a three-way tap on the arterial line and a small peristaltic pump draws blood with a flow of few milliliters per minute. The lithium concentration is measured versus time. The time integral of the measured IDC is used as given in equation 2.2 for the CO assessment.

The lithium dilution curve is usually used for calibration purposes. Based on the IDC CO measurement and the establishment of the relation pressure volume (compliance), continuous CO monitoring can be performed (see also Hamilton, Huber, & Jessen, 2002; Jonas & Tanzer, 2002). In more detail, an uncalibrated stroke volume is derived from the arterial pressure waveform by calculating the root-mean-square of the pressure wave after subtraction of the mean value. The cardiac cycle is easily derived from the same pressure waveform. The uncalibrated stroke volume divided by the cardiac cycle provides an uncalibrated flow that is linearly related to the real CO. The calibration factor is derived from the lithium IDC measurement of CO.

### 2.2.3. ULTRASOUND FLOWMETERS

Ultrasound flowmeters are based on at least one of two physical principles that occur where a (preferably narrow) beam of ultrasound interacts with matter such as biological tissues:

1. If the beam encounters moving reflecting particles, the frequency of the reflections differs from the frequency of the transmitted beam. The frequency difference parallels the velocity of the moving particles, such as red blood cells, whose velocity is that of the blood. This is the well-known Doppler effect.
2. If the beam encounters any change in acoustic impedance, reflections occur. Changes in acoustic impedance generally occur where tissue properties change, and the change is largest when tissue properties change abruptly and greatly, such as at the walls of blood vessels. The time delay after which reflected "echoes" are received denotes the depth of the reflecting tissue transition, because the ultrasound velocity in the tissues of interest does not vary appreciably.[2]

---

2   Ultrasound at clinical diagnostic frequencies (greater than 1 MHz) cannot pass bones and air (e.g., in the lungs). This may pose clinical problems.

Simple ultrasound flowmeters use only the first (Doppler) principle: they measure only the instantaneous blood velocity. Hence they are not really flowmeters, which is a never-ending source of confusion. If the blood flow is wanted, the blood velocity must be multiplied by the area of the cross section of the examined vessel, which can be estimated by the second (non-Doppler) method.

An ultrasound flowmeter is a noninvasive device for the measurement of instantaneous blood flow (or the instantaneous blood velocity, which is an uncalibrated measure of blood flow if the measurement takes place in a constant-diameter blood vessel). Usually it is embedded in a standard clinical ultrasound scanner that must be set to Doppler mode and equipped with a proper transducer. However, portable dedicated devices are also available for clinical use.

### 2.2.3.1. Ultrasound Generation

An ultrasound transducer is a device that generates ultrasonic waves by means of piezoelectric crystals whose oscillations are excited and controlled by electrical voltage. Ultrasonic waves are pressure waves whose frequency is higher than 20 kHz (audibility threshold). Usual frequencies in clinical applications range from 1 MHz to 10 MHz. The adopted piezoelectric crystals can be either natural (e.g., quartz) or synthetic (e.g., lead-zirconate-titanate, poly-vinylidene-di-fluoride, lead-magnesium-niobate, barium-lead-titanate or -zirconate) and are placed on the tip of a probe.

Each piezoelectric crystal makes an approximately linear conversion between electrical voltage and mechanical pressure. The crystal size determines the working frequency of the transducer, which is chosen to be equal to the resonant frequency of the crystal because this is the frequency at which the highest energy is transferred to the external medium. If $L$ and $v_c$ are, respectively, the crystal length and the velocity of ultrasound through the crystal, then the resonance frequency $f_0$ corresponds to

$$ f_0 = \frac{v_c}{2L}. \tag{2.19} $$

The parameter that characterizes different media with respect to ultrasonic waves is the acoustic impedance, $Z_a = \rho v$, where $\rho$ is the medium density and $v$ is the ultrasound velocity in the medium, which in tissue is about 1540 m s$^{-1}$. Variations of $Z_a$ produce reflections of the ultrasonic waves. Ultrasound signal interpretation (ultrasonography) is based on the detection and interpretation of the reflected waves. The characterization of pressure waves propagating through a medium is beyond the scope of this chapter, but detailed information can be found in other literature (Duck, Baker, & Starritt, 1998; Hedrick, Hykes, & Starchman, 1995; Szabo, 2004; Wells, 1977).

Because of the large acoustic impedance difference between piezoelectric crystals and skin, where most of the power would be reflected and thus not enter the body, ultrasound transducers are covered by an impedance-matching layer whose thickness is equal to one-fourth of the ultrasonic wavelength (in order to obtain constructive reflections) and whose impedance is between that of tissue and skin. Such layers are basically made of aluminum powder in an epoxy resin: the higher the concentration of aluminum, the higher the acoustic impedance. However, new transducers are being developed that do not require a matching layer. They are made by polyvinylidene fluoride (PVF$_2$) with acoustic impedance close to that of biological tissue (Hedrick et al., 1995).

### 2.2.3.2. Doppler Effect

A schematic representation of an ultrasound flowmeter is provided in Figure 2.8. A transmitter ($Tx$) and a receiver ($Rx$) are integrated in the same probe. Starting at a certain distance (explained by the

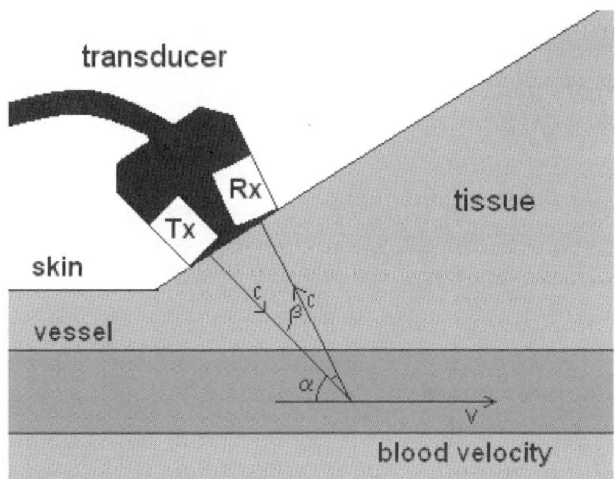


**Figure 2.8.** Doppler flowmeter for blood flow measurements. Ultrasonic waves are transmitted (*Tx*) and received (*Rx*) after being reflected by moving scatterers (red blood cells). The angle β, which determines the focal depth, is used in equation 2.21 together with the angle α for the determination of blood velocity *v*.

Huygens principle), the generated ultrasonic pressure waves can be approximated by planar waves (Fraunhofer approximation for distances larger than $r^2\lambda^{-1}$, where $r$ is the transducer radius and $\lambda$ is the ultrasound wavelength in the medium). The focal depth, where the blood velocity is measured, is determined by the angle β, which depends on the structure of the transducer and can be varied mechanically. The transducer transmits ultrasound pressure waves with frequency $f_t$. If $c$ and $v$ are the propagation velocity of ultrasound and the blood velocity, respectively, the red blood cells receive the signal with a frequency equal to $f_t(1 - vc^{-1}\cos\alpha)$ and the receiver *Rx* receives the signal reflected by the blood particles with a frequency $f_r$, as in equation 2.20:

$$f_r = f_t \left( \frac{c - v\cos\alpha}{c} \right) \left( \frac{c}{c + v\cos(\alpha + \beta)} \right) = f_t \left( \frac{c - v\cos\alpha}{c + v\cos(\alpha + \beta)} \right) \quad (2.20)$$

For small β and for $v \ll c$, the frequency shift $\Delta f = f_t - f_r$, known as the Doppler frequency (frequency of the Doppler signal), is given as

$$\Delta f = f_t \left( 1 - \frac{c - v\cos\alpha}{c + v\cos(\alpha + \beta)} \right) \cong v \left( \frac{2f_t}{c} \right) \cos\alpha. \quad (2.21)$$

Therefore, since $f_t$ and $c$ are known, the Doppler frequency $\Delta f$ is linearly related to the blood velocity. For instance, with blood velocity $v$ of 20 cm s$^{-1}$, a typical $f_t$ of 5 MHz, and $\alpha = 30°$, the Doppler frequency becomes $\Delta f = 1.1$ kHz. This is within the human audibility range and the reason why the user interface is often a loudspeaker. In order to obtain $\Delta f$, the received signal is demodulated by a mixer that multiplies it by the transmitted signal. Suppose that $S_t = a_t\cos(2\pi f_t t)$ is the transmitted signal and $S_r = a_r\cos(2\pi f_r t)$ is the received signal. Then the mixer multiplies $S_t$ by $S_r$ obtaining $S_t S_r = a_t a_r [\cos(2\pi(f_t - f_r)t) + \cos(2\pi(f_t + f_r)t)]/2$. Finally, by low-pass filtering, the high-frequency component $(f_t + f_r)$ is suppressed. The remaining part represents the Doppler signal with frequency $\Delta f = f_t - f_r$.

### 2.2.3.3. Basic Implementation

A quadrature demodulator distinguishes between forward and reverse flow (Evans & McDicken, 2000; Hedrick et al., 1995; Szabo, 2004). Each of the two quadrature components is multiplied by a 90-degree delayed version of the other component. This implementation yields two channels that represent the forward and reverse flow, respectively. A stereo audio output is then a suitable user interface in clinical practice. Figure 2.9 shows a schematic representation of this implementation. Other solutions make use of filters (single-sideband detectors) or frequency shifts (heterodyne detector) and are implemented in several systems (Evans & McDicken, 2000; Hedrick et al., 1995; Szabo, 2004).

As an alternative to the use of analog mixers, the signal can be analog-to-digital (A/D) converted and the signal processing can be implemented in software by means of the Hilbert transform and the fast Fourier transform (FFT). The FFT results in the spectrum of the demodulated signal, which corresponds with an estimate for $\Delta f$. A complex FFT can also be applied to the quadrature components to estimate the spectrum of the analytical signal (low-band components). As a result, the forward and the reverse flow will simply result in a translation of the energy spectrum to positive or negative frequencies. The resulting energy spectrum, scaled to indicate the velocity, is usually presented on a screen by a typical time–frequency representation. For each time sample ($x$ axis), the energy contribution of each frequency ($y$ axis) is gray-level coded. An example is given in Figure 2.10.

Because of the parabolic flow profile in the vessels, the frequency spectrum is broad, and it depends also on the ratio between the size of the focal zone of the ultrasound beam, referred to as the sample volume, and the diameter of the vessel (Hedrick et al., 1995). When these uncertainties must be eliminated and quantification of the blood velocity is required, several methods can be adopted that use, for example, the maximum, median, or mean frequency of the measured spectrum (Evans & McDicken 2000; Hedrick et al., 1995). The analysis can be improved by use of the time–frequency distribution to improve the compromise between time and frequency resolution (Evans & McDicken, 2000).

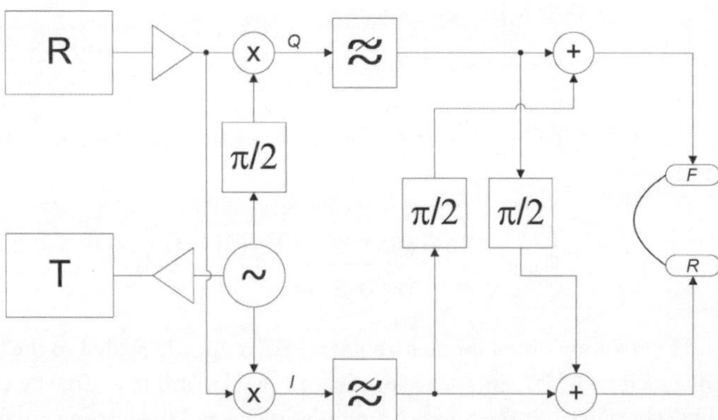


**Figure 2.9.** Scheme of a Doppler system based on a quadrature detector. The ultrasound signal is transmitted by block *T* and its echoes are received by block *R*. The in-phase (*I*) and quadrature (*Q*) components of the received signal are then low-pass filtered and added in a way that the Doppler signal related to the forward (*F*) and reverse (*R*) flow is directed to two different channels (e.g., the left and right loudspeaker of a headset).

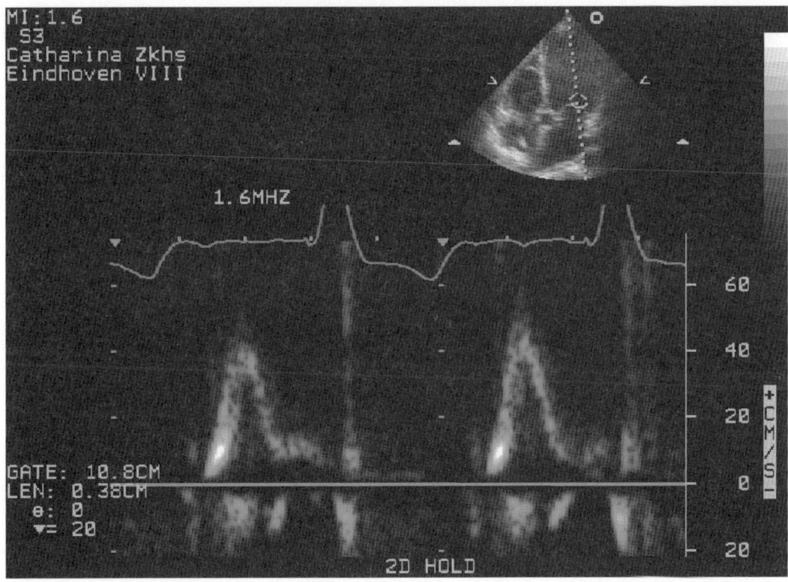


**Figure 2.10.** Video output showing a Doppler investigation of the left ventricle transmitral inflow. Courtesy of the Department of Cardiology, Catharina Hospital, Eindhoven, The Netherlands.

Thus far a transducer composed of two single crystals, a transmitter, and a receiver (as shown in Fig. 2.8) has been discussed. A more complex transducer is composed of two crystal arrays that allow steering of the beam (the focal area) over a plane. Ultrasonic beam steering is realized by applying a delay between the activation of successive array elements (see Fig. 2.27 in section 2.3.2.2). This is the technique used in ultrasound imaging, referred to as B-mode ultrasound, so that a multielement Doppler measurement can be performed with the same transducer that is adopted for ultrasound imaging. The resulting advantages consist of the possibility of observing the examined vessels in B-mode imaging in order to improve the focus and alignment (determination of the angle $\alpha$) of the Doppler measurement.

The system described is the simplest application of the Doppler effect for blood velocity estimation, and it is referred to as continuous wave (CW) or narrowband Doppler. The main disadvantage of this technique is the difficulty in distinguishing between different moving targets. Every movement within the ultrasonic sample volume provides a signal and contributes to the velocity estimation.

### 2.2.3.4. Pulsed Doppler Implementation

The difficulty in distinguishing between different moving targets is overcome by a different system, referred to as pulsed wave (PW) or wideband Doppler (Evans & McDicken, 2000; Feigenbaum, 1994; Szabo, 2004). Each element of the transducer is used both as a transmitter and a receiver, and a train of pulses is transmitted and received. As a consequence, it is possible to determine the position of the targets from the delays in the echoes using the same methods used in B-mode imaging. Knowing that the ultrasound propagation velocity in tissue is approximately 1540 m s$^{-1}$, the estimation of the depth of the detected echo with respect to the probe is straightforward. A time window applied to the received signal allows the signals of only a certain reception depth to be processed.

The use of the transducer in PW mode requires the generation of short pulses and thus a capability to stop the crystal vibrations as soon as the electric signal is turned off. To obtain this result, the internal surfaces of the crystals are covered by a thick damping layer made of epoxy. Figure 2.11 shows the structure of a monocrystal transducer. More details can be found in Wells (1977). The acoustic lens on the crystal improves the lateral resolution of the transducer by realizing a narrower ultrasonic beam.

To achieve good spatial resolution, the transmitted pulse duration should be as short as possible. On the other hand, the achievement of good frequency resolution, and thus good velocity resolution, requires the use of long bursts. This compromise is known as the uncertainty principle, which is well known in time–frequency analysis problems. A typical compromise is, for instance, a 5 MHz (carrier frequency) burst of 1 μs duration (5 cycles).

Figure 2.12 shows the principles of the PW Doppler assuming $\alpha = 0$. In (a), a train of pulses (bursts) is shown, reflected by a particle (red blood cell) that is moving away from the transducer (increasing depth) with a velocity equal to $(\Delta d/2)(PRF)$, where PRF stands for pulse repetition frequency.[3] The motion of the particle makes the echo of each pulse relatively delayed by the time required to travel $\Delta d$. In (b), the Doppler signal with frequency $\Delta f$ is shown, which is sampled with a frequency equal to the PRF, since the transmitting and receiving circuits are synchronized (they are connected to the same crystals).

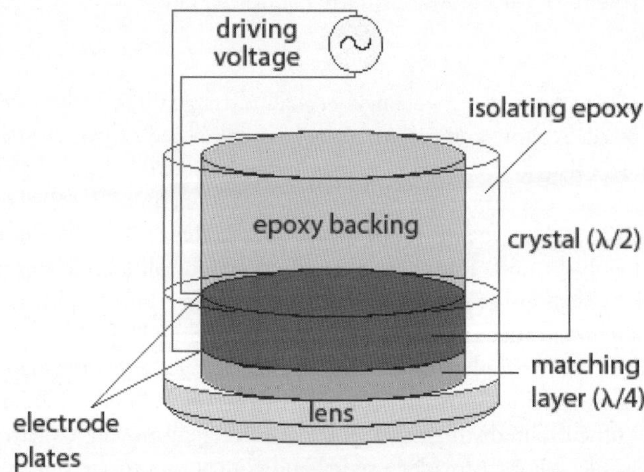


**Figure 2.11.** Simplified scheme of a single-element transducer. A driving voltage is connected to the electrode plates on the crystal. Epoxy is used to isolate the system as well as to dampen the back of the crystal for an accurate transmission of short pulses. Aluminum powder in epoxy is typically used for the matching layer. The acoustic lens permits a narrowing of the transmitted ultrasonic beam, thus improving lateral resolution.

---

3   Notice that $\Delta d$ is the displacement between two subsequent pulses, which is twice the distance covered by the moving target during one pulse repetition period. This is because the pulse covers twice (forward and backward direction) the distance covered by the moving target.

Based on the implementation of the PW Doppler system shown in Figure 2.12, it is obvious that this velocity measurement does not use the Doppler effect. In fact, the frequency shift of single pulses is not relevant to the measurement. Given a moving target, the resulting signal in Figure 2.12(b) at the frequency $f_b = \Delta f$ is simply the result of the combination of pulse transmission and sampling rates, which are equal. Despite this, an attempt can still be made to provide an intuitive interpretation of the relation between the frequency $f_b$ of the signal in (b) and the Doppler frequency.

The transmitted pulse is a spatial wave of length $\lambda = cf_t^{-1}$, where $f_t$ is the carrier frequency. The output signal in Figure 2.12(b) corresponds to the reception of this spatial wave (of fixed wavelength $\lambda = cf_t^{-1}$) propagating at a velocity equal to $2v$, with $v$ being the particle velocity. The factor 2 accounts for the fact that the pulse displacement $\Delta d$ during one pulse repetition period equals twice the particle displacement. Thus the received frequency corresponds to $f_b = 2v\lambda^{-1} = 2vf_t c^{-1}$, which corresponds to the expression for $\Delta f$ given in equation 2.21 when $\alpha = 0$. This is an interpretation in the continuous domain of the discrete system described in Figure 2.12. To consider the general case where $\alpha \neq 0$, it is sufficient to consider the projection $v_p$ of the blood velocity $v$ on the direction of the ultrasound propagation velocity, that is, $v_p = v\cos\alpha$ (refer to Fig. 2.8 with $\beta = 0$). As in the CW case, to obtain a distinction between forward and reverse flow requires the use of a quadrature sampler (Szabo, 2004).

Since the Doppler effect is not involved, the PW Doppler system can be viewed from a different perspective. Instead of focusing on the Doppler frequency, the phase shift $\Delta\varphi$ between two subsequent

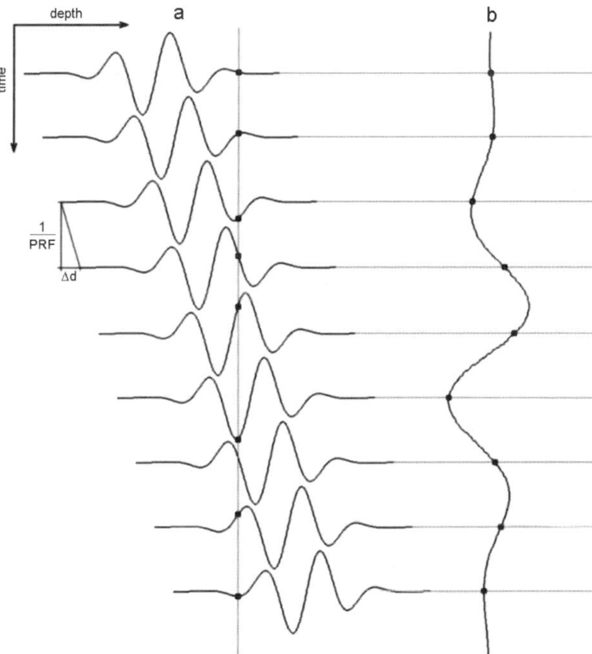


**Figure 2.12.** Pulsed wave Doppler example. In (a), the transmitted train of bursts is reflected by a target displaced by a distance $\Delta d/2$ for each pulse repetition. In (b), the sampled Doppler signal is shown. The sampling frequency equals the pulse repetition frequency (PRF).

received pulses could be estimated by their cross-correlation function (Szabo, 2004). The phase shift $\Delta\varphi$ equals $2\pi(\Delta d)\lambda^{-1}$ radians, where $\lambda = cf_t^{-1}$ is the pulse wavelength. Therefore, recalling that the blood particle is moving at velocity $(\Delta d/2)(\text{PRF})$, the blood velocity $v$ can be given as a function of the estimated $\Delta\varphi$ as

$$v = \text{PRF} \cdot \frac{c\Delta\varphi}{4\pi f_t}. \tag{2.22}$$

A new burst is not transmitted until the reflection from the deepest layer is received back. As a consequence, the maximum PRF equals $c(2d)^{-1}$, with $d$ equal to the distance between the transducer and the deepest layer. The PRF also represents the sampling frequency applied to the Doppler signal, since the whole system has to be synchronized (Fig. 2.12). Therefore the system must satisfy the Nyquist relation $\text{PRF} > 2\Delta f$, which combined with equation 2.21 defines the maximum detectable velocity $v_{max}$, as given in equation 2.23, where $f_t$ is now the carrier frequency within the single pulse:

$$v_{max} = \text{PRF}\left(\frac{c}{4f_t \cos\alpha}\right) = \frac{c^2}{8f_t d \cos\alpha}. \tag{2.23}$$

This equation shows that for a shorter distance $d$, and consequently a larger PRF, the maximum detectable velocity is higher. When the blood velocity is higher than $v_{max}$, aliasing occurs and the signal interpretation may fail. In modern devices, routines are implemented that detect and manage these errors in order to avoid wrong diagnoses.

Another important advantage of PW over CW Doppler is the possibility of determining the blood velocity profile. The delay between transmission and reception of a single burst is a direct indication of the depth from which the pulse has been reflected. Therefore, if the receiver decomposes the detected echoes into different time windows (referred to as gates, usually between six and thirty-two), each window selects the part of the echoes that are reflected from a specific depth interval. The received bursts can be processed concurrently in different channels. The velocity profile is obtained by simply combining the output from each channel. This technique is referred to as multigate pulsed Doppler (Evans & McDicken, 2000; Hedrick et al., 1995).

### 2.2.3.5. Major Limitations

Both CW and PW Doppler present the problem of clutter noise. Clutter noise is introduced by the slow motion of tissue, which adds low-frequency components to the Doppler signal, for example, the slow expansion and contraction of vessel walls. In order to remove clutter noise, a high-pass filter is implemented in every system (Evans & McDicken, 2000; Hedrick et al., 1995).

Another major problem of Doppler ultrasound measurements is the dependency of the computed result on the angle $\alpha$ between the transducer axis and the blood flow. This angle is often unknown or only an estimate, therefore a substantial uncertainty is introduced into the measurement and thus into the estimated value of the absolute velocity (and flow). The only medical application where $\alpha$ can be estimated approximately is in the measurement of laminar flow through a straight vessel. In this case, the angle can be estimated from the corresponding B-mode image of the same vessel. However, several methods have been developed to integrate a more accurate and quicker estimation of the angle $\alpha$ into the system (Jensen, 1996). The current development of transducers capable of spanning a three-dimensional (3D) space might open new possibilities for an accurate estimation of $\alpha$ (Ogura, Katakura, & Okujima, 1997).

In CW Doppler systems, the sample volume is determined by the frequency and geometry of the transducer, and it is larger than that for PW gated Doppler systems. A larger sample volume includes a larger number of different velocities that can be the result of a parabolic flow profile or turbulence. As a result, the measured Doppler frequency spectrum can be significantly broadened, and a specific Doppler frequency cannot be determined.

### 2.2.3.6. Latest Developments

A multigate PW can be applied in such a way that not only is one line analyzed, but an entire plane. To this end it is sufficient to translate the transducer in the lateral direction. When a multielement transducer is adopted, the beam translation can be performed electronically by activating the adjacent crystals in a temporal sequence. The field of view can be further expanded (beyond the physical dimensions of the transducer) by steering the ultrasound beam using phased array technology, that is, adding linear delays between the elements of the transducer in order to vary (steer) the direction of the generated ultrasonic plane wave (Evans & McDicken, 2000; Hedrick et al., 1995). The result is usually presented as a color-coded image, where the intensity and direction of the blood velocity have different colors. For this reason, this mode is referred to as color flow Doppler imaging (Feigenbaum, 1994). Forward and reverse flows are usually represented in red and blue, respectively. The signal intensity (the absolute velocity) is then given by the color intensity. The color-coding is usually presented as a color bar on the side of the image.

Very often a better view of the imaged area is desirable. To this end, a combination of color flow and B-mode imaging is implemented in so-called duplex scanners (Evans & McDicken, 2000). The scanner makes use of a multielement array to alternatively build a B-mode image, which shows the tissue structures, and a color flow image, which shows the blood flows (hemodynamics) in the same field of view. This solution, although providing a lower temporal resolution (fewer frames per second depending on the image size, that is, the depth and the aperture angle), allows a better interpretation of the Doppler signal as well as a more accurate alignment of the transducer.

Unfortunately, the presence of noise in the measured signals represents a serious problem, especially for the detection of blood flow direction. Therefore, weak signals, such as those received from small vessels, cannot be properly detected and interpreted. A solution for this problem is power Doppler imaging, where the color-coding is related to the total Doppler power rather than the frequency shift. This system is useful in the analysis of flow in smaller vessels (Desser, Jedrzejewicz, & Haller, 1998; Evans & McDicken, 2000; Szabo, 2004).

A measurement that is particularly important for patients that have cardiovascular dysfunctions, as well as for follow-up after surgical intervention, is CO, the total blood flow delivered by the heart into the aorta. The use of Doppler allows the estimation of CO by integrating the measured velocities (velocity profile) over one full cardiac cycle (time integration) and the cross-sectional area (spatial integration) of the ascending aorta or LV out-tract (Feigenbaum, 1994; Schiller et al., 1989). In practice, spatial integration is often replaced by a product of the cross-sectional area and the estimated velocity in one sample volume. Today the measurement of CO by ultrasound echo-Doppler is also performed with transesophageal probes, resulting in high-quality measurements whose correlation coefficient with the standard cold thermodilution is about 0.9 (Poelaert et al., 1999). A transesophageal probe is an ultrasound transducer on the tip of a flexible shaft (tube; Stoddard et al., 1992) that is so narrow it can be introduced into the esophagus through the mouth. The advantages of a transesophageal transducer compared to a transthoracic transducer are improved signal-to-noise ratio (SNR), due to the absence of disturbances from ribs and lungs, as well as a more stable orientation of the field of view over time. Because patients find their application unpleasant, transesophageal probes are mainly used during surgery in order to monitor cardiac function.

## 2.2.4. MAGNETIC RESONANCE METHODS

Magnetic resonance imaging is a noninvasive imaging technique that is used in medical settings to produce images of the interior of the human body. It provides excellent contrast between soft tissues and has a high spatial resolution (1–2 mm) in every direction.

Felix Bloch and Edward Purcell discovered the magnetic resonance phenomenon independently in 1946. In the beginning, MRI was developed and used for chemical and physical molecular analysis and it was usually referred to as nuclear magnetic resonance (NMR). In 1971 Raymond Damadian showed that the nuclear magnetic relaxation times of tissues and tumors differed. This motivated scientists to consider magnetic resonance for the detection of disease. Early in the 1970s Paul Lauterbur discovered that he could reconstruct an image by introducing gradients in the magnetic field. MRI is today a routine method for noninvasive diagnostics and is also suitable for noninvasive and accurate measurements of flow. This section provides an introduction to the basic principles of MRI in order to understand the basic techniques for flow visualization and quantification, referred to as magnetic resonance angiography (MRA). A more detailed presentation and explanation of all MRI techniques can be found in several dedicated books (e.g., Liang & Lauterbur, 2000; Vlaardingerbroek & den Boer, 2003).

### 2.2.4.1. MRI Principles

Magnetic resonance imaging is based on the phenomenon of nuclear magnetic resonance, which, as its name suggests, refers to the resonance of atomic nuclei. The human body is mainly constituted of water molecules and therefore contains many hydrogen atoms. A hydrogen atom consists of one proton in the nucleus and one electron. Each hydrogen nucleus shows an angular momentum $\vec{J}$, generally referred to as spin, which is due to the nucleus rotating around its own axis. Since the rotating nucleus has an electric charge, it generates a magnetic field, which can be represented by the magnetic dipole moment $\vec{\mu}$.[4] Therefore a nucleus can be considered a small magnet.

The magnetic moment is parallel and proportional to the spin angular momentum; the constant of proportionality is a physical constant, the gyromagnetic ratio $\gamma$, which is a proton property characterized by quantum mechanics and is equal to $2.675 \times 10^8$ rad s$^{-1}$ T$^{-1}$. Thus the relationship between the spin angular momentum and the magnetic moment is given as

$$\vec{\mu} = \gamma \cdot \vec{J}. \qquad (2.24)$$

The spinning protons, which have both angular momentum and magnetic moments, possess a specific spin quantum number that characterizes their orientations and corresponding energy levels. In the absence of an external magnetic field, the direction of the magnetic moments of spinning protons is completely random. When an external magnetic field of magnitude $\vec{B}_0$ is applied in the $z$ direction, the spins tend to align in the direction of the field. Two orientations of the nuclear magnetic moment relative to the field direction are possible: parallel and antiparallel (Fig. 2.13).

---

4    In the general case, for a current loop, the magnetic moment is $\vec{\mu} = A\,I_c\,\hat{n}$, where $A$ is the loop surface, $I_c$ is the electrical current intensity, and $\hat{n}$ is the normal vector with respect to $A$.

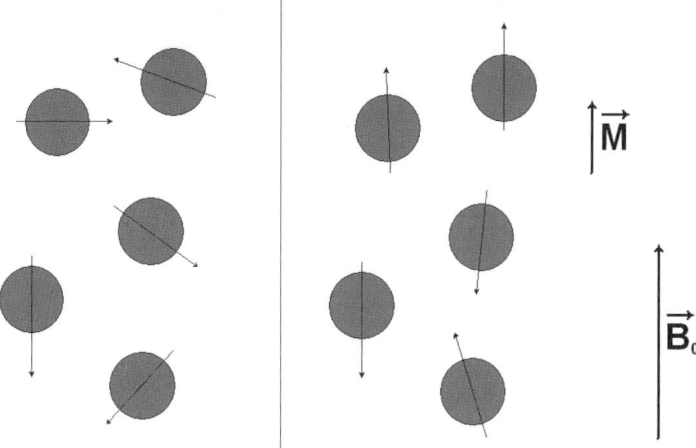



**Figure 2.13.** Magnetic moments of spinning protons without (left) and with (right) the presence of an external magnetic field $\vec{B}_0$. In the presence of the external magnetic field, the development of a net magnetization $\vec{M} = \sum \vec{\mu}_i$ can be noticed due to a prevalence of magnetic moments that align parallel to the external magnetic field.

These two states correspond to two allowed energy levels. The parallel orientation corresponds to a lower energy level. At equilibrium, the number of protons at the lower energy level exceeds that at the higher level. This leads to a net magnetization $\vec{M}$ in the direction of the field, which is the cumulative effect of the sum of all the magnetic moments of the nuclei in the object considered, and it is referred to as longitudinal magnetization (Fig. 2.13).

According to classical mechanics, the magnetic moment experiences a torque $\vec{\tau}$ from the external magnetic field that is equal to the rate of change of its angular momentum and is given by the equation of motion for isolated spins as

$$\vec{\tau} = \frac{d\vec{J}}{dt} = \vec{\mu} \times \vec{B}_0.  \tag{2.25}$$

Combining equations 2.24 and 2.25 gives

$$\frac{d\vec{\mu}}{dt} = \gamma\vec{\mu} \times \vec{B}_0  \tag{2.26}$$

As a result, the magnetic moment precesses around the axis of the external magnetic field at a special frequency referred to as the Larmor frequency, schematically shown in Figure 2.14. The relationship between the Larmor frequency $f_L$ and the applied magnetic field is the solution of equation 2.26, that is,

$$f_{\mathrm{L}} = \left(\frac{\gamma}{2\pi}\right)B_0.  \tag{2.27}$$

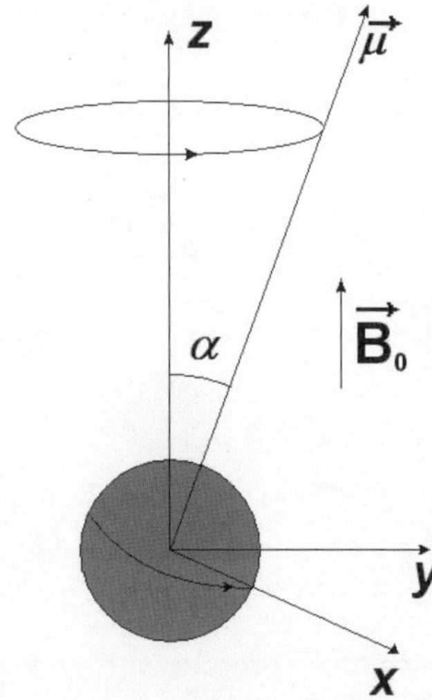



**Figure 2.14.** Precession of a nuclear spin around the external magnetic field $\vec{B}_0$ applied in the $z$ direction.

The value for $\gamma(2\pi)^{-1}$ is $42.58 \times 10^6$ Hz T$^{-1}$ in the case of protons. This is the frequency at which the nuclei can receive the radio frequency (RF) energy to change their states and exhibit nuclear magnetic resonance.

If an additional alternating field $\vec{B}_1$ is applied that is aligned along the $x$-axis and rotates around the $z$-axis with a frequency equal to the Larmor frequency, then the spins absorb energy. As a result, the population at the upper energy level increases while that at the lower level decreases. This is referred to as a resonance process. The net magnetization vector $\vec{M}$ is no longer in the direction of the external magnetic field, and it starts to move away from the $z$-direction. This net magnetization vector is flipped by a certain angle $\alpha$ that depends on the magnitude of the magnetic field $B_1$ and on the duration ($\Delta t$) of the applied RF pulse:

$$\alpha = \gamma B_1 \Delta t. \tag{2.28}$$

An RF energy pulse required to rotate the net magnetization into the transverse plane is referred to as a 90-degree pulse. If enough energy is supplied, the net vector can be completely flipped over with a 180-degree shift into the opposite direction with respect to the external magnetic field. Once the RF pulse is finished, the net magnetization vector returns to its original equilibrium state through a relaxation process. The previously absorbed energy is emitted at the same precession frequency and can be detected as an electrical signal by receiving coils perpendicular to the $z$-axis. The transient response magnetic resonance (MR) signal of a spin system after an RF pulse excitation is referred to as the free induction decay (FID) signal. A receiver coil perpendicular to the $z$-axis detects the electrical signal. The induced voltage can be derived by applying the principle of reciprocity and Faraday's law[5] as given in equations 2.29 and 2.30:

---

5   Faraday's law of induction states that a time-varying magnetic flux through a conducting loop induces in the coil an electromagnetic force (or voltage) that is equal to the rate at which the magnetic flux through the coil changes.

$$\Phi_{\mathrm{m}} = \int_{object} \vec{B}(\vec{r}) \cdot \vec{M}(\vec{r}) \, d\vec{r}, \qquad (2.29)$$

$$V(t) = -\frac{\partial \Phi_m}{\partial t} = -\frac{\partial}{\partial t} \int_{object} \vec{B}(\vec{r}) \cdot \vec{M}(\vec{r},t) \, d\vec{r} \qquad (2.30)$$

$\vec{B}$ is the magnetic field generated by the coil at location $\vec{r}$ and $\Phi_m$ is the magnetic flux through the coil. As the $M_z$ component varies much more slowly than the $M_{xy}$ component, it can be neglected, and the resulting expression is given as

$$V(t) \approx -\int_{object} \vec{B}_{xy} \cdot \frac{d}{dt}\left[\vec{M}_{xy}(r,t)\right] d\vec{r} . \qquad (2.31)$$

### 2.2.4.2. Magnetic Relaxation

Relaxation expresses the recovery toward equilibrium of nuclear dipoles that have been perturbed by RF excitations. The time-dependent behavior of the net magnetization vector $\vec{M}$ in the presence of an applied magnetic field $\vec{B}$ is described by Bloch's equation:

$$\frac{d\vec{M}}{dt} = \gamma \, \vec{M} \times \vec{B} - \frac{M_x \hat{i} + M_y \hat{j}}{T_2} - \frac{\left(M_z - M_0\right)\hat{k}}{T_1} , \qquad (2.32)$$

where $M_0$ is the equilibrium value for $M_z$ in the presence of $\vec{B}_0$ only. The vectors $\hat{i}, \hat{j}$, and $\hat{k}$ are the unit vectors along the Cartesian directions $x$, $y$, and $z$, respectively. $T_1$ and $T_2$ are the longitudinal and transverse relaxation times, respectively. They are relaxation parameters that are unique to each tissue.

Equation 2.32 can be decomposed into the three spatial coordinates as shown in equation 2.33:

$$\begin{pmatrix} \dfrac{dM_x}{dt} \\[2ex] \dfrac{dM_y}{dt} \\[2ex] \dfrac{dM_z}{dt} \end{pmatrix} = \begin{pmatrix} \gamma \, M_y B_0 - \dfrac{M_x}{T_2} \\[2ex] -\gamma \, M_x B_0 - \dfrac{M_y}{T_2} \\[2ex] \dfrac{M_0 - M_z}{T_1} \end{pmatrix} . \qquad (2.33)$$

The solutions of Bloch's equation are then given as

$$\left. \begin{array}{l} M_x(t) = M_0 e^{\frac{-t}{T_2}} \cos(\gamma B_0 t) \\[3ex] M_y(t) = -M_0 e^{\frac{-t}{T_2}} \sin(\gamma B_0 t) \end{array} \right\} M_{xy}(t) = \sqrt{M_x^2 + M_y^2} = M_0 e^{\frac{-t}{T_2}} \quad (2.34)$$

$$M_z(t) = M_0 \left( 1 - e^{\frac{-t}{T_1}} \right) \qquad (2.35)$$

Equations 2.34 and 2.35 represent the time-dependent behavior of the magnetization vector in the transverse and in the longitudinal plane, respectively.

An important parameter in MRI is the spin density $\rho$. The spin density is proportional to the effective number of hydrogen nuclei per unit volume contributing to the signal from each voxel (3D pixel) of the object. Therefore $M_0$ in equations 2.34 and 2.35 is proportional to $\rho$, which can be used together with $T_1$ and $T_2$ to distinguish different tissue types. A typical value for the blood $T_1$ at $1.5\,T$ is 1350 ms, while the blood $T_2$ varies between 50 and 200 ms, depending on the hematocrit (Bottomley et al., 1984; Hornak, 1996).

### 2.2.4.2.1. $T_1$ Relaxation

Longitudinal or spin-lattice relaxation time $T_1$ refers to the time that the magnetization takes to return to its equilibrium in the longitudinal direction of the external magnetic field after being flipped by an RF pulse excitation. The energy that is absorbed by the magnetic spin from the RF pulse is transferred back to the environment or lattice during the relaxation process. At equilibrium, the net magnetization vector lies along the direction of the external magnetic field and is referred to as the equilibrium magnetization $M_0$. In this configuration, the longitudinal component of magnetization $M_z$ equals $M_0$ and there is no transverse magnetization. However, when the energy transferred by the RF pulse is sufficient, it is possible to saturate the spin system and make $M_z$ equal to zero. Such an RF pulse is referred to as a 90-degree pulse (Fig. 2.15). The time constant that represents the return of $M_z$ to its equilibrium is the spin lattice relaxation time $T_1$. This relaxation dynamic is given in equation 2.35.

Since there is an exchange of energy between protons and the environment, $T_1$ relaxation times depend on the nature of the surrounding molecules. For instance, the magnetization associated with lipids relaxes faster than that associated with pure water or much larger molecules, such as proteins. Moreover, the magnetic field magnitude has influence on the $T_1$ relaxation time as well. In general, $T_1$ increases with the field magnitude for most tissues.

### 2.2.4.2.2. $T_2$ Relaxation

The second relaxivity property of tissue is the transverse or spin-spin relaxation, referred to as $T_2$ relaxation. In this relaxation process the magnetic moments of the spins turn out of phase as a result of their mutual interaction. Each spin experiences a slightly different magnetic field and rotates at its

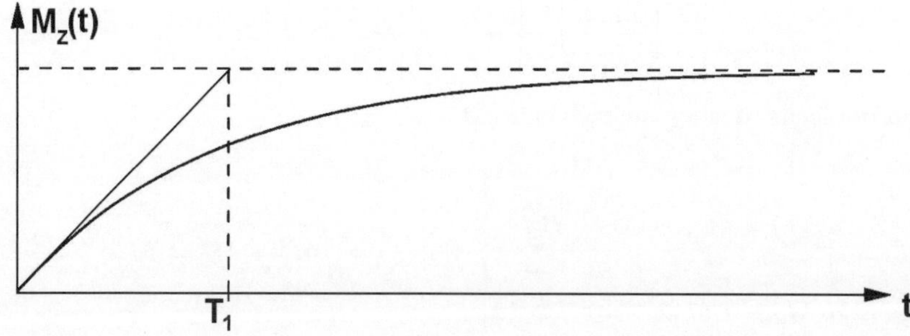


**Figure 2.15.** Longitudinal relaxation curve after applying a 90-degree pulse. The recovery time constant is equal to $T_1$.

own Larmor frequency, leading to loss of spin phase coherence (dephasing). As a result, the transverse magnetization $M_{xy}$ decays and therefore returns to its equilibrium state. Longer elapsed times lead to larger phase difference and smaller transverse magnetization, as shown in Figure 2.16. The time constant that describes this process is the relaxation time $T_2$. The transverse magnetization after an RF excitation pulse is described by equation 2.34.

Unlike the $T_1$ relaxation, no energy is transferred from the nuclei to the environment during the $T_2$ relaxation. Each tissue has a characteristic $T_2$ relaxation time that is not directly dependent on the magnetic field magnitude and is referred to as the decay of the transverse magnetization. However, the actual rate of signal decay is more rapid than the predicted decay (Fig. 2.17). The observed transverse relaxation time, referred to as $T_2{}^*$, is affected by local magnetic field inhomogeneities that cause the precessional rates of the individual spins to differ from each other and dephase.

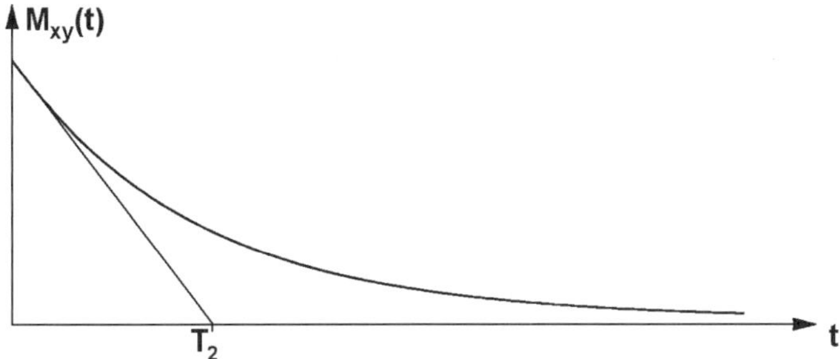


**Figure 2.16.** Transversal relaxation curve after applying a 90-degree pulse. The decay time constant is equal to $T_2$.

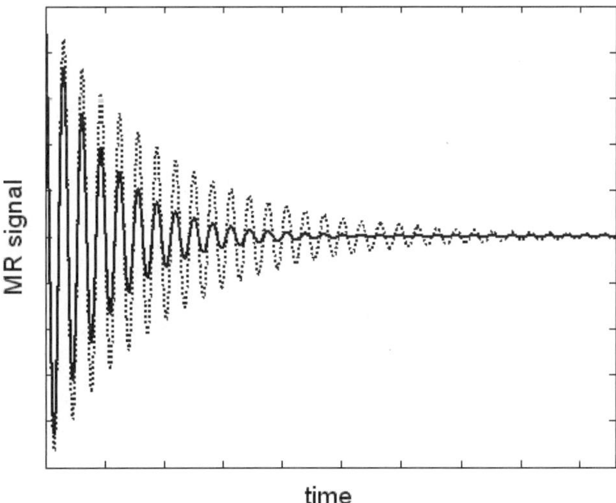


**Figure 2.17.** The actual signal decay with a $T_2{}^*$ relaxation time (solid line) is faster than that predicted according to the $T_2$ relaxation time (dotted line).

### 2.2.4.3. Spatial Localization

The measured MR signal does not contain localization information. Therefore, in order to reconstruct an image, it is necessary to perform a spatial encoding. Since the precession frequency is proportional to the magnetic field magnitude, if an additional magnetic field gradient $\vec{G}$ is superimposed on the static external magnetic field, the spatial locations within the object can be encoded with localized precession frequencies.[6]

The expression of the MR signal $S(t)$ detected by the receiving coil from an object with spin density $\rho(\vec{r})$ can therefore be derived from equations 2.31 and 2.34 as

$$S(t) \approx \int_{object} \frac{d}{dt} M_0(\vec{r}) e^{\frac{-t}{T_2}} e^{-i\gamma(B_0 + \vec{G}\cdot\vec{r})t} \, d\vec{r} \propto \int_{object} \frac{d}{dt}\rho(\vec{r}) \, e^{\frac{-t}{T_2}} e^{-i\gamma(B_0 + \vec{G}\cdot\vec{r})t} \, d\vec{r} \approx$$

$$\approx e^{-i\frac{\pi}{2}}\gamma B_0 \int_{object} \rho(\vec{r}) \, e^{\frac{-t}{T_2}} e^{-i\gamma(B_0 + \vec{G}\cdot\vec{r})t} d\vec{r}. \tag{2.36}$$

The exponential $\gamma\left(B_0 + \vec{G}\cdot\vec{r}\right)$ represents the precession angular frequency at the location $\vec{r}$. The derivative can be approximated by a coefficient (constant) $e^{-i\frac{\pi}{2}}\gamma B_0$ of the integral, as $\vec{G}\cdot\vec{r}$ and $(-T_2)^{-1}$ are negligible. After demodulation (i.e., removal of the carrier signal $e^{-i\gamma B_0 t}$ by a mixer), and neglecting the relaxation effect (i.e., removing the $e^{\frac{-t}{T_2}}$ factor), equation 2.36 can be rewritten as

$$S(t) \propto \int_{object} \rho(\vec{r}) \, e^{-i\gamma(\vec{G}\cdot\vec{r})t} \, d\vec{r}. \tag{2.37}$$

With the substitution

$$\vec{k} = \frac{\gamma t \vec{G}}{2\pi} \tag{2.38}$$

it becomes clear that the received signal in the so-called k-space is the Fourier transform of the spin density in the imaged volume. In fact,

$$S(\vec{k}) = \int_{object} \rho(\vec{r}) e^{-i2\pi\vec{k}\cdot\vec{r}} \, d\vec{r}. \tag{2.39}$$

Therefore an image can be reconstructed by a reverse Fourier transform. The difficulty and the distinguishing feature of several MRI methods is in the adopted strategy of filling the k-space by means of RF or gradient pulses. Typically a slice is selected by the gradient along the $z$-axis and the remainder of the pulse sequence is used to fill the two-dimensional (2D) k-space corresponding to the selected slice.

Depending on the adopted pulse sequence, the reconstructed image can be more sensitive to variations of $T_1$, $T_2$, or $\rho$. A discussion of the different pulse sequences is beyond the scope of this chapter, the goal of which is to provide the physical principles on which MRI is based in order for the

---

6   A magnetic field gradient is a magnetic field that increases linearly in strength along a particular direction ($x$, $y$, or $z$). The strength of a gradient refers to the rate at which its magnetic field changes with distance.

reader to understand how MRI can be used for flow measurement. A recent survey of the available pulse sequences can be found in Bernstein, King, & Zhou (2004).

### 2.2.4.4. Magnetic Resonance Angiography

The reconstruction of an image or volume requires filling the k-space by detecting the spin relaxation signals following an RF pulse. The available methods are mainly based on the assumption of a fixed target tissue where no motion is present. Motion produces artifacts in the reconstructed image. Triggering or gating the image acquisition can minimize common motion artifacts, such as those due to the heart beating. However, these techniques do not improve the artifacts introduced by the presence of flow. When flow is present, mainly due to blood flow in vessels, the spins move across different areas and receive different pulse sequences with respect to fixed tissue. This phenomenon produces artifacts in the image, which can also be exploited for a qualitative and quantitative analysis of flow.

A qualitative approach for the visualization of blood flow consists of the use of inflow artifacts by so-called time-of-flight imaging techniques. As a consequence of flow, unsaturated spins, which have not received any RF pulse, enter the field of view of the scanner during the RF pulse sequence. The total magnetization of these spins is parallel to the field $\vec{B}_0$, while the spins of tissue are flipped by an angle related to the RF pulse and their relaxation time. As a result, the spins related to unsaturated blood entering the field of view provide an MR signal that is much stronger than that provided by the fixed structures (e.g., tissue) in the image. By exploiting this effect, an image can be built such that all vessels are enhanced due to the presence of flow (Kouwenhoven et al., 1994; Pope & Yao, 1993; Vlaardingerbroek & den Boer, 2003). Moreover, the use of specific presaturation protocols allows the selective visualization of veins or arteries (Kouwenhoven et al., 1994).

Typically the MR slices are positioned perpendicular to the flow. The flow-related enhancement is therefore dependent on the blood velocity, the slice thickness $d$, and the pulse repetition time (TR; Kouwenhoven et al., 1994; Pope & Yao, 1993). In general, the minimal blood velocity $v_{min}$ for complete and homogeneous flow visualization is

$$v_{min} \geq \frac{d}{TR}. \tag{2.40}$$

Figure 2.18 shows an example of inflow MRA. Other time-of-flight techniques for flow visualization and analysis make use of presaturating pulses in orthogonal sets of planes. These tagging prepulses leave a label in the spins. If an imaging pulse sequence is applied after grid tagging, it is possible to detect the deformation of the grid and thus derive the velocity of the spins. This technique, also used in cardiac applications for myocardial strain analysis, allows the visualizing and quantifying complex flow patterns. However, limits in the tagging time, which must be short with respect to both $T_1$ and the displacement time of flowing spins, limit the suitability of this technique to applications in the presence of low flow (Pope & Yao, 1993). Figure 2.19 shows an example of a tagged image of the heart.

Another inflow-related effect is the phase accumulation of spins moving across different magnetic fields (Kouwenhoven et al., 1994; Pope & Yao, 1993; Vlaardingerbroek & den Boer, 2003). This effect can be used for a quantitative measurement of flow. This MRA modality is referred to as phase contrast angiography. Consider the only gradient $G_x(t)$ in the $x$ direction: according to equation 2.37, the phase accumulated during a gradient pulse of time duration $T$ by a spin moving along the $x$ direction with a constant velocity $v$ is given as

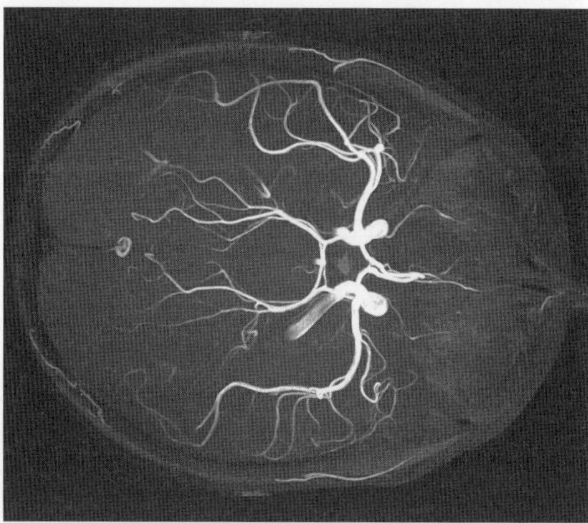

**Figure 2.18.** Example of a brain MRA at 3*T*. Courtesy of the Department of Radiology, Catharina Hospital, Eindhoven, The Netherlands.

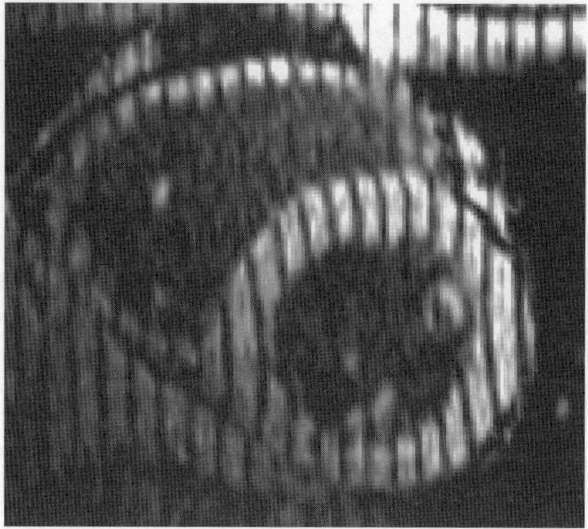

**Figure 2.19.** MR short-axis view of the heart. The vertical tagging lines are clearly visible. Courtesy of the Department of Radiology, Catharina Hospital, Eindhoven, The Netherlands.

$$\varphi = \gamma \int_0^T x(t) \cdot G_x(t) \ dt = \gamma \int_0^T \left( x_0 + v \cdot t \right) \cdot G_x(t) \ dt, \qquad (2.41)$$

where $x_0$ is the initial position of the spin. For a bipolar gradient pulse as given in Figure 2.20, the accumulated phase $\varphi$ is a linear function of the velocity $v$. Different gradient shapes are also possible as long as the time integral of $G_x(t)$ is zero. Based on this principle, MRA is a very useful and accurate method for velocity quantification. Attention must be paid to the MR settings in order to limit the phase so that $-\pi < \Phi \leq \pi$; beyond these limits phase warping and aliasing occur (Pope & Yao, 1993). It is also possible to design different gradient pulses that are insensitive to flow, that is, the first statistical moment of the gradient $G_x(t)$ reported in equation 2.41 is equal to zero. An example of such a gradient pulse is shown in Figure 2.20. When an image that is generated by a flow-insensitive acquisition is subtracted from a velocity-sensitive image, only the signal due to velocity is left. The measurement of flow can then be obtained by integrating the velocity over the surface of the vessel section (Franck et al., 2005; Hoogeveen, Bakker, & Viergever, 1997; Kouwenhoven et al., 1994; Mohiaddin & Pennell, 1998; Pope & Yao, 1993). Eventually accurate measurements of CO can also be obtained (Irarrázaval et al., 1999; Szolar, Sakuma, & Higgins, 1996).

### 2.2.4.5. MRI Hardware

An MRI scanner consists of complex hardware. The stationary external magnetic field $\vec{B}_0$ for MR imaging of the human body is provided by a large superconducting magnet with a typical strength of 0.5 to 3 T. Superconducting wires have approximately zero resistance when they are cooled to a temperature close to absolute zero (−273.15°C or 0 K) by submerging them in liquid helium. Generally, three orthogonal gradient coils at room temperature are used to add gradient magnetic fields to $\vec{B}_0$.

During the nuclear excitation phase, an RF coil with electronic circuitry is used to transmit time-varying RF pulses. The same RF coil with computerized programming and switching control is used for receiving the RF emissions during the nuclear relaxation phase. The FID signal is recorded by the RF coil at a selected RF. Computerized control of the electronic circuitry allows programming of the RF coil to transmit and receive specific RF pulses as required by the selected pulse sequence for image reconstruction. Today arrays of receiving coils are often used in order to improve the time resolution for real-time imaging of moving structures by smart parallel imaging methods (see the end of section 2.3.3.2).

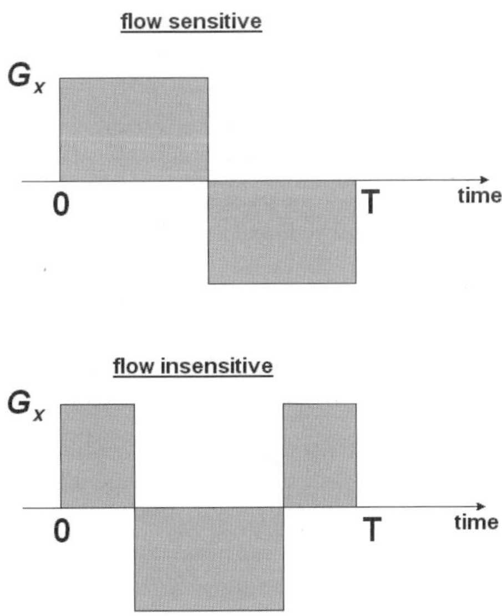


**Figure 2.20.** Examples of flow-sensitive (upper plot) and flow-insensitive (lower plot) gradients.

The RF transmitter section includes a wave synthesizer, RF modulator, RF amplifier, and a coupler that couples the RF signal to the RF coils. The RF receiver section uses the coupler to switch the signal from the RF coil to an assembly of preamplifiers and demodulators. The received FID signal is then sent to an A/D converter for recording the data in digital format.

Components that are sensitive to electromagnetic fields, such as computers or magnetic storage media, must be kept at a safe distance from the main magnet. As a result, the MRI acquisition scanner must be surrounded by a Faraday cage (usually made of copper) to isolate the electric fields from the surrounding departments and devices in the hospital. This limitation is of primary importance in some clinical applications, such as diagnostics in the intensive care unit or operating rooms.

## 2.2.5. THE ELECTROMAGNETIC FLOWMETER

The electromagnetic flowmeter is based on Faraday's law of induction (Webster, 1997, 1999). If a conductor of length $L$ moves with velocity $\vec{v}$ perpendicular to a magnetic field $\vec{B}$, then the inducted electromotive force (EMF) across the ends of the conductor is given by

$$\text{EMF} = \int_L \vec{v} \times \vec{B} \cdot dl = BLv. \qquad (2.42)$$

The electromagnetic flowmeter generates an EMF that depends on the movement of blood, which is a conductor with a conductance similar to that of saline. A schematic representation of the working principle of an electromagnetic flowmeter is depicted in Figure 2.21, which shows a section of a blood vessel with two applied electrodes. The magnetic field $\vec{B}$, the direction of movement of the electrical conductor (blood velocity $\vec{v}$), and the line $L$ between the electrodes (vessel diameter) must all be perpendicular to each other so that equation 2.42 is still valid. There is a linear relationship between the induced EMF and the blood velocity. When $L$ is known, the relation between the blood flow $\Phi = v\pi L^2/4$ and the inducted EMF is derived from equation 2.42 as

$$\Phi = \text{EMF} \cdot \left(\frac{\pi L}{4B}\right). \qquad (2.43)$$

If the ends of the conductor are connected to an external circuit, the induced EMF causes a current of intensity $I_c$ that can be processed (e.g., by a galvanometer) for the assessment of flow. The resistance of the moving conductor (the blood along the line $L$) can be represented by an internal resistance $R$, giving a terminal voltage $V = (\text{EMF}) - RI_c$. Thus the system has to be calibrated with the estimated $R$. As shown in equation 2.42, the quantity that is directly measured is the average velocity $v$ of the blood (an average along the line $L$ of the longitudinal component). The average value[7] is used because the blood velocity along the section of a vessel in the case of laminar flow is not constant, but shows a parabolic profile. To be able to measure the flow from equation 2.43, an estimate of the vessel section's length $L$ must be available.

Measurement errors may occur with the use of small electrodes, resulting in an inhomogeneous sensitivity of the system to blood velocities at different distances from the electrodes. The system is more sensitive to velocities near the electrodes, which may provide an average flow underestimation in the case of laminar parabolic flow. This problem can be overcome by adding sophisticated signal

---

7   A spatial average, not a temporal average.

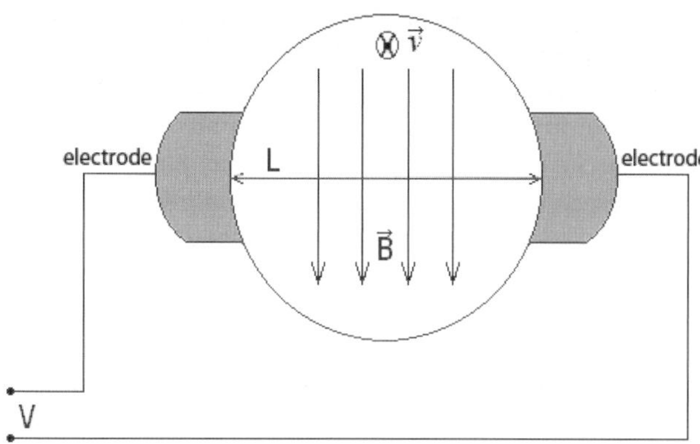


**Figure 2.21.** Scheme (section view) of a magnetic flowmeter surrounding the walls of a blood vessel. Two electrodes are placed on the opposite sides of a vessel with a distance *L* from each other. A magnetic field $\vec{B}$, perpendicular to the blood velocity $\vec{v}$, is applied for the flow measurement.

analysis to the electromagnetic flowmeter. Some methods use the weight function method, which involves a numerical integration of products between the bidimensional distribution of the magnetic density vector $\vec{B}$, a weight function, and the velocity profile function (Lim & Chung, 1998). Alternative techniques make use of the finite volume method (Lim & Chung, 1998). Another source of inaccuracy that should be considered is the dependency of the blood conductance on the hematocrit (Schwan, 1983).

The flowmeter design just discussed is referred to as a DC flowmeter, since the magnetic field $\vec{B}$ is constant. This design results in a series of errors mainly recognized as polarization of the electrodes (random voltage drift), low SNR due to the typical $1/f$ noise of the amplifier, and appearance of the harmonic components of the electrocardiographic signal, very similar to the harmonic components of flow near the heart (pulsatile flow).

Drift and polarization problems are mostly combated by the use of an alternating magnetic field (about 400 Hz), but this introduces a new source of noise. In fact, since EMF $= -\partial \Phi_m / \partial t$, where $\Phi_m$ is the magnetic flux through the circuit, the alternating magnetic field generates by induction an alternating EMF in the circuit of the electrodes. A common solution to this problem is the use of a quadrature filter in order to remove the undesired components. Similar to the strategy adopted for ultrasonic Doppler measurements, this type of design also allows determination of the flow direction. The use of higher frequencies also permits improvement of the time resolution of the measurement system, making it more suitable for pulsatile flow measurements (e.g., in the aorta).

In practice the system has two different applications. The first one, referred to as a perivascular probe, makes use of a toroidal structure for the transducer and has to be applied by surgery around the blood vessel, which is clinically undesirable. The second one, referred to as an intravascular probe, makes use of a catheter-tip probe. The probe can be inserted, for instance, through the femoral artery up to the ascending aorta in order to measure the instantaneous CO. Current technology allows constructing probes that are sufficiently small to be inserted through vessels 2 mm in diameter.

In in vitro measurements, the accuracy of the measurement can reach 0.25% (Webster, 1999), but in clinical (in vivo) applications it is often difficult to obtain correct measurements because the perpendicularities of all the vectors as well as estimation of the vessel diameter are influenced by several factors that are partly unknown and thus sources of error. In particular, when using the catheter-tip probe the transducer must be perfectly centered in the middle of the vessel.

Because of the poor accuracy and complexity of in-body measurements, the electromagnetic flowmeter is mostly used for measurements outside the body, where the accuracy of the flow measurement is the same as for in vitro applications. These applications mainly involve flow measurement in heart–lung machines, which are used during cardiac surgery to temporarily take over the functions of the heart and the lungs (i.e., the blood pumping and oxygenation [gas exchange]). Another possibility is the surgical placement of a shunt so that the blood flow takes a detour outside the body and is measured by an electromagnetic flowmeter. This method provides complete control of the factors that influence the measurement, such as vessel size and vector alignment.

## 2.2.6. PLETHYSMOGRAPHY

Plethysmography includes all those methods that measure the volume changes of an organ or a part of the body. Volume changes are related to the inflow and outflow of fluids or gasses, thus these methods can also be suitable for the evaluation of flow. The main applications relate to the assessment of cardiac stroke volume (SV), CO, and peripheral blood flow. These methods are suitable for the assessment of blood flows in major blood vessels, as described in this section, but they are also suitable for the assessment of peripheral flow (e.g., tissue and microcirculation perfusion).

The change of blood volume can be detected by several plethysmographic techniques. In general, these can be divided into three major groups of techniques:

- bioimpedance plethysmography
- strain-gauge plethysmography
- photoelectric plethysmography

### 2.2.6.1. Bioimpedance Plethysmography

The assumptions behind bioimpedance plethysmography are (1) that a body compartment consists of (a) tissues and (b) blood; and (2) that changes in the compartment's volume are due only to changes in the volume of blood, that is, blood flow.

Bioimpedance plethysmography is mainly used for cardiac monitoring (Malmivuo & Plonsey, 1995; Nyboer, 1970; Webster, 1999) and has the advantage of providing continuous CO measurement at no risk to the patient. A small current of 0.5 mA to 4 mA at a frequency of 50 kHz to 100 kHz is passed through the thorax from a pair of electrodes while another pair of sensing electrodes is used to measure the changes in impedance within the thorax using a high-impedance galvanometer. In practice, the thoracic impedance is measured by means of four band electrodes, as shown in Figure 2.22. In the physical arrangement of the external pair (current generator), one electrode is placed around the abdomen and the other around the upper part of the neck. For the internal electrode pair, one electrode is placed around the thorax at the level of the joint between the xiphoid and the sternum, and the other is placed around the lower part of the neck. More recently, band electrodes have sometimes been replaced by normal contact electrodes.

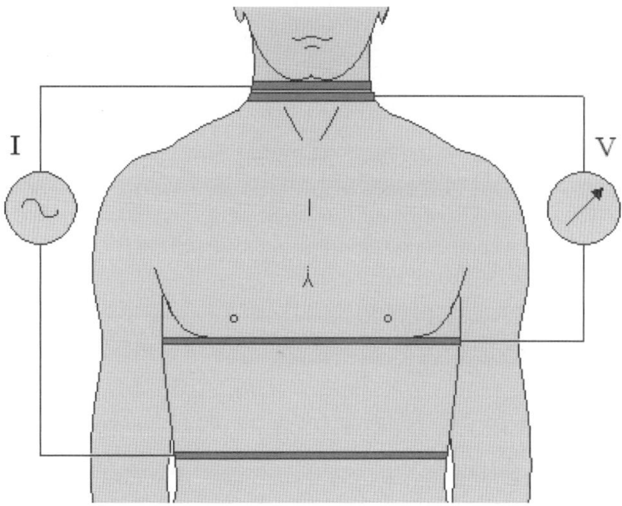


**Figure 2.22.** Electrode positioning during thoracic plethysmography.

A simplified model that is widely used to characterize thorax impedance is a double cylinder consisting of tissue and blood compartments, as shown in Figure 2.23 (Nyboer, 1970). As a consequence, the total thorax impedance $Z$ is given by the parallel connection of blood and tissue impedances $Z_b$ and $Z_t$. To investigate changes in $Z$, this may be differentiated with respect to $Z_b$, the resulting differential equation being

$$\frac{dZ}{dZ_b} = \frac{d}{dZ_b}\left(\frac{Z_t Z_b}{Z_b + Z_t}\right) = \left(\frac{Z}{Z_b}\right)^2 . \tag{2.44}$$

A biological impedance, especially skin impedance, is in general represented by a complex number. However, the blood impedance is mainly resistive and thus $Z_b$ can be represented by a real number. From the model in Figure 2.23, $Z_b = \rho_b L A_b^{-1}$, where $\rho_b$ is the blood resistivity (about 150 $\Omega$ cm), and $A_b$ and $L$ are the cross section and the length of the blood compartment (left cylinder in Fig. 2.23), respectively. By differentiating the blood volume $V_b = LA_b = \rho_b L^2 Z_b^{-1}$ with respect to $Z_b$ and substituting $Z_b$ with $Z$, as given in equation 2.44, the following equation can be derived:

$$dV_b = d(A_b L) = -\left(\frac{\rho_b L^2}{Z^2}\right) dZ. \tag{2.45}$$

For small impedance variations, the value of $Z$ in the denominator can be assumed constant and determined by the minimum impedance during the cardiac cycle $Z_0$, which corresponds to the minimum $V_b$. Equation 2.45 relates blood volume variations to total impedance variations, so that blood volumes can be assessed by means of electrical impedance measurements. Contraction of the ventricles produces a cyclical change in transthoracic impedance of about 0.5%. These changes are exploited by a specific equation, referred to as Kubicek's equation, to assess the stroke volume (SV; Kubicek

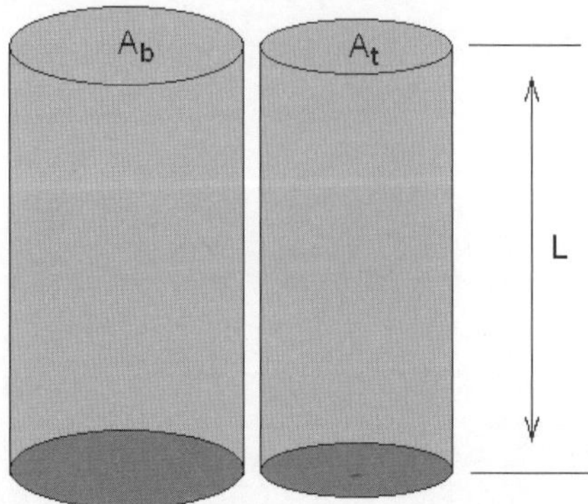



**Figure 2.23.** Cylindrical model for thorax tissue and blood impedance. $A_t$ and $A_b$ are the tissue and blood sections. $L$ is the cylinder length.

et al., 1966). Some assumptions are made concerning the relationship between SV and net change in the thorax blood volume. The impedance is assumed to mainly depend on the blood volume in the lungs. Moreover, it is assumed that no blood leaves the lungs during systole. As a consequence, the impedance should continuously decrease during systole. If the time derivative $Z'$ of the impedance during systole is estimated, the first-order approximation of the total impedance variation $\Delta Z$ during the ejection time $\tau_e$ is given as $\Delta Z = Z'\tau_e$. Usually the minimum value of the derivative is used.[8] Combining this result with equation 2.45, the SV can be derived as

$$SV = -\rho_b \frac{Z'L^2\tau_e}{Z_0^2}. \tag{2.46}$$

Eventually, once the SV is known, the CO can be obtained as the product of SV and the heart rate. The accuracy of this method is limited by several factors (Bronzino, 2000; Deng et al., 2002). First of all, the model in Figure 2.23 is an extreme simplification of the real system. Moreover, the blood impedance depends on several factors, such as the concentration of red blood cells (hematocrit) and their shape and orientation. In addition, the effects of blood flow are still unknown. Respiratory artifacts also affect the measurements.

Although the resistive and reactive components of the impedance are represented by a complex number, the measured total impedance $Z$ is the modulus of the complex impedance only and is a function of the adopted frequency. In some applications an impedance spectrum is determined at a number of different frequencies in order to distinguish between different tissues (Lorenzo et al., 1997). At low frequencies, for instance, the current flows mainly through the extracellular space, while at higher frequencies the current can pass across the cellular membranes, which behave like capacitors, so that the intracellular space is included in the measurement as well. It is worth mentioning that this method has also developed into a technology referred to as electrical impedance imaging. This technique uses

---

8   During ejection the impedance decreases, so that the minimum value of the derivative corresponds to the maximum slope of the impedance curve.

multiple electrodes and permits the construction of internal images of the body that are related to the impedance characteristics of different tissues (Newell, 1996).

### 2.2.6.2. Strain-Gauge Plethysmography

Equation 2.45 can also be used for the assessment of blood flow through body limbs such as arms and legs (Shankar & Webster, 1991). In particular, blood flow through the legs has an important prognostic value in the diagnosis of venous thrombosis.

Often the plethysmographic quantification of blood flow through body limbs is performed by strain gauges. The main application consists of measurement of the total blood flow through the limb, which can be assessed by venous occlusion. This method, shown in Figure 2.24, was first described by Whitney in 1953. An occluding cuff is inflated above venous pressure (about 60 mmHg) in order to block venous outflow while preserving arterial inflow. Simultaneously a strain gauge is used to measure the volume increase between the cuff and limb. The rate of volume increase is the arterial flow. After a few seconds the volume reaches a plateau, the value of which relates to the compliance of the venous system. If the cuff is then suddenly deflated, the volume shows an exponential decay whose time constant is related to the venous flow.

In order to interpret the volume variation that is measured by the strain gauge, a simple monocompartment model can be adopted. Once the veins are blocked, the blood pool experiences an increase of volume $V$ whose dynamics can be described as the inflation of an elastic monocompartment by the following differential equation:

$$\frac{dV}{dt} R_\mathrm{h} = \Delta P - \frac{V}{C_\mathrm{h}},\qquad(2.47)$$

where $\Delta P$ is the initial pressure drop between the arteries and the veins of the limb, and $R_h$ and $C_h$ are, respectively, the resistance and compliance of the hemodynamic system of the limb. By definition, the resistance of a fluid-dynamic system represents the ratio between the pressure drop and flow, while the compliance represents the ratio between the volume and pressure variations (in case of elastic walls). Solving equation 2.47 for initial volume $V = 0$, the volume variation as a function of time is obtained:

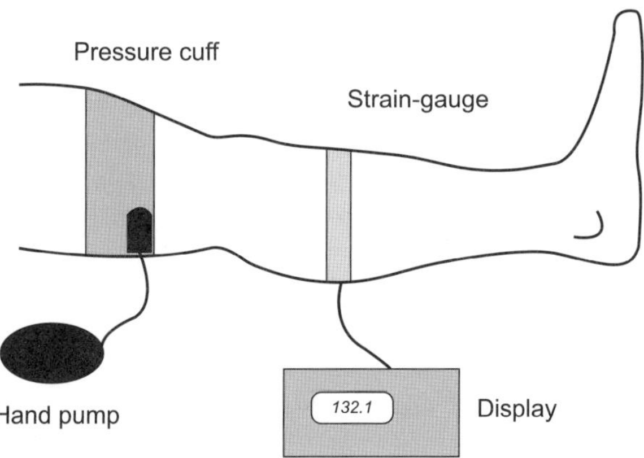


**Figure 2.24.** Clinical application of strain-gauge plethysmography.

$$V(t) = C_b \Delta P\left(1 - e^{-\frac{t}{\tau}}\right), \tag{2.48}$$

where $\tau$ is equal to $R_b C_b$. The time derivative of $V(t)$ in equation 2.48 for $t = 0$ is equal to $\Delta P R_b^{-1}$, which corresponds to the arterial flow. After a sufficiently long time, when no volume variations are observed anymore, the value of the volume increase is equal to $\Delta P C_b$.

When the cuff is suddenly deflated, the system can be modeled by a monocompartment outflow through the veins, since reverse flow is not possible because of the unidirectional valves that are present in the veins. If $P_0$ is the output venous pressure beyond the cuff, the volume dynamics can be represented similarly to equation 2.47:

$$-\frac{dV}{dt} R_b = \frac{V}{C_b} - P_0. \tag{2.49}$$

The solution for initial volume $V_i > P_0 C_b$ is

$$V(t) = \left(V_i - C_b P_0\right) e^{-\frac{t}{\tau}} + C_b P_0. \tag{2.50}$$

Obviously the strain-gauge measurement is relative to the initial condition (volume), so that the baseline $C_b P_0$ is not measured. Once again, $\tau$ is equal to $R_b C_b$ and it has a prognostic value for the diagnosis of venous thrombi, that is, it is larger in the presence of a venous thrombus. In summary, as a result of equations 2.49 and 2.50, the typical curve that is measured by a strain gauge is the combination of two exponentials, as shown in Figure 2.25. In measurements, oscillations due to the pulsatile character of the flow are visible as well.

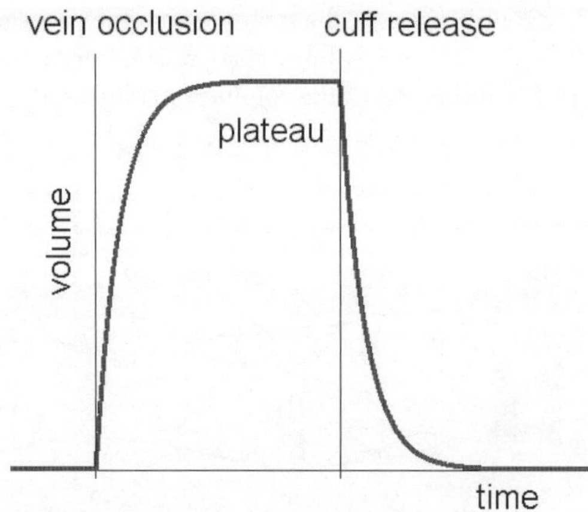


**Figure 2.25.** Strain-gauge plethysmographic volume curve. Venous occlusion induces the volume increase until a plateau is reached for a volume equal to $\Delta P C_b$, where $\Delta P$ is the pressure drop between the arteries and veins and $C_b$ is the vessel compliance. After the occlusion is removed (cuff release), the volume decreases with an exponential behavior until the initial volume (before occlusion) is reached.

A strain gauge is a sensor that is used to measure a deformation. In this application it is placed around the limb to measure its increase in circumference, which is related to the volume increase. Typically a strain gauge is a conductor whose electrical resistance varies depending on its elongation. In a wire strain gauge, for instance, the wire is composed of a uniform conductor of electric resistivity $\rho$ with length $L$ and cross-sectional area $A$. Its electrical resistance $R$ is a function of its geometry and is given by

$$R = \rho \frac{L}{A}. \tag{2.51}$$

The resistance variation is a combination of changes in length, cross-sectional area, and resistivity of the wire:

$$dR = \frac{\rho}{A} dL - \frac{\rho L}{A^2} dA + \frac{L}{A} d\rho \Rightarrow \frac{dR}{R} = \frac{dL}{L} - \frac{dA}{A} + \frac{d\rho}{\rho}. \tag{2.52}$$

Under the assumptions of linear elasticity theory, the wire radius $r$ is related to the wire length by the Poisson ratio $\upsilon$ as

$$\frac{dr}{r} = -\nu \frac{dL}{L}. \tag{2.53}$$

Combining equations 2.52 and 2.53, the strain-gauge sensitivity factor $S$ is derived:

$$S = \frac{\dfrac{dR}{R}}{\dfrac{dL}{L}} = \left(1 + 2\nu\right) + \left(\frac{\dfrac{d\rho}{\rho}}{\dfrac{dL}{L}}\right). \tag{2.54}$$

The first term in equation 2.54 is dominant in metals, while the second term is dominant in semiconductors. $S$ is known (provided by the vendors), and thus the relative elongation of the strain gauge can be derived by measuring $R$. Unfortunately the resistivity of a material depends on temperature, especially in semiconductors. Usually four strain gauges are combined together in a Wheatstone bridge configuration in order to increase the gain of the system and reduce measurement sensitivity to temperature variations (Webster, 1997).

The same measurement can be realized with any sensor that is able to measure displacement or elongation. A common solution used to be mercury strain gauges (not allowed anymore), whose measurement principle is based on the resistance variations in deformation of a flexible tube filled with mercury. Another solution is inductive plethysmography, where the displacement or elongation is measured as variations in inductive coupling (Webster, 1997).

A direct method for the measurement of volume variations is air/water plethysmography, where a chamber filled with air or water is fixed around the leg to directly measure volume variations. A cuff is also suitable for this measurement. In air plethysmography, the product of pressure and volume at constant temperature (Boyle's law) allows measuring pressure variations to derive volume variations.

### 2.2.6.3. Photoelectric Plethysmography

Another approach to the measurement of peripheral blood volumes, and therefore perfusion, makes use of the light absorption and reflection properties of blood. This technique is referred to as photoelectric plethysmography and was first introduced by Hertzman in the mid-1930s (Hertzman & Spealman, 1937). Blood absorbs light more than the surrounding tissues, so an increase in blood volume can be detected by a light absorption increase. In general, IR light with a wavelength greater than 700 nm is used. A light emitting diode (LED) or laser made of, for example, galium arsenide (GaAs; also used for CD players) is a suitable light source. The receiver can be a photodiode, a phototransistor, or a photo-resistor (light-dependent resistor). Absorption variations between 1% and 2% are associated with the pulsatile nature of the flow.

Instead of an absorption measurement, referred to as transmission plethysmography, where the transmitter and detector must be placed on opposite sides of a body part, such as a finger, a reflection measurement can be employed. This method is referred to as reflection plethysmography. The reflection is clearly correlated with flow variations, for example, oscillations related to the cardiac cycle. A good explanation has yet to be formulated: the reflection modulation seems to be related to the different orientation of the erythrocytes, but this explanation is still debated (Nijboer, Dorlas, & Mahieu, 1981).

## 2.3. SENSORS FOR FLOW IN TISSUES AND MICROCIRCULATION

The evaluation of blood flow in tissues and microcirculation is complicated by the reduced size of the vessels. In fact, tissue perfusion is performed by the microcirculation and eventually by capillaries whose diameters range from 5 µm to 10 µm. As a consequence, the invasive catheterization approaches that are used for flow measurements in larger vessels are not applicable. The only solution to study and possibly quantify blood flow in the microcirculation relies on imaging methods. However, the sensitivity of imaging methods such as Doppler ultrasound and MRA is often insufficient for an accurate evaluation of tissue perfusion. This is due to the limited velocities (less than 1 mm s$^{-1}$) and volumes of blood as well as to the limited sizes of the capillaries in the microcirculation. As a result, both the resolution and the sensitivity of the imaging systems are inadequate.

A solution to this problem is the use of contrast agents, which are usually introduced into the bloodstream by a peripheral intravenous injection. Unlike the indicator detection methods discussed in section 2.2.2, the detection of contrast agents does not require contact between the indicator and sensor, and can be performed noninvasively by contrast-specific imaging modalities.

The addition of contrast agents increases the SNR and makes the quantification of tissue perfusion more accurate. Several applications are currently in use in clinical practice, ranging from myocardial perfusion for the detection of coronary artery disease (ischemia) to perfusion of tissue for the detection of cancerous masses and brain perfusion for functional imaging.

Perfusion quantification (or semiquantification) is performed using several techniques. The type of contrast is obviously dependent on the adopted imaging technique. Some contrast imaging techniques for perfusion analysis are already well established and are discussed in this section. In particular, section 2.3.1 discusses nuclear imaging, section 2.3.2 discusses contrast echography, section 2.3.3 discusses contrast MRI, and section 2.3.4 discusses functional MRI (fMRI). Other emerging methods for tissue perfusion (e.g., based on light transmission or reflection) are very promising and interesting (Colak et al., 1999). However, they are still in their infancy and are not discussed in this chapter.

One important clinical procedure to visualize perfusion (e.g., in the myocardium) is not treated here. This is X-ray angiography, where an opaque contrast agent that absorbs X-rays is used to visualize the arteries and detect the presence of a stenosis or aneurism (Baim & Grossman, 2000). The agent is injected by catheterization, typically through the femoral artery, and consists of iodine-based compounds. Inorganic iodine, in fact, is toxic, so ratio 1.5 ionic compounds with sodium and a low concentration of calcium disodium ethylene diamine tetra-acetate (i.e., chelated with ethylene diamine tetra-acetic acid) are typically used in the traditional high-osmolarity ionic contrast media (HOCM). Ratio 3 or low-osmolarity ionic and nonionic contrast media (LOCM), which reduce hypertonicity side effects, were introduced in the late 1980s. However, LOCM has not yet been completely substituted for HOCM because of the cost, which is almost three times higher than that of HOCM. The reason why X-ray angiography is only briefly mentioned in this chapter relates to the lack of real quantification by this application, which is extensively used for visualization.

## 2.3.1. NUCLEAR SCINTIGRAPHY

Nuclear scintigraphic methods are based on the injection of radionuclides, often referred to as radiopharmaceuticals, in the bloodstream. Radionuclides are radioisotopes whose radioactive decay leads to the emission of $\alpha$- and $\beta$-particles as well as gamma and X-radiation. As a result, these contrast media are suitable for detection using sensors that measure radioactivity.

The measurement system consists of a scintillation camera that is usually referred to as a gamma camera. The gamma camera is a photon counter that can count (Mahan & Myers, 1987) particles with a minimal photon energy of about 50 keV. It consists of a scintillating thallium-activated sodium iodide crystal that covers a matrix of photomultiplier tubes. Only gamma and X-radiation can be detected with detectors that are outside the body. The gamma camera was first introduced by Hal Anger in the late 1950s (Anger, 1964) and was based on the findings of the physicist Robert Hofstadter (Nobel Prize in 1961) on scintillator crystals.

The crystal receives high-frequency radiation and the energy levels of its electrons change. Once a minimal energy state is again reached, the crystal emits a fluorescent light pulse that is detected by photomultiplier tubes. The number of photon flashes is then counted and used to construct an image whose local intensity is related to the number of counts at that location, and therefore the local radionuclide concentration. A filter is typically applied in order to count only those pulses whose energy matches the expected energy from the radionuclide gamma ray. Eventually the number of selected counts shows a linear relationship with the radionuclide concentration. This is guaranteed by a dose calibrator that must be tested daily.

A tungsten collimator is usually adopted in order to increase the spatial resolution of the imaging system. However, the resolution of a gamma camera is on the order of 0.5 cm. This is almost a factor ten worse than the resolution of other imaging systems such as MRI or echography.

Emission tomography systems are divided into two main groups, depending on the type of radiation that is emitted by the adopted radiopharmaceuticals: single photon emission computed tomography (SPECT) and positron emission tomography (PET). Here a short overview of these techniques is presented, mainly oriented toward quantification applications. A more detailed description of scintigraphic technology and measurements can be found in Ell and Gambhir (2004) and Mettler and Guiberteau (2006).

Single photon emission computed tomography systems make use of single photon gamma emitters such as $^{99m}$Tc, $^{131}$I, $^{123}$I, $^{67}$Ga, and $^{201}$Tl. They are generally designed to collect data from different angles (projections) by rotating the gamma camera. The acquired projections are then postprocessed to reconstruct a volume. The reconstruction requires a mathematical back-projection operation that can be viewed as the inverse of a radon transform. More information can be found in Dhawan (2003).

Typical SPECT applications involve the analysis of perfusion in the myocardium and brain. Myocardial perfusion testing is usually performed by a stress test protocol (see also section 2.3.2.3), with images taken before and after inducing stress in the patient. Stress is induced either by exercise or by administration of vasodilators such as adenosine or dipyridamole, which increase the level of perfusion. The time resolution of a SPECT system is very low. Typical imaging times might be 3 s per image for the first 40 s, followed by a lower time resolution period of about 2 minutes at six or fewer frames per minute (Bacharach, Libutti, & Carrasquillo, 2000).

Brain perfusion is important in the analysis of the cortex following a specific external stimulus. The signal intensity is related to the level of perfusion so that functional studies and diagnosis of diseases such as dementia or Alzheimer can be performed (Donnemiller et al., 1997).

In general, myocardial perfusion studies are more complicated than brain perfusion studies. This is because the myocardium, which is about 1 cm thick, moves more rapidly than SPECT imaging, with its low time resolution, can follow. Because of the limited resolution of SPECT both in time and space, the number of counts that should relate only to the myocardium's radionuclide concentration also includes counts that come from the ventricular cavity, which reduces the accuracy of the method.

Perfusion studies can also make use of a bolus injection. This resembles MRI (see section 2.3.3.2), where an input IDC is measured in the feeding artery and an output IDC or washout curve is measured in the region where the perfusion is to be analyzed. A deconvolution technique is then used for the identification of the dilution system between the input and output measurement regions (Jansson, 1997). A monocompartment model, such as that given in equation 2.3, is typically adopted to describe the system, and the flow is therefore related to the time constant $\tau$.

A PET system detects annihilation radiation from positron emitters such as $^{11}C$, $^{13}N$, $^{15}O$, $^{18}F$, and $^{68}Ga$. It consists of two or more opposed detectors that permit detection of the two 511 keV gamma photons that are emitted simultaneously in opposite directions by the annihilation process. Thus the line that intercepts the emission point can be determined.

The most advanced radionuclide technique for dynamic image analysis is multigate imaging, also referred to as a ventriculogram, where the gamma camera takes images triggered by the electrocardiographic signal.

Because they emit radiation, radionuclides must be used with caution, especially in women who are pregnant or breast-feeding.


## 2.3.2. CONTRAST ULTRASOUND

Flow in tissues and in the microcirculation can, in principle, be analyzed by an ultrasound Doppler technique (see section 2.2.3). However, the system resolution, which is on the order of 1 mm, and the SNR are not sufficient. Moreover, alignment problems (i.e., the estimation of $\alpha$ in equation 2.21) make quantification impossible. Therefore a different approach is taken that involves the addition of ultrasonic scatterers in the bloodstream. As a result, visualization of perfusion becomes possible even when the system resolution is not sufficient. These ultrasonic scatterers are microbubbles that can be injected into the bloodstream and easily visualized by an ultrasound transducer. In fact, when these microbubbles pass through an ultrasonic field, they oscillate and reirradiate (scatter) a large part of the received energy. This section provides a short overview of ultrasound contrast agents (section 2.3.2.1), visualization strategies (section 2.3.2.2), and applications for quantification of tissue perfusion (section 2.3.2.3).

### 2.3.2.1. Ultrasound Contrast Agents

An ultrasound contrast agent (UCA) is a solution of microbubbles with diameters ranging from less than 1 μm to about 20 μm (Becher & Burns, 2000; Feinstein, 2004). Their size is comparable to that of red blood cells (6–8 μm) and thus they can pass through the capillaries and microcirculation. Today commercial agents are made of a gas bubble encapsulated in a stabilizing shell. UCAs can therefore be distinguished by their shell and gas properties. The shell can be made of phospholipids, liposomes, albumin, fatty acids, or polymers. The inner gas is characterized by a large-size molecule and low diffusivity. Typical gases include sulfurhexafluoride ($SF_6$), air, and several fluorocarbons such as $C_3F_8$ and $C_4F_{10}$.

Due to the natural oscillations (contraction–expansion) of insonated bubbles, the interaction between contrast agents and ultrasound is a nonlinear process that adds several harmonics to the backscattered ultrasound. The oscillations of a single bubble are commonly characterized by the model developed by Plesset (Plesset, 1949; Plesset & Prosperetti, 1977) to describe the motion of vibrating spheres. Several adjustments to this model have been made to include, for instance, the effects related to the presence of a shell. The derivation of such models is beyond the scope of this chapter. More detailed information can be found in Brennen (1995), Hoff (2001), and Leighton (1994).

As an example, consider the model proposed by Nico de Jong under the assumption of a Newtonian fluid, ideal gas, and fixed shell thickness, whose formulation is given as (de Jong et al., 1992; Frinking & de Jong, 1998)

$$\rho r \ddot{r} + \frac{3}{2}\rho \dot{r}^2 = \left(\frac{2\sigma_t}{r_0} + P_0 - P_v\right)\left[\left(\frac{r_0}{r}\right)^{3k} - 1\right] - S_p\left(\frac{1}{r_0} - \frac{1}{r}\right) - 2\pi f \delta_t \rho r \dot{r} - P(t), \quad (2.55)$$

where $r$ is the bubble radius (assuming a symmetric spherical motion), $\rho$ is the fluid density, $\sigma_t$ is the surface tension coefficient (N m$^{-1}$), $P$ is the pressure, $P_v$ is the vapor pressure, $S_p$ is the shell elasticity parameter (N m$^{-1}$), $f$ is the frequency of the oscillation, and $k$ is the polytropic exponent, which equals 1 for an isothermal transformation and $\gamma$ for an adiabatic transformation ($\gamma = 5/3$ for a noble gas). The index 0 indicates the initial (rest) value. The term $\delta_t$ in equation 2.55 is the total damping factor and is the sum of four contributions: reradiation damping, viscosity damping, thermal damping, and shell friction damping (Hoff, 2001; Leighton, 1994).

As already mentioned, the literature describes several other models of bubble dynamics in an ultrasonic field. Many of them are derived from the Rayleigh–Plesset equation (Church, 1988; Hoff, 1996), but other useful models are also derived from the Herring and Gilmore equations (Flynn, 1975; Gilmore, 1952; Keller & Miksis, 1980; Morgan et al., 2000; Prosperetti, Crum, & Commander, 1988). These models are based on the enthalpy energy of the system and can describe oscillations with compressible (non-Newtonian) fluids. As a result, these models are more suitable for the characterization and prediction of large amplitude oscillations.

The amplitude of the oscillations depends on the pressure of the ultrasonic field. The interaction between ultrasound and UCAs is usually characterized by the mechanical index (MI), which is given as

$$MI = \frac{P_r}{\sqrt{f_0}}, \quad (2.56)$$

where $P_r$ is the peak rarefaction pressure (in MPa) and $f_0$ is the central frequency of the ultrasonic wave (in MHz).

The adopted MI is an important factor in designing proper contrast imaging modes. At low MI (MI < 0.1) microbubbles behave almost linearly and their dynamics can be characterized by a second-order linear system that approximates equation 2.55 for small oscillations. In this case a resonance frequency can be well defined and exploited for optimized contrast detection. At higher MIs, the non-linear behavior of the oscillations is no longer negligible and can be used to distinguish between UCA and tissue. For MIs greater than 0.7, most bubbles collapse, offering another possibility for specific release burst imaging modes (Frinking et al., 2001). The violent bubble collapse, referred to as inertial cavitation, is also associated with a considerable release of energy that can be used for advanced medical treatment (targeted drug and gene delivery; Unger et al., 2004). However, because of the energy levels involved, cavitation can also cause undesired bioeffects (permanent cell damage), especially in the microcirculation (Hwang et al., 2005).

The efficacy of a UCA depends on its echogenicity, and therefore on its ability to be readily detected by an ultrasound transducer. This characteristic is defined by the backscatter coefficient, which is the scattering cross section ($cm^2$) per unit volume ($cm^3$) and per scattering angle (sr). The scattering cross section of a bubble is the ratio of the power scattered in all directions and the incident acoustic intensity (Frinking & de Jong, 1998; Hoff, 2001).

Another important parameter that characterizes the echogenicity and efficacy of UCAs is the attenuation coefficient, which represents the loss of acoustic pressure along the distance that the ultrasound beam travels through the contrast dispersion. It is mainly related to the scattering of acoustic energy in multiple directions, and the viscous, thermal, and friction damping, already included in the damping factor $\delta_t$ in equation 2.55. An exponential attenuation of the intensity $I$ (usually expressed in W m$^{-2}$) of ultrasonic waves is also present when they propagate through tissue (expressed in Neper cm$^{-1}$ and MHz$^{-1}$) as

$$I = I_0 e^{-2adf}, \tag{2.57}$$

where $I_0$ is the transmitted intensity, $d$ is the distance from the transducer, $f$ is the central ultrasonic frequency, and $a$ is the attenuation coefficient; the coefficient 2 takes into account the fact that ultrasonic waves cover the distance $d$ two times (incident and reflected wave; Wells, 1977). Thus the attenuation increases with the distance and the central frequency of the pulses. However, the attenuation coefficient through UCAs can be much higher, since it is proportional to the UCA concentration (Hoff, 2001). As a result, the efficacy of a UCA can be viewed as the ratio between backscattering and attenuation (Frinking & de Jong, 1998). In fact, for large UCA concentrations, the attenuation effect can be such that a total shadowing of the structures to be visualized occurs because the ultrasonic waves cannot penetrate through the UCA dispersion. A typical example is the "half moon" effect shown in Figure 2.26. For higher concentrations, the ultrasonic waves cannot penetrate through the UCA dilutions and only the first intercepted layer can be visualized.

### 2.3.2.2. Ultrasound Contrast Imaging

Based on the same technology discussed for color flow Doppler (see section 2.2.3.6), images that are related to the acoustic impedance and scattering properties of the medium can be realized. Short ultrasonic pulses are transmitted and their reflections are received by the same crystals using appropriate time windows. Since the velocity of ultrasound in tissue and blood is known, for each pulse, a line can be reconstructed that represents the acoustic discontinuities and scatterers along the distance traveled by the pulse. The shorter the pulse, the higher the longitudinal resolution, which is typically on the

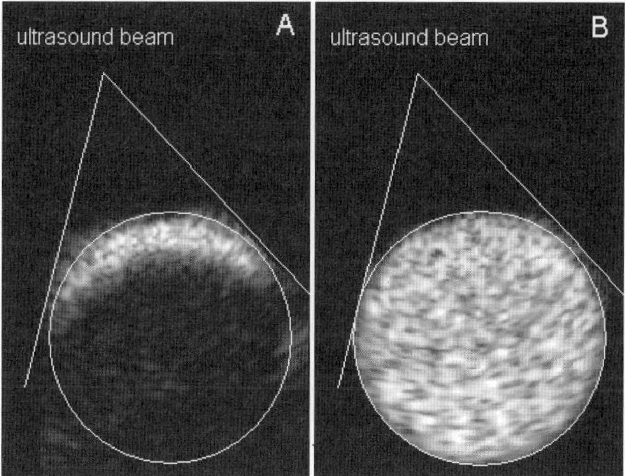


**Figure 2.26.** A cylindrical sample of diluted UCA is insonated through its section by an ultrasound transducer. (A) The "half moon" effect can be seen due to a higher UCA concentration that does not permit ultrasonic wave penetration. At a lower concentration, (B) the ultrasonic waves can penetrate and the full UCA sample ("full moon") can be visualized.

order of 1 mm. Higher frequencies allow shortening the pulse, however, they also cause higher attenuation, as in equation 2.57. Common frequencies range from 2 MHz to 7 MHz. The lateral resolution is regulated by the principle of Huygens, and reaches its maximum at a distance from the crystal equal to $r^2/\lambda$, where $r$ is the crystal radius (assuming a circular surface) and $\lambda$ is the ultrasound wavelength in the tissue.

Any ultrasound modality that aims at realizing an image is referred to as B-mode, where B stands for brightness. Typically an array transducer is used to reconstruct an image from inside the body. A linear array transducer with, for instance, 128 elements (crystals) allows building an image whose lateral size is limited by the probe size. Today, especially for cardiac applications where the probe has to fit between the ribs, phased array probes are used in order to steer the ultrasonic beam by varying the delay between the activation of the elements of the transducer (see Fig. 2.27). Proper delays between the activation of the elements also allow implementing dynamic focusing, so that the user can choose the focal region in the image. Further developments concern the use of a 2D matrix of elements (crystals) so that the ultrasonic beam can be steered in two directions (elevation and lateral plane) to reconstruct volumes from inside the body (3D echography; see Fig. 2.28).

An important application of echography makes use of a miniaturized probe (diameter of about 1 mm) that can be placed on the tip of a catheter and inserted into blood vessels. The employment of this technology is referred to as intravascular ultrasound (IVUS). The IVUS probe can image a plane that is perpendicular to the catheter and the vessel by spanning 360 degrees in a circular fashion (see Fig. 2.29). These transducers are commonly used to visualize plaques (Kakadiaris et al., 2006; Nair et al., 2002), but recently they are also being employed for perfusion assessment in the vessel tissue, and, in particular, to detect the presence of angiogenesis and vasa vasorum, which is related to the formation of atherosclerotic plaques (Goertz et al., 2006). These studies require the infusion of contrast agents.

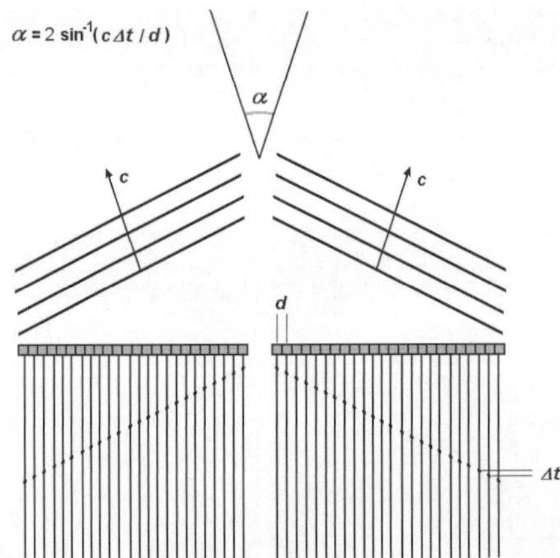



**Figure 2.27.** Beam-forming scheme. A sector of angle $\alpha$ can be spanned, provided that the adjacent crystals, which have a distance $d$ between each other, are excited with a proper delay, $\Delta t$, in order to steer the direction of the generated planar waves. The angle $\alpha$ depends also on the ultrasound velocity $c$.

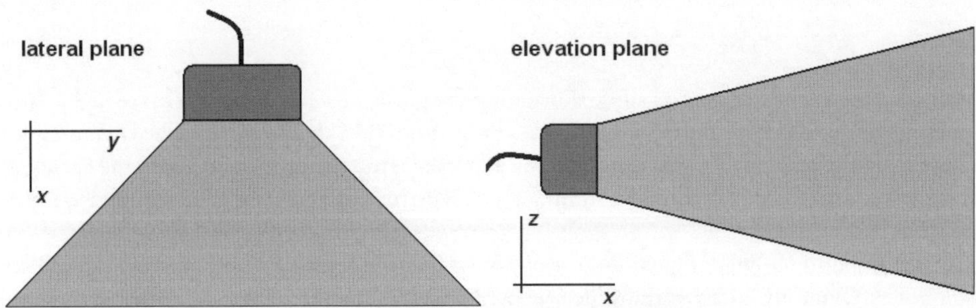



**Figure 2.28.** Three-dimensional imaging by beam steering along the lateral and elevation planes.

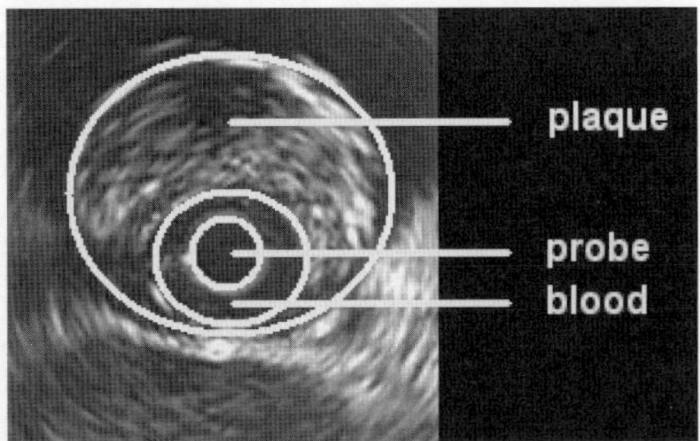



**Figure 2.29.** Example of an intravascular ultrasound (IVUS) image in the presence of an atherosclerotic plaque (hyperechoic area above the ultrasound probe). The probe is the small circle in the middle of the image. The hypoechoic area around the probe is the part of the vessel lumen where blood can still flow.

Since the transducer is miniaturized (small crystals) and must focus at short distances (a few millimeters), the resonance frequency is higher than for normal transducers and can reach 40 MHz.

Typically the ultrasonic pulses are transmitted and received at the same frequency. In fact, the behavior of tissue can be well approximated by a linear function, and frequencies that are not present in the transmitted ultrasonic beam cannot be generated. A different characterization, discussed in section 2.3.2.1, considers UCAs that show nonlinear behavior and provide an opportunity for the development of specific imaging modes to preferentially detect the echoes from the agent while suppressing those from other structures, such as tissue, that have a linear behavior (de Jong, Bouakaz, & Ten Cate, 2002; de Jong et al., 2000; Frinking et al., 2000).

The fundamental mode is when the ultrasound scanner is set to transmit and receive at the same (fundamental) frequency. Today contrast detection modes, referred to as harmonic modes, are also widely available in ultrasound scanners. The objective of these harmonic imaging modes is to maximize the contrast-to-tissue ratio (CTR; Bouakaz et al., 2002; de Jong et al., 2002). In harmonic mode, the system transmits at one frequency but is tuned to receive echoes preferentially at a different frequency. These applications require a broadband transducer.

The frequencies that are commonly used for contrast detection are distinguished in subharmonic (about half of the fundamental harmonic), ultraharmonic (between the fundamental and the second harmonic), second and higher harmonics, and superharmonic (between higher harmonics; Bouakaz et al., 2002; de Jong et al., 2000, 2002; Frinking et al., 2000). For these frequencies, the signals coming from the contrast show larger amplitudes than those coming from tissue, which shows a mechanically linear response to ultrasound.

Apart from the use of filters that are tuned to receive at specific frequencies, other strategies have been developed in order to distinguish between linear and nonlinear media. These techniques involve modulation of the amplitude and phase of the transmitted pulses (Shen & Li, 2003; Eckersley, Chin, & Burns, 2005) and are referred to as power modulation imaging and phase modulation imaging, respectively. These techniques do not require the employment of expensive broadband transducers.

The most common phase modulation technique is referred to as pulse inversion. Two pulses $p_1(t)$ and $p_2(t) = -p_1(t)$ are transmitted in rapid succession. The sum of the received echoes results in the cancellation of the echoes from linear structures (i.e., tissue), while the echoes from microbubbles do not cancel, resulting in a selective detection of UCAs. Amplitude modulation (or power modulation) techniques directly quantify the nonlinearity of the ultrasound transmission-detection channel (i.e., the medium), which is related to the presence of UCAs. If $h(p)$ represents the channel response to a pressure pulse of amplitude $p$ and the channel is nonlinear, then $2h(p)$ differs from $h(2p)$. Figure 2.30 shows an echocardiographic long-axis view of the LV during UCA infusion in fundamental mode and in power modulation mode, where the CTR enhancement can be recognized visually. Several implementations combine power modulation and pulse inversion (PMPI) with a number of different pulse sequence schemes. A combination of power modulation with band-pass filters at frequencies that are different from the fundamental is also used. New methods focusing on the employment of specific frequency codes are still being developed (Eckersley, Chetty, & Hajnal, 2006) that permit the use of longer pulses to achieve a better SNR without a significant loss in longitudinal resolution.

### 2.3.2.3. Ultrasound Perfusion Quantification

The most common use of UCAs is for the opacification of the vascular bed in order to increase the visualization of particular structures. For instance, opacification of the LV permits a more accurate

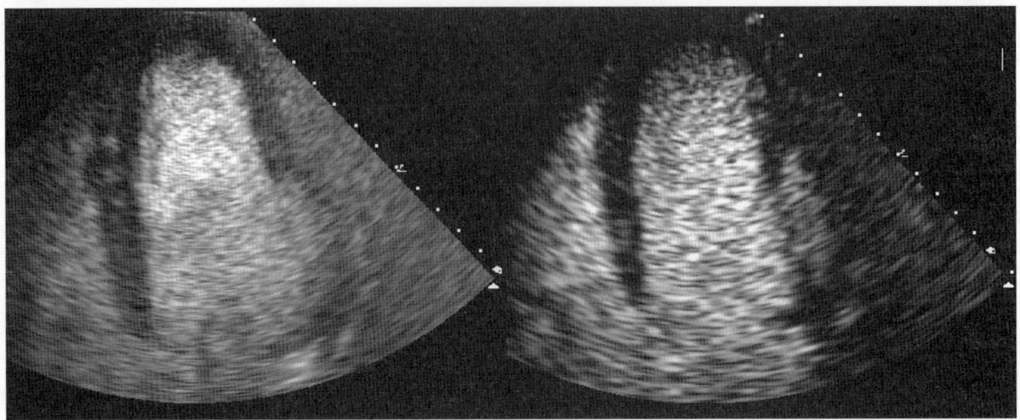

**Figure 2.30.** Opacification of the left ventricle in fundamental imaging (left frame) and power modulation imaging (right frame). A higher CTR ratio can be seen in the frame on the right. Courtesy of the Department of Cardiology, Catharina Hospital, Eindhoven, The Netherlands.

delineation of the endocardium. Apart from these visual applications, contrast echography also permits the quantitative analysis of dynamic processes, such as tissue perfusion. Since UCAs are only intravascular (no extravasations through the vessel wall are present), the analysis of UCA dynamics is purely related to hemodynamics. Quantification of flow or perfusion is difficult because of the unstable absolute relation between contrast concentration and acoustic intensity measured by an ultrasound scanner. However, although the absolute relation is unstable, it can be approximated by a linear function (Mischi, Kalker, & Korsten, 2004a, 2004b), permitting the evaluation of the impulse response of hemodynamic systems of interest (Mischi, Jansen, & Korsten, 2007).

The estimation of the response to a step function is particularly easy, as the microbubbles can be destroyed along the transducer imaging plane by transmitting a series of high-MI ultrasonic pulses. This technique, which is implemented in all recent ultrasound scanners, is referred to as replenishment (Wei et al., 1998). It consists of the destruction of microbubbles followed by a low-MI imaging phase during UCA infusion. This technique was initially used for quantification of myocardial perfusion in order to detect ischemic regions. The replenishment curve is detected by recording the acoustic intensity versus time curves in specific regions of interest in the myocardium. The fit of these replenishment curves by proper models allows the quantification of myocardial perfusion.

In practice, a simple monocompartment model is adopted to represent the dilution system of the myocardium as shown in Figure 2.31. Therefore the replenishment curve $C(t)$ is modeled by the step response of a monocompartment model as

$$C(t) = C_0\left(1 - e^{-\frac{t}{\tau}}\right), \tag{2.58}$$

where $C_0$ is the steady level of concentration that is reached at the measurement site for large $t$ and $\tau$ is the time constant of the monocompartment model. The flow and the perfusion level are proportional to $C_0\tau^{-1}$, so that an image of the myocardium can be generated where the gray level (or color coding) corresponds to the perfusion level (Vogel et al., 2005).

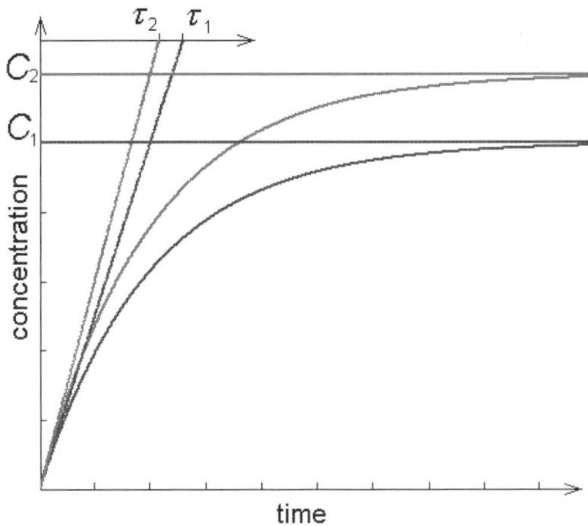


**Figure 2.31.** Two replenishment curves representing a lower and higher level of perfusion (blood flow per unit of tissue volume) corresponding to the time constants $\tau_1$ and $\tau_2$ and the steady levels $C_1$ and $C_2$, respectively.

The replenishment technique is used in combination with a stress test. The patient must exercise immediately before the analysis. In patients that are unable to exercise, the stress test is performed by the injection of vasodilator drugs, such as adenosine or dipyridamole, that increase the level of perfusion. Other drugs that induce a heart rate increase, such as dobutamine, may also be used. An important parameter that can be estimated by means of these methods is the coronary flow reserve, that is, the increase of myocardial blood flow under stress conditions. It corresponds to the ability of the cardiovascular system to increase coronary blood flow in response to vasoactive mechanisms.

Developed for myocardial quantification, the replenishment technique is now also applied for detection of vascularization and angiogenesis processes related to cancerous tissues (Schor & Schor, 1983). Interesting studies are presented for the detection of liver metastases (Ferrara & Meritt, 2000). A limitation of this technique for these applications is due to the different vascular system, where a single input function cannot be defined and a monocompartment model is not very representative either.

The use of intermittent imaging has been introduced in order to avoid microbubble destruction during the imaging phase (Ferrara & Meritt, 2000). Destructive pulses are sent more than once with sufficient delays to permit a full replenishment after each pulse. Between every two destructive pulses only one imaging frame is recorded and the delay from the preceding destructive pulse increases each time. The result is again a replenishment curve, but each measurement is performed at the first imaging frame after bubble destruction.

Another interesting application of this method combines the intermittent replenishment technique with an UCA bolus injection (Krix et al., 2003). During the bolus's first pass (IDC), a series of destructive pulses with a fixed repetition time is transmitted. After each pulse a single frame is recorded (intermittent imaging) with different, increasing delays. The replenishment curve is then extracted with reference to the IDC fit. The plateau level is therefore predicted on the basis of the IDC fit, which can be performed by, for instance, a gamma model (see section 2.2.1.2). The advantage of this method is the limited dose of injected contrast, which is significantly lower for a bolus injection than for a continuous infusion. This also avoids UCA pooling in the liver parenchyma that can occur during perfusion (Krix et al., 2003).

The use of IVUS in combination with contrast infusion permits the visualization of neovascularization around the vessels, which is correlated with atherosclerotic plaque formation, and the assessment of plaque perfusion (Goertz et al., 2006). These are novel studies aimed at the establishment of a relation between plaque perfusion and plaque instability (Feinstein, 2006). However, a method to grade the level of perfusion has not yet been established.

In general, as UCAs are basically dispersed particles (such as red blood cells), they are also used for SNR improvement in Doppler or power Doppler imaging. Improved results are reported for the detection of angiogenesis and neovascularization related to prostate cancer growth by contrast-enhanced power Doppler (Wijkstra, Wink, & de la Rosette, 2004).

## 2.3.3. CONTRAST MRI

As discussed in section 2.2.4.2, the MR signal that is used to reconstruct images and volumes of the body depends on the relaxation times $T_1$ and $T_2$. Differences in these values allow distinguishing between different tissues. The use of so-called $T_1$-weighted or $T_2$-weighted imaging sequences makes the resulting images depend more on $T_1$ or $T_2$, respectively.

When the analysis involves dynamic processes, for example, due to the presence of flow, the addition of specific agents that are injected into the bloodstream may improve the visualization, and therefore the analysis. In fact, although MRA permits accurate measurements of flow in large vessels, the same measurement methods are significantly more difficult in the microcirculation due to the small size of vessels (smaller than the resolution of the MRI system) and the limited velocities. In this context, MRI contrast agents play an increasingly important role.

### 2.3.3.1. Magnetic Resonance Contrast Agent Principles

Magnetic resonance contrast agents are molecular constructs containing paramagnetic atoms such as gadolinium ($Gd^{3+}$) or manganese ($Mn^{2+}$) ions that alter the relaxation times of blood and therefore the MR signal (Atkinson, Burstein, & Edelman, 1990; Vallee et al., 1999; Schreiber et al., 2002; Ivancevic, 2003a, 2003b; Nakajima et al., 2004; Perrin et al., 2004). As a result, they are easily detectable by MRI. Paramagnetic substances are characterized by large magnetic susceptibilities. All materials placed in a magnetic field affect that field by their magnetic susceptibility $\chi$, which defines the ratio between the magnetization $\vec{M}$ (net magnetic dipole moment per unit volume in the material) and the external magnetic field strength $\vec{H}$ as

$$\vec{M} = \chi\,\vec{H}. \tag{2.59}$$

The relationship between the total magnetic field in the material $\vec{B}$ and the external magnetic field strength $\vec{H}$ is

$$\vec{B} = \mu\,\vec{H}, \tag{2.60}$$

where $\mu$ is the permeability of the material (likewise $\mu_0$, the permeability of free space), which is related to the susceptibility as

$$\mu = \mu_0(1 + \chi). \tag{2.61}$$

As a result, the total magnetic field in the material $\vec{B}$ can be written as

$$\vec{B} = \mu_0 \cdot (\vec{H} + \vec{M}). \tag{2.62}$$

A large susceptibility results, therefore, in the ability to become magnetized in an external magnetic field.

Magnetic resonance imaging contrast agents are molecules that contain atoms with permanent dipole moments, even without an applied magnetic field. When no external magnetic field is applied, these atomic dipoles do not present a mutual interaction and are randomly oriented, resulting in a zero net moment. In contrast, when an external magnetic field is applied they act like magnets and the atomic dipoles tend to align with the magnetic field and, as a result, contribute to it (strengthen it). As the external magnetic field is removed, thermal motion disrupts the magnetic alignment very quickly. In general, paramagnetic effects are small, with a magnetic susceptibility on the order of $10^{-3}$ to $10^{-5}$.

The effect of such contrast agents can be the shortening of $T_1$ as a result of dipole–dipole interaction. In this case they are referred to as positive contrast agents, as the effect results in increased MR signal intensity. This provides high sensitivity for detection of hypervascular tissues (e.g., tumors) and permits the evaluation of brain perfusion. More recently, superparamagnetic contrast agents (such as iron [$Fe^{2+}$, $Fe^{3+}$]) have become available. These contrast agents predominantly affect $T_2$ or $T_2^*$ relaxation and are referred to as negative relaxation agents. The effect is, in fact, a decreased MR signal intensity. These agents appear very dark on $T_2$-weighted images and can be used, for instance, for liver imaging, since normal liver tissue retains the agent, whereas abnormal areas, like scars and tumors, do not.

The relaxivities $R_1$ and $R_2$ are the parameters that describe the contrast agent effectiveness to reduce $T_1$ and $T_2$ as a function of its concentration $C$, which are given, respectively, as

$$T_1^{-1} \, (observed) = T_1^{-1} + R_1 C \tag{2.63}$$

$$T_2^{-1} \, (observed) = T_2^{-1} + R_2 C. \tag{2.64}$$

Therefore the inverse of the observed relaxation times are linearly dependent on the concentration $C$ of the paramagnetic species.

### 2.3.3.2. Magnetic Resonance Contrast Agent Applications

Despite the flexibility of MRI measurements, which can be employed for a range of recognized clinical diagnostic problems, the use of contrast agents is required for several important emerging applications (Yuh, 1999). The combination of MRI with the infusion of contrast media permits improved evaluation (usually qualitative) of several dysfunctions, including perfusion defects (e.g., in the myocardium, brain, kidney, and liver) and extravasations in suspected infarcts and tumors. As a consequence, the clinical use of contrast media in MRI is rapidly increasing. Of greatest interest are exogenous paramagnetic compounds, for example, gadolinium ($Gd^{3+}$), iron ($Fe^{2+}$, $Fe^{3+}$), and manganese ($Mn^{2+}$), but especially gadolinium, which is currently used in several MRI studies for perfusion imaging. Its toxicity is reduced to an acceptably low level by chelation to molecules such as diethylenetriamine pentaacetic acid (DPTA). As already discussed, the intravascular infusion of paramagnetic contrast agents leads to a reduction of blood magnetic relaxation time and enhancement of the MR signal (Fig. 2.32).

Several recent studies confirm that the relation between MRI signal enhancement and gadolinium concentration is approximately linear for low concentrations (Henderson et al., 2000; Ivancevic

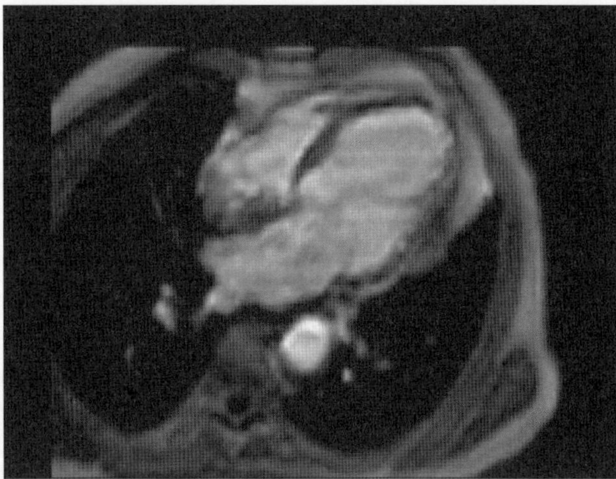

**Figure 2.32.** Enhancement of the MR signal in the cardiac cavities and the aorta by $T_1$-weighted imaging after an intravenous injection of a bolus of gadolinium DPTA. Courtesy of the Department of Radiology, Catharina Hospital, Eindhoven, The Netherlands.

et al., 2003a; Morkenborg et al., 2003). This finding permits novel perfusion imaging applications. Therefore, although the use of contrast MRI mainly aims at qualitative diagnostics, some studies are available that provide more quantitative measurements of blood perfusion and vascular leakage. Local studies in the myocardium, brain, kidney, liver, and lungs have been reported (Buonocore & Katzberg, 2005; Carroll, Rowely, & Haughton, 2003; Detre et al., 1992; Elkington et al., 2005; Nakajima et al., 2004; Nikolaou et al., 2004; Ostergaard et al., 1996). Often an arterial input function is derived in the feeding artery and a deconvolution method is used for the dilution system identification (Anderesen et al., 2002; Wirestam et al., 2000).

Focusing on myocardial perfusion, which is of major importance in the detection of coronary artery ischemia (perfusion defect), the input function is the IDC that is measured in the LV and the output function is the IDC that is measured at any location in the myocardium. The IDC measurement in the LV and the myocardium follow a peripheral intravenous injection of an MR contrast bolus. Typically the dilution system between the LV and the myocardium is represented by a monocompartment model (see equations 2.3 and 2.4 in section 2.2.1.2). Therefore a deconvolution technique may be employed to estimate the time constant $\tau$ of the model (exponential decay). This time constant represents the mean transit time (MTT) of the contrast bolus between the LV and the selected measurement site in the myocardium. A short MTT identifies a larger flow and perfusion. Parametric images can also be generated on the basis of the estimated MTT so that perfusion defects and ischemic areas can be detected.

Some additional problems for the use of deconvolution methods relate to the different signal intensities (contrast relaxivity) in the arterial lumen, where the arterial input function is measured, and in the perfusion area (microcirculation). The latter shows a low SNR, requiring the injection of a larger contrast agent dose, leading to saturation and distortion effects on the measured arterial input function. These complex problems have been approached by the injection of a prebolus with a lower contrast dose (Kostler et al., 2004).

The study of vascular leakage in tumors is feasible because of the small size of gadolinium molecules, which can diffuse through the capillary wall into the interstitial space. Several models have been tested that describe this diffusion process (Cao et al., 2005; Henderson et al., 2000; Paran et al., 2004; Ruediger et al., 1999; Tofts, 1997; Tofts et al., 1999). However, for some cardiovascular studies, the use of purely intravascular contrast agents is more suitable. New opportunities for perfusion are now provided by novel blood pool agents, such as gadolinium-based albumin-bound agents (e.g., gadofosveset trisodium, also known as MS-325) and dendritic gadolinium complexes (e.g., Gadomer). These agents show a longer intravascular life time (slow clearance) due, respectively, to albumin binding and to larger molecular size, which limit contrast extravasations (Henderson et al., 2000; Jerosch-Herold et al., 2003; Kraitchman et al., 2002; Troughton et al., 2004).

It is important to note that contrast MRI for perfusion imaging, usually referred to as dynamic contrast-enhanced (DCE) MRI, requires a higher temporal resolution than other MRI applications where a single volume reconstruction is typically needed and produced. In general, MRI is a relatively slow technique. The reconstruction of an image requires the repetition of several excitation pulses to fill the k-space and reconstruct an image by Fourier back-transformation (Bernstein et al., 2004; Kuperman, 2000; Liang & Lauterbur, 2000; Nitz & Reimer, 1999; Vlaardingerbroek & den Boer, 2003). For rapid dilution processes, a fast scanning technique is a fundamental requirement. Recent technical developments have increased the time resolution of MRI, which is now approaching that of X-ray computed tomography (CT) and ultrasound echography. These improvements consist mainly of advanced strategies to fill the k-space with a reduced number of excitation pulses. To this end, several different pulse sequences have been proposed whose names vary depending on the manufacturer (Bernstein et al., 2004; Brown & Semelka, 1999; Nitz, 2002; Nitz & Reimer, 1999). Alternative techniques to boost the time resolution of MRI based on smart k-space construction strategies consist of filling the k-space with radial or spiral trajectories and exploiting the symmetry of the Fourier transform of a real signal (Bernstein et al., 2004; Nitz, 2002; Semelka et al., 1996).

The latest developments to increase temporal resolution consist of the use of arrays of receiving coils, referred to as parallel MRI. Several techniques have been developed for the reconstruction of the imaged volume by integrating the information derived by the different coils. Well known among these techniques are the simultaneous acquisition of spatial harmonics (SMASH), parallel imaging with localized sensitivities (PILS), generalized autocalibrating partially parallel acquisition (GRAPPA), and sensitivity encoding (SENSE; Griswold et al., 2002; Griswold et al., 2000; Pruessmann et al., 1999; Sodickson & Manning, 1997; Weiger, Pruessmann, & Boesiger, 2000). Frequency-temporal interpolation of the k-space can also lead to an increase in temporal resolution. The most advanced developments in spatio-temporal k-space interpolation make use of the k-t BLAST (or k-t SENSE if combined with the SENSE technique) method, where a least squares approach is used to treat aliasing problems due to simultaneous down-sampling in frequency and time (Tsao, Boesiger, & Pruessmann, 2003).

## 2.3.4. FUNCTIONAL MRI

The addition of paramagnetic contrast agents is not the only possibility that MRI offers in order to evaluate and quantify hemodynamic processes. In fact, another modality of imaging is possible that provides quantitative information on the level of perfusion. This is possible because of the presence in blood of a natural (referred to as endogenous) MR contrast, deoxyhemoglobin. Deoxyhemoglobin is deoxygenated hemoglobin, in contrast to oxyhemoglobin. Since deoxyhemoglobin has paramagnetic properties, the level of blood oxygenation can be detected by MRI (Ogawa et al., 1990). The resulting MR technique is referred to as functional MRI (fMRI), and it has a clear advantage over similar scintigraphic measurements (see section 2.3.1) because it does not require contrast infusion. The use of fMRI is typically aimed at the assessment of perfusion and activation levels in different areas of the brain cortex.

The underlying principles of fMRI are based on the balloon model, which is a nonlinear model that links the level of oxygenation to the level of perfusion (Buxton, Wong, & Frank, 1998). Both are then linked to neuronal stimulation and activation. The model is given as

$$
\begin{cases}
\ddot{\Phi} = \varepsilon u(t) - \dfrac{\dot{\Phi}}{\tau_s} - \dfrac{\Phi - 1}{\tau_f} \\[2ex]
\dot{V} = \dfrac{1}{\tau}\left( \Phi - V^{\frac{1}{\alpha}} \right) \\[2ex]
\dot{C} = \dfrac{1}{\tau}\left( \Phi \dfrac{1 - \left(1 - E_0\right)^{\frac{1}{\Phi}}}{E_0} - C \cdot V^{\frac{1}{\alpha} - 1} \right),
\end{cases}
\tag{2.65}
$$

where $\Phi$ is the blood flow into the venous compartment, $\varepsilon$ is the neuronal efficacy, $u(t)$ is the neuronal input, $\tau_s$ is the signal decay time constant, $\tau_f$ is the feedback autoregulation time constant, $V$ is the venous blood volume, $C$ is the deoxyhemoglobin concentration, $\tau$ is the transit time through the balloon, $\alpha$ is the stiffness parameter, and $E_0$ is the resting extraction fraction of $O_2$. All the values are typically expressed as fractions of the resting value.

The fMRI measurement can then be represented by a state-space formulation:

$$
\begin{cases}
\dot{x}(t) = f_p\big(x(t), u(t)\big) \\[1.5ex]
y(t) = g_p\big(x(t)\big) \\[1.5ex]
x(t) = \begin{pmatrix} \Phi & \dot{\Phi} & V & C \end{pmatrix},
\end{cases}
\tag{2.66}
$$

where $g_p(x(t))$ is a nonlinear function of the hidden state $x(t)$ and the subscript p indicates dependency on the balloon model parameters. The measured (observed) MR signal $y(t)$ is referred to as the blood oxygenation level dependent (BOLD) signal. The input signal $u(t)$ is typically an auditory or visual input to the subject that will stimulate perfusion of specific areas in the cortex and therefore produce changes in the hidden state $x(t)$ (Fox & Raichle, 1985). The quantification of perfusion and cortex activation is thus performed by identification of equation 2.66, which is not trivial. Several methods have been proposed in the literature for the identification of this and other nonlinear models describing brain cortex perfusion and oxygenation (Friston et al., 2000).

In general, also according to the balloon model, the increase in blood flow occurs without a corresponding increase in $O_2$ extraction. As a result, the concentration of deoxyhemoglobin decreases. Since deoxyhemoglobin is paramagnetic, it alters the $T_2$-weighted MRI signal (see sections 2.3.3.1 and 2.2.4.2). In particular, it makes the MRI signal decay faster on a $T_2$-weighted pulse sequence (due to loss of spin phase coherence). Therefore there is an inverse relationship between deoxyhemoglobin content and fMRI signal: during activation, deoxyhemoglobin decreases, and thus the MRI signal increases. As with all perfusion imaging techniques (see the end of section 2.3.3.2), fMRI also requires a fast imaging technique (Bandettini et al., 1992).

After the fMRI images have been acquired, the dynamics of each voxel are analyzed to identify the activated regions of the cortex. The voxels where there is a close correlation between the time course of fMRI signal intensity and the time course of task performance are considered activated. Eventually a 3D activation map is produced (Ogawa et al., 1993).

## 2.4. SENSORS FOR FLOW IN OTHER FLUIDS

So far the major techniques and sensors for the measurement of blood flow, which is certainly the most important flow measurement in clinical practice, have been considered. Similar principles can also be used, in general, for flow measurement in other fluids. The fact that blood recirculates in a closed fluid-dynamic circuit may make blood flow measurements particularly complicated. This complication does not occur for flow measurement in other fluids, which are typically produced and expelled (open fluid dynamic circuit). The flow measurement thus reduces to the quantification of the expelled volume of fluid.

Of particular interest are the flow rates of urine, saliva, tears, and gastric acids. As these fluids are produced and expelled, their measurement reduces to the quantification of the volume of the expelled fluid.

The measurement of urinary flow, referred to as uroflowmetry, is a simple diagnostic measurement for the assessment of the flow rate of urine over time. Uroflowmetry is performed by having a person urinate into a special funnel that is connected to an instrument that measures the urine volume and derives the flow rate. This information is converted into a graph and interpreted by a physician. Several methods can be adopted for such flow measurements, the simplest being the gravimetric method, where the urine passes into a container that is continuously weighed. However, such techniques may suffer from inaccurate measurements due to vibrations.

Information about urinary flow helps in evaluating the function of the lower urinary tract or determining whether there is an obstruction of normal urine outflow. Many other pathologic conditions, such as urinary incontinence, prostate cancer (or hyperplasia), bladder cancer, and infections, can influence urinary flow.

Draining and spitting methods have been commonly employed for the assessment of salivary production, using collections of unstimulated or stimulated whole saliva. The stimulated whole saliva flow rate can be assessed by means of masticatory and gustatory methods. Reduced production of saliva is a symptom of Sjogren syndrome or Stevens–Johnson syndrome. A reduction of salivary flow rates is also related to a flow reduction of lachrymal fluid, as both lachrymal and salivary fluids are produced by exocrine glands. The flow of lachrymal fluid is typically measured by Shirmer paper strips, where strips of absorbing paper are inserted into the lower conjunctival sac of each eye. The eyes are then closed. After 5 minutes the strips are removed and the lengths of the wet portions are measured. A normal value is about 15 mm. Recently measurement based on fluorescent photography has been proposed (Kawai et al., 2007).

The assessment of the secretion of gastric acid in the stomach is an important clinical measurement. A lack or excess of acidity is related to difficult digestion and may be a symptom of an infection or some other disease. The measurement is performed by the standard intubation test with a gastric tube. The gastric juice is aspirated for several minutes. A second measurement is then performed after administration of pentagastrine, a synthetic polypeptide that stimulates the secretion of gastric acid. The acidity (determined by the negative logarithm of the concentration of hydrogen ions in solution, referred to as pH) of the two samples is then compared. The lowest pH of secreted acid is between 0.8 and 1, but after dilution in the stomach lumen it increases about three times. Because of the discomfort of performing this measurement, several alternatives have been proposed that are better for the patient. One of these involves the variation of fluid electrical resistivity at different acidity levels. The measurement can be obtained by electrical impedance methods (Sarker et al., 1997).

## REFERENCES

Anderesen, I. K., Szymowiak, A., Rasmussen, C. E., Hanson, L. G., Marstrand, J. R., . . . & Hansen, L. K. (2002). Perfusion quantification using Gaussian process deconvolution. *Magnetic Resonance in Medicine, 48*, 351–361.

Anger, H. O. (1964). Scintillation camera with multichannel collimators. *Journal of Nuclear Medicine, 5*, 515–531.

Atkinson, D. J., Burstein, D., & Edelman, R. R. (1990). First-pass cardiac perfusion: Evaluation with ultrafast MR imaging. *Radiology, 174*, 757–762.

Bacharach, S. L., Libutti, S. K., & Carrasquillo, J. A. (2000). Measuring tumor blood flow with $H_2^{15}O$: Practical considerations. *Nuclear Medicine and Biology, 27*(7), 671–676.

Baim, D. S., & Grossman, M. D. (2000). *Grossman's cardiac catheterization, angiography, and intervention* (1st ed.). Philadelphia, PA: Lippincott Williams & Wilkins.

Bandettini, P. A., Wong, E. C., Hinks, R. S., Tikofsky, R. S., & Hyde, J. S. (1992). Time course EPI of human brain function during task activation. *Magnetic Resonance in Medicine, 25*, 390–397.

Becher, H., & Burns, P. N. (2000). *Handbook of contrast echocardiography* (1st ed.). Frankfurt, Germany: Springer Verlag.

Bernstein, M. A., King, K. F., & Zhou, X. J. (2004). *Handbook of MRI pulse sequences* (1st ed.). Burlington, MA: Elsevier Academic Press.

Blom, J. A. (2003). *Monitoring of respiration and circulation* (1st ed.). Boca Raton, FL: CRC Press.

Bogaard, J. M., Jansen, J. R. C., von Reth, E. A., Versprille, A., & Wise, M. E. (1986). Random walk type models for indicator-dilution studies: Comparison of a local density random walk and a first passage times distribution. *Cardiovascular Research, 20*(11), 789–796.

Bogaard, J. M., Smith, S. J., Versprille, A., Wise, M. E., & Hagemeijer, F. (1984). Physiological interpretation of skewness of indicator-dilution curves: Theoretical considerations and practical application. *Basic Research in Cardiology, 79*, 479–493.

Bottomley, P. A., Forster, T. H., Argersinger, R. E., & Pfeifer, L. M. (1984). A review of normal tissue hydrogen NMR relaxation times and relaxation mechanisms for 1–100 MHz: Dependence on tissue type, NMR frequency, temperature, excision and age. *Medical Physics, 11*, 425–448.

Bouakaz, A., Frigstad, S., Ten Cate, F. J., & de Jong, N. (2002). Improved contrast to tissue ratio at higher harmonics. *Ultrasonics, 40*, 575–578.

Brennen, C. E. (1995). *Cavitation and bubble dynamics* (1st ed.). New York, NY: Oxford University Press.

Bronzino, J. D. (2000). *The biomedical engineering handbook* (2nd ed.). Boca Raton, FL: CRC Press.

Brown, M. A., & Semelka, R. C. (1999). MR imaging abbreviations, definitions, and descriptions: A review. *Radiology, 213*, 647–662.

Buonocore, M. H., & Katzberg, R. W. (2005). Estimation of extraction fraction (EF) and glomerular filtration rate (GFR) using MRI: Considerations derived from a new Gd-chelate biodistribution model simulation. *IEEE Transactions on Medical Imaging, 24*(5), 651–666.

Buxton, R. B., Wong, E. C., & Frank, L. R. (1998). Dynamics of blood flow and oxygenation changes during brain activation: The balloon model. *Magnetic Resonance in Medicine, 39*, 855–864.

Cao, Y., Brown, S. L., Knight, R. A., Fenstermacher, J. D., & Ewing, J. R. (2005). Effect of intravascular-to-extravascular water exchange on the determination of blood-to-tissue transfer constant by magnetic resonance imaging. *Magnetic Resonance in Medicine, 53*, 282–293.

Carroll, T. J., Rowely, H. A., & Haughton, V. M. (2003). Automatic calculation of the arterial input function for cerebral perfusion imaging with MR imaging. *Radiology, 227*, 593–600.

Chen, X., Schwarz, K. Q., Phillips, D., Steinmetz, S. D., & Schlief, R. (1998). A mathematical model for the assessment of hemodynamic parameters using quantitative contrast echocardiography. *IEEE Transactions on Biomedical Engineering, 45*(6), 754–765.

Church, C. C. (1988). Prediction of rectified diffusion during nonlinear bubble pulsations at biomedical frequencies. *Journal of the Acoustic Society of America, 83*(6), 2210–2217.

Colak, S. B., van der Mark, M. B., 't Hooft, G. W., Hoogenraad, J. H., van der Linden, E. S., & Kuijpers, F. A. (1999). Clinical optical tomography and NIR spectroscopy for breast cancer detection. *IEEE Journal of Selected Topics in Quantum Electron, 5*, 1143–1158.

de Jong, N., Bouakaz, A., & Ten Cate, F. J. (2002). Contrast harmonic imaging. *Ultrasonics, 40*(1), 567–573.

de Jong, N., Frinking, P. J. A., Bouakaz, A., & Ten Cate, F. J. (2000). Detection procedures of ultrasound contrast agents. *Ultrasonics, 38*, 93–98.

de Jong, N., Hoff, L., Skotland, T., & Bom, N. (1992). Absorption and scatter of encapsulated gas filled microspheres: Theoretical considerations and some measurements. *Ultrasonics, 30*(2), 95–103.

Deng, A. L. H., Karagiannoglou, S. H., Sakkas, W. I., Lowe, G. D. O., & Barbenel, J. C. (2002). The impedance measurement of human blood in relations to the hemorheological determinants. *International Journal of Bioelectromagnetism, 4*(2), 167–168.

Desser, T. S., Jedrzejewicz, T., & Haller, M. I. (1998). Color and power Doppler sonography: Techniques, clinical applications, and trade-offs for image optimization. *Ultrasound Quarterly, 14*(3), 128–149

Detre, J. A., Leigh, J. S., Williams, D. S., & Koretsky, A. P. (1992). Perfusion imaging. *Magnetic Resonance in Medicine, 23*(1), 37–45.

Dhawan, A. P. (2003). *Medical image analysis* (1st ed.). New York, NY: John Wiley & Sons.

Donnemiller, E., Heilmann, J., Wenning, G. K., Berger, W., Decristoforo, C., Moncayo, R., . . . Ransmayr, G. (1997). Brain perfusion scintigraphy with 99mTc-HMPAO or 99mTc-ECD and 123I-β-CIT single-photon emission tomography in dementia of the Alzheimer-type and diffuse Lewy body disease. *European Journal of Nuclear Medicine and Molecular Imaging, 24*(3), 320–325.

Duck, F. A., Baker, A. C., & Starritt, H. C. (1998). *Ultrasound in medicine* (1st ed.). Philadelphia, PA: Institute of Physics Publishing.

Eckersley, R. J., Chetty, K., & Hajnal, J. V. (2006). Investigating the nonlinear microbubble response to chirp encoded, multipulse sequences. *Ultrasound in Medicine and Biology, 32*(12), 1887–1895.

Eckersley, R. J., Chin, C.-T., & Burns, P. N. (2005). Optimising phase and amplitude modulation schemes for imaging microbubble contrast agents at low acoustic power. *Ultrasound in Medicine and Biology, 31*(2), 213–219.

Elkington, A. G., He, T., Gatehouse, P. D., Prasad, S. K., Firmin, D. N., & Pennell, D. J. (2005). Optimization of the arterial input function for myocardial perfusion cardiovascular magnetic resonance. *Journal of Magnetic Resonance Imaging, 21*, 354–359.

Ell, P. J., & Gambhir, S. S. (2004). *Nuclear medicine in clinical diagnosis and treatment* (3rd ed.). London, England: Churchill Livingstone.

Evans, D. H., & McDicken, W. N. (2000). *Doppler ultrasound: Physics, instrumentation and signal processing* (2nd ed.). New York, NY: John Wiley & Sons.

Fegler, G. (1954). Measurement of cardiac output in anaesthetised animals by a thermodilution method. *Quarterly Journal of Experimental Physiology, 39*, 153–164.

Feigenbaum, H. (1994). *Echocardiography* (5th ed.). Philadelphia, PA: Lippincott Williams & Wilkins.

Feinstein, S. B. (2004). The powerful microbubble: From bench to bedside, from intravascular tracer to therapeutic delivery system, and beyond. *American Journal of Physiology, 287*, H450–H457.

Feinstein, S. B. (2006). Contrast ultrasound imaging of the carotid artery vasa vasorum and atherosclerotic plaque neovascularization. *Journal of the American College of Cardiology, 48*(2), 236–243.

Ferrara, K. W., & Meritt, C. R. B. (2000). Evaluation of tumor angiogenesis: Imaging, Doppler, and contrast agents. *Academic Radiology, 7*, 824–839.

Flynn, H. G. (1975). Cavitation dynamics I: A mathematical formulation. *Journal of Acoustic Society of America, 57*, 1379–1396.

Fox, P. T., & Raichle, M. E. (1985). Stimulus rate determines regional brain blood flow in striate cortex. *Annals of Neurology, 17*(3), 303–305.

Franck, A., Selby, K., Tyen, R. V., Nordell, B., & Saloner, D. (2005). Cardiac-gated MR angiography of pulsatile flow: k-space strategies. *Journal of Magnetic Resonance Imaging, 5*(3), 297–307.

Frinking, P. J. A., Bouakaz, A., Kirkhorn, J., Ten Cate, F. J., & de Jong, N. (2000). Ultrasound contrast imaging, current and new potential methods. *Ultrasound in Medicine and Biology, 26*(6), 965–975.

Frinking, P. J. A., Cespedes, E. I., Kirkhorn, J., Torp, H. G., & de Jong, N. (2001). A new ultrasound contrast imaging approach based on the combination of multiple imaging pulses and a separate release burst. *IEEE Transactions on Ultrasonics, Ferroelectrics, and Frequency Control, 48*(3), 643–651.

Frinking, P. J. A., & de Jong, N. (1998). Acoustic modeling of shell encapsuled gas bubbles. *Ultrasound in Medicine and Biology, 24*(4), 523–533.

Friston, K. J., Mechelli, A., Turner, R., & Price, C. J. (2000). Nonlinear responses in fMRI: The balloon model, Volterra kernels, and other hemodynamics. *Neuroimage, 12*(4), 466–477.

Gefen, N., Barnea, O., Abramovich, A., & Santamore, W. P. (1999). Experimental assessment of error sources in thermodilution measurements of cardiac output and ejection fraction. *IEEE Proceedings of the First Joint BMES/ EMBS Conference Serving Humanity, Advancing Technology, 2*, 796.

Gilmore, F. R. (1952). The collapse and growth of a spherical bubble in a viscous compressible liquid. *California Institute of Technology, Hydrodynamics Lab, Report 26*(4), 1–40.

Gödje, O., Höke, K., Fischlein, T., Vetter, H., & Reichart, B. (1996). Less invasive, continuous cardiac-output measurement through pulse contour analysis versus conventional thermal dilution. *Critical Care in Medicine, 22*(1), S58.

Goertz, D. E., Frijlink, M. E., de Jong, N., & van der Steen, A. F. W. (2006). Nonlinear intravascular ultrasound contrast imaging. *Ultrasound in Medicine and Biology, 32*(4), 491–502.

Griswold, M. A., Jakob, P. M., Heidemann, R. M., Nittka, M., Jellus, V., Wang, J., . . . & Haase, A. (2002). Generalized autocalibrating partially parallel acquisition (GRAPPA). *Magnetic Resonance in Medicine, 47*, 1202–1210.

Griswold, M. A., Jakob, P. M., Nittka, M., Goldfarb, J. W., & Haase, A. (2000). Partially parallel imaging with localized sensitivities (PILS). *Magnetic Resonance in Medicine, 44*, 602–609.

Hamilton, T. T., Huber, L. M., & Jessen, M. E. (2002). Pulse CO: A less-invasive method to monitor cardiac output from arterial pressure after cardiac surgery. *Annals of Thoracic Surgery, 74*, S1408–S1412.

Hamilton, W. F., Moore, J. W., Kinsman, J. M., & Spurling, R. G. (1928), Simultaneous determination of the pulmonary and systemic circulation times in man and of a figure related to cardiac output. *American Journal of Physiology, 84*, 338–334.

Hedrick, W. R., Hykes, D. L., & Starchman, D. E. (1995). *Ultrasound Physics and Instrumentation* (3rd ed.). St. Louis, MO: Mosby.

Henderson, E., Sykes, J., Drost, D., Weinmann, H. J., Rutt, B. K., & Lee, T. Y. (2000). Simultaneous MRI measurement of blood flow, blood volume, and capillary permeability in mammary tumors using two different contrast agents. *Journal of Magnetic Resonance Imaging, 12*, 991–1003.

Hertzman, A. B., & Spealman, C. R. (1937). Observations on the finger volume pulse recorded photoelectrically. *American Journal of Physiology, 119*, 334.

Hoff, L. (1996). Acoustic properties of ultrasound contrast agents. *Ultrasonics, 34*, 591–593.

Hoff, L. (2001). *Acoustic characterization of contrast agents for medical ultrasound imaging* (1st ed.). Dordrecht, Netherlands: Kluwer Academic.

Hornak, J. P. (1996). *The basics of MRI* (1st ed.). Rochester, NY: Author.

Hoogeveen, R. M., Bakker, C. J. G., & Viergever, M. A. (1997). Phase-derivative analysis in MR angiography: Reduced Venc dependency and improved vessel wall detection in laminar and disturbed flow. *Journal of Magnetic Resonance Imaging, 7*, 321–330.

Hwang, J. H., Brayman, A. A., Reidy, M. A., Matula, T. J., Kimmey, M. B., & Crum, L. A. (2005). Vascular effects induced by combined 1-MHz ultrasound and microbubble contrast agent treatments in vivo. *Ultrasound in Medicine and Biology, 31*(4), 553–564.

Irarrázaval, P., Santos, J. M., Guarini, M., & Nishimura, D. (1999). Flow properties of fast three-dimensional sequences for MR angiography. *Magnetic Resonance Imaging, 17*, 1469–1479.

Ivancevic, M. K., Zimine, I., Foxall, D., Lecoq, G., Righetti, A., Didier, D., & Vallee, J. P. (2003a). Inflow effect in first-pass cardiac and renal MRI. *Journal of Magnetic Resonance Imaging, 18*, 372–376.

Ivancevic, M. K., Zimine, I., Montet, X., Hyacinthe, J. N., Lazeyras, F., Foxall, D., Vallee, J. P. (2003b). Inflow effect correction in fast gradient-echo perfusion imaging *Magnetic Resonance in Medicine, 50*, 885–891.

Jansen, J. R. C. (1995). The thermodilution method for clinical assessment of cardiac output. *Intensive Care Med, 21*, 691–697.

Jansson, P. A. (1997). *Deconvolution of images and spectra* (2nd ed.). London, England: Academic Press.

Jensen, J. A. (1996). *Estimation of blood velocities using ultrasound: A signal processing approach* (1st ed.). New York, NY: Cambridge University Press.

Jerosch-Herold, M., Hu, X., Murthy, N. S., Rickers, C., & Stillman, A. E. (2003). Magnetic resonance imaging of myocardial contrast enhancement with MS-325 and its relation to myocardial blood flow and perfusion reserve. *Journal of Magnetic Resonance Imaging, 28*(5), 544–554.

Jonas, M., Hett, D., & Morgan, J. (2002). Real time, continuous monitoring of cardiac output and oxygen delivery. *International Journal of Intensive Care, 9*(1), 33–44.

Jonas, M. M., & Tanzer, S. J. (2002). Lithium dilution measurements of cardiac output and arterial pulse waveform analysis: an indicator dilution calibrated beat-by-beat system for continuous estimation of cardiac output. *Current Opinion in Critical Care, 8*, 257–261.

Kakadiaris, I. A., O'Malley, S. M., Vavuranakis, M., Carlier, S., Metcalfe, R., Hartley, C. J., . . . Naghavi, M. (2006). Signal-processing approaches to risk assessment in coronary artery disease. *IEEE Signal Processing Magazine, 23*(6), 59–62.

Kawai, M., Yamada, M., Kawashima, M., Inoue, M., Goto, E., Mashima, Y., & Tsubota, K. (2007). Quantitative evaluation of tear meniscus height from fluorescein photographs. *Cornea, 26*(4), 403–406.

Keller, J. B., & Miksis, M. (1980). Bubble oscillations of large amplitude. *Journal of the Acoustic Society of America, 68*, 628–633.

Kostler, H., Ritter, C., Lipp, M., Beer, M., Hahn, D., & Sandstede, J. (2004). Prebolus quantitative MR heart perfusion imaging. *Magnetic Resonance in Medicine, 52*, 296–299.

Kouwenhoven, M., Bakker, C. J. G., Hartkamp, M. J., & Mali, W. P. T. M. (1994). Current MR angiographic imaging techniques, a survey. In: P. Lanzer and J. Rosch (Eds.), *Vascular diagnostics*. Heidelberg, Germany: Springer-Verlag.

Kraitchman, D. L., Chin, B. B., Heldman, A. W., Solaiyappan, M., & Bluemke, D. A. (2002). MRI detection of myocardial perfusion defects due to coronary artery stenosis with MS-325. *Journal of Magnetic Resonance Imaging, 15*(2), 149–158.

Krix, M., Kiessling, F., Vosseler, S., Kiessling, I., Le-Huu, M., Fusenig, N. E., & Delorme, S. (2003). Comparison of intermittent-bolus contrast imaging with conventional power Doppler sonography: Quantification of tumor perfusion in small animals. *Ultrasound in Medicine and Biology, 29*(8), 1093–1103.

Kubicek, W. G., Karnegis, J. N., Patterson, R. P., Witsoe, D. A., & Mattson, R. H. (1966). Development and evaluation of an impedance cardiac output system. *Aerospace Medicine, 37*(12), 1208–1212.

Kuperman, V. (2000). *Magnetic resonance imaging. Physical principles and applications* (1st ed.). London, England: Academic Press.

Kurita, T., Morita, K., Kato, S., Kawasaki, H., Kikura, M., Kazama, T., & Ikeda, K. (1999). Lithium dilution cardiac output measurements using a peripheral injection site: comparison with central injection technique and thermodilution. *Journal of Clinical Monitoring and Computing, 15*, 279–285.

Leighton, T. G. (1994). *The acoustic bubble* (1st ed.). London, England: Academic Press.

Liang, Z.-P., & Lauterbur, P. C. (2000). *Principles of magnetic resonance imaging: A signal processing perspective* (1st ed.). Piscataway, NJ: IEEE Press.

Lieshout, J. J. V., & Jansen, J. R. C. (2007). Continuous cardiac output monitoring by blood pressure analysis. *Journal of Applied Physiology, 102*, 826.

Lim, K. W., & Chung, M. K. (1998). Relative errors in evaluating the electromagnetic flowmeter signal using the weight function method and the finite volume method. *Flow Measurement and Instrumentation, 9*(4), 229–235.

Linton, R. A., Band, D. M., Chir, B., & Haire, K. M. (1993). A new method of measuring cardiac output in man using lithium dilution. *British Journal of Anaesthesia, 71*(2), 262–266.

Linton, R. A. F., Linton, N. W. F., & Band, D. M. (1995). A new method of analysing indicator dilution curves. *Cardiovascular Research, 30*, 930–938.

Lopatatzidis, A., & Millard, R. K. (2001). Empirical estimators of gamma fits to tracer dilution curves and their technical basis and practical scope. *Physiological Measurements, 22*, N1–N5.

Lorenzo, A. D., Andreoli, A., Matthie, J., & Withers, P. (1997). Predicting body cell mass with bioimpedance by using theoretical methods: a technological review *Journal of Applied Physiology, 82*(5), 1542–1558.

Lu, Z., & Mukkamala, R. (2006). Continuous cardiac output monitoring in humans by invasive and noninvasive peripheral blood pressure waveform analysis. *Journal of Applied Physiology, 101*, 598–608.

Mahan, B. J., & Myers, R. J. (1987). *University chemistry*. London, England: Addison-Wesley.

Malmivuo, J., & Plonsey, R. (1995). *Bioelectromagnetism* (2nd ed.). New York, NY: Oxford University Press.

Mettler, A. F. A., & Guiberteau, M. J. (2006). *Essentials of nuclear medicine imaging* (5th ed.). Philadelphia, PA: W. B. Saunders.

Mischi, M., Jansen, A. H. M., & Korsten, H. H. M. (2007). Identification of cardiovascular dilution systems by contrast ultrasound. *Ultrasound in Medicine and Biology, 33*(3), 439–451.

Mischi, M., Kalker, A. A. C. M., & Korsten, H. H. M. (2004a). Contrast echocardiography for pulmonary blood volume quantification. *IEEE Transactions on Ultrasonics, Ferroelectrics, and Frequency Control, 51*(9), 1137–1147.

Mischi, M., Kalker, A. A. C. M., & Korsten, H. H. M. (2004b). Videodensitometric methods for cardiac output measurements. *EURASIP Journal on Applied Signal Processing, 2003*(5), 479–489.

Mohiaddin, R. H., & Pennell, D. J. (1998). MR blood flow measurement: Clinical application in the heart and circulation. *Cardiology Clinics, 16*(2), 161–187.

Morgan, K. E., Allen, J. S., Dayton, P. A., Klibanov, A. L., Chomas, J. E., Ferrara, K. W., Medwin, H. (2000). Experimental and theoretical evaluation of microbubbles behavior: Effect of transmitted phase and bubble size. *IEEE Transactions on Ultrasonics, Ferroelectrics, and Frequency Control, 47*(6), 1494–1509.

Morkenborg, J., Pederson, M., Jensen, F. T., Jorgensen, H. S., Djurhuus, J. C., & Frokier, J. (2003). Quantitative assessment of Gd-DTPA contrast agent from signal enhancement: An in-vitro study. *Magnetic Resonance Imaging, 21*, 637–643.

Nair, A., Kuban, B. D., Tuzcu, E. M., Schoenhagen, P., Nissen, S. E., & Vince, D. G. (2002). Coronary plaque classification with intravascular ultrasound radiofrequency data analysis. *Circulation, 106*(17), 2200–2206.

Nakajima, T., Oriuchi, N., Tsushima, Y., Funabasama, S., Aoki, J., & Endo, K. (2004). Noninvasive determination of regional myocardial perfusion with first-pass magnetic resonance (MR) imaging. *Academic Radiology, 11*(7), 802–808.

Newell, J. C. (1996). A status report for medical impedance imaging. *IEE Colloquium on Advances in Electrical Tomography (Digest No: 1196/143)*, 1/1–1/3.

Nijboer, L. A., Dorlas, J. C., & Mahieu, H. F. (1981). Photoelectric plethysmography: Some fundamental aspects of the reflection transmission method. *Clinical Physics and Physiological Measurement, 2*(3), 205–215.

Nikolaou, K., Schoenberg, S. O., Brix, G., Goldman, J. P., Attenberg, U., Kuehn, B., . . . & Reiser, M. F. (2004). Quantification of pulmonary blood flow and volume in healthy volunteers by dynamic contrast enhanced magnetic resonance imaging using a parallel imaging technique. *Investigative Radiology, 39*(9), 537–545.

Nitz, W. R. (2002). Fast and ultrafast non-echo-planar MR imaging techniques. *Magnetic Resonance, 12*, 2866–2882.

Nitz, W. R., & Reimer, P. (1999). Contrast mechanisms in MR imaging. *European Radiology, 9*, 1032–1046.

Norwich, K. H. (1977). *Molecular dynamics in biosystems* (1st ed.). Oxford, England: Pergamon Press.

Nyboer, J. (1970). *Electrical impedance plethysmography* (2nd ed.). Springfield, IL: C. C. Thomas.

Ogawa, S., Lee, T. M., Nayak, A. S., & Glynn, P. (1990). Oxygenation sensitive contrast in magnetic resonance image of rodent brain at high magnetic fields. *Magnetic Resonance in Medicine, 14*, 68–78.

Ogawa, S., Menon, R. S., Tank, D. W., Kim, S.-G., Merkle, H., Ellermann, J. M., & Ugurbil, K. (1993). Functional brain mapping by blood oxygenation level-dependent contrast magnetic resonance imaging. *Biophys Journal, 64*(3), 803–812.

Ogura, Y., Katakura, K., & Okujima, M. (1997). A method of ultrasonic 3-D computed velocimetry. *IEEE Transactions on Biomedical Engineering, 44*(9), 823–830.

Ostergaard, L., Soresen, A. G., Kwong, K. K., Weisskoff, R. M., Gyldensted, C., & Rosen, B. R. (1996). High resolution measurement of cerebral blood flow using intravascular tracer bolus passages. Part II: Experimental comparison and preliminary results. *Magnetic Resonance in Medicine, 36*(5), 726–736.

Paran, Y., Bendel, P., Margalit, R., & Degani, H. (2004). Water diffusion in different microenvironments of breast cancer. *NMR in Biomedicine, 17*, 170–180.

Perrin, R. L., Ivancevic, M. K., Kozerke, S., & Vallee, J. P. (2004). Comparative study of FAST gradient echo MRI sequences: Phantom study. *Journal of Magnetic Resonance Imaging, 20*, 1030–1038.

Plesset, M. S. (1949). The dynamics of cavitation bubbles. *ASME Journal of Applied Mechanics, 16*, 228–231.

Plesset, M. S., & Prosperetti, A. (1977). Bubble dynamics and cavitation. *Annual Review of Fluid Mechanics, 9*, 145–185.

Poelaert, J., Schmidt, C., van Aken, H., Hindler, F., & Molloff, H. M. L. T. (1999). A comparison of transoesophageal echocardiographic Doppler across the aortic valve and the thermodilution technique for estimating cardiac output. *Anaesthesist, 54*(2), 128–136.

Pope, J. M., & Yao, S. (1993). Quantitative NMR imaging of flow. *Concepts in Magnetic Resonance, 5*, 281–302.

Prosperetti, A., Crum, L. A., & Commander, K. W. (1988). Nonlinear bubble dynamics. *Journal of the Acoustic Society of America, 83*, 502–514.

Pruessmann, K. P., Weiger, M., Scheidegger, M. B., & Boesiger, P. (1999). SENSE: Sensitivity encoding for fast MRI. *Magnetic Resonance in Medicine, 42*, 952–962.

Ruediger, E. P., Knopp, M. V., Hoffmann, U., Milker-Zabel, S., & Brix, G. (1999). Multicompartment analysis of gadolinium chelate kinetics: Blood–tissue exchange in mammary tumors by dynamic MR imaging. *Journal of Magnetic Resonance Imaging, 10*, 233–241.

Sakka, S. G., Reinhart, K., & Meier-Hellmann, A. (1999). Comparison of pulmonary artery and arterial thermodilution cardiac output in critically ill patients. *Intensive Care Medicine, 25*(8), 843–846.

Sarker, S. A., Mahalanabis, D., Bardhan, P. K., Alam, N. H., Rabbani, K. S., Kiber, A., . . . & Gyr, K. (1997). Noninvasive assessment of gastric acid secretion in man (application of electrical impedance tomography (EIT)). *Journal Digestive Diseases and Sciences, 42*(8), 1804–1809.

Schiller, N. B., Shah, P. M., Crawford, M., DeMaria, A., Devereux, R., Feigenbaum, H., . . . Tajik, A. J. (1989). Recommendations for quantitation of the left ventricle by two-dimensional echocardiography. *Journal of the American Society of Echocardiography, 2*, 358–367.

Schor, A. M., & Schor, S. L. (1983). Tumor angiogenesis. *Journal of Pathology, 141*, 385–413.

Schreiber, W. G., Schmitt, M., Kalden, P., Mohrs, O. K., Kreitner, K. F., & Thelen, M. (2002). Dynamic contrast-enhanced myocardial perfusion imaging using saturation-prepared TrueFISP. *Journal of Magnetic Resonance Imaging, 16*, 641–652.

Schwan, H. P. (1983). Electrical properties of blood and its constituents: Alternating current spectroscopy. *Journal Annals of Hematology, 46*(4), 185–197.

Semelka, R. C., Kelekis, N. L., Thomasson, D., Brown, M. A., & Laub, G. A. (1996). HASTE MR imaging: Description of technique and preliminary results in the abdomen. *Journal of Magnetic Resonance Imaging, 6*(4), 698–699.

Shankar, R., & Webster, J. G. (1991). Noninvasive measurement of compliance of human leg arteries. *IEEE Transactions on Biomedical Engineering, 38*(1), 62–67.

Shen, C.-C., & Li, P.-C. (2003). Pulse-inversion-based fundamental imaging for contrast detection. *IEEE Transactions on Ultrasonics Ferroelectrics and Frequency Control, 50*(9), 1124–1133.

Sheppard, C. W. (1962). *Basic principles of tracer methods: Introduction to mathematical tracer kinetics* (1st ed.). New York, NY: John Wiley & Sons.

Sodickson, D. K., & Manning, W. J. (1997). Simultaneous acquisition of spatial harmonics (SMASH): Fast imaging with radiofrequency coil arrays. *Magnetic Resonance in Medicine, 38*, 591–603.

Stewart, G. N. (1897). Researches on the circulation time and on the influences which affect it. *Journal of Physiology, 22*, 159–183.

Stoddard, M. F., Liddell, N. E., Longaker, R. A., & Dawkins, P. R. (1992). Transesophageal echocardiography: Normal variants and mimickers. *American Heart Journal, 124*(6), 1587–1598.

Swan, H. J. C., Ganz, W., Forrester, J., Marcus, H., Diamond, G., & Chonette, D. (1971). Catheterization of the heart in man with use of a flow-directed, balloon-tipped catheter. *New England Journal of Medicine, 283*, 447–451.

Szabo, T. L. (2004). *Diagnostic ultrasound imaging* (1st ed.). Burlington, MA: Elsevier.

Szolar, D. H., Sakuma, H., & Higgins, C. B. (1996). Cardiovascular applications of magnetic resonance flow and velocity measurements. *Journal of Magnetic Resonance Imaging, 6*(1), 78–89.

Thompson, H. K., Starmer, C. F., Whalen, R. E., & McIntosh, H. D. (1964). Indicator transit time considered as a gamma variate. *Circulation Research, 14*, 502–515.

Tofts, P. S. (1997). Modeling tracer kinetics in dynamic Gd-DPTA MR imaging. *Journal of Magnetic Resonance Imaging, 7*(1), 91–101.

Tofts, P. S., Brix, G., Buckley, D. L., Evelhoch, J. L., Henderson, E., Knopp, M. V., . . . & Weisskoff, R. M. (1999). Estimating kinetic parameters from dynamic contrast-enhanced T1-weighted MRI of a diffusible tracer: standardized quantities and symbols. *Journal of Magnetic Resonance Imaging, 10*, 223–232.

Troughton, J. S., Greenfield, M. T., Greenwood, J. M., Dumas, S., Wiethoff, A. J., Wang, J., . . . & Caravan, P. (2004). Synthesis and evaluation of a high relaxivity manganese(II)-based MRI contrast agent. *Inorganic Chemistry, 43*(20), 6313–6323.

Tsao, J., Boesiger, P., & Pruessmann, K. L. (2003). k-t BLAST and k-t SENSE: Dynamic MRI with high frame rate exploiting spatiotemporal correlations. *Magnetic Resonance in Medicine, 50*, 1031–1042.

Unger, E. C., Porter, T. R., Culp, W., Labell, R., Matsunaga, T., & Zutshi, R. (2004). Therapeutic applications of lipids-coated microbubbles. *Advanced Drug Delivery Reviews, 56*, 1291–1314.

Vallee, J. P., Lazeyras, F., Kasuboski, L., Chatelain, P., Howarth, N., Righetti, A., Didier, D. (1999). Quantification of myocardial perfusion with FAST sequence and Gd bolus in patients with normal cardiac function. *Journal of Magnetic Resonance Imaging, 9*, 197–203.

Vlaardingerbroek, M. T., & den Boer, J. A. (2003). *Magnetic resonance imaging* (3rd ed.). Heidelberg, Germany: Springer.

Vogel, R., Indermühle, A., Reinhardt, J., Meier, P., Siegrist, P. T., Namdar, M., Kaufmann, P. A. (2005). The quantification of absolute myocardial perfusion in humans by contrast echocardiography, algorithm and validation. *Journal of the American College of Cardiology, 45*(5), 754–762.

Webster, J. G. (1997). *Medical instrumentation: Application and design* (3rd ed.). New York, NY: John Wiley and Sons.

Webster, J. G. (1999). *Measurement, instrumentation and sensors handbook* (1st ed.). Boca Raton, FL: CRC Press.

Wei, K., Jayaweera, A. R., Firoozan, S., Linka, A., Skyba, D. M., & Kaul, S. (1998). Quantification of myocardial blood flow with ultrasound-induced destruction of microbubbles administrated as a constant venous infusion. *Circulation, 97*, 473–483.

Weiger, M., Pruessmann, K. P., & Boesiger, P. (2000). Cardiac real-time imaging using SENSE. *Magnetic Resonance in Medicine, 43*, 177–184.

Wells, P. N. T. (1977). *Biomedical ultrasonics* (1st ed.). London, England: Academic Press.

Whitney, J. R. (1953). The measurement of volume changes in humans limbs. *Journal of Physiology, 121*, 1–27.

Wijkstra, H., Wink, M. H., & de la Rosette, J. J. (2004). Contrast specific imaging in the detection and localization of prostate cancer. *World Journal of Urology, 22*(5), 346–350.

Wirestam, R., Andersson, L., Ostergaard, L., Bolling, M., Aunola, J. P., Lindgren, A., . . . Stahlberg, F. (2000). Assessment of regional cerebral blood flow by dynamic susceptibility contrast MRI using different deconvolution techniques. *Magnetic Resonance in Medicine, 43*, 691–700.

Wise, M. E. (1966). Tracer dilution curves in cardiology and random walk and lognormal distributions. *Acta Physiol Pharmacol Neerl, 14*, 175–204.

Yelderman, M. (1990). Continuous measurement of cardiac output with the use of stochastic system identification techniques. *Journal of Clinical Monitoring, 6*, 322–332.

Yuh, W. T. C. (1999). An existing and challenging role for the advanced contrast MR imaging. *Journal of Magnetic Resonance Imaging, 10*, 221–222.

Zierler, K. (2000). Indicator dilution methods for measuring blood flow, volume, and other properties of biological systems: A brief history and memoir. *Annals of Biomedical Engineering, 28*, 836–848.

## SYMBOLS AND UNITS

$a$:               ultrasound attenuation coefficient [m$^{-1}$ Hz$^{-1}$]

$A$:               cross-sectional area [m$^2$]

$A_t$ and $A_b$:   cross-sectional area [m$^2$] of tissue and blood compartments, respectively

$B_0$ or $\vec{B}_0$:   static magnetic induction [T]

$B_1$ or $\vec{B}_1$:   time-varying magnetic induction [T]

$B_{xy}$:          transverse magnetic induction [T]

$c$:               ultrasound propagation velocity in water or in tissue [m s$^{-1}$]

$C$:               concentration [kg m$^{-3}$]

$C_n$:             concentration in the $n$th compartment [kg L$^{-1}$]

$c_b$:             specific heat of blood [J kg$^{-1}$ K$^{-1}$]

$C_b$:             blood vessel compliance [Pa m$^{-3}$]

$d$:               distance [m]

$D$:               diffusion coefficient [m$^2$ s$^{-1}$]

$E$:               electric potential [V]

$E_0$:             extraction fraction of oxygen in the brain capillaries at rest [dimensionless]

$F$:               Faraday constant 96485 [C mol$^{-1}$]

$f$:               frequency [Hz]

$f_0$:             central frequency of ultrasonic pulses [Hz]

$f_L$:             Larmor frequency [Hz]

$f_r$:             receiving frequency [Hz]

$f_t$:             transmitting frequency [Hz]

$\vec{G}$:         magnetic induction gradient [T m$^{-1}$]

$G_x$:             magnetic induction gradient in the $x$ direction [T m$^{-1}$]

$H$:               magnetic field strength [A m$^{-1}$]

$i$:               $(-1)^{0.5}$

$\hat{i}$:         unit vector along the $x$-direction of a Cartesian coordinate system [dimensionless]

$I$:               acoustic intensity [W m$^{-2}$] or in phase component of a signal

$I_0$:             initial acoustic intensity [W m$^{-2}$]

$I_c$:             electrical current intensity [A]

$\hat{j}$:         unit vector along the $y$-direction of a Cartesian coordinate system [dimensionless]

$\vec{J}$:         angular momentum [kg m$^2$ s$^{-1}$]

$k$:               polytropic gas exponent [dimensionless]

$\vec{k}$:         three-dimensional coordinate in the k-space [m$^{-1}$]

$\hat{k}$:         unit vector along the $z$-direction of a Cartesian coordinate system [dimensionless]

$K$:               scale factor [dimensionless]

$L$:               length [m]

$m$:      mass [kg]

$\hat{k}$:      net magnetization [A m$^2$]

$M_0$ or $\vec{M}_0$:      net magnetization at equilibrium in presence of $B_0$ alone [A m$^2$]

$M_{xy}$:      transversal magnetization [A m$^2$]

$M_z$:      longitudinal magnetization [A m$^2$]

$n$:      numerical index $\in N$ or ion valence [dimensionless]

$\hat{n}$:      normal unit vector [dimensionless]

$P$:      pressure [Pa]

$P_0$:      resting or initial pressure [Pa]

$P_e$:      external pressure [Pa]

$P_i$:      internal pressure [Pa]

$P_r$:      peak rarefactional pressure [Pa]

$P_v$:      vapor pressure [Pa]

$P_{H_2O}$:      pressure of water vapor [Pa]

$Q$:      heat [J] or in quadrature component of a signal

$Q'$:      heat flow [W]

$r$:      radius [m]

$\vec{r}$:      coordinates of a point in a three-dimensional space [m]

$R$:      electrical resistance [$\Omega$] or gas constant 8.314 [J mol$^{-1}$ K$^{-1}$]

$R_h$:      hemodynamic resistance [Pa s m$^{-3}$]

$R_1$ and $R_2$:      longitudinal and transverse relaxivity [m$^3$ kg$^{-1}$ s$^{-1}$], respectively

$S(t)$:      magnetic resonance signal [V]

$S$:      strain-gauge sensitivity factor [dimensionless]

$S_p$:      shell elasticity parameter [N m$^{-1}$]

$S_t$ and $S_r$:      transmitted and received signals by an ultrasound transducer [V]

$\Phi$:      volumetric flow [m$^3$ s$^{-1}$]

$\Phi_m$:      magnetic flux [Wb]

$t$:      time [s]

$t_0$:      initial time [s]

$T$:      temperature [K]

$T_1$ and $T_2$:      longitudinal and transverse relaxation time [s]

$T_2^*$:      observed transverse relaxation time [s]

$T_e$:      external temperature [K]

$T_i$:      internal temperature [K]

$u(t)$:      neuronal input; multiplied by the neuronal efficacy $\varepsilon$, it gives [m$^3$ s$^{-3}$]

$v$:      velocity [m s$^{-1}$]

$V$:      volume [m$^3$]

$v_c$:          velocity of ultrasound through the piezoelectric crystal [m s$^{-1}$]

$Z$:          electrical impedance [$\Omega$]

$Z_a$:          acoustic impedance [rayl (kg m$^{-2}$ s$^{-1}$)]

$Z_b$ and $Z_t$:          blood and tissue electrical impedance [$\Omega$], respectively

$\alpha$:          plane angle [rad] or stiffness parameter in the balloon model [dimensionless]

$\beta$:          plane angle [degrees]

$\gamma$:          gyromagnetic ratio, $2.685 \times 10^8$ [rad s$^{-1}$ T$^{-1}$]

$\Gamma$:          gamma function

$\delta_t$:          total damping factor [dimensionless]

$\Delta$:          prefix to indicate a variation in a quantity

$\varepsilon$:          neuronal efficacy; multiplied by the neuronal input $u(t)$, it gives [m$^3$ s$^{-3}$]

$\lambda$:          wavelength [m]

$\mu$:          magnetic permeability [N A$^{-2}$]

$\mu_0$:          magnetic permeability of free space, $4\pi \times 10^{-7}$ [N A$^{-2}$]

$\vec{\mu}$:          magnetic dipole moment [A m$^2$]

$\mu^1$:          first statistical moment

$\upsilon$:          Poisson ratio [dimensionless]

$\pi$:          pi, approximately 3.14159 [dimensionless]

$\rho$:          mass density [kg m$^{-3}$] or [mol m$^{-3}$]

$\rho_b$:          mass density of blood [kg m$^{-3}$] or blood resistivity [$\Omega$ m$^{-1}$]

$\sigma_t$:          surface tension coefficient [N m$^{-1}$]

$\tau$:          time constant [s]

$\vec{\tau}$:          torque [N m]

$\tau_e$:          ejection time [s]

$\tau_f$:          feedback autoregulation time constant [s]

$\tau_s$:          signal decay time constant [s]

$\phi$:          phase [rad]

$\chi$:          susceptibility [dimensionless]


## LIST OF ABBREVIATIONS

A/D:          analog to digital

B-mode:          brightness mode

BOLD:          blood oxygenation level dependent

CO:          cardiac output

CT:          computed tomography

CTR:          contrast-to-tissue ratio

CW:          continuous wave

DC:        direct (continuous) electrical current
DCE MRI:  dynamic contrast-enhanced magnetic resonance imaging
DPTA:     diethylenetriamine pentaacetic acid
EMF:      electromotive force [V]
FFT:       fast Fourier transform
FID:        free induction decay
fMRI:      functional magnetic resonance imaging
FPT:       first passage time (model)
Gd:        gadolinium
GRAPPA:  generalized autocalibrating partially parallel acquisition
HOCM:   high osmolarity contrast media
IDC:       indicator dilution curve
IVUS:     intravascular ultrasound
LDRW:    local density random walk (model)
LED:      light emission diode
LOCM:    low osmolarity contrast media
LV:        left ventricle
MI:        mechanical index
MR:        magnetic resonance
MRA:      magnetic resonance angiography
MRI:       magnetic resonance imaging
MTT:      mean transit time
MUGA:    multi-gate
NIR:       near infrared
PET:       positron emission tomography
pH:        acidity or alkalinity of a solution
PILS:     parallel imaging with localized sensitivities
PMPI:    power modulation phase inversion
PRF:      pulse repetition frequency [Hz]
PW:       pulsed wave
RA:        right atrium
RF:        radio frequency
RV:        right ventricle
SENSE:    sensitivity encoding
SMASH:   simultaneous acquisition of spatial harmonics
SNR:      signal-to-noise ratio
SPECT:    single photon emission computed tomography

SV:          stroke volume [L]

TR:          repetition time [s]

UCA:         ultrasound contrast agent

## ABOUT THE AUTHORS

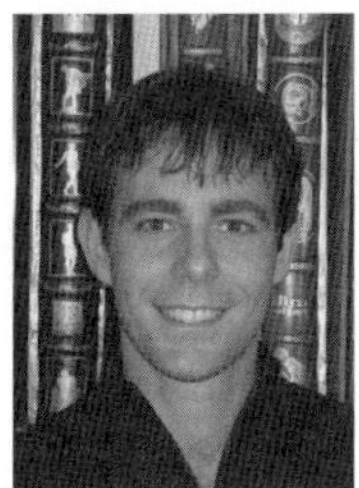

**Dr. Massimo Mischi** was born in Rome (Italy) in 1973. In 1999 he received an MSc degree in electrical engineering at La Sapienza University of Rome. In 2000 he became a research assistant at the Eindhoven University of Technology (the Netherlands), where in 2002 he completed a two-year postmaster program in technological design, information, and communication technology. In 2004 he received his PhD for the development of cardiovascular diagnostic methods by contrast-enhanced ultrasonography. Since 2007, he has been an assistant professor at the Eindhoven University of Technology. His research topics include biomedical measurements and signal processing, with special interests in electromyography, magnetic resonance imaging, and ultrasound imaging. Massimo Mischi is a Senior Member of the IEEE and is currently secretary of the Benelux Chapter of the IEEE Engineering in Medicine and Biology Society.

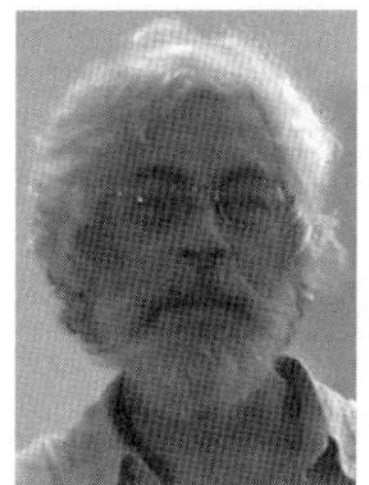

**Professor J. A. Blom** (born 1944) finished his electrical engineering studies at the Eindhoven University of Technology in 1970, specializing in measurement and control. In 1971 he joined the TNO Institute of Medical Physics in Utrecht to work on applications in anesthesia and intensive care and became an assistant professor in the measurement and control group in 1972. From 1974 to 1975 he was at the Department of Surgery, University of Alabama, researching control of blood infusion in patients after heart surgery. In 1975 he returned to the Eindhoven University of Technology, where his research interests included signal processing, the extraction of information from physiological systems, patient monitoring in intensive care, optimal control of drug delivery, and expert systems for clinical decision support. He retired from the university in 2007.

# CHAPTER 3

# FLOW SENSORS FOR RESPIRATORY GASES

G. Kim Prisk

*Departments of Medicine and Radiology*
*University of California, San Diego, La Jolla, CA, USA*

## 3.1. INTRODUCTION

### 3.1.1. WHAT TO MEASURE: FLOW OR VOLUME?

The earliest measurements of respiratory flows were accomplished by measurement techniques that utilized volume sensors, as opposed to flow sensors. In their simplest incarnation, these were balanced, water-filled spirometers in which air was introduced beneath inverted drums of known dimensions (counterbalanced to account for weight). The vertical displacement then became a measure of volume change. John Hutchinson used such a device in the mid-1800s to measure the vital capacity (VC) of more than 4000 subjects (Spriggs, 1977), although such volumetric measurements go back to Lavoisier (circa 1789) and further (Spriggs, 1978). Subsequently other devices such as dry-bellows wedge spirometers were also developed.

Measuring volume changes is of course conceptually and, to a degree, technologically simple, and to this day volume measurement remains a gold standard technique for many measurements in respiratory medicine. Spirometers have been updated using dry rolling seal designs with the incorporation of electronic differentiators, so that today, with readily available computer technology, flow measurements can be obtained by differentiation of volume as a function of time.

However, measuring volume, and hence deriving flow, presents numerous technological and practical challenges, so there is a clear impetus to directly measure flow in numerous circumstances. Spirometers contain elements that are massive, and so, even if properly counterbalanced, present an inertance to the flow that alters the dynamics. Spirometers are, by design, closed systems and thus are of limited applicability when trying to make measurements over a period of time as opposed to single breath studies. Further, spirometers are bulky and require considerable space, which in many experimental circumstances can be limiting. Thus it is often desirable to directly measure flow (and when necessary, integrate to provide volume).

## 3.1.2. THE CHALLENGES OF RESPIRATORY FLOW MEASUREMENT

While it is obvious that the flow sensor represents a desirable measuring device in respiratory physiology and pulmonary medicine, it is initially less obvious that there are significant technical challenges that abound in the design and use of such sensors. These challenges make for difficult measurement conditions and are perhaps best explored by considering the most common measurement performed in pulmonary medicine today, forced spirometry. A brief examination of this deceptively simple test of pulmonary function serves as a good example for understanding the problems inherent in the accurate measurement of respiratory flow.

### 3.1.2.1. The Maximum Expiratory Flow Volume Curve

By far the most commonly performed measurement in the diagnosis of pulmonary disease is forced spirometry. Almost any person referred to a pulmonary physician will undergo this diagnostic procedure and the results have been repeatedly shown to be of considerable diagnostic value. Beginning as far back as the 1850s, VC was measured using spirometers (see section 3.1.1 and Spriggs [1977]). Conceptually VC is a simple measurement defined as the volume between maximal inspiration and maximal expiration. These two lung volumes, total lung capacity (TLC) and residual volume (RV), represent the extremes of the voluntary excursions of lung volume. However, it should be noted that at RV the lungs are not emptied of all gas, but retain a considerable volume that is approximately 15% to 20% of TLC in normal subjects. Clearly, as pointed out in the section 3.1.1, spirometers represent an almost ideal means of measuring VC.

It became clear that not only did the VC change as pulmonary disease progressed, but the rate at which gas could be exhaled from the lungs also changed, at least in some disease processes. Furthermore, the rate at which gas could be exhaled often fell more sharply than did the actual VC. However, inspiratory flow did not exhibit the same reduction as disease progressed. This led to the development of the forced expiratory maneuver by Robert Tiffeneau in the 1940s (Yernault, 1997). The understanding of such a mechanism came from the seminal work of Hyatt (1983), who showed that during expiration, the positive pleural pressure generated by the expiratory effort limits the expiratory flow by creation of a choke point in the airways at the point at which pressure inside the airway falls below that outside. The effect is readily observable when releasing a child's rubber balloon that has been inflated. Flow is limited by the collapsing neck of the balloon (often resulting in a fluttering of the neck), resulting in a reduction in the pressure in the neck of the balloon below atmospheric pressure (the pressure surrounding the balloon) because of the flow of escaping gas (the Bernoulli effect). This phenomenon also occurs in the lungs and results in a process called dynamic compression of the airways. The consequence is that an increase in expiratory effort (an increase in pleural pressure) does not result in an increase in expiratory flow—that is, the expiratory flow is "effort independent." Because during inspiration the pleural pressure is decreased rather than increased, the airways are held open and dynamic compression does not occur. The equal pressure point concept is illustrated in Figure 3.1.

Because dynamic compression is a function of airway elasticity and airway tethering (which tends to hold airways open), any disease that results in a loss of this elasticity results in an increase

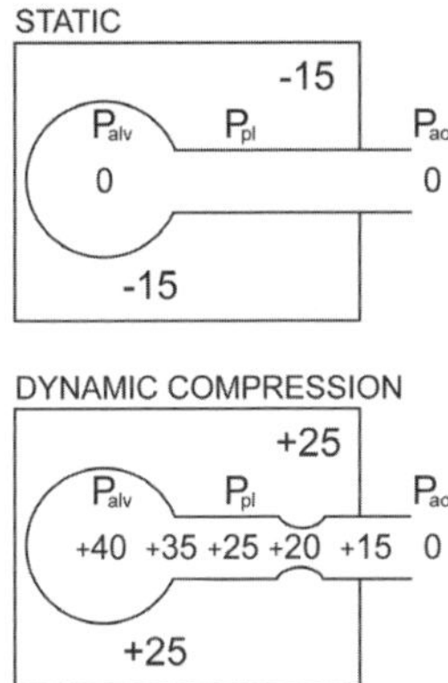



**Figure 3.1.** The equal pressure point concept of expiratory flow limitation. At the end of inspiration (labeled STATIC), pleural pressure ($P_{pl}$) is subatmospheric and alveolar pressure ($P_{alv}$) is zero (there is no flow). During expiration (labeled DYNAMIC COMPRESSION), $P_{pl}$ is increased by muscular effort that is transmitted to the alveolus. There is a pressure drop between the alveolus and the mouth ($P_{ao}$) that generates a flow. At some point along the airway, pressure inside the airway falls below that outside, and the airway collapses, limiting further increases in flow. Because of this mechanism, expiratory flow from the lungs becomes "effort independent" above a certain degree of effort. Units of pressure shown are $cmH_2O$.

in dynamic compression. Similarly diseases that tend to narrow airway caliber result in larger pressure drops with an attendant increase in dynamic compression. Many diseases of this type exist, for example, emphysema (in which lung parenchymal tissue is destroyed) and asthma (in which airways are narrowed), and so the measurement of reductions in forced expiratory flow are a useful diagnostic tool.

Initially this was accomplished by using a spirometer and including in the measurement the volume that could be exhaled in a short (usually 1 second) period of time at the beginning of expiration. This volume, which is still considered one of the principal parameters of forced spirometry, is termed the forced expiratory volume in 1 second ($FEV_1$). Often, it is reported as a fraction of the forced vital capacity (FVC). $FEV_1$/FVC, expressed as a percentage, is typically in the 70% to 80% range in normal subjects and shows a progressive decrease with age as elastic tissue in the lungs degrades. Figure 3.2 shows a tracing from a spirometer measurement in which the subject was asked to exhale as forcefully as possible, starting from TLC and continuing to RV. It is easy to see that $FEV_1$ can readily be determined from the trace. Similarly, at any point in time along the trace of volume as a function of time, instantaneous flow can be taken as the tangent (assuming an adequate dynamic response of the spirometer system) and the data can then be transformed to a plot of flow as a function of volume, as seen on the right in Figure 3.2.

More typically, the flow-volume curve, or when considering forced spirometry, the maximum expiratory flow-volume (MEFV) curve, is plotted as shown in Figure 3.3 with flow on the *y*-axis and volume on the *x*-axis. The inspiratory portion of a forced maneuver is also shown Figure 3.3, which serves to illustrate graphically the difference between expiratory flow (in which dynamic compression limits flow rate over much of the expiration) and inspiratory flow (in which flow is essentially limited

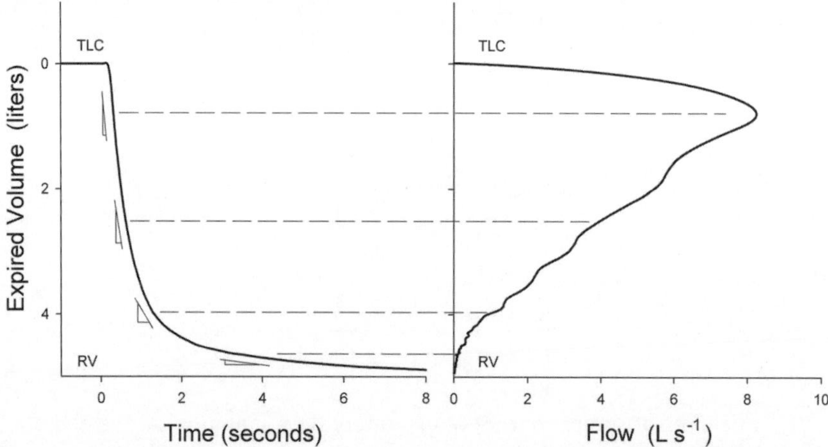

**Figure 3.2.** Volume spirogram and the conversion to flow-volume format. On the left, volume, beginning at TLC, is plotted as a function of time. The expiratory maneuver continues for several seconds, even in normal subjects. The tangent at any point to the volume-time curve gives the flow, which can be plotted against volume, giving the flow-volume curve.

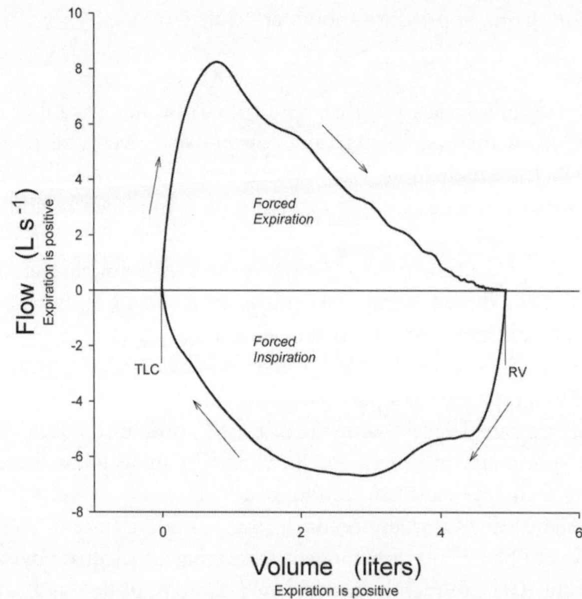

**Figure 3.3.** The maximum expiratory flow-volume and maximum inspiratory flow-volume (MEFV/MIFV) curve. Flow (expiration positive) is plotted on the vertical axis and volume is plotted on the horizontal axis. The maneuver starts at zero flow at TLC (the point of zero flow and volume) and flow shows a rapid rise as expiratory effort is made. However, dynamic compression then limits expiratory flow, and by RV, flow is reduced to zero. In contrast, during a subsequent forced inspiration there is no dynamic compression and flow is largely determined by effort.

by the ability of the respiratory muscles to generate the flow-driving pressures required). So-called obstructive lung diseases, such as emphysema and asthma, result in a reduced VC and a significant and obvious limitation of expiratory flow, or a "scooping out" of the expiratory portion of the MEFV curve as dynamic compression becomes more prevalent. As a consequence, much of the expired volume results from gas leaving the lungs at rather low flow rates.

The very nature of the MEFV curve highlights the challenges faced by respiratory flow sensors, the conditions under which the gas is measured, the composition of the gas being measured, the range of flows over which measurements need to be made with considerable accuracy, and the dynamics of flow changes.

### 3.1.2.2. Measuring Conditions

The measuring conditions are an important aspect of respiratory flow measurement. Within the lungs, gases are warm (normal human body temperature being approximately 37°C) and saturated with water vapor (with a water vapor pressure of 6.3 kPa or 47 mmHg at 37°C). These conditions are referred to as body temperature and pressure, saturated (BTPS). In contrast, surrounding air is at ambient temperature (which is assumed to be 20°C in this discussion) and, for the most part, is fairly dry. These conditions are often referred to as ambient temperature and pressure, dry (ATPD).

Consider the inspiration of 1 L of gas under ATPD conditions. The resulting lung volume change depends on the volume of that gas as it is warmed and moistened to reach BTPS conditions. By the ideal gas law, $PV/T$ = constant, 1 L of gas under ATPD conditions at 1 atmosphere absolute pressure (101.32 kPa, or 760 mmHg) occupies

$$[(760)/(20 + 273)]/[(760 - 47)/(37 + 273)]\ \text{L},$$

or approximately 1.13 L under BTPS conditions. Thus if one is interested in the lung volume change resulting from an inspiration of gas under ATPD conditions, then clearly the change in gas condition must be taken into account in order to reconcile that with the resulting change in lung volume.

Expiration is even more complex. If the flowmeter is at ambient temperature, then the gas must cool to that temperature, with an attendant decrease in the water vapor pressure (and the resultant condensation of exhaled water vapor in the flowmeter itself). Thus a first approximation, assuming a sufficiently large heat-sink capability of the flowmeter itself, is that expired gas is measured under ambient temperature and pressure, saturated (ATPS) conditions. This will, of course, change the scaling factor of 1.13 calculated in the previous paragraph, and so, even for a lung volumetric change in which inspiration and expiration are exactly matched, the indicated volume change (the integral of the flow over time) will be different for inspiration and expiration. In circumstances in which the flowmeter has insufficient thermal mass to allow the assumption of ambient temperature, some assumption (often little more than a guess) must be made as to actual flowmeter temperature during the measurement, and this can even change over the course of a single expiration, and almost certainly changes as breathing frequency is altered (as is often the case with exercise tests). One common means of minimizing these problems is to heat the flowmeter to 37°C, which has the added advantage of minimizing condensate collection.

In the example of the MEFV curve described earlier, in which a maximal inspiration follows a maximal expiration (Fig. 3.3), the ability of a system to provide a closed loop (i.e., equal expiratory and inspiratory volumes; something that is often used for quality control of patient effort) critically depends on adequately dealing with the issue of gas conditions within the flowmeter.

### 3.1.2.3. Gas Composition

The second and obviously related problem to that of measuring conditions is the composition of the gas itself. The purpose of the lungs is to provide the gas exchange necessary to support life by providing an input pathway for oxygen and an output pathway for carbon dioxide. For a subject breathing room air, the inspired gas is approximately 21% oxygen, 78% nitrogen, and 1% argon. Expired gas has a composition of approximately 16% oxygen, 5% carbon dioxide, with the balance being nitrogen and argon (ignoring the issue of water vapor discussed previously). Carbon dioxide has a different density, viscosity, thermal conductivity, heat capacity, and molecular mass than oxygen, and so any flowmeter technology that relies on one or more of these properties is subject to error because inspired and expired gas composition varies. Further, as gas exchange by the body is altered (e.g., during a progressive exercise test), the amount of oxygen and carbon dioxide in each exhaled breath will change, making the use of correction factors determined under one set of circumstances inapplicable.

The situation is even more complex during the performance of many other tests of pulmonary function. Beyond the direct measurement of lung volume and flow (e.g., an MEFV test), foreign gases with differing physical and chemical properties can be used to probe various aspects of lung function. Of particular relevance are the insoluble gases, used to measure absolute lung volume (recall that the lung never completely empties). A gas commonly used in this capacity is helium, which, with an atomic mass of only 4, is very different from oxygen (32) or carbon dioxide (44). Besides the difference in density, helium also possesses very different thermal conductivity properties and viscosity. A test that has been used on occasion to study the degree of heterogeneity of lung ventilation is the multiple breath washout (Fig. 3.4). In this test the subject breathes through a nonrebreathing valve system and washes out a tracer gas that has previously been equilibrated throughout the lung. Thus the end-expiratory concentration falls toward zero in a quasi-exponential fashion.

If the gas flow is measured with a flowmeter (as opposed to a bag-in-box and spirometer system, for example; see section 3.3.4) then this flowmeter must be capable of accurately measuring the volume of each breath of the test during which each expiration has a different concentration of foreign gas. In some circumstances it is desirable to accurately control both the volume and end-expiratory volume of each breath of the test (inhomogeneity of lung ventilation, which this test measures, changes as absolute lung volume is altered). In this case the overall system must maintain a constant end-expiratory lung volume in the face of alterations in gas measuring conditions and composition that is stable to within approximately 100 mL over the course of twenty breaths (Prisk et al., 1995), a challenge that could not be met by this author using a breathe-through flowmeter system (also see section 3.3.4 on bag-in-box systems).

### 3.1.2.4. Ranges of Flows

Another challenge in the development of a good respiratory flow sensor is that of dynamic range. The MEFV curve from a large normal subject requires that the flowmeter must measure flows of approximately 12 L s$^{-1}$ for expiratory flow, and perhaps a little less for inspiratory flow. However, equally important as having a high upper flow limit is the performance of the flowmeter at low flows. In a subject with obstructive pulmonary disease, expiratory flow rapidly becomes limited by dynamic compression, and so the lung empties very slowly. In a subject with very severe obstructive disease, a significant portion of the total FVC is exhaled at flows of only a few hundred milliliters per second over periods lasting several seconds. Since the FVC is an important parameter in respiratory medicine, it is therefore necessary that the flowmeter be accurate in this low range, which can be about

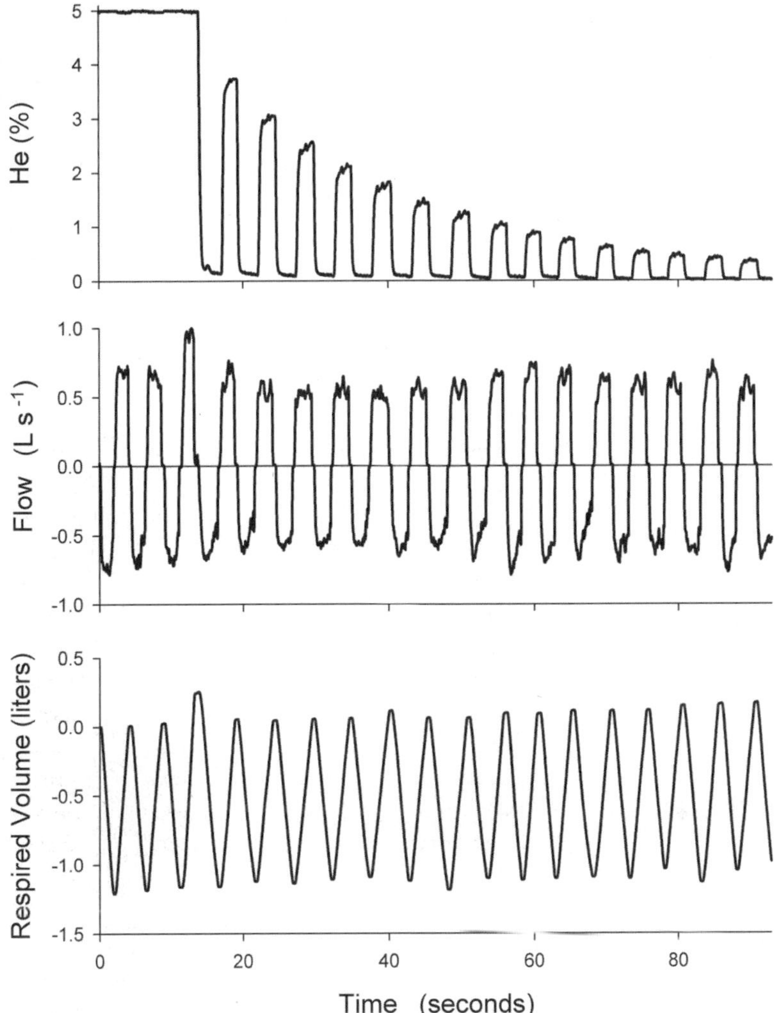

**Figure 3.4.** Multiple breath washout of an inert insoluble gas (helium). Having previously equilibrated the lungs with 5% helium, the subject breathes helium-free gas during a period of controlled breathing. A constant inspiratory concentration (0%) results, while expiratory concentration approaches zero in a quasi-exponential fashion. Note the regularity of flow and volume in this well-controlled experiment, and that for every expiration the helium concentration changes.

one-hundredth that of the upper range required. This requirement is often not met by many flowmeters, limiting their use in some circumstances.

### 3.1.2.5. Flow Dynamics

The MEFV curve also shows the other major challenge that respiratory flow can create—a rapid change in flow. Because the MEFV display format eliminates the time axis, it may be easier to consider

Figure 3.2, which shows the transformation from a volume-time plot to a flow-volume plot. At the beginning of the forced expiration, flow changes in an almost steplike fashion from zero to the peak expiratory flow rate (which can be around 12 L s⁻¹). Performance of an adequate forced expiratory maneuver requires a rapid flow acceleration to peak flow within 5% of FVC (which typically means within approximately 0.2 seconds; American Thoracic Society, 1994). If a flowmeter is to be used to measure this, then it is important that the dynamic response of the instrument be both adequate for following this abrupt change and appropriately damped so as not to introduce oscillation artifacts into the measured flow signal.

## 3.2. PNEUMOTACHOGRAPHY

### 3.2.1. FLEISCH PNEUMOTACHOGRAPH

One of the most common forms of respiratory flowmeter is the Fleisch pneumotachograph, originally developed by Adolph Fleisch in 1925. In essence this is simply a device placed in the airstream that provides a very slight resistance to flow, generating a small pressure drop across it when flow occurs. The device exists in numerous forms with various designs for the resistive element, but in all cases the principle of operation is the same (Fig. 3.5).

In the example in Figure 3.5, the resistive element consists of a series of tubes, each about 0.8 mm in diameter and about 32 mm in length, collected into a bundle that forms the flow path. The outer tubes of this bundle are perforated near each end and connect to annular pressure ducts around the circumference of the bundle. These ducts are connected to the two pressure-sensing ports. These devices typically include electrical heating elements for raising the temperature to 37°C if desired. As flow occurs through the device, the upstream pressure exceeds the downstream pressure, and assuming the flow is laminar (discussed later), Poiseuille's equation describes the pressure drop along any channel as

$$\Delta p = p_1 - p_2 = 8\eta \dot{V} L/\pi r^4, \tag{3.1}$$

where $(p_1 - p_2)$ is the pressure drop along the tube, $\eta$ is the viscosity of the gas, $\dot{V}$ is the volume flow rate, $L$ the length of the tube, and $r$ is the radius of the tube.

Clearly the design of the device must be such that any one of the tubes within the bundle must have an individual flow rate sufficiently low that the condition of laminar flow is met. In typical use the pressure drop across a Fleisch pneumotachograph does not exceed 1 cmH$_2$O (0.098 kPa) pressure.[1] In practice, this translates to a flow per tube of not more than approximately 1.6 mL s⁻¹ (assuming air is the gas flowing through the tube), which results in a Reynolds number in the vicinity of 155. Thus it is clear that the range of flows for which a particular size Fleisch may be used is limited at the upper end by the necessary condition of laminar flow within it, and it is for this reason that a range of devices with differing sizes are available. To use the example given previously of a forced expiration measurement, the minimum diameter of the flow-resistive element for such a measurement is somewhere in the vicinity of 45 mm to 50 mm.

---

1 The pressure unit of cmH$_2$O, while clearly not an SI unit, is still commonly used in the field of pulmonary physiology and provides some sense of physiological meaning. For that reason it will be used here. The pressure difference generated by the diaphragm in a normal breath at rest (a tidal breath) is approximately 5 cmH$_2$O. Thus the pressure drop across a Fleisch pneumotachograph is considerably less than that seen during normal breathing. For comparison, 1 atm is a pressure of 1033.2 cmH$_2$O.

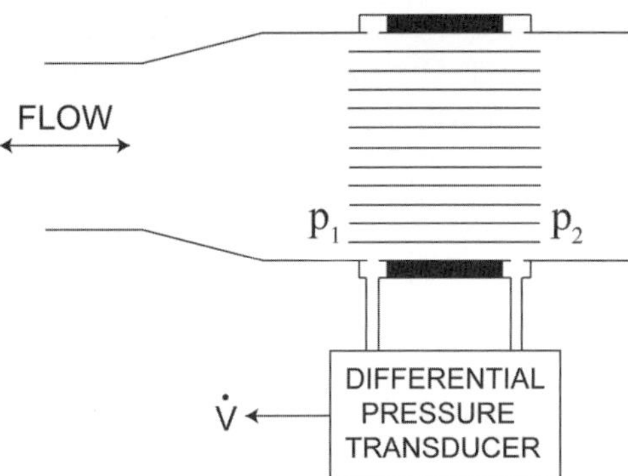



**Figure 3.5.** A schematic of a Fleisch pneumotachograph. The cluster of small tubes provides a very slight resistance to flow. The outer tubes of the cluster are perforated and connect to annular pressure-sensing channels around the device. The pressure drop across the flow-sensing head is described by Poiseuille's equation (equation 3.1) provided that flow is in the laminar range. The pressure drop is sensed with a differential pressure transducer. In order to accommodate all flow ranges, sensor heads with different numbers of flow channels are produced.

While in strict parlance the flow-sensing element is the Fleisch pneumotachograph itself, in practical terms the pressure sensor that detects the pressure drop across the flow sensor is also a critical part of the system. Although a detailed treatment of pressure sensors is beyond the scope of this chapter, a brief description of one in common use is appropriate here because it is the combined behavior of the flow-sensing element, the pressure sensor, and the coupling between the two that determines the performance of the flowmeter system as a whole.

While there are obviously a large number of differential pressure sensors that can be used with a Fleisch pneumotachograph, one, the Validyne air-filled variable reluctance transducer (MP-45), has been the subject of numerous studies in terms of performance and thus is described here. The device consists of a metal diaphragm (of varying thickness, providing different measurement ranges) sandwiched between two halves of the sensor body, each of which contains a sense coil that forms part of an alternating current (AC) bridge system. As the diaphragm is displaced, the reactances of the two coils are altered. This arrangement is usually coupled to the Fleisch pneumotachograph head by flexible tubing. With the advent of solid-state pressure transducer technologies, there are now numerous other differential pressure sensors that can be used with pneumotachographs.

In the 1970s there were extensive studies of the response characteristics of such systems. The important outcome of those studies was the realization that many of the dynamic characteristics of the systems were due to the response characteristics of the pressure transducer and interconnecting tubing, as opposed to the characteristics of the flow sensor head itself. These elements are mentioned in the section on dynamic response (see section 3.3.3).

### 3.2.2. MESH-SCREEN PNEUMOTACHOGRAPHS

The concept of using a pressure drop across a resistance element is not limited to the Fleisch pneumotachograph design. For the continuous measurement of respiratory flow, another design in routine use is the mesh-screen pneumotachograph. As shown in Figure 3.6, the design consists of a fine mesh screen (a 400 mesh size is typical) stretched across the flow path. In order not to introduce too large a resistance to the flow, the surface area is often considerably larger than the size of the connecting tubes (see Fig. 3.6). One advantage of such a design is the simpler engineering and manufacturing of the flow head and the ability to easily disassemble and clean the flow-sensing element. However, screen flowmeters are not vastly different in operation from the Fleisch pneumotachograph, although they often exhibit a degree of nonlinearity that is greater than that in the Fleisch pneumotachograph, as the flow through the sensor head is not as well-developed as in the long, straight tubes of the Fleisch system. Typically the same styles of differential pressure transducers are used as with the Fleisch pneumotachograph.

### 3.2.3. TURBINE FLOWMETERS

Turbine flowmeters have found common use in ventilation measurement during exercise and in forced spirometry, often for the measurement of peak expiratory flow rate (PEFR). The theory behind a turbine flowmeter is described under ideal conditions as a function of turbine geometry. Figure 3.7 provides a brief outline. With a pitch angle $\beta$, $r\omega_i = v \tan \beta$, where $r$ is the rotor radius, $v$ the velocity of the fluid, and $\omega_i$ is the ideal rotational speed. Converting this to a volumetric flow formulation gives

$$\omega_i = [\tan \beta/(r_{bar}A)]\dot{V}, \tag{3.2}$$

where $\dot{V}$ is the volumetric flow rate, $A$ is the area of the annular cross-section, and $r_{bar}$ is the root-mean-square of the inner and outer blade radii. Equation 3.2 shows that the ideal rotational speed is proportional to the volumetric flow rate.

Turbine flowmeters have found favor in the field of exercise testing principally because they are simple and offer minimal resistance to flow, an important consideration when the addition of resistance

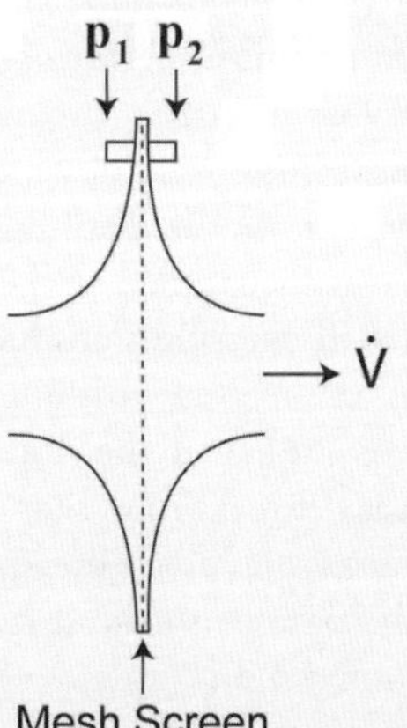


**Figure 3.6.** A typical design for a mesh-screen pneumotachograph. The flaring of the inlet and outlet tubes provides an increased surface area for the mesh, reducing overall resistance and giving better conditioning of the flow through the mesh. As with the Fleisch pneumotachograph, the devices are produced in varying sizes to accommodate different flow ranges.

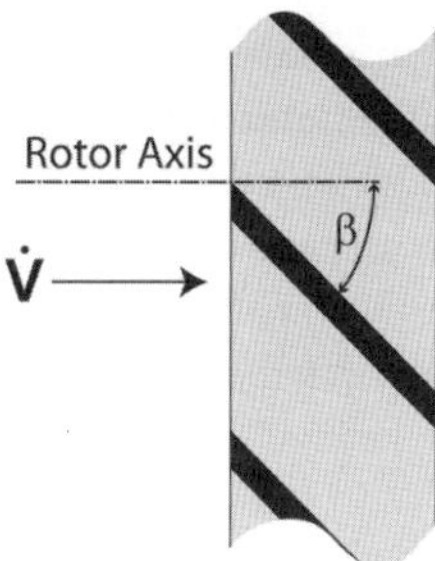


**Figure 3.7.** Consider flow parallel to the rotor axis that is everywhere uniform. With no forces acting to slow down the rotor, it will rotate at a speed that exactly maintains the fluid flow velocity vector at the blade surfaces (see equation 3.2).

to a flow circuit can alter the work of breathing and the maximum level of ventilation that can thus be obtained. The design commonly in use is that of an axial turbine contained in a clear plastic module that can be placed in the breathing circuit. It is generally claimed (at least by the manufacturers) that such devices are minimally affected by changes in gas composition and the presence of condensation. A sensor unit is placed around this with an optical counting system that counts the turbine rotation and thus (strictly) the volume that passes in a given time. The turbine itself is a lightweight metal vane resembling a two-bladed propeller. As with most flowmeters, the devices have a range over which they are optimally used and the sensor head (the turbine itself) is made in a range of sizes. One manufacturer quotes measurements of 0.5 mL, 1 mL, and 2 mL per pulse (corresponding to a half turn of the turbine) for each of three different-size flow heads.

While the turbine flowmeters are conceptually simple, their use raises various practical issues that must be considered in their application. Turbines exhibit a generally poor performance at low flow rates due to the inertia of the rotating element, leading to an underestimation of very low flows (especially in circumstances in which flow acceleration is very low). In essence this introduces a "lag-before-start" error, and so there is a time delay inherent in the turbine signals (Yeh et al., 1987). While this is not an issue in steady-state flow conditions, the majority of turbine flowmeters have been used in exercise testing, which results in large flow changes with time. The other issue is a "spin-after-stop" process, in which the turbine continues to rotate after the cessation of flow. This problem is especially prevalent in situations where flow is unidirectional, for example, when inspired and expired flows are separated by a nonrebreathing valve, or at low breathing frequencies in which there may be an end-expiratory pause in the flow. The problem can be minimized to some extent by placing the turbine on the subject side of the nonrebreathing valve so that with each breath there is an abrupt flow reversal as flow transitions from inspiration to expiration. In addition, there are often "corrections" for both lag-before-start and spin-after-stop incorporated into the counting electronics. However, at least to this author's knowledge, these "correction algorithms" are typically considered proprietary by the manufacturer, leaving the user with little choice but to assume some sort of black-box behavior. In any case, there is a time delay in the signal from a turbine flowmeter that must be accounted for in situations such as exercise testing, where integration of flow with the gas concentration signal is required. To complicate matters, this time delay, because it arises from the lag-before-start and spin-after-stop effects, tends to vary as a function of the flow rates being measured, a problem of considerable magnitude in situations such as progressive exercise testing.

Geometries other than the a simple axial turbine described earlier are used in several settings. These devices are quite commonly used in the field of flow monitoring during anesthesia. A sketch of two commonly used geometries is shown in Figure 3.8. The rotating vane design has been used extensively in the Wright respirometer, which has been used for volumetric measurement in numerous circumstances. However, none of these devices typically exhibits great accuracy, and they certainly do not possess the dynamic response characteristics that are desirable in many cases.

## 3.2.4. PITOT TUBE FLOWMETERS

Pitot tubes are occasionally used in measuring respiratory flow. However, these devices tend to exhibit poor linearity (even taking into account their $v^2$ dependence) and a high degree of sensitivity to gas composition. As is the case with rotating vane flowmeters, their use is often limited to anesthetic monitoring or other circumstances in which a high degree of accuracy and large dynamic range are not required. However, more sophisticated designs are now finding their way into respiratory function testing hardware. Manufacturers have been drawn to such devices because their inherently simple geometric design allows fabrication using injection-molded plastics, allowing these devices to be manufactured at low cost. These devices can use disposable flow sensor heads or sensor heads that are readily sterilized. A pitot tube flowmeter is shown in Figure 3.9. The pressure drop is defined by

$$\Delta p = 0.5\rho v^2, \tag{3.3}$$

where $\rho$ is the density of the gas (which varies with gas composition) and $v$ is the velocity of the gas. Provided the cross-sectional area of the tube is known and some assumptions are made about flow characteristics, velocity $v$ can be converted to flow $\dot{V}$.

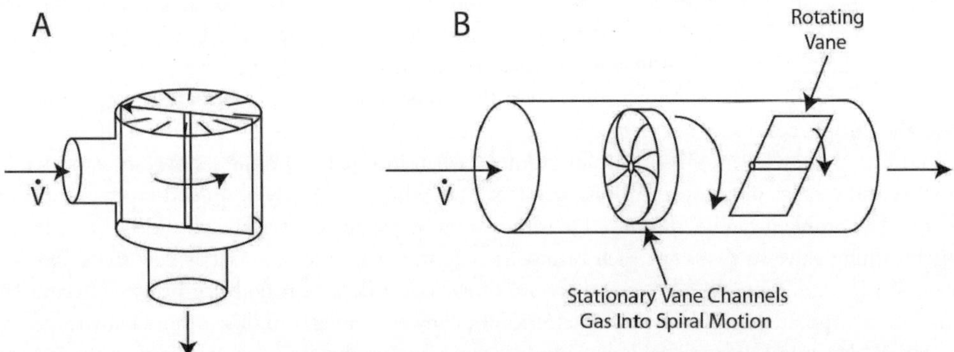


**Figure 3.8.** Sketch of two rotating vane flow sensors (variants of turbine flow sensors). (a) The design used in the Wright respirometer. This design has been extensively used for measuring exhaled volume. (b) The axial design includes a stationary device to impart a spiral motion to the gas flow upstream of the rotating vane. Both devices are unidirectional in design and are commonly used in anesthesiology.

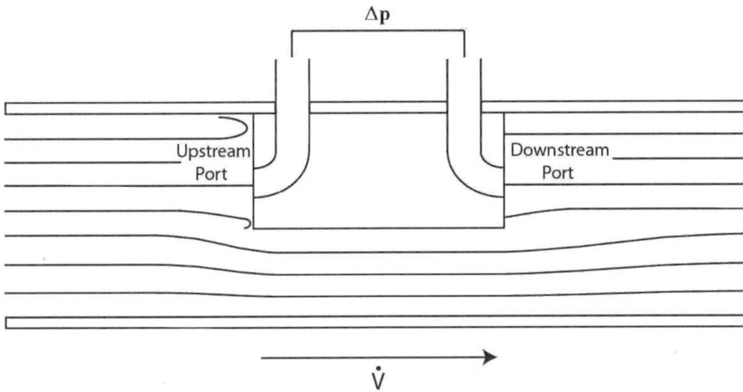



**Figure 3.9.** Schematic of the pitot tube flowmeter concept. The difference between the upstream and downstream pressures ($\Delta p$) is measured using a differential pressure transducer (see section 3.2.1). The pressure differential is given by equation 3.3.

## 3.2.5. VARIABLE ORIFICE FLOWMETERS

Variable orifice flowmeters represent another design that finds occasional use in situations not requiring a high degree of accuracy, such as anesthetic monitoring. The devices typically consist of a fixed orifice covered by a flexible plastic flap (Fig. 3.10). As flow increases, the flap opens. The $\Delta p$ across the orifice is then taken as an indication of the flow. The device characteristics depend critically on the orifice geometry and the mechanical properties of the flap itself. There are few theoretical methods to describe these devices, and calibration and characterization are achieved principally by empirical means. By design, the devices are unidirectional in nature.

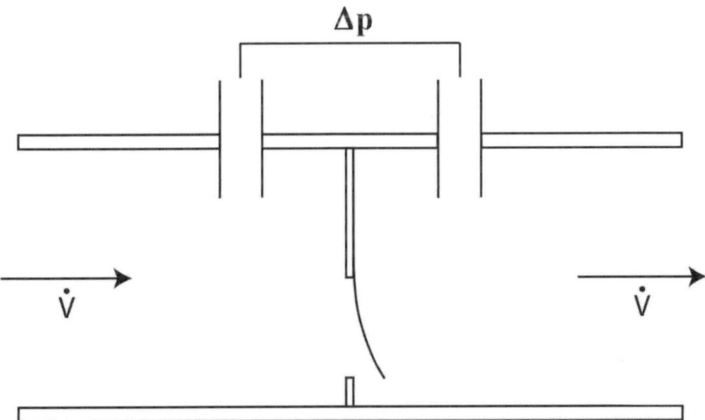



**Figure 3.10.** The concept of a variable orifice flowmeter. Gas flow pushes open the plastic flap to varying degrees. The $\Delta p$ across the flowmeter is used as an index of flow velocity (and thus flow).

The other common use of variable orifice design flowmeters is in home-use peak flow monitoring for asthma sufferers. Clinical experience has shown that when a patient suffers an asthma attack (characterized by a narrowing of the airways due to bronchoconstriction as their airway smooth muscle shortens and by increased mucus secretions within the airways), the peak expiratory flow the patient can produce from a forced expiration decreases. Variable orifice flowmeters have been developed in which the $\Delta p$ generated across the orifice is used to shift a mechanical pointer along a scale, giving the patient an indication of peak expiratory flow. These devices have become the standard of care in many regions of the world (less so in the United States than in Europe and Australasia), allowing patients to tailor their drug therapy to prevent or minimize their asthma attacks.

## 3.2.6. HOT-WIRE ANEMOMETERS

Hot-wire anemometers have been used quite extensively in respiratory flow measurement. The most common design involves a constant-temperature hot-wire element. Flow is determined based on the power needed to maintain an electrically heated wire inside the sensor head at a constant temperature in spite of the cooling effects of a moving gas. The loss of heat from the wire depends on the gas composition since different gases have different thermal conductivities. In some designs the thermal conductivity of the gas is taken into account by including a second hot-wire within the flowmeter head, allowing some degree of compensation for alterations in gas composition.

From a conceptual standpoint, these devices are attractive because they present virtually no impediment to flow and have a large dynamic range. A schematic of one design for a hot-wire anemometer is shown in Figure 3.11. In this design, a pair of tungsten sense wires surround the platinum flow-sensing wire, providing directional information.

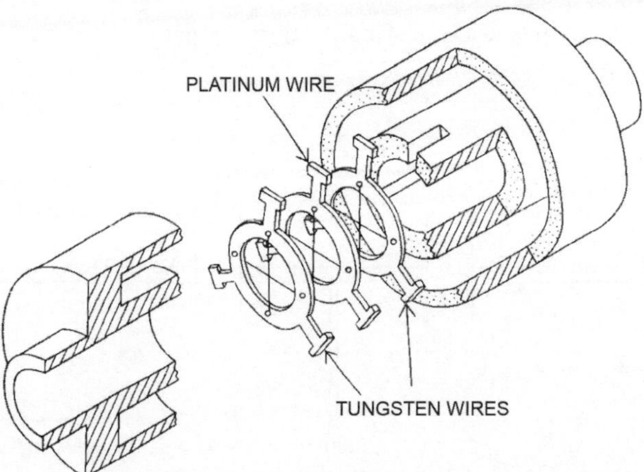



**Figure 3.11.** Schematic of a hot-wire anemometer incorporating three sensor wires. The constant-temperature platinum wire (heated to 375°C) measures flow. This is positioned between two tungsten wires that sense the heated gas after it flows over the platinum wire, giving flow direction information. Reproduced from "A Bidirectional Respiratory Flowmeter Using the Hot-wire Principle," by I. Yoshiya, T. Nakajima, I. Nagai, and S. Jitsukawa, 1975, *Journal of Applied Physiology, 38*(2), pp. 360–365, with permission.

Problems with hot-wire anemometers primarily center around sensitivity to gas composition (and, in particular, to the water vapor content of the gas, which changes greatly between inspiration and expiration; see section 3.1.2.2) and the highly nonlinear nature of the output of the device as a function of flow rate (Yoshiya et al., 1975; Yoshiya, Shimada, & Tanaka, 1979). The latter issue is of particular importance at low flow rates. Further, the theory behind the devices is not well understood and thus calibration strategies are largely empirical. Finally, the practical issue of fragility is a major problem. In order to have a rapid response the sense wire must have a very small thermal mass; as a consequence, it tends to be very fragile and prone to failure.

### 3.2.7. ULTRASONIC FLOWMETERS

More recently, ultrasonically based flowmeters have been developed. Like hot-wire anemometers, these have the advantage of providing little impediment to flow (in general the flow path is completely unobstructed). In addition, unlike the hot-wire design, there are no fragile wires in the flow path.

There are two basic designs for ultrasonic flowmeters: a continuous transmission phase-shift design and a pulsed time-of-flight design (Buess et al., 1986). A typical design uses frequencies in the 20 kHz to 30 kHz range with a pulse rate of approximately 500 Hz. The principle behind both designs is the same: for a situation in which the medium between a pair of ultrasonic transmit–receive pairs moves with a velocity $v$, the transmit–receive times for the upstream and downstream paths ($t_u$ and $t_d$) differ (see Fig. 3.12).

Figure 3.13 shows conceptual schematics of a phase-shift ultrasonic flowmeter and a time-of-flight flowmeter. In the phase-shift design, a continuous transmitted signal of frequency $f$ is produced by the transmit element and received at two equidistantly placed receivers, one upstream, the other down stream. The phase difference $\alpha$ between the two received signals is proportional to the difference in the transmit–receive times ($t_d - t_u$). From this, flow velocity $v$ can be calculated, assuming $L$ is the path length between the transmit–receive pairs, $c$ is the speed of sound in the medium, and $\phi$ is the angle between the signal path and the direction of flow:

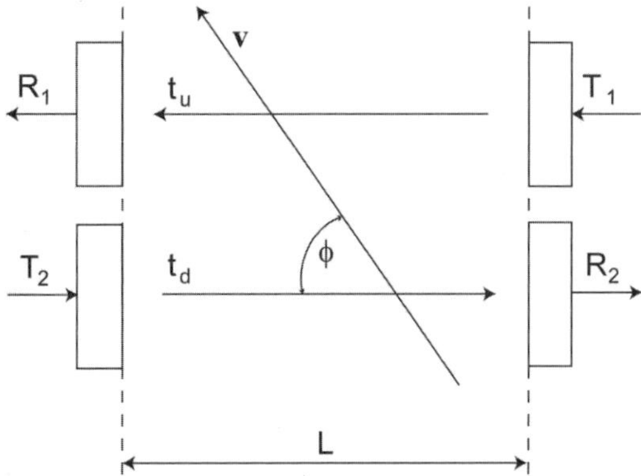


**Figure 3.12.** The fundamental measurement principle of an ultrasonic flowmeter. R: receiver; T: transmitter.

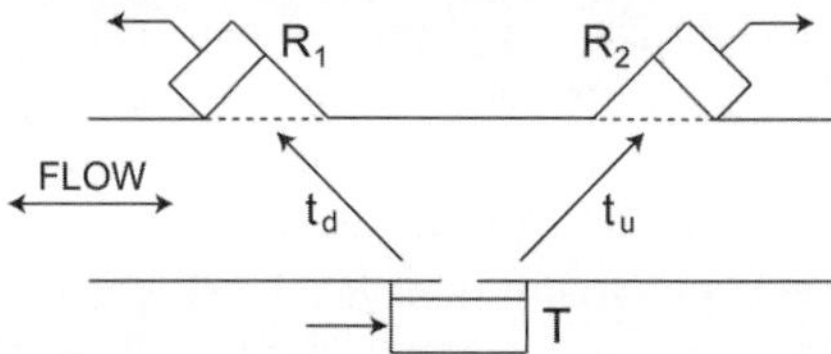


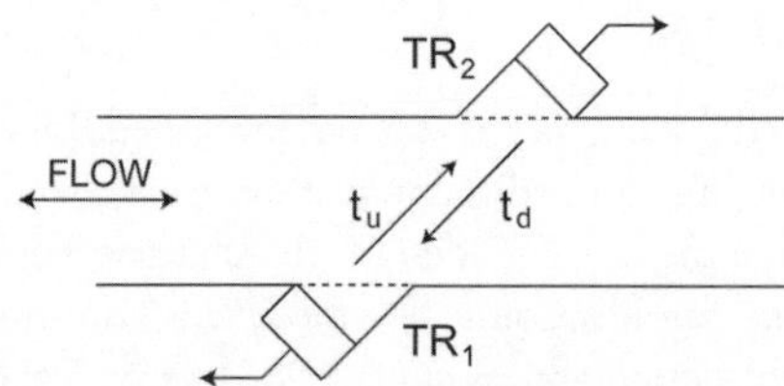


**Figure 3.13.** Representative configurations for a continuous wave phase-shift design (upper) and a pulsed time-of-flight design ultrasonic flowmeter (lower). R: receiver; T: transmitter.

$$\alpha = 2\pi f(t_d - t_u), \tag{3.4}$$

and so

$$\alpha = 4\pi f L v \cos(\phi)/[c^2 - v^2 \cos^2(\phi)], \tag{3.5}$$

and, assuming $v \ll c$,

$$\alpha = 4\pi f L v \cos(\phi)/c^2, \tag{3.6}$$

and so

$$v = \{c^2/[2L \cos(\phi)]\}[\alpha/2\pi f]. \tag{3.7}$$

Thus, in approximation, $v$ is proportional to the phase difference $\alpha$. However, in practice, difficulties with ambiguity in the phase shift (0° and 360° are indistinguishable) and with differences in the temperature of the gas within the flowmeter (gas temperature changes over the course of an expiration), which results in differences in the velocity of sound in the two different transmission paths, present problems.

In contrast to the phase-shift design, the pulsed time-of-flight design does not suffer from the problem of different measurement conditions over the two transmission paths because the paths are identical. In this design, short ultrasound pulses are simultaneously transmitted from both transducers, which then switch to receive mode. The system is then able to measure the difference between the upstream and downstream transmission times, providing flow velocity, and, based on the sign of the difference, flow direction. In the upstream direction the transit time is

$$t_u = L/[c + v \cos(\phi)], \tag{3.8}$$

where $L$ is the path length between the transmit–receive pair, $c$ is the speed of sound in the medium, $v$ the velocity of the medium, and $\phi$ is the angle between the signal path and the direction of flow. Similarly for the downstream direction,

$$t_d = L/[c - v \cos(\phi)]. \tag{3.9}$$

Given the equations for $t_u$ and $t_d$, the average flow velocity is then

$$v = [L/2 \cos(\phi)][t_d - t_u]/[t_d t_u]. \tag{3.10}$$

Note that this is a measure of the average flow over the transmission path. Of importance in understanding the behavior of a flowmeter of this design is understanding the effects of the flow profile within the device on the transmission times. If flow is laminar, then a parabolic profile is present (depending of course on upstream geometry leading to the flowmeter), and the average velocity registered will be approximately 1.33 times the actual average velocity of the gas (Plaut & Webster, 1980). If the flow rate is sufficiently high that flow is turbulent, then the flow is more uniform across the profile of the tube and the velocity registered by the device more closely approximates the true average velocity. However, such calculations are difficult to perform in practice because it is not entirely clear what the area of illumination of the ultrasonic pulses is across the tube.

A further parameter that can be derived from the time-of-flight design is the equivalent molecular weight of the gas, since the speed of sound in the gas depends on both temperature and molecular weight. Thus if the temperature of the gas is known, the average molecular weight of the gas can be determined. While the concept appears simple, in practice difficulties with temperature measurement in the face of ever-changing water vapor loads, the need to add a fragile, rapidly responding temperature sensor to the system, and the limited practicality of knowing the average molecular weight of the gas have all restricted the usefulness of this approach.

## 3.2.8. OTHER FLOW SENSORS

In addition to the measurement of respired flow covered in sections 3.2.1–3.2.7, there are common flow-sensing devices that are used to monitor the delivery of gases, especially in the field of inhalation anesthesia. While these do not strictly fall into the category of "respiratory flow sensors," it seems appropriate to provide brief comments on them in this chapter.

### 3.2.8.1. Rotameters

Rotameters are variable area flowmeters with a simple principle of operation: air flow passes through a vertical, tapered tube and pushes a ball or float having a diameter slightly less than the smallest diameter of the tube (Fig. 3.14). As the ball rises, the clearance between the ball and the tube wall increases. The ball becomes stationary when the diameter of the tube is large enough to allow the total air flow to move past the ball. The flow rate is determined by noting the position of the ball on an engraved scale on the tube. Because they are nonelectrical and relatively simple to manufacture, they have found wide use in areas such as inhalation anesthesia and in delivering varying levels of oxygen ($O_2$) and carbon dioxide ($CO_2$) during anesthesia, and they can be found in virtually any hospital. Because they are dependent on the gas characteristics for their operation, they are usually calibrated for a specific gas composition.

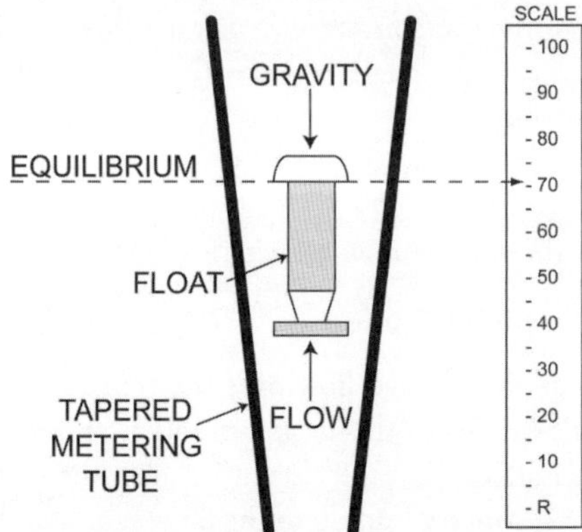


**Figure 3.14.** The concept of a rotameter. Flow up the tapered tube passes around the float. At equilibrium, the flow can be read from the scale. The devices are gas-composition specific.

### 3.2.8.2. Mass Flow Controllers

An electronic alternative to rotameters for the accurate delivery of gas are mass flow controllers. These have now become readily available and provide a means of accurately delivering a known mass of a specific gas via a delivery system. They are finding use in control systems in, for example, the study of ventilatory control and in the accurate delivery of known volumes (strictly masses) of gas to breathing systems, such as those used for the measurement of cardiac output. Because they are computer controlled they are ideal for automated or semiautomated systems. The concept is shown in Figure 3.15.

Gas enters the flow body and divides into two flow paths (see Fig. 3.15). Most of the flow goes through the laminar-flow bypass, creating a pressure drop that forces a known fraction of the flow through the sensor tube. In the sensor tube, two resistance temperature detector coils direct a constant amount of heat into the gas stream. Heat transfer between these elements results from interaction with

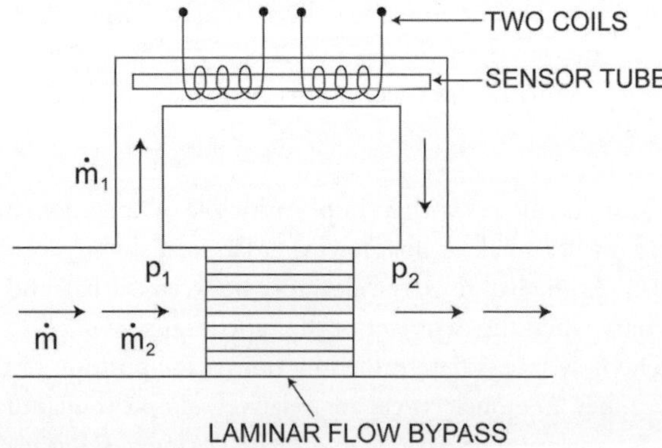


**Figure 3.15.** A schematic of a mass flow controller. The laminar flow element forces a known fraction of the flow through the sensor tube. Mass flow through the tube is inversely proportional to the temperature difference between the coils.

the molecules of the flowing gas, independent of pressure or temperature fluctuations. In operation, the mass flow of the gas carries heat from the upstream coil to the downstream coil. The downstream coil thus has a higher temperature and hence more resistance than the upstream coil. These coils form the legs of a bridge circuit with an output voltage proportional to the difference between the coils' resistances, which in turn is proportional to the mass flow rate in the capillary tube.

## 3.3. CALIBRATION

### 3.3.1. CALIBRATION STRATEGIES: FLOW VERSUS VOLUME

While it might seem obvious that calibration of a flowmeter should be done with a reference flow source, that procedure is, in practical terms, difficult to achieve. Generating a single calibrated flow rate source is not particularly difficult, but the practicalities of generating multiple calibrated flow rates is, in practice, very difficult. Further, while at times respiratory measurements are directly concerned with flow, they are more often focused on the measurement of volume by way of integrated flow. Fortunately it is a relatively simple matter to manufacture a volume displacement device with an accurate, reproducible, and known swept volume. Thus the majority of calibration strategies employ a fixed-volume syringe.

### 3.3.2. NONLINEARITIES

While all the flow sensors described in section 3.2 have some degree of nonlinearity and asymmetry to flow, the circumstances in which they are used provide a source of considerable difficulty in terms of calibration. There are no hard and fast rules for the geometry of tubing leading to the flow sensor head. However, unless the connecting tubing is straight, smooth walled, and of sufficient length (a rule of thumb is five times the diameter of the flow-sensing element), then the system geometry will influence the linearity and calibration of the system. It is often difficult, if not impossible, to satisfy flow condition requirements because the inclusion of such tubing into the system introduces dead space into that system. Often the only approach is to accept the nonlinearities in the system and characterize them.

#### 3.3.2.1. Bidirectional Calibration

Unless the upstream and downstream geometries of the plumbing leading to a flowmeter are identical, the output will almost certainly be asymmetrical. For this reason, calibration is often performed in such a way as to allow for separate calibration factors based on flow direction. Also, the issues of altered gas composition between inspiration and expiration (see section 3.1.2.2) contribute to the problems of asymmetry.

#### 3.3.2.2. Look-up Tables

With the now widespread use of computerized data acquisition systems, the use of look-up tables to linearize otherwise nonlinear and asymmetric flow sensors has become common. While numerous calibration strategies have been used over the years, one of the major advances was the technique developed by Yeh et al. (1982) permitting characterization of a flow sensor using only a calibrated syringe. By sampling many syringe strokes, each of differing average flow rate, a table describing the nonlinearity (and, if desired, the asymmetry) of a flowmeter can be established. Figure 3.16 shows such a table for a Fleisch pneumotachograph with and without an upstream linearizing screen.

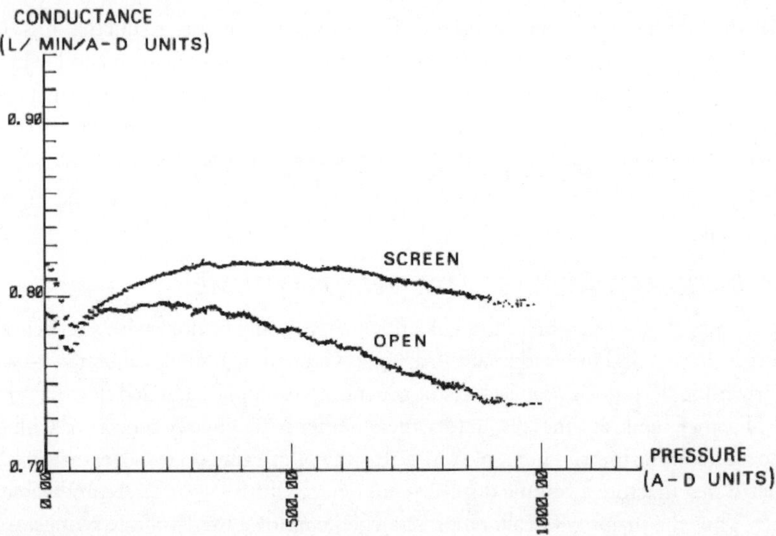


**Figure 3.16.** Conductance curves for a Fleisch pneumotachograph with and without an upstream linearizing screen. The difference emphasizes the importance of in situ calibration of respiratory flowmeters. Reproduced from "Computerized Determination of Pneumotachometer Characteristics Using a Calibrated Syringe," by M. P. Yeh, R. M. Gardner, T. D. Adams, and F. Yanowitz, 1982, *Journal of Applied Physiology, 53*, pp. 280–285, with permission.

The table shows the conductance of the flowmeter as a function of flow through it. A completely linear device would have a conductance curve that is straight and horizontal (corresponding to the slope of a perfectly linear conventional calibration curve). There is a marked difference in the shape of the conductance curve between the case with an upstream linearizing screen and an open Fleisch pneumotachograph, emphasizing the importance of characterizing the linearity of the flowmeter in situ. One advantage of this approach is that conductance curves have a tendency to move in parallel, so if measurement conditions change (e.g., because of a change in gas composition) recalibration simply involves determination of a new overall scaling factor as opposed to determination of the overall shape of the curve (Yeh et al., 1984).

## 3.3.3. DYNAMIC RESPONSE ISSUES

As alluded to several times before, the issue of dynamic response of the flowmeter may be important in respiratory flow because flow accelerations can occasionally be quite large. Several studies have extensively examined this matter, at least in relation to the Fleisch pneumotachograph (Finucane, Egan, & Dawson, 1972; Jackson & Vinegar, 1979; Proulx et al., 1979). It turns out that most of the important aspects of the dynamic response of the flowmeter result from the dynamics of the differential pressure transducer used and, importantly, the characteristics of the tubing between the flow sensing head and the pressure transducer. Once again this emphasizes the need for characterization of the particular system as opposed to some generalized solution.

### 3.3.3.1. Standardized Waveform Generators

The widespread use of forced spirometry has lead to the extensive development and publication of standards for the measurements inherent in the test both by the American Thoracic Society (American Thoracic Society, 1994) and by thoracic societies in other countries (Quanjer et al., 1993). These address the means by which flowmeters (and spirometers) should be tested, and now include twenty-four separate waveforms specifically designed to adequately test for the appropriate dynamic response of the flow instrument under test. Compliance with these guidelines goes a long way toward ensuring accurate calibration and setup of a flowmeter system for work in respiratory physiology.

### 3.3.4. BAG-IN-BOX SYSTEMS

As mentioned in the section on nonlinearities (section 3.3.2), flowmeters are sensitive to the geometry of the connecting tubing leading to them. One means by which long, straight, smooth-walled tubes can be utilized without adding large amounts of dead space to a system is through the use of a bag-in-box system. In this system the subject breathes from flexible bags contained within a box, the only outlet is via a flowmeter through which air is displaced as the bags in the box inflate or deflate. Because the subject is not breathing directly through the flowmeter, the addition of flow-conditioning tubes does not contribute to the dead space. Further, only dry air passes through the flowmeter, avoiding issues pertaining to water condensation and changes in gas composition. However, consideration of gas conditions (ATPS, BTPS) is still required. The use of such a method in a spaceflight experiment produced a system in which the cumulative error from twenty bidirectional strokes of a 1 L calibration syringe was only 16 ± 37 mL, an error of approximately 0.1% (Prisk et al., 1995), far beyond the level of accuracy the author could achieve using a breathe-through system. However, the disadvantages of such a system are the large volume of the box and a slower dynamic response (Bates et al., 1984), which is a function of box volume. Nevertheless, bag-in-box systems remain in use in certain circumstances when high accuracy is required.

## REFERENCES

American Thoracic Society. (1994). Standardization of spirometry, 1994 update. *American Journal of Respiratory and Critical Care Medicine, 152,* 1107–1136.

Bates, J. H. T., Prisk, G. K., Tanner, T. E., & McKinnon, A. E. (1984). Characterizing and correcting for the dynamic response of a bag-in-box system. *Journal of Applied Physiology, 56,* 254–258.

Buess, C., Pietsch, P., Guggenbuhl, W., & Koller, E. A. (1986). Design and construction of a pulsed ultrasonic air flowmeter. *IEEE Transactions on Biomedical Engineering, 33*(8), 768–774.

Finucane, K. E., Egan, B. A., & Dawson, S. V. (1972). Linearity and frequency response of pneumotachographs. *Journal of Applied Physiology, 32*(1), 121–126.

Fleisch, A. (1925). Der Pneumotachograph: ein Apparat zur Geschwindigkeits—registierung der Atemluft. *Pflugers Archives, 209,* 713–722.

Hyatt, R. E. (1983). Expiratory flow limitation. *Journal of Applied Physiology, 55,* 1–7.

Jackson, A. C., & Vinegar, A. (1979). A technique for measuring frequency response of pressure, volume, and flow transducers. *Journal of Applied Physiology, 47*(2), 462–467.

Plaut, D., & Webster, J. (1980). Ultrasonic measurement of respiratory flow. *IEEE Transactions on Biomedical Engineering, 27*(10), 549–558.

Prisk, G. K., Guy, H. J. B., Elliott, A. R., Paiva, M., & West, J. B. (1995). Ventilatory inhomogeneity determined from multiple-breath washouts during sustained microgravity on Spacelab SLS-1. *Journal of Applied Physiology, 78*, 597–607.

Proulx, P. A., Harf, A., Lorino, H., Atlan, G., & Laurent, D. (1979). Dynamic characteristics of air-filled differential pressure transducers. *Journal of Applied Physiology, 46*(3), 608–614.

Quanjer, P. H., Tammeling, G. J., Cotes, J. E., Pedersen, O. F., Peslin, R., & Yernault, J.-C. (1993). Lung volumes and forced ventilatory flows. Report Working Party. Standardization of lung function tests. *European Respiratory Journal, 6* (Suppl. 16), 5s–40s.

Spriggs, E. A. (1977). John Hutchinson, the inventor of the spirometer—His north country background, life in London, and scientific achievements. *Medical History, 21*, 357–364.

Spriggs, E. A. (1978). The history of spirometry. *British Journal of Diseases of the Chest, 72*, 165–180.

Yeh, M. P., Adams, T. D., Gardner, R. M., & Yanowitz, F. G. (1984). Effect of $O_2$, $N_2$, and $CO_2$ composition on nonlinearity of Fleisch pneumotachograph characteristics. *Journal of Applied Physiology, 56*, 1423–1425.

Yeh, M. P., Adams, T. D., Gardner, R. M., & Yanowitz, F. G. (1987) Turbine flowmeter vs. Fleisch pneumotachometer: A comparative study for exercise testing. *Journal of Applied Physiology, 63*(3), 1289–1295.

Yeh, M. P., Gardner, R. M., Adams, T. D., & Yanowitz, F. G. (1982). Computerized determination of pneumotachometer characteristics using a calibrated syringe. *Journal of Applied Physiology, 53*, 280–285.

Yernault, J. C. (1997). The birth and development of the forced expiratory manoeuvre: A tribute to Robert Tiffeneau (1910–1961). *European Respiratory Journal, 10*, 2704–2710.

Yoshiya, I., Nakajima, T., Nagai, I., & Jitsukawa, S. (1975). A bidirectional respiratory flowmeter using the hot-wire principle. *Journal of Applied Physiology, 38*(2), 360–365.

Yoshiya, I., Shimada, Y., & Tanaka, K. (1979). Evaluation of a hot-wire respiratory flowmeter for clinical applicability. *Journal of Applied Physiology, 47*, 1131–1135.

## ABOUT THE AUTHOR

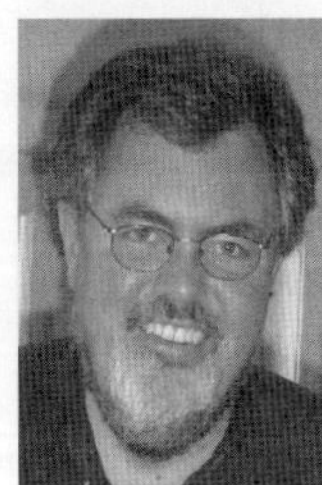

**Professor G. Kim Prisk**, PhD, DSc is a professor of medicine and radiology at the University of California, San Diego (UCSD). He received his PhD in respiratory physiology from the University of Otago, New Zealand in 1983, and since then has been at UCSD. He has studied the effects of gravity on the respiratory system, the deposition of aerosol in the human lung, and quantitative functional imaging of the lung. He has flown experiments on seven space shuttle flights and on the International Space Station. He has been active in developing several systems for studying pulmonary function in weightlessness. In 2003 he received a doctor of science degree from the University of Otago, New Zealand.

# CHAPTER 4

# Biomedical Sensors of Ionizing Radiation

Robert Speller, Alessandro Olivo, Silvia Pani, and Gary Royle

*Department of Medical Physics and Bioengineering*
*University College, London, UK*

## 4.1. BASIC REQUIREMENTS FOR SENSING IONIZING RADIATION

### 4.1.1. GENERAL INTRODUCTION

To understand the performance of a sensor or make a choice between different sensors for a detection task it is important to have an understanding of how the recorded signals are generated. In the case of sensing ionizing radiation, signals are generated after the incoming radiation has undergone interactions within the sensor material. The types of interactions and the subsequent resultant particles depend upon the type of incident radiation, its energy, and the material that makes up the sensing medium. This introductory section deals with these interactions and discusses the processes that lead to detectable signals.

There are many textbooks that deal with these aspects in depth. For more details than are given in this introductory section, the interested reader should consult Evans (1955), Heitler (1954), ICRU (1984, 1992), Kember (1994), Knoll (2000), and Smith (2000).

### 4.1.2. BASIC REQUIREMENTS

Table 4.1.1 lists the possible mechanisms for the detection of different radiations that are relevant to biomedical applications.

**Table 4.1.1.** Radiation types and the mechanisms for their detection

| | Classification | Type of radiation | Detection requirements |
|---|---|---|---|
| 1 | Electromagnetic | X-rays, γ-rays | Must interact to produce a directly ionizing particle. |
| 2 | Directly ionizing particles | α-particle, β-particle, protons | Energy is transferred to the detection medium through interactions with the electrons or nucleons of the medium. |
| 3 | Indirectly ionizing particles | Neutron | Must interact to produce a directly ionizing particle. |

Note that for all radiations, the only mechanism for detectable effects in a material is the transfer of energy to the medium.

From Table 4.1.1 it can be seen that unless incident energy is transferred first to ionizing particles and then to the detection medium, an event will not be sensed. It is therefore clear that if electromagnetic or indirectly ionizing radiations are to be detected, it is important that the detection material have a significant cross section for interaction with those radiations so that secondary, directly ionizing particles are produced. Directly ionizing particles will always interact with the detection medium. To maximize the detection probability, it is important that the resultant transfer of particle energy to some method of detection be as efficient as possible. There are two principal methods: chemical changes and collection or movement of charges. Chemical changes have been used in many imaging techniques, although modern methods are now based on the collection of charges. Most quantitative techniques are based on the collection or movement of charges.

If a charge is to be collected or its movement controlled and monitored, then a detector bias will be required. This collection or movement of charge represents the signal that will be used to register the detection of ionizing radiation. The relationship between how much charge is created, that is, the magnitude and development of the signal, and some property of the incident radiation (energy, particle type, location of the interaction, etc) is an important relationship. To understand this relationship it is essential to appreciate the details of how radiation interacts with the sensor material.

### 4.1.2.1. Sensor Materials

The material of which a sensor is made plays a significant role. Table 4.1.2 presents a range of materials and outlines the reasons why they make good choices as active components for sensors.

**Table 4.1.2.** Materials used in sensors for ionizing radiation

| Material | Applications |
|---|---|
| Argon | Fill gas for high-pressure gas detectors |
| BaF | A phosphor used in intensifying screens |
| CaW | A phosphor used in intensifying screens |
| CsI | A scintillator usually doped with Tl or Na |
| CdTe | A compound semiconductor used to make compact sensors |
| CdZnTe | An improved version of CdTe by the introduction of Zn to help with charge trapping |
| GaAs | |
| Ge | Used in high-quality spectroscopy systems for photons |

## 4.1.3. INTERACTIONS OF CHARGED PARTICLES

For the majority of interactions that are of interest in biomedical sensors for ionizing radiation, the interaction will be a Coulomb interaction between the incident charged particle and the electrons of the medium making up the active volume of the sensor. With this in mind, it is convenient to place these interactions into two categories:

1. Heavy charged particle interactions—protons, ions. In this case, the mass of the incident particle is far greater than the mass of the particle in the material. The form of energy transfer is restricted to multiple small depositions of energy and little change in the path of the incident particle (see Fig. 4.1.1).
2. Light charged particles—electrons, positrons. In this case, the mass of the incident particle matches that of the particle in the material. Energy transfers can be significant and will certainly cause large changes in the incident particle trajectory. Again, the total loss of particle energy will be made up of a very large number of individual interactions (see Fig. 4.1.1).

Other mechanisms of interaction are possible, but rarely have any relevance to the detection of ionizing radiation except in the case of neutron detection. One of the important characteristics of the mechanism of energy transfer is the distance travelled during this process. To discuss this property it is important to distinguish the distance travelled along the track (pathlength) and the distance that the particle penetrates into the material (range). There are a number of different definitions for range.

### 4.1.3.1. Particle Range

If the number of particles transmitted through a material, $N$, is counted in an experiment, as shown in Figure 4.1.2, then the plot of $N$ versus the thickness of the material, $x$, can be characterized by several parameters. The most important quantity is the mean range, $r_0$, the thickness to reduce the number of particles by half. The continuous curve plot in Figure 4.1.2 applies to heavy charged particles and exhibits a nearly constant fraction of transmission for a considerable thickness of material. For light charged particles (shown as the broken curve plot in Fig. 4.1.2), the tortuous path leads to a different

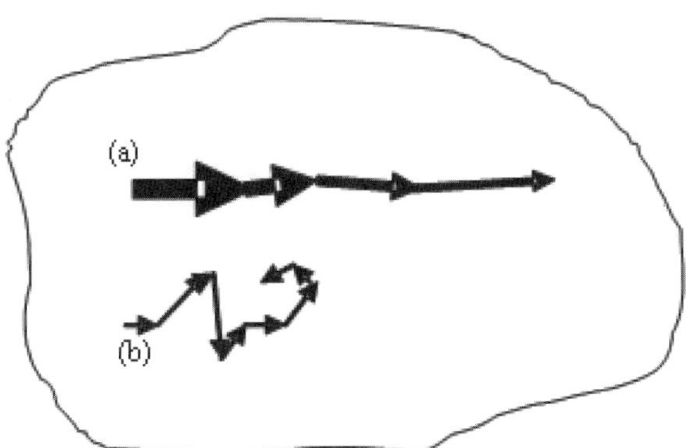


**Figure 4.1.1.** Particle tracks within the medium of a sensor. The heavy charged particle track (a) is almost straight, whereas the light charged particle (b) follows a very tortuous track.

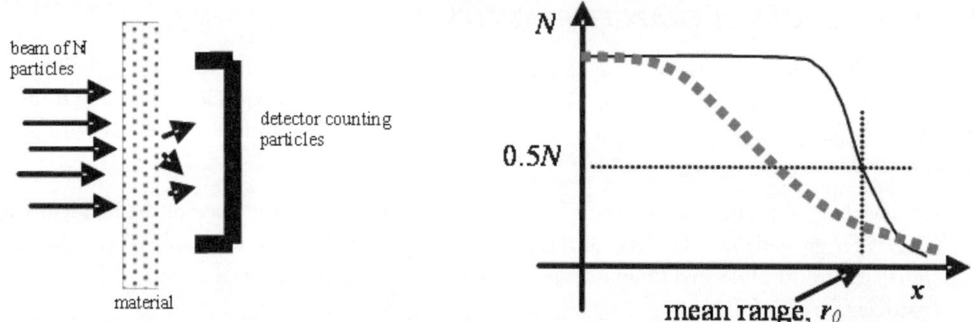



**Figure 4.1.2.** Experiment depicting a beam of particles passing through a material of thickness *x*. The detector used in this experiment is able to count the number of particles transmitted, *N*.

shape for the transmission curve. However, the same definition of mean range can be applied. Typical values for $r_0$ are given in Table 4.1.3.

### 4.1.3.2. Relevance of Particle Range in Selecting a Sensor

When selecting a sensor it is important that the thickness or volume of the sensor is large enough to ensure that most, if not all of the energy associated with an ionizing photon or particle is deposited within the active part of the sensor. Clearly the range of the incident particle or the secondary electrons created by an incident photon plays an important role in selecting the thickness. In general, if photons are being detected, the major consideration for the detector volume is to provide enough material to ensure that the probability of interaction is acceptably high. Any volume chosen on this basis will be more than sufficient to cover the range of the secondary charged particles, particularly in a solid-state detector material. However, particle beams can use much smaller volumes for detection, as can be seen from Table 4.1.3.

### 4.1.3.3. Collisional and Radiative Energy Transfer

Energy loss mechanisms within a medium can be split into two broad categories: *radiative*, where energy is transferred to electromagnetic radiation, and *collisional*, where the transferred energy creates excitations and ionizations of the medium. Radiative loss is only significant for energetic electrons

**Table 4.1.3.** Range values for different sensor materials for electrons of different energies

| Energy (keV) | Carbon | Silicon | Germanium | Cesium Iodide (CsI) | Sodium Iodide (NaI) | Photoemulsion |
|---|---|---|---|---|---|---|
| 10 | 1.66 | 1.49 | 0.92 | 1.39 | 1.53 | 1.22 |
| 100 | 94.2 | 78.2 | 44.7 | 60.2 | 69.2 | 58.8 |
| 1000 | 2920 | 2312 | 1230 | 1605 | 1879 | 1650 |

All values are in micrometers.

Data from ICRU Report 37 (1984).

passing through high atomic number materials. Since most biomedical sensing applications involve relatively low-energy secondary charged particle creation, collisional losses are the major mechanism for transferring energy to the material of the sensor. The rate at which energy is transferred as the particle moves through the sensor is another important property of the particle and the medium that makes up the sensor. This quantity is called the stopping power.

### 4.1.3.4. Stopping Power and Its Relevance to Selecting a Sensor

Stopping power $\left(dE/ds\right)$ is defined as the rate of energy loss per unit path length, $s$. Developing a theoretical model to describe this process has been successfully undertaken for both classical as well as quantum mechanical approaches. The quantum mechanical result is often referred to as the Bethe equation and is given as

$$dE/ds = \frac{4\pi r_e^2 mc^2}{u}\frac{\rho}{\beta^2}\frac{Z}{A}z^2\left[\ln\left(\frac{2mc^2\beta^2}{\left(1-\beta^2\right)I}\right)-\beta^2\right]$$

for heavy charged particles and

$$dE/ds = \frac{2\pi r_e^2 mc^2}{u}\frac{\rho}{\beta^2}\frac{Z}{A}\left[\ln\left(T/I\right)^2 + \ln\left(1+\tau/2\right)+F^-\left(\tau\right)-\delta\right]$$

for electrons. Here, $r_e$ is the classical radius of the electron and $\beta$ is the ratio of the particle velocity to the speed of light. Also in these equations, $u$ is the atomic mass unit, $Z$ is the atomic number of the medium, $A$ is the atomic weight, $I$ is the mean excitation energy (describing the average energy lost to the medium at each Coulomb interaction), $T$ is the kinetic energy of the incident particle, and $\tau = T/(mc^2)$. $\delta$ is a correction for the so-called density effect, and $F$ is a factor that allows for the difference in behavior between electrons and positrons. All quantities in the square brackets are slowly changing functions of energy, and hence the major behavior is governed by the nonconstant values in front of the square brackets. It can be seen that for both heavy charged particles and electrons, the rate of loss of energy per unit path length is proportional to $\rho\left(\dfrac{z}{v}\right)^2$, where $z$ is the charge on the particle (1 for electrons), $v$ is the velocity of the particle, and $\rho$ is the density.

### 4.1.3.5. Bragg Curve

One of the effects of the dependence of stopping power on particle velocity is that energy loss is not uniformly distributed along the path length, but is much less when the particle first moves through the material than when it is near the end of its path. This observation, shown graphically in Figure 4.1.3, is called the Bragg curve. Note that if all the energy associated with an event is to be deposited within a given sensor, it is most important that the end of the Bragg curve be included, as this may constitute a significant proportion of the total energy.

### 4.1.3.6. Minor Effects of Charged Particle Interactions

There are several interesting features of charged particle interactions that occur at low energies. As particles (primary events or secondary charged particles) lose energy along their path, a point will come

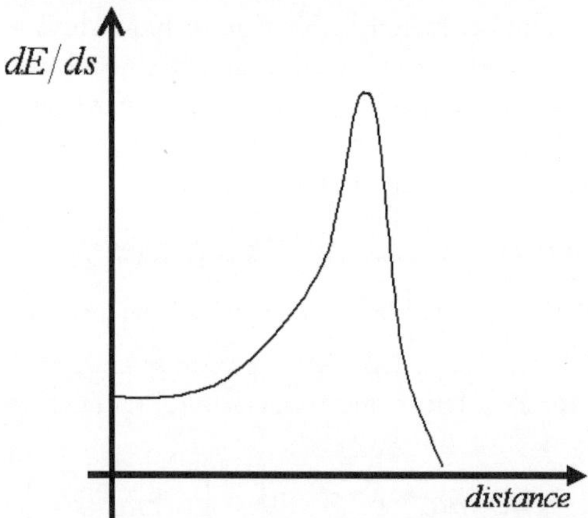



**Figure 4.1.3.** The Bragg curve for a heavy charged particle. Electrons do not exhibit such a pronounced peak in the Bragg curve because of their tortuous path.

when their energy is either insufficient to ionize atoms effectively or their velocity becomes comparable to the orbital velocity of the atomic electrons in the medium of the sensor. Both of these will affect the total charge created by an event. The results of these effects are discussed in the appropriate sections on dosimetry.

### 4.1.3.7. Summary of Charged Particle Interactions

The following are important points:

- Ionizing radiation can only be detected or sensed by the effects of charged particle interactions.
- If the radiation to be detected is electromagnetic (X- or $\gamma$-rays), then the energy associated with the quanta must first be converted to charged particles—generally electrons or positrons in the case of biomedical applications.
- Important parameters such as range and stopping power (and to a lesser extent the Bragg curve) contribute to the choice of a suitable material for a sensor.
- For biomedical applications, charged particles will travel only short distances within a sensor material.

## 4.1.4. INTERACTIONS OF X- AND GAMMA RAYS

X- and gamma rays are part of the electromagnetic spectrum and are generally referred to as photons, so it is assumed that most of their behavior is best described by particle-like characteristics. This is true for the important interactions insofar as biomedical sensors are concerned. In biomedical applications, the energy range of interest is usually from 1 keV to 25 MeV, and within this range there are four processes by which the photon can interact. Some, but not all, of these processes result in the creation of secondary charged particles that can lead to detection of the photon.

When a beam of many photons enters a material, some of the photons will be transmitted and some will interact. This process is described by considering the *absorption* and *scattering* of the beam leading to the concept of *attenuation*. If the material being considered is a sensor, then the attenuation provided by the sensor will lead to the concept of efficiency, usually referred to as *quantum efficiency*. Consider the sensor in Figure 4.1.4. The incident beam provides an intensity (energy passing through unit area in unit time) of $I_0$. Some of the photons in the beam do not interact in the sensor and pass through as intensity $I$. Some interact and deposit all their energy in the sensor. Others interact and may or may not deposit some energy in the sensor, but will have their direction of travel changed and thus become scattered photons. An ideal sensor has properties that produce no transmitted beam, with all the scattered photons being reabsorbed within the sensor. This would lead to 100% quantum efficiency if all the deposited energy could be measured.

Transmitted and incident intensity are related by $I = I_0 e^{-\mu x}$, where $\mu$ is the total linear attenuation coefficient of the sensor material and $x$ is the thickness. Note that this relation does not describe the level of scattered radiation. However, it is clear that thick, large-volume sensors decrease the level of both transmitted and scattered radiation and increase the quantum efficiency. To fully understand the different contributions to the energy deposited in the sensor, and hence its output, it is necessary to consider the different types of interactions. For each interaction type there are two aspects to consider. First, the energetics of the interaction; that is, if an interaction takes place, what actually happens? Second, a discussion about the factors that govern the probability of the interaction taking place.

### 4.1.4.1. Photoelectric Interaction

#### 4.1.4.1.1. Energetics of Photoelectric Interactions

When an incident photon interacts with a bound electron in the sensor material, the energy associated with that photon is transferred to the electron. This energy is used to overcome the binding energy so as to eject the electron. The ejected electron, known as a photoelectron, has energy equal to the incident photon energy minus the binding energy it had when in the atomic structure. This energetic secondary electron loses energy, as described in section 4.1.3. The atom from which the electron has been removed is unstable, having an inner shell electron missing, and so rearranges its electron structure to maintain stability. This is achieved by an electron from another shell or subshell moving

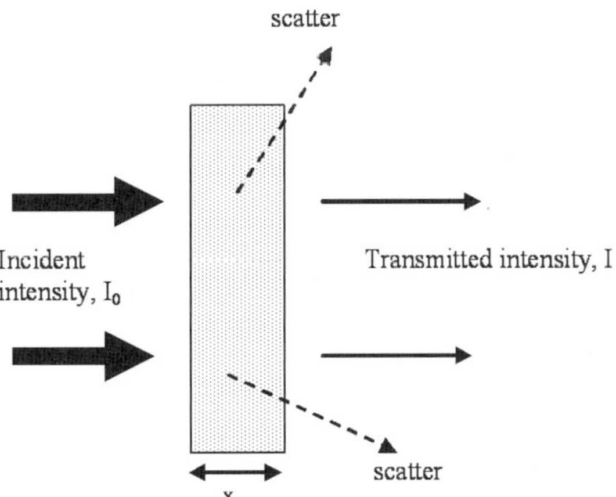


**Figure 4.1.4.** A sensor irradiated by photons of intensity $I_0$, creating both a transmitted beam as well as scattered photons.

into the vacancy: this move is governed by quantum mechanical selection rules. The result of this rearrangement means that further energy becomes available when the energy of the electron states is taken into account. This energy can either give rise to a characteristic X-ray (usually the case when the nucleus of the atom concerned has a high atomic number) or an Auger electron. An Auger electron is an intershell vacancy transfer that is produced when the energy made available is given directly to one of the outer shell electrons, causing it to be ejected by the atom. Since most sensors are made of high-$Z$ materials (see Table 4.1.2), characteristic X-ray generation is the most likely outcome of a photoelectric interaction in the sensor. In order for all the energy associated with the photon to be captured within the sensor, it means that either these characteristic X-rays must be stopped in the sensor or the result of the primary interaction must be to produce an Auger electron. If neither of these conditions is met, then only part of the energy will be deposited.

The effects of this are most significant when considering spectroscopy (see section 4.4). If all the energy is left in the sensor, the signal generated will be directly related to the incident photon energy. It is worth noting that as characteristic photons are created in high-$Z$ materials, they are not likely to travel great distances in such a material. Furthermore, if the interaction is in a low $Z$ material, the "excess" energy appears as an Auger electron. Thus, whether the interaction is in a high or low $Z$ material, the secondary radiations are quickly stopped. This often leads to the assertion that, provided the volume of the material in which a photoelectric interaction takes place is on the order of a few cubic millimeters, the photoelectric interaction is one of total absorption. However, this statement should not be interpreted to say that a sensor needs to be only a few cubic millimeters in volume to be an effective detector.

### 4.1.4.1.2. Probability of Interaction

Theoretical descriptions of the photoelectric interaction can be used to develop the dependence of the interaction upon the atomic number of the sensor medium $Z$, the incident photon energy $E$, and the physical density of the sensor medium $\rho$. For the energy range of interest in biomedical sensors, the relationship is often simplified as $\tau \propto \dfrac{Z^3}{E^3}\rho$, where $\tau$ is the photoelectric linear attenuation coefficient (the probability that a photoelectric interaction will take place per unit thickness of the sensor material). In practice, noninteger powers are required that also have a dependence on $E$ and $Z$ (White, 1977). Clearly, if the probability increases, then so does the quantum efficiency of the sensor. It can be seen that higher-$Z$ materials and materials with high density will produce a high probability of interaction, and hence detection. It is also clear that lower energy photons are easier to detect.

The relationship given in the previous paragraph for $\tau$ is true for the interaction of an incident photon and a given shell or subshell electron that takes part in the interaction. When interactions from a beam of photons of differing energies are considered, the effect of *absorption edges* must be taken into account. Figure 4.1.5 plots the value of $\tau/\rho$ for different sensor materials over the energy range of 10 keV to 100 keV. These data have been taken from XCOM (see http://www.nist.gov). The effects of absorption edges are clear in this figure. Silicon (Si) and germanium (Ge) have similar values of $\tau/\rho$ at 10 keV, but because of the absorption edge for Ge at 11 keV, Ge has a value of $\tau/\rho$ an order of magnitude greater above 11 keV. Similar effects can be noticed for CsI above 35 keV. The performance of a sensor can be significantly altered by the presence or otherwise of an absorption edge; hence, for increased sensitivity it is always advisable to choose a sensor material with an absorption edge below the photon energy to be detected.

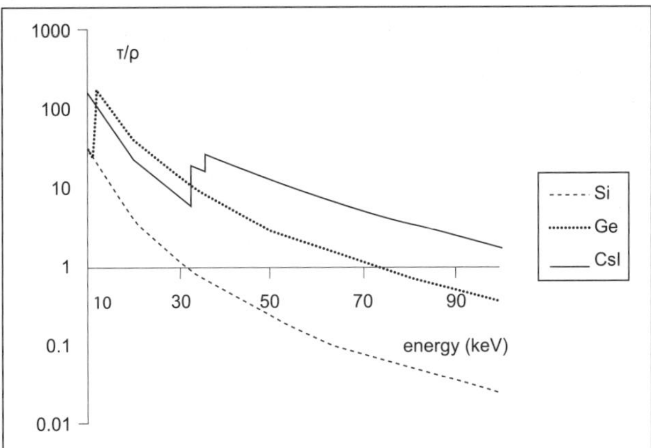


**Figure 4.1.5.** Photoelectric attenuation data demonstrating the increase in probability at particular energies. These are called absorption edges. Data taken from XCOM (http://www.nist.gov).

## 4.1.4.2. Rayleigh Scattering

Rayleigh scattering is an interaction process whereby no energy is deposited in the material and hence, in itself, does not allow a photon event to be detected. However, it can play an important role if absolute measurements of event rates are to be determined because it will need to be taken into account in any such measurement.

## 4.1.4.3. Compton Effect

### 4.1.4.3.1. Energetics of Compton Scattering

Compton scattering is an inelastic scattering process whereby a photon loses part of its energy to the medium of the sensor and the reduced energy photon is scattered in a new direction. For this event to take place, the incident photon energy must significantly exceed the binding energy of the electron in the medium. This condition is satisfied in many sensor materials for incident photons greater than 50 keV, and above this energy, this will become significant. The process is usually described as a "billiard ball" type of collision, where the incident photon, energy $E$, scatters off the atomic electron at an angle $\phi$. The scattering event imparts energy $T$ to the electron, which leaves in some direction $\theta$. There are various relationships that can be derived from these energetics, but for understanding the performance of a sensor, the most important is that $E = T + E'$, where $E'$ is the scattered photon energy. This simple result indicates that not all the incident photon energy is deposited in the medium. If $E'$ is significant, the scattered photon may have sufficient energy to leave the volume of the sensor. Under these conditions only part of the incident photon energy is recorded. This can have two consequences. It may mean that insufficient energy is deposited for the event to be recognized above the noise of the system, or, if spectroscopy is to be undertaken, the event will be registered with the wrong energy.

### 4.1.4.3.2. Probability of Compton Scattering

Theoretical understanding of the Compton interaction was developed by Klein and Nishina (1929). Their work developed differential collision and scattering cross sections that must be integrated to obtain Compton attenuation coefficients. The result of these integrations is that $\sigma \propto f(E)\rho$, where $\sigma$ is the linear Compton attenuation coefficient, $\rho$ is the physical density of the sensor medium, and $f(E)$ is a function that describes the variation of $\sigma$ with $E$. $f(E)$ is a slowly varying function of $E$, falling faster as $E$ increases. Up to values of 100 keV it is often assumed to take on a constant value of approximately $0.2\,\rho\ \text{cm}^{-1}$ when $\rho$ is measured in grams per cubic centimeter ($\text{g cm}^{-3}$). This simplification can be useful to estimate the sensor thickness required to ensure adequate quantum efficiency.

### 4.1.4.4. Pair Production

#### 4.1.4.4.1. Energetics of Pair Production

Pair production is an event that only occurs at incident photon energies in excess of 1.02 MeV. The process involves the incident photon energy being converted into matter within the favorable conditions offered by the electrostatic force of the nucleons. This force is sensed close to the nucleus and its magnitude can be modified by inner shell electron effects in large, complicated nuclei. The conversion into matter requires at least sufficient rest mass energy to create the resultant particles. At energies in the biomedical range of interest, this means the creation of an electrically neutral pair of low-mass particles, that is, an electron and a positron. Each has a rest mass energy of 0.511 MeV, hence the threshold for this effect to be observed is 1.02 MeV. Energy in excess of this threshold is divided approximately equally between the particles. Both particles move off through the medium, undergoing Coulomb interactions and losing energy, as described in section 4.1.3. At very low, almost zero energy there is a marked difference in the behavior of the electron and positron. The electron takes up a position in the outer shell of an atom. The positron, on the other hand, does not exist naturally and is annihilated with an electron in the medium, turning matter back into energy. If the positron had effectively zero kinetic energy, and likewise the electron with which it is annihilated, the result of the annihilation is two 0.511 MeV photons traveling in opposite directions. These are relatively energetic photons and therefore have a finite probability of escaping the confines of the detector. If this is the case, their energy will not be deposited within the detector, affecting the magnitude of any detected signal.

#### 4.1.4.4.2. Probability of Interaction

Theoretical models developed to study the pair production interaction draw parallels with those describing the photoelectric interaction. In the case of the photoelectric interaction, an electron (the photoelectron) is ejected from a positive energy state. In the case of pair production, the electron is ejected from a negative energy state. This gives rise to the electron, and the vacancy left in the negative energy state appears as a positron in the laboratory frame of reference. Hence the pair is produced. This allows the interaction to be handled in a similar way to the photoelectric interaction. The result is that $\kappa \propto Z\rho\ln E$, where $\kappa$ is the probability of pair production per unit thickness of material, $\rho$ is the physical density of the material, and $E$ is the incident photon energy. It is important to note that as the energy increases, so does the probability of interaction. Clearly high $Z$ and high $\rho$ will increase the quantum efficiency of a detector in this energy range.

### 4.1.4.5. Summary of Photon Interactions

The following points are most important to remember:

- Detection of photons requires conversion of the photon into charged particles. Thus only those interactions that create charged particles are useful for event detection.

- Only if all the photon energy is converted to charged particles can the energy of the photon be determined.
- Secondary photons that escape the detector reduce the detected signal.
- Photoelectric interactions provide the best opportunity for full energy deposition.
- Too many Compton interactions generally lead to poor detector performance.
- Combining all the interactions that can take place gives the overall energy response that can be expected from a given sensor material.

## 4.1.5. NEUTRON INTERACTIONS

### 4.1.5.1. Energetics of Neutron Interactions

There are three possible mechanisms for neutron interactions:

- The neutron is scattered by the nuclear potential of the medium through which it is passing (*direct scattering*).
- The neutron enters the nucleus to form a compound nucleus and the subsequent deexcitation can be either *elastic* (a neutron of the same energy is emitted), *inelastic* (a neutron of lower energy and one or more gamma rays or particles are emitted), or *radiative* (only gamma rays are emitted, often leaving an unstable nucleus that will decay).
- Breakup of the nucleus can occur at very high energies—this is not relevant to biomedical sensors.

Of these, the most useful for neutron detection are reactions such as (n,α) and (n,p), where part of the neutron energy is converted to heavy charged particles. Reactions leaving gamma rays are not so useful because the gamma rays can be difficult to detect due to their energies. These reactions only occur at "slow" neutron energies (i.e., less than 0.5 eV), so it is often necessary to slow down (moderate) higher energy neutrons using hydrogenous materials.

### 4.1.5.2. Probability of Interaction

Entering a nucleus to form a compound nucleus is a resonance phenomenon that occurs with greater probability when the incident neutron energy matches the rest-mass energy plus the excitation energy of one of the resonance states. Outside this region it can be shown that $\sigma_{n,\gamma}(E) \propto \dfrac{1}{v}$, where $\sigma_{n,\gamma}$ is the probability that radiative capture will take place and $v$ is the velocity of the incident neutron.

## 4.1.6. EFFECTS OF INTERACTIONS ON SENSOR OPERATION

The output from a sensor is governed by the mechanisms that have deposited energy within the sensor volume. Whether the primary radiation consists of charged particles or electromagnetic radiation, interactions within the sensor create further charged particles that are then responsible for forming the signal. This process of forming the detector response can be chemical or a mechanism to either directly or indirectly sense the charge. If quantitative estimates of the energy deposited are required, then important parameters need to be considered. The amount of energy it takes to create ionization describes the *ionization potential* of the sensor material. The *average* energy required to form an ion pair or charge pair is usually the most relevant parameter when considering how the detected signal might be used in dosimetry. This quantity is usually called the *W*-value in gases or the *w*-value in semiconductor materials.

### 4.1.6.1. Ion Pair or Electron-Hole Creation

An important parameter when selecting a sensor is how much energy, on average, is required to produce an ion or charge pair. Knowledge of this quantity is essential in dosimetry, but it also dictates the statistical precision with which the event can be characterized. This translates into the energy resolution in spectroscopy and the low contrast performance of imaging detectors.

A further effect to be considered is when light charged particles are responsible for creating the sensor response (as in most cases). The value of $w$ (or $W$) changes as the charged particle energy falls to low values (because there is a greater probability of creating excitation rather that ionization) and hence needs to be considered.

### 4.1.6.2. Charge Collection

Sensors whose output depends upon charge collection can usually be operated in one of two basic configurations: integrating or pulse mode. In an integrating detector, the total charge created by all events that occur in the detector in a given time is summed to form the output. Thus instantaneous evaluation of this current gives an output expressed as a rate (e.g., dose rate or exposure rate). In pulse mode, the charge associated with each event is recorded.

Charge is collected by forming an electric field gradient within the sensor and allowing the charge to drift under its influence. Alternatively, and sometimes in conjunction with drift, a potential well is created within the sensor to hold charge within a region. If operating with drift, at the point when the ion or charge pair is formed, the positive and negative components induce signals on the anode and cathode of the sensor. If operated in pulse mode, the rates at which the charges drift to their respective electrodes create the temporal response of the sensor. If operated in integrating mode, a near steady state of charge flow is set up, and only at the start and finish of the total exposure are any effects due to drift differences noticeable.

The shape of the electric field distribution within the sensor is critical to the detector output. In some gas detectors (ion chambers, for example) a uniform electric field strength is desirable. On the other hand, the rapidly changing electric field strength inside a Geiger-Mueller tube or proportional counter enables the moving charge to gain energy, create further charge through collisions, and hence increase the output of the sensor. This increase can either be controlled and predictable (proportional gas counter) or in the form of an avalanche (Geiger-Mueller). Similar considerations apply to solid-state detectors, although only recently have multiplying effects within the sensor been used. Generally, uniform fields are used to maintain good charge collection efficiency, leading to excellent spectroscopic performance.

### 4.1.6.3. Photon Counting, Spectroscopy, and Integration

If the sensor signal is derived from the collection of charge, then the signal processing electronics as well as the electrical characteristics of the sensor govern the final signal used to derive the output (see Fig. 4.1.6). Processing electronics with a fast time constant ($R \times C$) compared to the charge collection time within the sensor can effectively follow the temporal development of the charge in the sensor.

Alternatively, a long time constant allows the full charge packet associated with the event to be presented to the electronics before any part of the signal transits through any processing stages. The former case is called an integrating system and the latter is called a pulse counting or photon counting

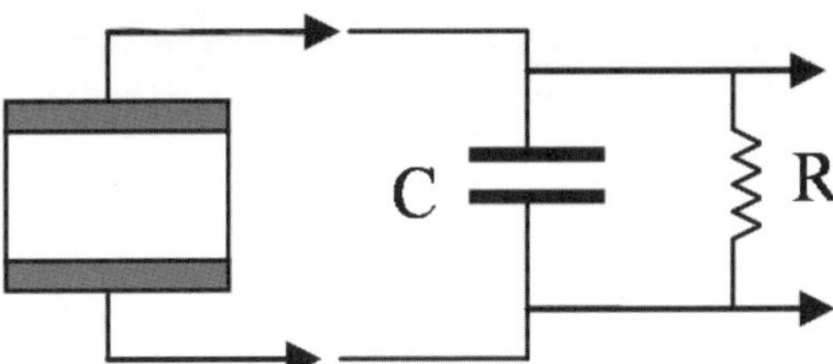

**Figure 4.1.6.** Schematic diagram of a sensor and processing electronics. The value of $C$ includes any capacitance associated with the sensor. The output of the sensor appears as a voltage across the load resistance $R$.

system. The temporal responses are shown in Figure 4.1.7. The total deposited energy is converted to charge, as described in sections 4.1.3 to 4.1.5. This charge forms an instantaneous current $i(t)$ that is presented to the processing electronics. Two cases are shown for the output from the processing electronics, where the value of the time constant is short or long compared to the time to collect charge, $t_c$. When $RC \gg t_c$ it is possible to relate the value of $V_{max}$ to the total energy deposited in the sensor. If the sensor is carefully chosen, this value should represent the total energy of the event.

## 4.1.7. DEFINITION OF QUANTITIES RELATED TO RADIATION DOSIMETRY

Since the beginning of research in both radiotherapy and X-ray imaging, an attempt has been made to identify quantities that could be related to the risk for the patient and to develop methods for

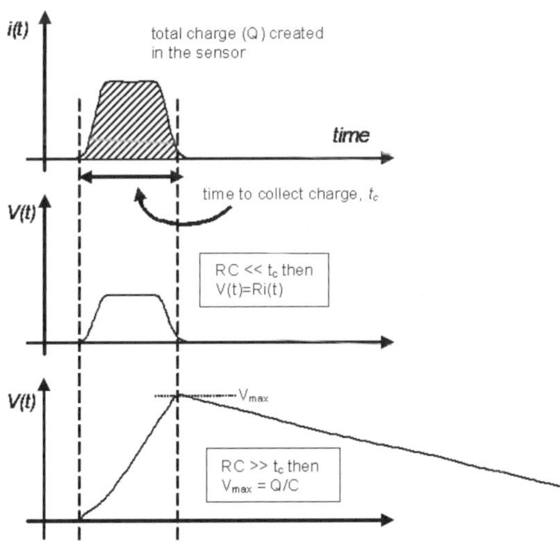


**Figure 4.1.7.** The top figure represents the current flowing in the sensor during the charge collection period. The other graphs show the output from the processing electronics with different values of $RC$.

measuring them. Delivered dose—the energy imparted per unit mass—is currently believed to be the most effective quantity for estimating patient risk. The need for high-precision dosimetry is particularly relevant in radiotherapy, the goal of which is to maximize the damage to the neoplastic tissue while minimizing the damage to healthy tissue.

It is well known that tumor control probability (TCP) and normal tissue complication probability (NTCP) are both increasing functions of the delivered dose, but they have different increase rates, the slope being steeper for normal tissue (AAPM, 2004), as shown in Figure 4.1.8. A correct estimation of the delivered dose is therefore crucial for effective tumor control without severely damaging healthy tissue. An underestimation of delivered dose can result in a complete control of the tumor, but also in damage to normal tissue, while an overestimation of the delivered dose can result in inadequate tumor control.

As for imaging dosimetry, there are less stringent guidelines stating that the delivered dose to the patient must be kept "as low as reasonably achievable" (ALARA), but correct dosimetry can still be of crucial importance because of the risk of radiation-induced carcinogenesis. This is particularly the case in screening procedures, such as mammography, aimed at identifying lesions in asymptomatic and thus potentially healthy subjects. In such cases the risk of the procedure has to be carefully balanced against the expected benefits.

This section focuses mainly on photon and electron radiotherapy dosimetry and on diagnostic dosimetry, although some applications to other fields, such as environmental dosimetry, will occasionally be mentioned. The main quantities of dosimetric interest will be introduced and the main requirements for dosimetric measurements will be discussed.

### 4.1.7.1. Quantities of Dosimetric Interest

#### 4.1.7.1.1. Photon Fluence and Energy Fluence

Photon fluence is a measure of the number of photons impinging on a unit area. The definition of photon fluence (ICRU, 1980) is

$$\Phi = \frac{dN}{da},\qquad(4.1.1)$$

where $dN$ is the number of photons incident on a sphere of cross-sectional area $da$.

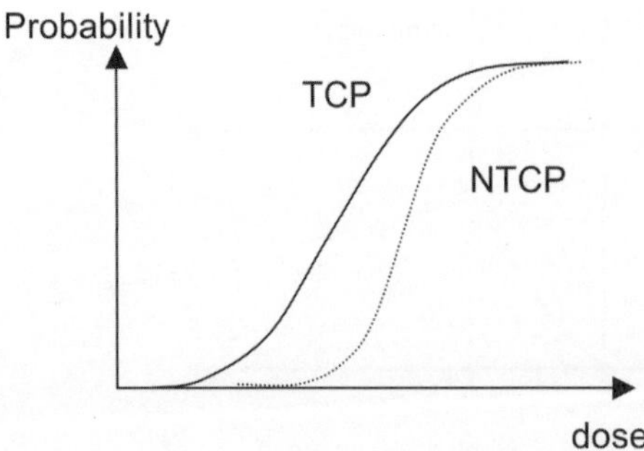


**Figure 4.1.8.** Tumor control probability (TCP) and normal tissue complication probability (NTCP) as a function of dose.

A quantity related to photon fluence is energy fluence, which is defined in a similar way as

$$\Psi = \frac{dR}{da},$$

(4.1.2)

where $dR$ is the radiant energy entering a sphere of cross-sectional area $da$ (ICRU, 1980).

### 4.1.7.1.2. Exposure

Since the earliest interest in dosimetric issues, it appeared a good idea to measure a beam by the charge it created in a medium. In particular, the first dosimetric quantity—exposure—was related to the charge released in air. This was convenient because air, with an atomic number of 7.6, is a tissue equivalent (tissue has an atomic number of 7.4). Another obvious advantage was the availability of air.

Exposure is defined as

$$X = \frac{dq}{dm},$$

(4.1.3)

"where the value of $dq$ is the absolute value of the total charge of the ions of one sign produced in air when all the electrons (negatrons and positrons) liberated by photons in air of mass $dm$ are completely stopped in air" (ICRU, 1980).

Consider this definition. As discussed in section 4.1.4, photons interact with air, producing electrons by photoelectric and Compton effects and, at energies above 1.022 MeV, by electron/positron pair production. These charged particles travel across the medium, in turn producing further ionization. The "total charge" referred to in the definition is the total charge produced by them along their path before they are stopped. They may also produce bremsstrahlung[1] photons, which are subsequently reabsorbed in the medium. The ionization produced by charged particles deriving from bremsstrahlung photons must not be taken into account: in other words, the interaction coefficient related to exposure is the energy absorption coefficient, not the energy transfer coefficient.

The SI unit for exposure is coulomb per kilogram (C kg$^{-1}$), but the historical unit roentgen (R) is still accepted: 1 R = 2.58 × 10$^{-4}$ C kg$^{-1}$.

### 4.1.7.1.3. Kerma

The acronym kerma stands for "kinetic energy released per unit mass." Kerma for a nondirectly ionizing beam (i.e., photons and neutrons) in a given material is given by

$$K = \frac{dE_{tr}}{dm},$$

(4.1.4)

where $dE_{tr}$ is the sum of the kinetic energies of all charged particles initially released in a given mass and $dm$ is the mass itself.

---

1    Bremsstrahlung, or "braking radiation," is the process by which charged particles moving in a medium lose energy, as electromagnetic radiation, through interaction with the nuclei of the medium. The power emitted is proportional to the effective atomic number of the medium and to the particle energy; hence, for soft tissue, characterized by low $Z$, it is negligible up to a few megaelectron volts. On the other hand, it is the main process involved in the production of diagnostic X-rays, where electrons of 10 keV to 150 keV are accelerated onto a high-$Z$ material such as tungsten or molybdenum.

The main conceptual difference between kerma and exposure lies in the fact that kerma is related to the initial kinetic energy of the charged particles released by noncharged particles: that is, it takes into account the energy that could subsequently be lost in the bremsstrahlung process. For a beam of energy fluence $\Psi$, $K = \Psi\mu_{tr}/\rho$, where $\mu_{tr}/\rho$ is defined as the mass energy transfer coefficient of the material of interest. Kerma is not completely defined unless a material is specified. Finally, kerma is not only defined for a photon beam, but also for a neutron beam. The SI unit for kerma is the gray (Gy): 1 Gy = 1 J kg$^{-1}$.

### 4.1.7.1.4. Absorbed Dose

Absorbed dose was introduced for measuring the effects of radiation in neutron beams because the initially defined quantity—exposure—referred only to photons. It is also used for directly ionizing radiation.

Absorbed dose at a point is defined as

$$D = \frac{d<\varepsilon>}{dm} \, , \tag{4.1.5}$$

where $d<\varepsilon>$ is the mean energy imparted by ionizing radiation to a material of mass $dm$. The presence of a mean value is due to the peculiar mechanism of energy deposition, which for photons and neutrons is a discrete process. The SI unit for absorbed dose is the gray (Gy). The gray has replaced the rad: 1 rad = 100 erg g$^1$ = 10$^{-2}$ Gy.

Consider the differences between kerma and absorbed dose. Kerma describes the energy initially released when the radiation beam interacts with matter, regardless of the processes that take place afterward, whereas absorbed dose describes the energy absorbed from the secondary particles created by the radiation beam in the medium in question.

To better understand this mechanism, consider a photon beam entering a medium and assume first that the beam is not attenuated by the medium and that the fraction of energy lost in bremsstrahlung is negligible (Fig. 4.1.9a). In this case, kerma is constant across the thickness of the material because the number of electrons produced per unit length is constant. Before producing ionization, and hence contributing to absorbed dose, secondary electrons travel a distance related to their range in the medium. For this reason, dose is small close to the entrance surface of the beam and increases with the depth in the medium. This mechanism is called dose buildup. At a certain depth the ionization produced within a layer of material by electrons generated outside it is equal to the ionization produced outside the layer by electrons generated within the layer, and the absorbed dose is equal to kerma. This is the condition of charged particle equilibrium.

When the beam is attenuated by the medium (Fig. 4.1.9b), kerma decreases exponentially. Dose buildup occurs until the secondary electron fluence is high enough to provide an energy deposition larger than the energy transfer described by kerma. At greater depth, dose buildup is compensated for by attenuation of the photon beam, and absorbed dose starts decreasing at the same rate as kerma. This regime is called transient charged particle equilibrium.

The distinction between kerma and dose is more relevant for therapy beams than for diagnostic beams, as dose buildup is negligible for diagnostic beams.

If the fraction of energy lost in the bremsstrahlung process is not negligible, the relationship between kerma and dose at charged particle equilibrium is

$$D = K(1 - g) = \frac{\mu_{en}}{\rho}\Psi \, , \tag{4.1.6}$$

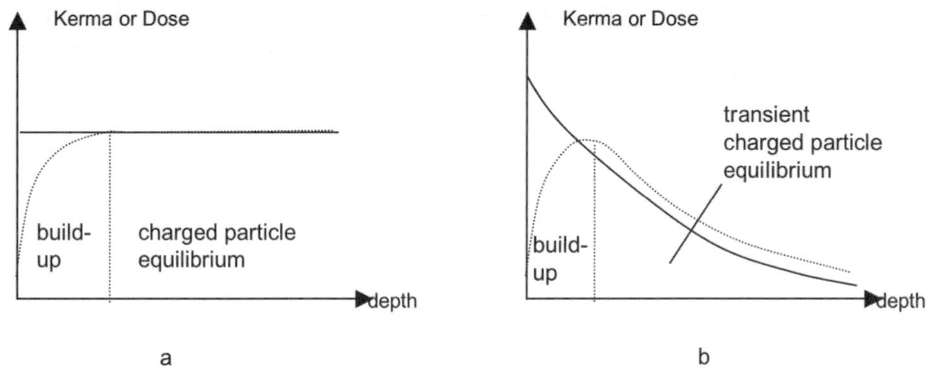



**Figure 4.1.9.** Kerma and dose as functions of depth in the cases of (a) charged particle equilibrium and (b) transient charged particle equilibrium.

where $g$ is the fraction of energy lost in the bremsstrahlung process, and the mass energy absorption coefficient, $\mu_{en}/\rho$, is correlated to the mass energy transfer coefficient by $\mu_{en}/\rho = (1 - g)\mu_{tr}/\rho$.

At charged particle equilibrium

$$D_{air} = X \frac{W_{air}}{e},$$ (4.1.7)

where $W_{air}$ is the mean energy required to produce an electron-ion pair in air, and $e$ is the electronic charge.

### 4.1.7.1.5. Dose Equivalent

Absorbed dose is ineffective for describing the actual biological effects of radiation. For this purpose, dose equivalent is defined as

$$H = Dw_R,$$ (4.1.8)

where $D$ is the absorbed dose and $w_R$ is the so-called radiation weighting factor, taking into account the beam type. Table 4.1.4 summarizes the values of $w_R$ for different types of radiation. It can be seen that dose and dose equivalent are numerically the same only for photon and electron irradiation, and that the biological effect is greater for all other beam types.

Although $w_R$ is a dimensionless quantity, the unit for the dose equivalent is not the same as the unit for dose (i.e., Gy), but is the sievert (Sv): 1 Sv = 1 J kg$^{-1}$.

## 4.1.8. DEFINITION OF QUANTITIES RELATED TO RADIATION IMAGING

This section considers the main parameters that should be taken into account when evaluating an imaging detector. Only the basic concepts will be discussed, as a comprehensive analysis is far beyond the scope of this chapter and a vast amount of literature is available on the subject.

**Table 4.1.4.** Radiation weighting factors for different radiation beams

| Type of radiation | $w_R$ |
|---|---|
| Photons | 1 |
| Electrons | 1 |
| Neutrons, energy | |
| < 10 keV | 5 |
| 10 keV to 100 keV | 10 |
| >100 keV to 2 MeV | 20 |
| >2 MeV to 20 MeV | 10 |
| >20 MeV | 5 |
| Protons, energy > 2 MeV | 5 |
| α particles | 20 |

ICRU, 1980.

### 4.1.8.1. Overall Detector Characteristics: Area Coverage, Uniformity, Stability, and Linearity

Before addressing some specific quantities in detail, it is worth discussing some general features that apply to all detectors and provide the primary lines along which the choice of a detector should be made, according to the targeted application. Among these, area coverage, uniformity, and stability are rather obvious but nonetheless primary issues. Regarding area coverage, not only the size of the sample that has to be imaged must be taken into account, but also the expected degree of magnification, in case a nonnegligible distance between the sample and detector is foreseen. This is often the case, as scattering rejection techniques can be based on air-gap methods, and magnification itself is frequently employed to increase the system spatial resolution. Area coverage values are standardized for most radiological applications ($35 \times 43$ cm$^2$ for chest radiography, $18 \times 24$ cm$^2$ for mammography, etc.), while in the biological field they are much more application driven.

Uniformity refers to the ability of each detector element (pixel) to provide the same response when exposed to the same amount of radiation. A nonuniform response results in fixed pattern noise (FPN), that is, the image obtained by exposing the system to a uniform radiation field is not perfectly flat. Different systems have different degrees of uniformity (for instance, complementary metal-oxide semiconductor [CMOS]-based sensors are historically regarded as more subject to FPN than charge-coupled devices [CCDs]), but a certain degree of nonuniformity is encountered in practically all systems. This is usually corrected by means of simple algorithms, and the higher the system stability, the more effective the result of the correction procedure. System stability is the ability of the system to provide the same response to the same input over different times, which is clearly a basic requirement in order to effectively apply the above corrections.

Correction algorithms depend on another basic property of the system, namely its linearity, which refers to the direct proportionality between the radiation input and the detector response. If the system is linear, the correction requires the acquisition of a flat field (i.e., the system response to a uniform radiation field, or simply to a uniform object if one wants to correct for the nonuniformities due to the radiation source) and a dark field image (i.e., an image without any radiation impinging on the detector), providing slope and intercept values, respectively, to the (linear) correction function, which is then applied on a pixel-by-pixel basis. If the system is not linear, more images have to be taken at intermediate exposure levels, and the appropriate (nonlinear) correction function is obtained by interpolating or fitting the acquired data.

### 4.1.8.2. Dynamic Range and Related Topics

The dynamic range is usually defined as the ratio between the maximum signal achievable in the individual detector pixel and the amount of signal that is stored in the individual pixel because of noise. Both the noise due to the detector and that due to the X-ray source have to be taken into account, and they are usually summed in quadrature. The phenomena of X-ray emission and interaction are subject to fluctuations described by Poisson statistics, in which the variance on a number of quanta is equal to the number of quanta. Hence this is an intrinsic limit that cannot be overcome and to which any further source of noise due to the detector system has to be added (in quadrature). Details on detector noise modeling are provided later, but it should be noted at this point that the dynamic range properties of a system benefit substantially from the design of detectors with optimum noise performance.

The maximum achievable signal depends on the specific detector design, for example, on the well capacity (i.e., how many electrons the single potential well can contain) in a CCD detector. However, with digital detectors it is possible to take two subsequent exposures and sum the resulting images, thus increasing this value; this possibility is clearly not available in film imaging.

In this framework it should be noted that in photon counting devices, in order to enable a proper counting of every single photon, any source of noise due to the detector system has to be eliminated by proper threshold settings. In such systems the only source of noise is due to the statistical nature of X-ray interaction, which means that the noise performances are kept at their theoretical maximum. Moreover, as each single photon is counted, there are no restrictions related to the pixel capacity, as occurs in integrating systems, and the maximum achievable signal depends only on the number of bits in the integrated counter (usually $2^{16}$, but higher capacities can be implemented). As a consequence, in counting systems the dynamic range can be pushed to the maximum values. Nevertheless, many applications are still based on integrating devices, as the ability of counting systems to handle high photon fluxes is still a subject of discussion. Moreover, many recently developed integrating systems feature a level of detector noise so small that it can be considered almost negligible when summed in quadrature with the X-ray Poisson values.

Finally, it should be mentioned here that, for practical purposes, the main image quality parameter is the signal-to-noise ratio (SNR), which in an image is defined as the contrast of a detail divided by the average noise surrounding it, the contrast being the difference between the average number of counts outside and within the detail. According to Rose (1973), the minimum SNR that the human eye can perceive ranges between 4 and 5. As a consequence, a more "practical" minimum for the dynamic range should be 4 or 5, while in the definition given above, the minimum possible value is 1. Moreover, if a detail has to be detected within a noisy background, the number of pixels forming the detail plays a major role: the higher this number (i.e., the greater the detail in the pixel scale), the higher the visibility. As a consequence, Yaffe proposed a modified definition of the dynamic range in which, before the ratio is evaluated, the maximum achievable signal is multiplied by the number of detail pixels and the overall noise level is multiplied by 4 or 5 according to the Rose criterion (Yaffe & Rowlands, 1997). This definition takes SNR requirements correctly into account but has less generality, as it depends on the specific imaging task.

### 4.1.8.3. Spatial Resolution

Before discussing spatial resolution in detail, it is worth clarifying the distinction between pixel aperture and spacing. Digital sensors are usually matrices of elements arranged in a regular array, and in many cases the entire surface of the single element is not sensitive to radiation (Fig. 4.1.10). The dimension of the active part of the element is called the aperture, while the dimension of the entire element, that is, the distance between the same point in two adjacent elements, is called spacing (for simplicity's sake, assume here that the elements are square). The aperture defines the intrinsic spatial resolution of the system, while the spacing determines the sampling frequency. The ratio between the active portion and the overall detector surface is called the fill factor. For an efficient use of radiation, the fill factor should be as close as possible to unity. For a single detector device, it is equal to the ratio between the square of the aperture and the square of the spacing, provided that any further nonsensitive area along the outer edges (guard rings, front-end electronics, etc.) is not irradiated. If the overall detector is obtained by tiling several devices, the fill factor can be further reduced.

The active part of a detector pixel is effectively described by the point spread function (PSF), which expresses the relative sensitivity of each point within the active surface (Fig. 4.1.11). Ideally one could measure it by finely scanning the entire active surface with a pencil beam of extremely small cross section and registering the response corresponding to each position. As this solution is clearly impractical, many alternative possibilities have been proposed, all of which basically measure the line spread function (LSF). The LSF is the response of the pixel to a blade of radiation, uniform in one direction and infinitely narrow in the other, which ideally should be scanned over the pixel in one direction only, as shown in Figure 4.1.11. In other words, the LSF is the PSF integrated along one direction. As in most practical cases, square pixels are employed, an isotropic behavior is assumed with respect to the pixel center, and the LSF is considered sufficiently representative of the spatial resolution properties of the device.

A simple approach to LSF measurement consists of covering the pixel with an absorbing edge and recording the pixel response as the edge is scanned in a direction orthogonal to the edge, thus progressively exposing to radiation larger portions of the pixel. The curve obtained is the integral of the LSF along the scanning direction, called the edge response function (ERF), and the LSF is then obtained by numerically differentiating the ERF (Fig. 4.1.12). This technique has the advantage of measuring individually the LSFs of all pixels in a row, but has the drawback of being time consuming.

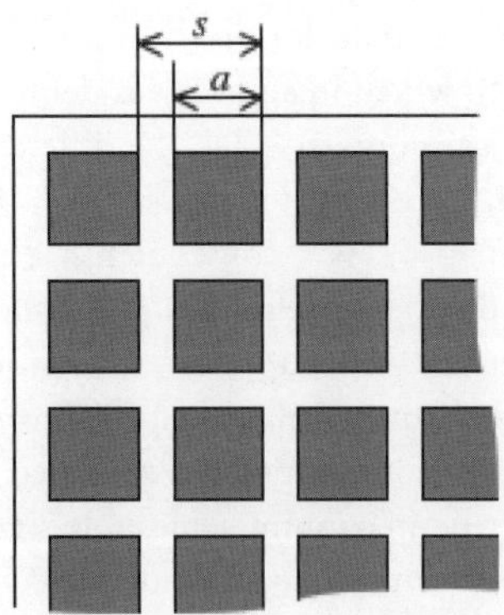


**Figure 4.1.10.** Aperture (*a*) and spacing (*s*) in a digital detector (sensitive area in grey).

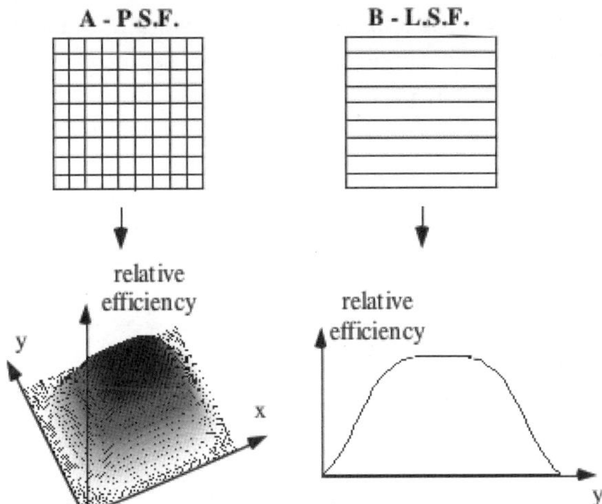



**Figure 4.1.11.** (A) PSF and (B) LSF of a detector pixel. In (A), the pixel is ideally subdivided into squarelets and the relative efficiency of each squarelet is given as a function of the squarelet position $(x, y)$. In (B), the pixel is ideally subdivided into stripes and the relative efficiency of each stripe is given as a function of position in the direction orthogonal to the stripes.

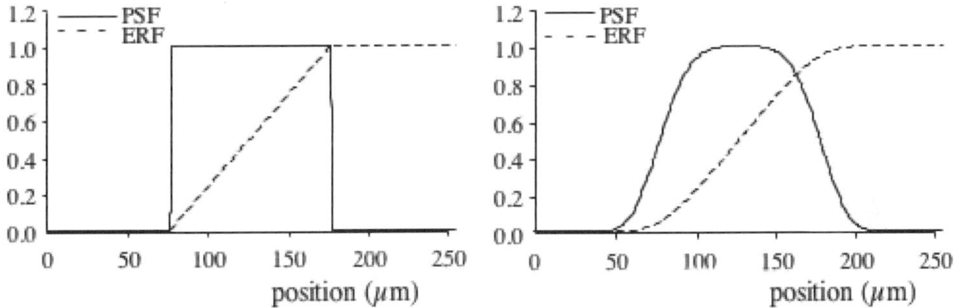



**Figure 4.1.12.** A PSF (solid line) and ERF (dashed line) for an ideal (left) and a real (right) 100 μm pixel. In the ideal case, every point in the pixel would have the same efficiency and the PSF would be a box function. In real cases, the relative efficiency often has its maximum in the pixel center and decreases near the edges.

A faster possibility, involving taking an image of an edge placed at a very small angle with respect to the pixel orientation, was proposed by Cunningham and Fenster (1987). An image profile taken along the orientation of the pixels, thus forming a small angle with the edge, provides the ERF (averaged over a number of pixels). The LSF is then obtained by numerical differentiation. A similar method, proposed by Fujita et al. (1992), employs a slightly tilted narrow slit instead of an edge, and makes possible a direct measurement of the LSF by combining the response of several rows of pixels taken in a direction (almost) orthogonal to the slit.

The modulus of the Fourier transform of the LSF provides the modulation transfer function (MTF), which is the most commonly employed quantity for expressing the spatial resolution of an imaging system. The MTF provides the relative amplitude with which each single spatial frequency is transferred by the system to the acquired image (Fig. 4.1.13). Actually, bar pattern test objects featuring progressively narrowing bar patterns of transmitting and absorbing materials make possible a direct determination of the MTF by measuring the decreasing amplitude of the patterns in the image as a function of the increasing frequency. However, this solution has two drawbacks: first, square rather than real sinusoidal functions are input into the system, and second, it allows the measurement of MTF values only at some predetermined spatial frequencies. Converging or diverging bar patterns may allow finer MTF sampling, but in this case a precise assessment of the spatial frequencies in which the MTF values are actually taken is important.

The MTF obtained with any of the previously mentioned techniques is actually the presampling MTF. As discussed earlier, in image acquisition, the sampling is determined by the pixel spacing. This means that the acquired image can be undersampled, as the presampling MTF may contain frequencies above the Nyquist limit ($[2s]^{-1}$ if $s$ is the spacing) imposed by the sampling. This results in the well-known phenomenon of aliasing. Without going into details (see, for instance, Bracewell, 1986), all frequencies higher than $(2s)^{-1}$ will not be reproduced in the image, and an overestimation of all Fourier coefficients may occur at frequencies lower than $(2s)^{-1}$. In order to avoid aliasing, the image should be "band limited" to frequencies below the Nyquist limit. In some cases, image blurring due to the focal spot size or light diffusion in the phosphor screen in indirect detection devices can help in fulfilling this requirement, although it cannot prevent aliasing effects from high-frequency noise. A safer solution may be to increase the sampling step rather than band-limiting the image, which can be achieved by taking several images while shifting the detector to different positions and then appropriately combining the acquired data (dithering). It was also demonstrated that under certain conditions, this technique can provide images with enhanced spatial resolution, determined by the scanning step rather than by the pixel size, provided that appropriate deconvolution algorithms are applied (Olivo et al., 2000).

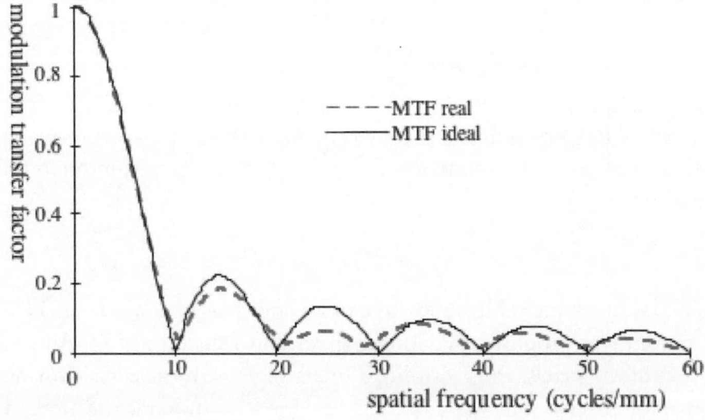


**Figure 4.1.13.** The MTF of an ideal 100 μm pixel (solid line) and a real one (dashed line). The PSFs of the same pixels are shown in Figure 4.1.12.

### 4.1.8.4. Noise Performance

As mentioned previously, the intrinsic statistical nature of X-ray emission and interaction, described by the Poisson statistic, imposes a lower limit to the noise performance of any X-ray imaging system. The fact that only a photon counting device, in which all noise apart from the Poisson fluctuations is cut by a threshold, can reach this theoretical limit was also mentioned.

Although the issue of efficiency is discussed in the next subsection, it is worth stressing here that if $\varepsilon$ is the quantum efficiency of a device, which means that $N_1 = \varepsilon N$ photons will be detected out of the $N$ quanta impinging on the detector, $N_1$ is still a Poisson-distributed variable; that is, the variance of $N_1$ is still equal to $N_1$ itself. Hence a limited efficiency does not prevent a counting system from reaching its theoretical limit in terms of noise performance.

In integrating systems, X-ray interaction is usually followed by one or more gain stages (e.g., the large number of visible photons created for each X-ray interaction in indirect detection techniques, or the electron multiplication in photomultiplier tubes). Following these gain stages, the new number of quanta will therefore be $N_2 = GN_1 = G\varepsilon N$ (where, for simplicity's sake, all gain factors are condensed into the single factor $G$). This has relevant consequences. First, the variance of $N_2$ will be increased, as fluctuations on $G$ have to be taken into account when the uncertainty propagation is carried out (Rabbani, Shaw, & Van Metter, 1987). Second, in general $N_2$ will not be Poisson distributed, even in those cases in which $G$ is Poisson distributed.

In order to describe systems in which several stages of gain and loss of quanta are encountered, the method of quantum accounting diagrams (QADs) was devised (Cunningham, Westmore, & Fenster, 1994; however, the authors declare in their paper that the term QAD was previously used by M. J. Yaffe). The system is described as a sequence of cascaded stages in which quanta are transferred from one stage to another and gains or losses occur at each transfer. An example is shown in Figure 4.1.14. In order to describe an indirect detection system (for instance, a CCD coupled with a phosphor screen via fiber optics) with the QAD method, the following steps are needed:

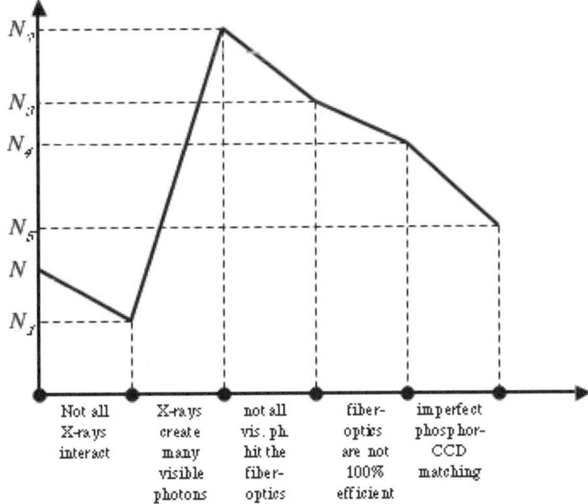


**Figure 4.1.14.** Example of a QAD for a CCD coupled to a phosphor via fiber optics.

1. $N$ photons impinge on the phosphor and $N_1 = \varepsilon N$ interact (obviously $N_1 < N$: a first loss has occurred). $N_1$ is the "primary quantum sink" representing the intrinsic noise limit: the ultimate SNR will be lower (or equal, in ideal counting systems) than the square root of $N_1$.

2. Each interacting X-ray gives rise to a large number of visible photons, hence the number of quanta created in the phosphor is $N_2 = GN_1$, with $N_2 > N_1$ (in the given example, $N_2$ is also much larger than $N$, as $G$ can be on the order of $10^3$).

3. A percentage of visible photons escape and are not collected by the fiber optics; hence, a loss is encountered: $N_3 = l_1 N_2$, $N_3 < N_2$.

4. The non-100% efficient transfer of visible photons through the fiber optic results in another loss: $N_4 = l_2 N_3$, $N_4 < N_3$.

5. A further loss arises from the nonperfect matching between the spectra of the visible photons emitted by the phosphor and the sensitivity curve of the CCD: $N_5 = l_3 N_4$, $N_5 < N_4$.

If $N_2$, $N_3$, $N_4$, and $N_5$ are all larger than $N_1$, the limit in the noise performances of the system is still determined by the primary quantum sink—that is, the SNR will not be higher than $(N_1)^{1/2}$—and the smaller the fluctuations in each single step of the chain, the closer it will be to this limit.

On the other hand, if, for example, $N_5$ (which in the example is the smallest of the four) is smaller than $N_1$, this represents a secondary quantum sink in the system, and the overall SNR will be smaller or equal to the square root of $N_5$. In general, if the quanta are transferred through $K$ subsequent stages, the smallest number between $N_1$ and $N_K$ will determine the ultimate limit in the noise performances of the system.

It should be noted, however, that the QAD method outlined here, although extremely helpful, is an approximate one, and is subject to two major limitations: no additive noise sources are taken into account, and perfect localization is assumed at every creation/collection of secondary quanta (i.e., the effects of scattering and diffusion are not considered). As a consequence, its use may result in an underestimation of the overall system noise.

In order to evaluate the effect that noise has on each single spatial frequency, the noise power spectrum (NPS) or Wiener spectrum has to be evaluated. If $I(x,y)$ is the data set, the NPS is defined as the Fourier transform of its autocorrelation function (Blackman & Tukey, 1958). However, using the properties of the Fourier transform, it can be demonstrated that the same result can be obtained by directly calculating the square modulus of the Fourier transform of the data itself (see, for instance, Williams, Mangiafico, & Simoni, 1999). This allows an easier approach to NPS calculation, and in fact is referred to as the "direct method" of NPS calculation, the autocorrelation-based technique being called the "indirect method." In fact, Dainty and Shaw (1974) define the NPS (for a continuous variable) as

$$NPS(u,v) = \lim_{X,Y \to} \frac{1}{4XY} \left\langle \left| \int_{-X}^{X} \int_{-Y}^{Y} [I(x,y) - \bar{I}]e^{-2\pi i(xu+yv)}\, dx\, dy \right|^2 \right\rangle, \qquad (4.1.9)$$

where $I(x,y)$ is the two-dimensional image intensity and $\bar{I}$ is the average background intensity. The angled brackets indicate that averaging over data ensembles is required. In order to apply the definition to digital detectors, discrete Fourier transform algorithms are employed in which the integrals are replaced with sums (see, for instance, Brigham, 1974). A comprehensive treatment can be found in the third chapter (by Dobbins) of the *Handbook of Medical Imaging* edited by Beutel, Kundel, and Van Metter (2000).

It should be noted, however, that many nontrivial practical problems are encountered when the NPS has to be measured experimentally. In general, the necessity of using a finite range of noise data affects the results at high frequencies and determines the frequency sampling of the NPS itself, and a large number of measurements has to be averaged in order to reduce the fluctuations. Some of these practical problems are discussed by Dobbins et al. (1995), while a somewhat "classical" theoretical description and experimental method can be found in Giger, Doi, and Metz (1984).

As already discussed in the case of the MTF, when square pixels are used, an isotropic behavior is assumed and a one-dimensional NPS is considered sufficient to describe the noise performance of the system. This is usually achieved by selecting a slice of the two-dimensional NPS close to the $\upsilon$ or $v$ axis, where $\upsilon$ and $v$ are the spatial frequency axes conjugated to the spatial coordinates $x$ and $y$, respectively.

### 4.1.8.5. Detection Efficiency

The first step in all X-ray imaging detectors is X-ray interaction, in the sensor material for direct detection systems or in the phosphor screen for indirect systems. The probability of interaction for the single X-ray, or quantum efficiency ($\varepsilon$), is thus determined by the thickness ($t$) and by the attenuation coefficient ($\mu$) of the material in which the interaction takes place:

$$\varepsilon = 1 - e^{-\mu(E)t}, \tag{4.1.10}$$

where the energy dependence of the attenuation coefficient on the X-ray energy ($E$) is explicitly expressed. Equation 4.4.10 holds only when monochromatic radiation is used, which is true only in a limited number of cases. When a polychromatic spectrum is used, equation 4.1.10 should be replaced with

$$\varepsilon' = \frac{\displaystyle\int_0^{E_{max}} \Phi(E)(1 - e^{-\mu(E)t})\,dE}{\displaystyle\int_0^{E_{max}} \Phi(E)\,dE}, \tag{4.1.11}$$

where $\Phi(E)$ is the X-ray spectrum impinging on the detector (i.e., beyond the imaged sample), which means that beam-hardening effects due to the sample must be taken into account. In noncounting detectors, since the detected signal actually depends on the energy absorbed by the detector rather than on the number of photons, the concept of energy absorption efficiency ($\varepsilon''$) is introduced in some cases:

$$\varepsilon'' = \frac{\displaystyle\int_0^{E_{max}} \Phi(E)E\,\frac{\mu_{en}(E)}{\mu(E)}(1 - e^{-\mu(E)t})\,dE}{\displaystyle\int_0^{E_{max}} \Phi(E)E\,dE}, \tag{4.1.12}$$

where the ratio between the energy absorption coefficient $\mu_{en}$ and the attenuation coefficient accounts for the amount of absorbed energy per interacting X-ray photon.

In counting devices, the concepts of quantum efficiency and MTF are sufficient to describe the system performance at all spatial frequencies, while for integrating detectors, the concept of detective quantum efficiency (DQE) has to be introduced. Before discussing the DQE, it is worth introducing the concept of noise equivalent quanta (NEQ).

As in a counting device, the only noise source is X-ray Poisson fluctuations, if $N$ is the number of interacting X-rays, $\sigma_N = N^{1/2}$, and $SNR_{ideal} = N/\sigma_N = N^{1/2}$. In an integrating device, the recorded signal $S$ is different from the number of interacting quanta, and thus in general $SNR_{nonideal} = S/\sigma_S < N^{1/2}$. As in the ideal (counting) behavior one has $(SNR_{ideal})^2 = N$, in the nonideal behavior it is useful to define the quantity $N' = (S/\sigma_S)^2 < N$, which establishes a direct comparison between the nonideal case and the ideal case. The quantity $N' = (SNR_{nonideal})^2$ is called the NEQ.

The DQE is defined as the ratio between the square of the SNR in the image and the square of the SNR input to the detector:

$$DQE = \frac{(SNR_{out})^2}{(SNR_{in})^2}, \tag{4.1.13}$$

where the numerator is, in practice, the NEQ. (In fact, using the previous definition for $N'$, it is possible to write $DQE = N'/N$). Although this definition might seem rather straightforward, it is important to notice that while $(SNR_{out})^2$ can be measured on the acquired image, the determination of $(SNR_{in})^2$ is not easy. If the beam is monochromatic, this corresponds to the number of photons impinging on the detector, but, as mentioned previously, this is the case only in a restricted number of cases. Strictly speaking, the DQE is referred to a number of photons; hence, when a polychromatic beam is used, the variances of the number of quanta should be individually evaluated at each energy (in practice, in each energy bin) and then summed to give the overall variance. According to some authors, however, since the effective signal in the detector depends on the deposited energy, emphasis should be placed on the energy variance rather than on the variance in the number of counts, and an energy-weighted balance should thus be used to estimate $(SNR_{in})^2$.

Although thus far the DQE has been treated as a scalar quantity (for simplicity's sake), its frequency dependence should already be clear as the MTF, which accounts for the decrease in the achievable image contrast with increasing spatial frequencies, as already discussed. Hence the DQE is actually a $DQE(\nu)$, where $\nu$ is the spatial frequency. (Again, although the DQE is actually a function of two independent variables, it is often approximated with a single-variable dependent function when the system is made of square pixels and an almost isotropic behavior is expected.)

Different ways of practically evaluating the NEQ (e.g., $(SNR_{out})^2$) are reported in the literature. Here, referring to the previously quoted work of Dobbins et al. (1995), in which a "normalized" noise power spectrum (NNPS) is evaluated as

$$NNPS(\nu) = \frac{NPS(\nu)}{(large \quad area \quad signal)^2}, \tag{4.1.14}$$

the NEQ or $(SNR_{out})^2$ as a function of spatial frequency is given by

$$NEQ(\nu) = \left(SNR_{out}(\nu)\right)^2 = \frac{(MTF(\nu))^2}{NNPS(\nu)}. \tag{4.1.15}$$

This approach is rather straightforward: the MTF provides the response of the system (i.e., the signal) at each frequency and the (normalized) NPS gives its variance (the noise). Finally, by dividing the result provided by equation 4.1.15 by $(SNR_{in})^2$, the frequency-dependent DQE is obtained.

## 4.2. SENSORS FOR DOSIMETRY

### 4.2.1. SPECIAL REQUIREMENTS FOR DOSIMETRIC MEASUREMENTS

#### 4.2.1.1. Characteristics of an "Ideal" Dosimeter

Dosimeters make possible the measurement of a delivered dose via a dose-related effect such as the temperature increase in a calorimeter, the current in an ionization chamber, or the optical density of a radiographic film. The required general characteristics for dosimetry detectors include the following:

##### 4.2.1.1.1. Linear Response

The output of the detector (current, analog-to-digital converter counts, etc.) should increase linearly with the absorbed dose and have no zero offset. Clearly this would make calibration as simple as possible. Ideally the range of linearity should be infinite, but saturation and other nonlinear behavior will occur in practice.

To a certain extent, and excluding the saturation regime, calibration can be performed in cases of nonlinear response. Figure 4.2.1 shows the response characteristics of different dosimetric systems.

##### 4.2.1.1.2. Tissue Equivalence

In order to reproduce correctly the mechanisms of energy release in tissues, the atomic number of an ideal dosimeter must be as close as possible to that of the tissue ($Z_{tissue}$ = 7.4). This implies a flat energy response across the range of use of the dosimeter.

Tissue equivalence is a major issue when a depth dose distribution or a three-dimensional (3-D) dose distribution has to be measured (for instance, for validating a treatment planning system). A change in the spectrum, typically occurring for photon beams, causes measurements made with a dosimeter that is not tissue equivalent to be unreliable. Tissue equivalence is even more relevant when performing neutron dosimetry, as the cross section for neutron interactions has very sharp changes, such as resonance peaks in elastic scattering.

On the other hand, tissue equivalence is a less stringent requirement in electron dosimetry because of the slow variation of the mass stopping power as a function of the beam energy (see section 4.2.1.2.1). Moreover, it is not important when measuring dose in one position because a calibration as a function of the beam energy against a tissue equivalent dosimeter can be performed. Most commercial devices are provided with calibration data for the most typical range of use.

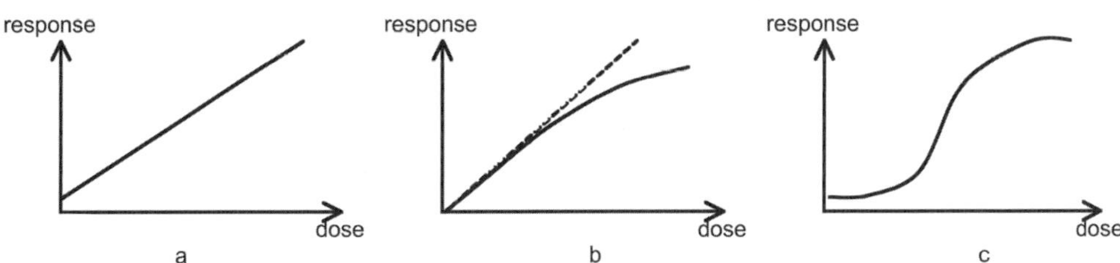



**Figure 4.2.1.** Examples of typical responses of dosimetric systems: (a) linear response; (b) sublinear response (the dotted line shows the linear behavior); (c) limited range of linearity, with a region of underexposure and a saturation region.

### 4.2.1.1.3. Independence of Dose Rate

An integrating dosimeter—that is, a device measuring the total dose deposited within a certain time interval—should not depend on the dose rate. In other words, it should measure the same dose independently of the time over which the dose has been delivered.

### 4.2.1.1.4. Independence of Ambient Parameters

The response of a dosimeter should not be affected by ambient parameters such as temperature and humidity, but few dosimeters satisfy this condition completely. In order to limit the effects of ambient parameters, storage and operating conditions must be controlled, otherwise a calibration as a function of these parameters must be carried out.

### 4.2.1.1.5. Independence of Beam Direction

An ideal dosimeter should always give the same output, independent of the direction of incidence of the beam, but this does not usually happen because of the geometry and the material of the dosimeter. This is a major issue when performing depth dose measurements because the angular distribution of radiation on the detector depends on scattered radiation, which is in turn dependent on the position in the material. Typical depth dosimeters, such as silicon (Si) diodes, are calibrated for the same geometry as that in which they are used.

### 4.2.1.1.6. Long-Term Stability of Calibration

It is clearly more convenient to use a dosimeter with a constant response over time, however, this is not always achieved. For instance, whereas the calibration of ion chambers is constant over time, other dosimeters, such as thermoluminescence (TL), devices show a change in sensitivity depending on their radiation and readout histories, and hence need periodic recalibration.

### 4.2.1.1.6. Precision and Accuracy

Precision is the spread in the distribution of repeated measurements and describes random uncertainties. To estimate the actual difference between the measured value and the "true" value, systematic uncertainties resulting from several factors, such as uncertainties in the calibration or in the estimation of the physical constants, also need to be taken into account. Accuracy describes the systematic uncertainties and is a less objective quantity, depending on the judgment of the experimenter. Both inaccuracy and imprecision need to be as small as possible.

Other desirable characteristics for a dosimeter are related to the specific application and will be discussed case by case. Some characteristics that can be desirable depending on the type of application include the following:

- Long-term information storage
- Possibility of 2-D and 3-D dosimetry
- Reusability
- Portability
- No need for high voltage

## 4.2.1.2. Specific Requirements for Dosimetry of Different Beams

### 4.2.1.2.1. Electron Dosimetry

Electrons are directly ionizing particles. At relatively low energy, they only produce other electrons, while at higher energies they start losing energy by the bremsstrahlung process. For instance, the radiation yield (i.e., the fraction of kinetic energy of the primary electron converted into bremsstrahlung) for electron beams in soft tissue is about 0.3% at 1 MeV and exceeds 10% only above 25 MeV (Berger, Coursey, & Zucker, 2000).

Electrons lose energy very quickly when passing through a material, so charged particle equilibrium (see section 4.2.3.2) is very seldom reached. In order to limit this effect as much as possible, dosimeters for electrons are usually designed to be very thin in the direction orthogonal to the incoming beam.

The tissue dose for an electron beam can be determined from the dose deposited in another material as follows:

$$D_{tissue} = D_m s_{tissue,\,m},\qquad(4.2.1)$$

where $D_{tissue}$ is the tissue dose, $D_m$ is the dosimetric material dose, and $s_{tissue,\,m}$ is the stopping power ratio of water to that of the dosimetric material.

Tissue equivalence is not as great an issue as it is in photon and neutron dosimetry because the ratio of the mass stopping power of two materials is a slowly varying function of the electron energy, and no sharp peaks, as for resonances in neutron interactions or for K-edges in photon interactions, are present. For example, Figure 4.2.2 shows the ratio of the collision mass stopping power of electrons in air and in Si to that in water.

### 4.2.1.2.2. Photon Dosimetry

Photons are indirectly ionizing particles, that is, they first interact with matter to produce charged particles (electrons and, at energies above 1022 keV, positrons). These charged particles produce ionization along their tracks.

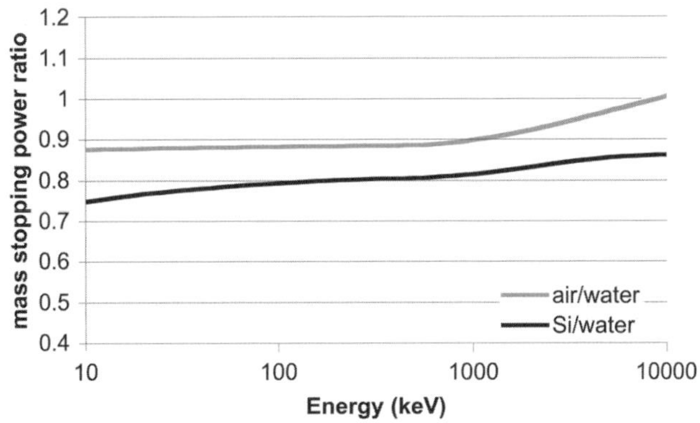


**Figure 4.2.2.** Collision mass stopping power ratio for electrons for two dosimetric materials compared to water (data from Berger, Coursey, & Zucker, 2000).

As previously mentioned, a good material for photon dosimetry must have an atomic number as close to that of the tissue as possible. This implies that the ratio of the interaction coefficients of the material to those of the tissue is a slowly varying function of the photon energy. In this way, the conversion from the material dose to the tissue dose can easily be performed, even when dealing with polychromatic beams (i.e., in the most common case), by means of equation 4.2.2:

$$D_{tissue} = D_m \frac{\overline{\left(\mu_{en}/\rho\right)}_{tissue}}{\overline{\left(\mu_{en}/\rho\right)}_m} , \qquad (4.2.2)$$

where $D_{tissue}$ is the tissue dose, $D_m$ is the detector material dose, and $\overline{\left(\mu_{en}/\rho\right)}_{tissue}$ and $\overline{\left(\mu_{en}/\rho\right)}_m$ are the average mass energy absorption coefficients of the beam for the tissue and dosimetric material, respectively.

Figure 4.2.3 shows a comparison of the ratio of the mass energy absorption coefficients for photons for two typical dosimetric materials to that of water.

Unlike in electron dosimetry, charged particle equilibrium can be achieved relatively easily in photon dosimetry by appropriately selecting the dimensions of the sensitive volume or the dimension and the composition of the outer walls of the instrument.

### 4.2.1.2.3. Neutron Dosimetry

As previously pointed out in section 4.2.1.1, tissue equivalence is even more relevant for neutron dosimeters than for photon dosimeters, as the interaction probabilities for neutrons do not have a smooth dependence on energy or atomic number of the material. Hence a dosimetric material for neutrons must have an atomic composition as close as possible to the tissue. In particular, the hydrogen content must be the same, as the contribution of hydrogen to delivered dose in soft tissue is predominant, although the weight fraction of the hydrogen content is only around 10% (Greening, 1985). However, when greater sensitivity is needed, neutron dosimeters are constructed with materials that have cross sections capable of neutron reactions, such as boron or lithium.

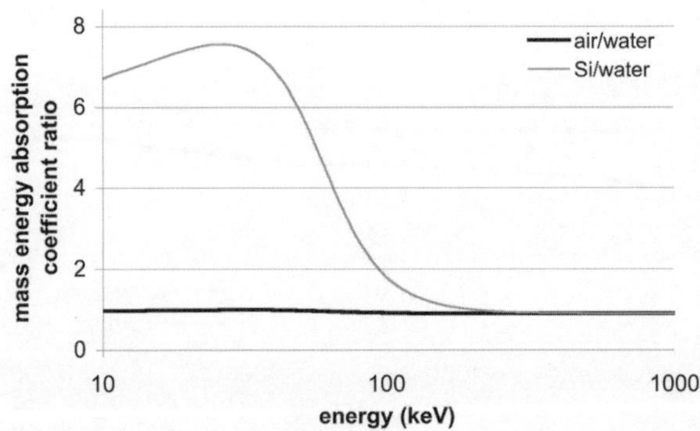


**Figure 4.2.3.** Mass energy absorption coefficient ratio for two different dosimetric materials compared to water (data from Nowotny, 1998).

## 4.2.2. THE CALIBRATION CHAIN

An absolute dosimeter is a detector that provides a signal from which the dose (or a related quantity such as kerma or exposure) can be determined based on physical constants derived independently. The only devices that can be regarded as absolute dosimeters are calorimeters, ionization chambers, and Fricke dosimeters.

A relative dosimeter needs to be calibrated against an absolute instrument or in a known radiation field. Examples of the output of a relative dosimeter are the optical density of a film dosimeter and the light yield of the readout system for a TL dosimeter.

The main steps for the correct calibration of a dosimeter are shown in Figure 4.2.4.

The key elements of the calibration chain are the primary standard dosimeters. These instruments, ion chambers, or calorimeters, depending on the national protocol, are permanently located in the national standards laboratories. Secondary standards, maintained by regional calibration laboratories, are transfer instruments used for calibrating local hospital standards. A calibrated local standard can then be used for calibrating beams or other local dosimeters. A local standard must be recalibrated periodically against a regional standard. The overall accuracy of the final calibration is thus dependent on the accuracy of the intermediate steps.

## 4.2.3. IONIZATION CHAMBERS

### 4.2.3.1. General Principles

The ionization chamber is the most typically used instrument for beam monitoring and calibration. It can be used as an absolute dose monitor, provided its geometry is known with high precision.

The working principle of the ionization chamber is based on detection of the ionization created in a gas by directly or indirectly ionizing particles. The number of electron-ion pairs indirectly created by a particle is equal to the energy deposited divided by the average energy needed to create an electron-ion pair. The average energies required for electrons to create an electron-ion pair ($W$-value) in different gases are shown in Table 4.2.1.

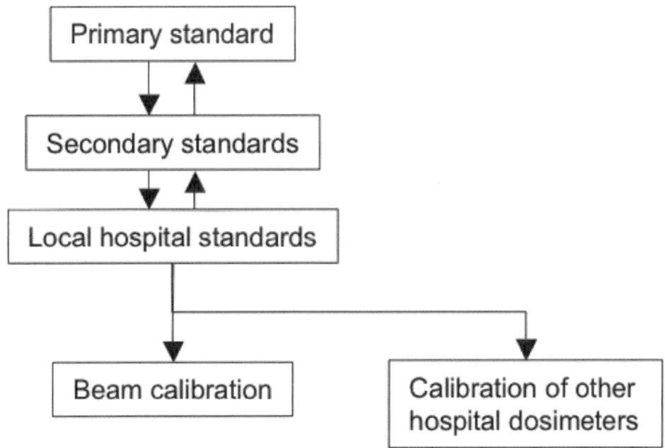


**Figure 4.2.4.** Schematic diagram of a dosimetry calibration chain (update of Planskoy, 1983).

**Table 4.2.1.** *W*-values for electrons in different gases

| Gas | *W*-value (eV) |
| --- | --- |
| Air | 33.8 |
| $N_2$ | 34.8 |
| Ar | 26.4 |
| $O_2$ | 30.8 |
| $CH_4$ | 27.3 |

ICRU, 1979.

If an external voltage is applied to the volume in which the ionization takes place, the electrons will drift toward the positive electrode and the positive ions will drift toward the negative electrode. Thus a current can be measured in an external circuit by means of an electrometer.

Air-filled ionization chambers are particularly suitable for measuring exposure, the definition of exposure being related to the charge created in air. The dose in air can then be calculated from exposure, as discussed in section 4.1.

The main issues related to the use of an ion chamber for dose-in-air measurements are discussed in sections 4.2.3.2 through 4.2.3.5.

### 4.2.3.2. Charged Particle Equilibrium

Exposure at a point is defined by the total charge of one sign created when all the electrons liberated by photons in air at that point are completely stopped, thus the tracks of all secondary electrons created at that point should be followed. This condition is equivalent to the condition of charged particle equilibrium, as explained in Figure 4.2.5. Let A be the volume of interest, and consider a volume B of air surrounding A large enough to completely stop any electron produced in A. Provided that every point in B is subject to the same exposure (i.e., that the beam attenuation in B is negligible), the ionization produced in A by electrons produced by photons interacting in B (track marked "b" in the figure) is

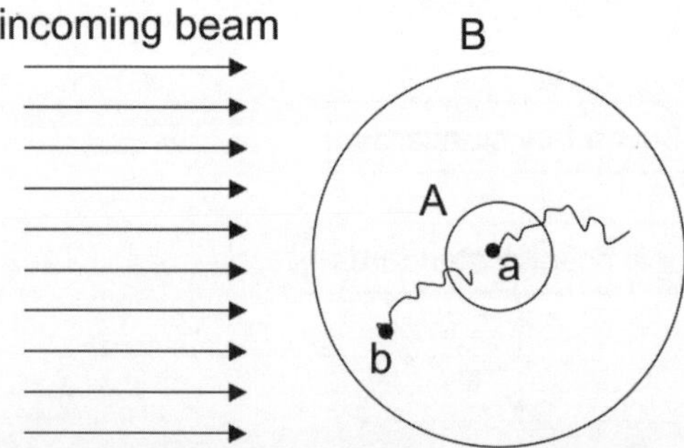



**Figure 4.2.5.** Charged particle equilibrium. The number of secondary electrons (b) produced in the outer volume B and stopped in the sensitive volume A is equal to the number of secondary electrons (a) produced in A and stopped in B.

exactly equal to the ionization produced in B by electrons produced by photons interacting in A (track marked "a" in the figure).

In order to achieve charged particle equilibrium, the sensitive volume of an air-filled ionization chamber must be surrounded by a large enough volume of air. Charged particle equilibrium is more easily reached for low-energy beams, such as diagnostic beams, because of the shorter range of low-energy electrons. More complex geometries must be adopted for reaching charged particle equilibrium for higher energy beams, as discussed in section 4.2.3.4.

### 4.2.3.3. Saturation Voltage

A major issue related to ion chambers is the selection of the correct voltage depending on the beam energy and the beam flux. A qualitative example of the voltage-current characteristic is shown in Figure 4.2.6 for two different energy fluxes of the incoming beam, $\Psi_1$ and $\Psi_2 > \Psi_1$.

At low voltages the electron-ion pairs have a high probability of recombination before reaching the electrodes and thus are not completely collected. Upon increasing the voltage, the probability of recombination decreases until all electron-ion couples have sufficient acceleration to reach the electrodes without recombining. The ionization current then reaches a plateau. The minimum value of the voltage at which a plateau is reached is called the saturation voltage. It is intuitive that the higher the energy flux of the incoming beam, the higher the number of electron-ion pairs produced per unit volume, and thus the higher the probability of recombination; therefore the saturation voltage is higher for more intense or more energetic beams. Saturation voltage also depends on the chamber geometry and on the gas used. More details about recombination can be found in Boutillon (1998).

### 4.2.3.4. Geometries for Ion Chambers

#### 4.2.3.4.1. The Free Air Chamber

The simplest ion chamber is called a free air ionization chamber, shown in Figure 4.2.7.

Here, the cross section of the sensitive volume is defined by means of an entrance collimator, while its length corresponds to the length of the volume delimited by the guard electrodes.

Since exposure is defined as the charge deposited per unit mass in air, the exposure rate for a photon beam, provided the geometry of the system is known, can be calculated as follows:

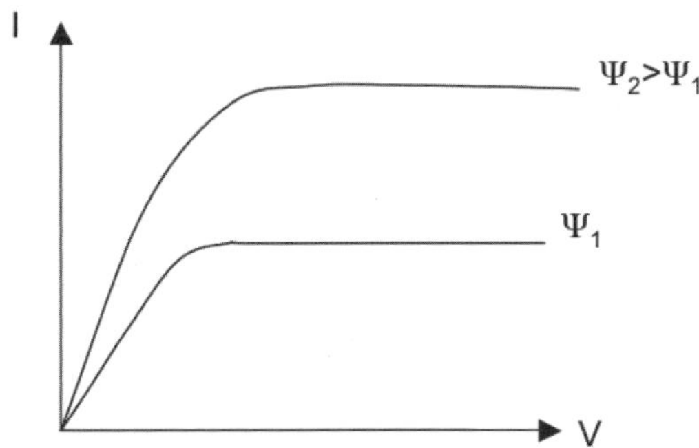


**Figure 4.2.6.** Voltage-current characteristic of an ion chamber for two different incoming beam energy fluxes.

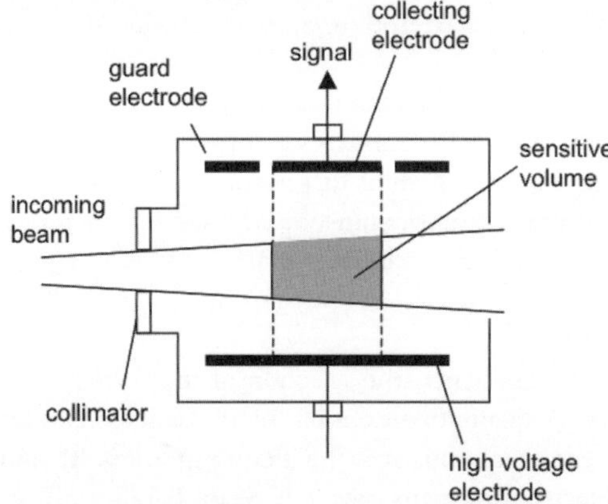


**Figure 4.2.7.** Schematic of a free air ion chamber. The sensitive volume is defined by the entrance collimator, the beam divergence, and the dimensions of the collecting electrode. Absolute dosimetry is only possible when all these quantities are known with high precision (Knoll, 2000).

$$\dot{X} = \frac{I}{m} = \frac{I}{\rho_{air}V}, \tag{4.2.3}$$

where $I$ is the ionization current measured by an electrometer, $\rho$ is the density of air, and $V$ is the sensitive volume of the chamber.

Since the air density depends on both temperature and pressure, equation 4.2.3 can be written more precisely as

$$\dot{X} = \frac{I}{\rho_{air}^{st}V}\frac{p_0}{p}\frac{T}{T_0}, \tag{4.2.4}$$

where $p$ and $T$ are the pressure and the absolute temperature of the gas; $T_0 = 273.15$ K, the standard temperature; $p_0 = 760$ mmHg, the standard pressure; and $p_{air}^{st} = 1.293$ kg m$^{-3}$, the density of air under the standard conditions $p_0$ and $T_0$. The dose rate can then be derived from the exposure rate according to equation 4.1.7.

However, unless the geometry of the system (thickness of the sensitive volume, collimator size, and beam divergence) is very well known, calibration with an absolute instrument is recommended rather than the use of equation 4.2.4. Corrections for temperature and pressure are always needed.

The free air chamber is used only in calibration laboratories as a calibration standard for X-rays generated at less than 300 kV; other geometries are more convenient for clinical practice.

### 4.2.3.4.2. The Cavity Chamber

In practice it is not always possible to achieve conditions of charged particle equilibrium in air, and in particular, when high-energy beams ($E > 300$ keV) have to be monitored. For example, the range for 200 keV electrons in air is 0.4 m (Berger, Coursey, & Zucker, 2000). However, the same condition can be achieved by "compressing" the outer volume B (needed to ensure charged particle equilibrium) into a thinner, denser volume by replacing it with a proper thickness of a solid material with an effective atomic number as close as possible to that of air but with a higher density (see Fig. 4.2.8). Carbon, for example, is a good candidate, and is used for the most common ion chambers in clinical use.

Because it is difficult to know with high precision the dimensions of the air volume and, above all, to what extent the outer wall material can be regarded as air equivalent, a cavity chamber needs to be calibrated against a free air chamber.

Theoretical issues regarding cavity chambers have been widely discussed and more details can be found in Greening (1985).

### 4.2.3.4.3. The Parallel Plate (Plane Parallel) Ion Chamber

The parallel plate ion chamber is, together with the Farmer chamber (see section 4.2.3.4.4), the most frequently used ion chamber in clinical practice. A typical application of this type of chamber is in the calibration of low-energy photon beams and electron beams of less than 10 MeV. According to the International Atomic Energy Agency (IAEA, 1997), they must actually be used below 5 MeV.

In the parallel plate ion chamber (sketched in Figure 4.2.9), the beam direction is orthogonal to the electrodes. One of these electrodes also acts as an entrance window and typically consists of a tissue

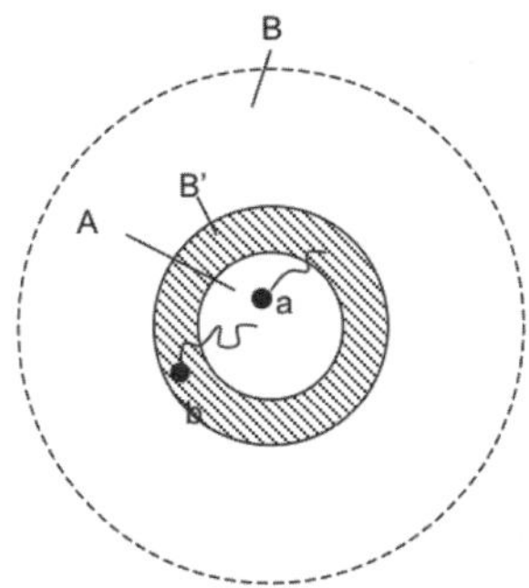


**Figure 4.2.8.** Principle of a cavity chamber: A is the volume of interest, B is the air volume needed for charged particle equilibrium, and B' is a volume with an atomic number close to that of air, but with a higher density.

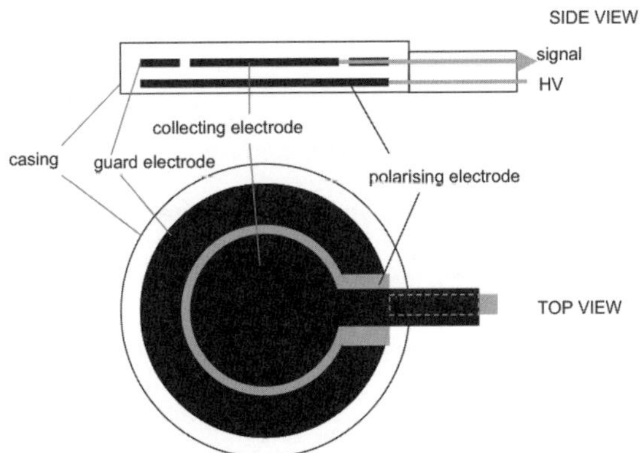


**Figure 4.2.9.** Parallel plate ion chamber (IAEA, 1997).

equivalent polymer (Kapton, Mylar) coated with a thin layer of conductive material. Typical materials for the coating are aluminum or graphite, although the latter is preferable due to its tissue equivalence. The back side of the chamber is either a conducting plastic material or a graphite-coated insulating material. A guard ring is also present.

Several commercial parallel plate chambers are reversible and equipped with two different entrance windows designed for high-energy and low-energy applications. Because of their thin collecting volume, some parallel plate chambers are suitable for depth dose measurements with good depth resolution.

### 4.2.3.4.4. The Cylindrical Ion Chamber (Thimble Chamber/Farmer-Type Chamber)

This geometry, shown in Figure 4.2.10, is typically adopted for beam calibration in radiotherapy. The chamber consists of a hollow cylinder made of low atomic number material (typically graphite) acting as an electrode and an aluminum central electrode about 1 mm in diameter. The presence of a strong electric field near the central electrode increases the charge collection efficiency, thus allowing the use of a lower voltage than in planar geometry.

Cylindrical ion chambers can be manufactured in very small sizes, with active volumes down to about 0.01 cm³. Small cylindrical chambers are suitable for use in radiation fields with strong gradients in one direction or for in vivo measurements in brachytherapy, although other devices, such as Si diodes, are more frequently used for such applications.

Usually, cylindrical chambers are used in the calibration of medium energy X-ray beams generated at greater than 80 kV, high-energy photon beams, and electron beams above 10 MeV. They are also suitable for proton dosimetry (IAEA, 2000).

### 4.2.3.4.5. Sealed Ion Chambers

In a sealed ion chamber, the gas pressure is controlled and no correction for air density changes is required. Moreover, it can be filled with a gas other than air or at a higher pressure, thus ensuring a higher sensitivity for low dose rate applications. Typical filling gases are argon, xenon, and nitrogen. Nitrogen is used for removing any dependence on air humidity rather than for increasing the sensitivity of the chamber, because the energy required for producing an electron-ion pair is very close to that required in air. High-pressure chambers are usually used as radiation survey meters.

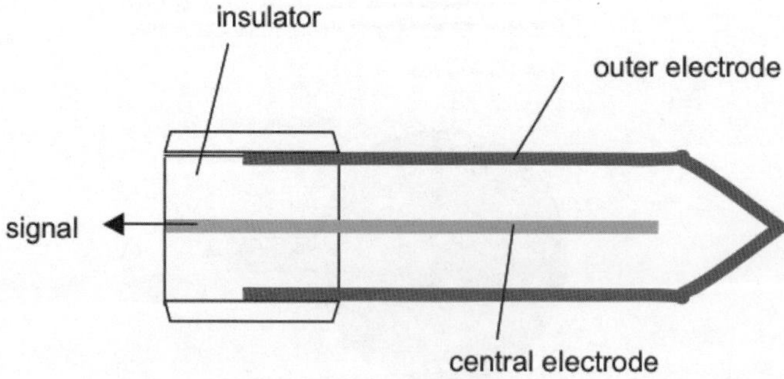


**Figure 4.2.10.** Cylindrical ion chamber (Aird & Farmer, 1972).

### 4.2.3.4.6. Brachytherapy Chamber

When a low dose rate brachytherapy source has to be calibrated, maximum sensitivity must be achieved, thus a well-shaped geometry for this operation is necessary, as shown in Figure 4.2.11. An appropriate active volume is about 1 L. The chamber is usually sealed, and therefore does not require any correction for air density. The source can be placed in a holder within the cavity, thus ensuring an approximately $4\pi$ geometry.

### 4.2.3.4.7. The Compensated Ion Chamber

This type of chamber is designed for neutron dosimetry and consists of two separated ion chambers, one neutron-sensitive, being coated with boron or with another material with a large cross section for neutron interactions, while the other is sensitive to photons. If the polarities are arranged so that the currents in the two chambers have opposite directions, the reading obtained from the electrometer indicates the difference between these two currents, thus allowing the contribution of photons to be separated from that of neutrons.

### *4.2.3.5. Advantages and Disadvantages*

Because ion chambers can have many different structures and applications, it is not easy to summarize their general characteristics. It must be pointed out that for precise beam calibration, several corrections must be made, including for radiation field perturbation caused by the chamber itself, the effects of ion recombination, chamber polarity effects, and other factors. Several protocols for the evaluation of such corrections have been proposed and are currently applied in clinical practice (see, for example, Almond et al., 1999; IAEA, 2000).

Some of the main advantages of ion chambers, which make them useful as one of the standards for beam calibration, are the following:

- They can be designed to be tissue equivalent.
- They are nearly impervious to radiation damage.

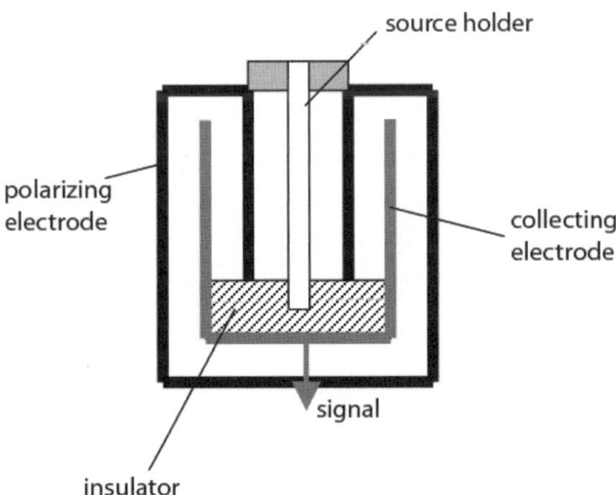


**Figure 4 2.11.** The brachytherapy chamber.

- They have long-term calibration stability.
- Although each type of chamber is designed for a specific application, the range of applications can be extended by adding suitable buildup layers or buildup caps.
- Provided their geometric characteristics are known with high precision, some types of ion chambers are suitable for absolute measurements of dose.
- They can be made sensitive to neutrons by adding a boron or lithium compound to the entrance window.

On the other hand, they do have some disadvantages:

- Because of the need for high voltages, the portability of ion chambers is limited.
- Apart from small volume cylindrical chambers, they are not usually suitable for in vivo measurements because of their large volume.

## 4.2.4. LUMINESCENCE DOSIMETRY

Luminescence dosimetry is a well-established solid-state method based on the use of materials with a small number of impurities. This principle is explained in Figure 4.2.12.

The presence of an impurity introduces traps for electrons at intermediate energies between the valence band and the conduction band. When the material is irradiated, the following occurs:

- A number of electrons is created.
- Each electron can excite a number of electrons from the valence band to the conduction band.
- Each excited electron migrates through the conduction band until it falls into a trap.

During the readout process, if the trap is deep enough to avoid simple thermal excitation at room temperature, the trapped electron can be excited, by means of light or heat, to jump into the conduction band, from where it can either fall into a trap or fall into the valence band, thus emitting light. The light yield, which can be measured using proper instrumentation, is proportional to the number of excited photons and, ideally, to the dose deposited in the material.

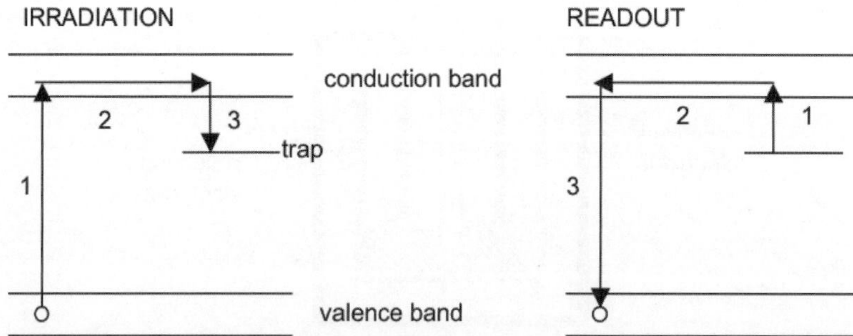


**Figure 4.2.12.** The thermoluminescence or optically stimulated luminescence process. During irradiation, an electron (1) is excited into the conduction band, (2) migrates through it, and (3) falls into a trap. During readout, the electron (1) is excited into the conduction band by means of light or heat, (2) migrates through the conduction band, and (3) falls into the valence band emitting light.

Two dosimetric techniques are based on this effect: TL dosimetry and optically stimulated luminescence (OSL) dosimetry.

### 4.2.4.1. Thermoluminescence Dosimetry

Thermoluminescence dosimeters, in particular lithium fluoride (LiF) dosimeters, are among the most commonly used dosimeters in clinical practice.

### 4.2.4.1.1. General Principles

As already mentioned, TL dosimetry is based on the excitation of trapped electrons by means of heat and on the detection of the light emitted during de-excitation. The microdosimetric mechanisms of TL dosimetry are not fully understood and produce a nonlinear response; however, the physical aspects involved are widely discussed in the literature (see, e.g., Cameron, Sunthralingham, & Kenney, 1968; Horowitz, 1981; and McKinlay, 1981).

### 4.2.4.1.2. Characteristics of TL Dosimeters

A TL dosimetry system consists of the following:

- A set of TL dosimeters, available in different forms (powder, pellet, chip, rod).
- A readout system consisting of a heated element where the TL dosimeters are placed, ensuring uniform thermal contact, and a photomultiplier tube that detects the light emitted during the heating process (see Fig. 4.2.13).
- A high temperature oven for heating the TL dosimeters at the end of the readout process in order to free any electrons still trapped in a metastable state. This process is called annealing. This operation is not necessary for all dosimeters, but it is commonly used in practice to ensure stability of the readout.

Although LiF dosimeters are most commonly used because of their near tissue equivalence ($Z = 8.14$) and wide range of use ($10^{-5}$ to $10^3$ Gy) (Johns & Cunningham, 1983), many TL materials and combinations of dopants have been evaluated in order to find the most suitable one for each application.

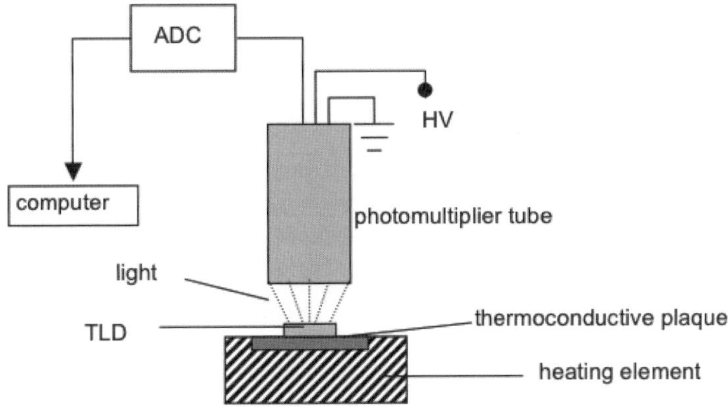


**Figure 4.2.13.** Schematic diagram of a TL dosimeter reader.

In general, highly sensitive materials such as LiF in combination with manganese (Mg), copper (Cu), or phosphorus (P), or aluminum oxide ($Al_2O_3$) are recommended for low-dose dosimetry, for example, for diagnostic beams, personal, and even environmental dosimetry (Duggan et al., 1999; Saez-Vergara et al., 1999). Moreover, TL compounds of boron or lithium (having a large cross section for neutron capture) are particularly suited to neutron dosimetry (Horowitz, 1981; Toivonen et al., 1998).

*The readout process.* After irradiation, TL dosimeters are placed in a reader and the temperature is increased at a steady rate. During the readout process, a nitrogen flow is used in some cases to prevent chemoluminescence emissions caused by reactions with oxygen or water vapor, which may alter the readout.

A plot of the light yield as a function of temperature (the glow curve) shows several peaks at fixed values of temperature (see Fig. 4.2.14).

These peaks are caused by the emptying of the different traps in the forbidden band and the subsequent emission of light when the electrons fall back into the valence band: the smaller the energy gap between the trap and the conduction band, the lower the temperature at which the peak will appear. The lower temperature peaks are usually rejected, as they can be more easily affected by fluctuations due to thermal excitation at room temperature.

Typical TL dosimeter readers allow the user to choose between different settings related to different readout system gains, offering either high sensitivity or wide range.

A major issue affecting TL dosimetry is fading, that is, the loss of information due to light excitation, thermal excitation at room temperature, or other imperfectly understood mechanisms. The fading phenomenon varies strongly from one material to another and depends on both the readout and the storage conditions (light, temperature, humidity). For some TL materials it is negligible, while for others materials it is extremely relevant (Horowitz, 1981).

Unless the fading of the selected TL material is negligible over long periods, when a precise comparison of measurements has to be performed, it is recommended that the readout be observed after the same time interval in all cases. Moreover, the dosimeters must be kept under the same conditions of temperature, light, and humidity before the readout.

*Calibration.* The response of TL dosimeters within the same set may vary because of small differences in the weights of the chips, small variations in their composition, or their individual radiation

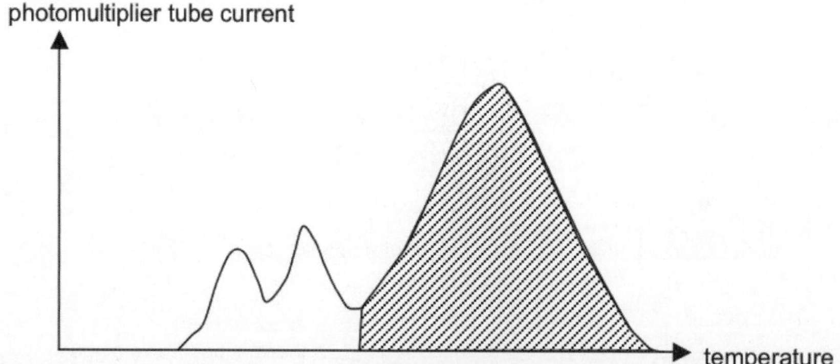


**Figure 4.2.14.** Schematic of a glow curve for a TL dosimeter material. It is usually good practice to reject the low temperature peaks and to integrate only the area under the higher temperature peaks, as highlighted in the graph.

histories. Thus, ideally, individual calibrations must be performed periodically, especially when relative dose measurements (e.g., depth dose distribution) have to be carried out. Alternatively, TL dosimeters can be grouped in batches according to their sensitivities.

*Advantages and disadvantages.* The main advantage of TL dosimeters is their small size. This provides a high degree of portability, allowing for off-site measurements and in vivo dosimetry. It also implies a small perturbation of the radiation field, thus on-patient measurements or depth dose measurements in tissue equivalent materials become feasible.

For these reasons, and also because of the wide range of available TL materials, allowing the selection of the most suitable one for each application, TL dosimetry is one of the most used dosimetry methods. However, other issues must be taken into account in order to avoid imprecise and misleading results:

- First, and most obvious, TL dosimeters must be handled with care, avoiding scratches that may alter their weight and dust that may mask the light emitted during the readout process. Moreover, a TL dosimeter can be damaged and lose sensitivity if exposed to either a very high dose during the irradiation process or excessive temperatures during the readout or annealing process. A recalibration is recommended every time any of these conditions occurs.
- For similar reasons, TL dosimeters are not recommended for use in water phantoms unless they are properly protected.
- Nonlinear behavior occurs above a certain energy (typically a few Gy). Typical behavior consists (Horowitz, 1981) of a region of supralinearity up to about 100 Gy, followed by a decrease of the readout–dose ratio until reaching a sublinear regime at dose levels of $10^3$ to $10^5$ Gy, as shown in Figure 4.2.15. Because the width of the supralinearity region depends on both the beam energy and the particles studied, apart from the TL material used and the composition and density of dopants, a calibration over the entire energy range of interest and for all the beam types involved must be performed.
- Some TL materials are not tissue equivalent. This may give rise to the problems previously discussed in section 4.2.1. Figure 4.2.16 shows a comparison of the photon mass energy absorption coefficient for several TL materials.

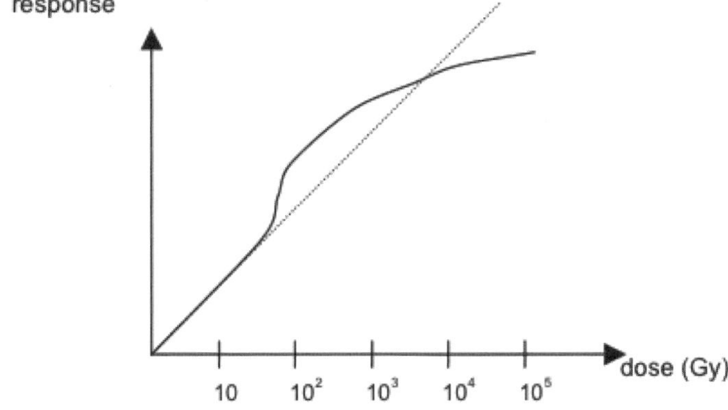


**Figure 4.2.15.** Generic diagram of the response of a TL dosimeter.

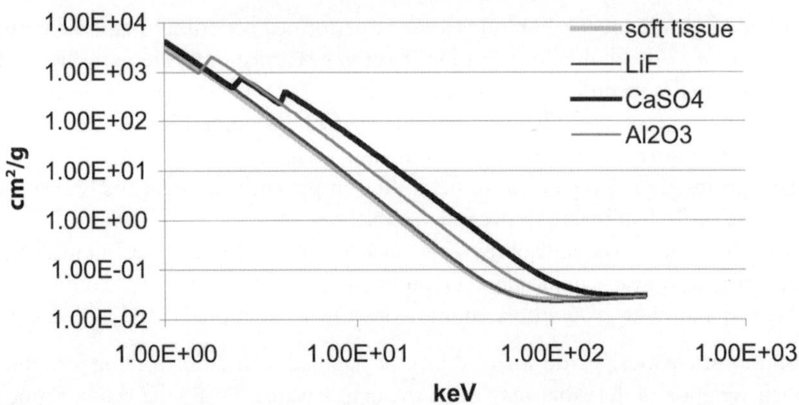


**Figure 4.2.16.** Mass energy absorption coefficients of some TL dosimeter materials (data from Nowotny, 1998).

- Although TL dosimeters are suitable for depth dose measurements, they are in general not very suitable for use in the presence of a strong radiation field gradient because their response depends on the depth at which the dose is deposited. Thus, unless they are uniformly irradiated, the result of a measurement may be misleading. Uniform irradiation in the presence of a strong radiation field gradient is possible only with small-size dosimeters, but a very small-size dosimeter is less reliable because of the large uncertainties that can affect the measurement. Better performances are obtained in this case with TL dosimeters in powder form.
- Reproducibility of the heating cycle is mandatory for good reproducibility of the results. This is normally achieved with modern readout systems.

### 4.2.4.2. Optically Stimulated Luminescence Dosimetry

The use of OSL dosimeters has developed only in recent years and is not yet competitive with TL dosimetry. However, its main advantage is that the processes involved are purely optical, so the readout system is simple compared with that for TL dosimetry, and the number of control parameters is reduced.

As the physical mechanisms involved are related, most of the issues discussed for TL dosimetry also apply to OSL dosimetry, including the relevance of fading and the necessity for both an average and individual calibration. Moreover, OSL dosimeters and TL dosimeters share ease of portability and convenience of use.

An OSL dosimetry readout system consists of a laser for stimulating the dosimeter and a photomultiplier tube for detecting the light emitted. A similar process to annealing can be useful in depleting the traps completely after the readout, although it is less important for a good result than is the annealing of TL dosimeters.

The dosimeter can be equipped with optical fibers for channeling both the stimulating and emitted light. In this case, "near-real-time" measurements are possible. Currently the most commonly used OSL material is $Al_2O_3$:C (Aznar et al., 2004; Bøtter-Jensen et al., 1997; Gaza, McKeever, & Akselrod, 2005), which has TL properties, but its OSL properties are more appealing for dosimetry. These include high sensitivity, high reproducibility, and linearity over a wide range. It has been shown (Bøtter-Jensen et al., 1997) that a standard $Al_2O_3$:C chip is sensitive to doses below 1 μGy and that its range of linearity with dose is about 0.05 to 50 Gy. Moreover, it is less subject to fading than typical TL dosimeters.

Because of its higher sensitivity, an OSL dosimeter can be built in smaller sizes than can a TL dosimeter, allowing reliable dose measurements in the presence of a strong radiation field gradient. Another advantage resulting from the use of OSL is the presence of a phenomenon called radioluminescence (RL), which consists of immediate and continuous luminescence during the irradiation. Although RL increases with irradiation time (Aznar et al., 2004), it can provide information about the delivered dose during the irradiation if the dosimeter is coupled with optical fibers. Another recently proposed method for obtaining near-real-time dose measurements in radiotherapy is to stimulate the dosimeter during the irradiation by using the same optical fiber for both the stimulation and the emission (Gaza et al., 2005).

The use of OSL dosimeters has been proposed in mammography (Aznar et al., 2005) and in vivo radiotherapy (Aznar et al., 2004; Yukihara et al., 2005). Currently, although TL dosimetry is a more established technique, OSL dosimetry is becoming competitive, and commercial systems are now available.

## 4.2.5. SEMICONDUCTOR DOSIMETERS

### 4.2.5.1. Silicon Diodes

#### 4.2.5.1.1. General Principles

A Si diode can be thought of as a solid-state equivalent of an ion chamber, consisting basically of two Si structures in contact, a p-doped one and an n-doped one. The p-doped Si has an excess of holes, while the n-doped Si has an excess of electrons.

If the two structures are in contact, the electrons migrate from the n-doped to the p-doped region, recombining with holes and leaving behind fixed positive charges in the form of ionized donor impurities. Conversely, holes will migrate to the n-doped region, leaving behind fixed acceptor sites that have acquired extra electrons. The net effect of this charge distribution is a potential gradient.

The junction region remains "depleted," that is, the density of the remaining charge carriers is negligible. When radiation hits the depleted zone, a number of electron-hole pairs proportional to the dose deposited in the chip are created. Because of the electric field created by charge displacement, electrons are attracted toward the n side and holes are attracted toward the p side.

This effect can be enhanced if the structure is reverse-biased, that is, if the n side is connected to a positive voltage. The potential gradient is enhanced and so is the charge collection efficiency when radiation hits the chip. Moreover, the thickness of the depleted region increases, increasing the efficiency of the diode.

The most typical Si diodes are called p-type and n-type diodes. A p-type Si diode consists of p-doped Si with a thin layer of n-doped Si diffused on the surface. An n-type Si diode consists of a p-doped layer diffused on the surface of an n-doped substrate.

Another diode used in dosimetry is the so-called p-i-n diode (positive-intrinsic-negative), consisting of an intrinsic Si layer with p-doped and n-doped Si diffused on opposite sides (see Fig. 4.2.17). P-i-n diodes have a higher charge collection efficiency than p-n diodes (Knoll, 2000).

#### 4.2.5.1.2. Characteristics of Si Diode Dosimeters

Both n-type and p-type Si diodes are available for dosimetry, p-type diodes being suitable for radiotherapy because they are more radiation resistant and have a smaller dark current (Grusell & Rikner, 1993). Typical Si diode dosimeters can be manufactured in very small sizes (a few hundred microns in size). They are usually sealed to allow measurements in vivo or in water and are provided with suitable buildup caps for different applications.

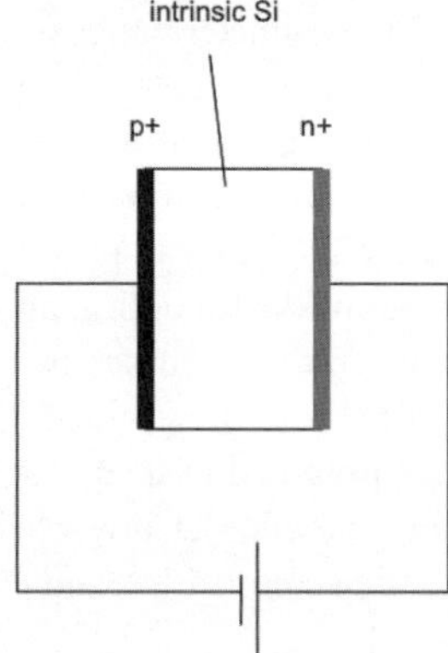



**Figure 4.2.17.** A p-i-n diode.

In clinical practice, Si diodes are frequently unbiased in order to limit as much as possible the leakage current, and hence the noise, allowing the measurement of low doses despite a loss in sensitivity because of the smaller size (a few tens of micrometers) of the depleted region. This also makes "in vivo" use very convenient.

Although they are more suitable for electron dosimetry than for photon and neutron dosimetry—not being tissue equivalent—Si diodes have become a standard in radiotherapy because of their ease of use.

The performance of Si diode dosimeters is well documented, and typical response characteristics include the following:

- Linearity—until radiation damage occurs (see below) Si diodes are linear with dose.
- Dependence on dose rate—the sensitivity of most Si diode dosimeters appears to be independent of dose rate for continuous irradiation, while it is an increasing function of the dose per pulse when irradiated with pulsed beams (Grusell & Rikner, 1985; Jornet, Ribas, & Eudaldo, 2000; Marre & Marinello, 2004; Rikner & Grusell, 1983). This effect is more relevant in n-type diodes.
- Radiation damage—the sensitivity of both p-type and n-type Si diodes has been shown to decrease sharply initially as a function of dose and decreases at a slower rate (Rikner & Grusell, 1983). Thus frequent calibration is recommended, especially in the initial stages. As previously pointed out, this effect is less important for p-type diodes than for n-type diodes. In order to limit the initial sharp decrease of sensitivity, many commercially available Si diodes are preirradiated with a dose of about 5 kGy to 10 kGy. Another effect related to radiation damage is the loss of linearity with respect to dose rate when Si diodes are used in pulsed radiation beams. This effect is more relevant to n-type Si diodes (Grusell & Rikner, 1985).
- Angular dependence—a certain angular dependence related to beam quality and diode geometrical characteristics has been shown, with typical maximum variations as functions of the beam angle ranging from about 2% to 3% to more than 20% (Eveling, Morgan, & Pitchford, 1999; Jornet et al., 2000; Marre & Marinello, 2004).

- Temperature dependence—operating temperature affects the response of Si diodes. Typical changes in sensitivity due to increases in temperature are about 0.2% to 0.3% per degree Celsius (Grusell & Rikner, 1986; Jornet et al., 2000; Saini & Zhu, 2002; Welsh & Reinstein, 2001). This may slightly affect in vivo dose measurements.

### 4.2.5.1.3. Typical Applications

Silicon diodes are widespread in clinical dosimetry. They are typically used for in vivo measurements of entrance and exit doses, but their small size also allows intracavity use as well as precise measurements of small beams and large gradients in the radiation field. Online measurements are also possible. 2-D arrays can also be built (Jursinic & Nelms, 2003), allowing 2-D dose mapping.

Large area diodes (a few millimeters on a side) are used for measuring low doses, but are not usually used in diagnostic dosimetry because diagnostic X-ray beams are easily monitored by means of tissue-equivalent detectors such as ion chambers or some types of TL dosimeters.

### 4.2.5.2. MOSFETs

#### 4.2.5.2.1. General Principles

A metal oxide semiconductor field-effect transistor (MOSFET) is a very well-known electronic device, the use of which has been well established in radiation dosimetry since the early 1990s, although it was originally proposed in 1974 (Holmes-Siedl, 1974).

A p-MOSFET, the most frequently used type (see Fig. 4.2.18), consists of an n-doped Si substrate, p-doped Si source and drain, and a metallic gate separated from the substrate by a thin oxide layer. When a gate bias is applied (negative in the case of p-MOSFETs) with an absolute value larger than a value $V_t$, the area below the oxide is converted into a channel that allows the flow of a source-drain current.

When the chip is irradiated, electron-hole pairs are created in the oxide. A fraction of them recombine, but some of the holes are trapped in the oxide-substrate interface, creating an electric field that increases the absolute value of $V_t$. The variation in $V_t$ is directly proportional to the dose delivered in the detector.

Two modes of operation are possible:

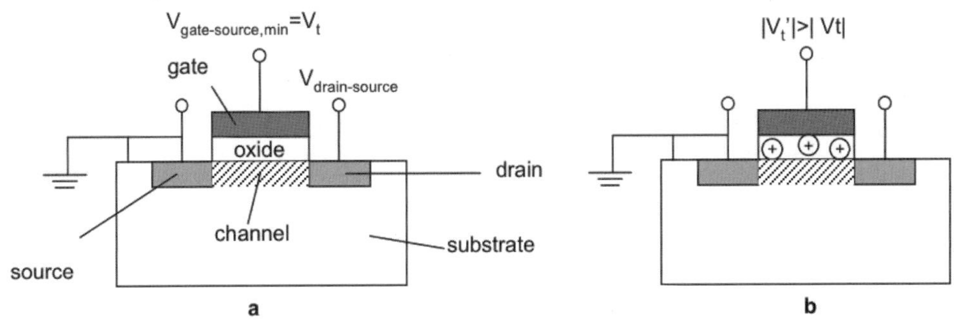


**Figure 4.2.18.** A MOSFET dosimeter: (a) before irradiation and (b) after irradiation.

- Biased mode—a gate-source bias is applied, limiting the recombination of electrons and holes. The variation in $V_t$ is thus increased and the resulting device is more sensitive.
- Unbiased mode—during the irradiation the chip is kept unbiased. It is read "offline" by measuring the shift in $V_t$ with respect to the nonirradiated system.

The most obvious advantage of the unbiased operation mode with respect to the biased mode is greater portability and the possibility of in vivo use. However, fading occurs in the unbiased mode because of the recombination of electrons and holes.

Conversely, a major issue in the biased mode is the fluctuation in $V_t$ caused by changes in external temperature. A possible solution to this problem was proposed by Soubra et al. (1994) and consists of the coupling of two MOSFETs, each with a different initial value of $V_t$. The difference between the values of $V_t$ after the irradiation in the two chips is related to the absorbed dose; the response of the device has been shown to be constant for doses up to 50 Gy to 60 Gy.

### 4.2.5.2.2. Characteristics of MOSFET Dosimeters

Metal oxide semiconductor field-effect transistor dosimeters share many characteristics with Si diode dosimeters. In particular, because they are not tissue equivalent, they are more suitable for electron dosimetry.

If they are operated in biased mode, MOSFETs offer the possibility of online dose readouts, and commercial systems are available for this task. However, they cannot be used in intensity modulated radiotherapy (IMRT) because of the so-called creep-up effect, which consists of an increase in $V_t$ in consecutive readings depending on the time interval between readings. This effect decreases after a few minutes and occurs for doses above 20 Gy (Ramani, Russell, & O'Brien, 1997). The effect of too short an interval between consecutive readouts is an overestimate of the dose.

The response characteristics of MOSFET dosimeters are the following:

- Linearity: The main advantage of MOSFET dosimeters is the large range of linearity (from a few mGy to tens of Gy).
- Radiation damage: The sensitivity of MOSFETs decreases steadily with accumulated dose, thus frequent calibration is required. Their lifetimes, depending on the beam quality and the operating parameters, have been estimated to be as low as 50 Gy for low-energy X-rays and about 200 Gy for high-energy photon and electron beams (Ehringfeld et al., 2005).
- Angular dependence: Angular dependence values vary significantly from author to author. The maximum reported variation as a function of the beam incidence angle is between 2.5% and 26%, depending on the dosimeter type and beam quality (Chuang, Verhey, & Xia, 2002; Ehringfeld et al., 2005; Ramani et al., 1997; Scalchi & Francescon, 1998).
- Temperature dependence: This is particularly relevant when performing in vivo measurements because the response will depend on the patient skin or internal temperature (Welsh & Reinstein, 2001).

Because of individual variability, MOSFETs need individual calibration.

### 4.2.5.2.3. Typical Applications

Metal oxide semiconductor field-effect transistors are suitable for conventional radiotherapy, and because of their small size they are particularly appealing when a high spatial resolution is required.

The use of implanted unbiased MOSFETs has been recently proposed (Beddar et al., 2005), allowing long-term use in radiotherapy treatment. Also, because of their linearity over a wide range, MOSFETs are suitable for use in quality assurance programs.

## 4.2.6. FILM DOSIMETRY

### 4.2.6.1. Radiographic Films

#### 4.2.6.1.1. General Principles

The use of radiographic films as dosimeters is well established. A radiographic film comprises a thin layer of polyethylene or other plastic material coated with a layer of emulsion. The emulsion typically consists of silver halide grains (in most cases silver bromide [AgBr]) dispersed in gelatin. Exposure to radiation causes ionization of the halide, forming a so-called latent image. The development process makes the image visible: the darker the area on the film, the higher the dose received.

The image can then be evaluated by means of a densitometer, an instrument capable of measuring the transmission of a small visible-light beam through the film. The output of a densitometer is the optical density (OD), defined as $OD = \log_{10}(I_0/I)$, where $I_0$ is the incident light intensity and $I$ is the transmitted light intensity. The response plot of a radiographic film is called a sensitometric curve (or HD curve, from Hurter and Driffield, who originally investigated it), and it shows the OD as a function of the exposure or the dose.

When a sensitometric curve is plotted, a logarithmic $x$-axis results in the sigmoid shape shown in Figure 4.2.19, and features five typical zones:

- Fog—the optical density corresponding to no exposure, which is usually subtracted from measurements
- Toe—a sublinear variation of OD for low exposures
- Linear—the useful portion of the exposure curve

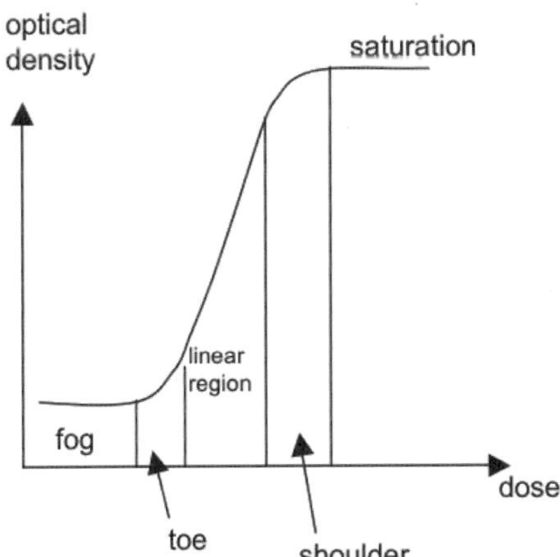


**Figure 4.2.19.** A typical response for a radiographic film. This characteristic ("HD") curve plots the OD against the logarithm to the base 10 of the relative exposure.

- Shoulder—the end of linear region
- Saturation—the region of constant OD for high exposure

As is clear from the figure, the expected exposure range must be known in advance in order to make sure that it falls within the linearity range.

The parameters characterizing a sensitometric curve are the following:

- Latitude—the ratio between the two extremes of the linearity region. For instance, if the maximum exposure within the linearity region is 10 Gy and the minimum is 1 Gy, the latitude is 10:1.
- Gamma—the slope of the linear portion of the curve
- Speed or sensitivity—the exposure required to produce a density of 1.0 over the fog level

### 4.2.6.1.2. Characteristics of Radiographic Film Dosimeters

A radiographic film provides a 2-D distribution of dose with a spatial resolution that can be down to a few micrometers. Characteristic parameters of a radiographic film include the size of the AgBr grains, the number of grains per unit area, and the thickness of the emulsion. The combination of these parameters affects the sensitivity and the spatial resolution of the film.

The main characteristics of radiographic film dosimeters are the following:

- *Tissue equivalence*: Radiographic films are not tissue equivalent, thus they must be carefully calibrated as a function of the beam energy, especially when used with photons. The result of a change in energy is a change in the slope of the sensitometric curve (Cheng & Das, 1996; Muench et al., 1991).
- *Linearity*: Although there are significant variations from one type of film to another, the typical range of use for film dosimeters is in tenths of grays (Bos et al., 2002; Cheng & Das, 1996).
- *Dose rate dependence*: Unlike diagnostic radiographic films, the response of most dosimetry films is nearly dose-rate independent because the energy is deposited by photons and electrons in a single hit, not allowing fading as occurs for visible light. However, a dependence on dose rate has recently been reported for new films (Martens et al., 2002).
- *Angular dependence*: The angular dependence of a film is limited, unless it is nearly parallel to the radiation beam.
- *Sensitivity to ambient parameters*: Variations from one batch to another, which are typically related to storage conditions, have been reported (Bos et al., 2002; Childress, Dong, & Rosen, 2002). Thus it is essential that a calibration film be exposed along with each series of films. Film dosimeters are also sensitive to visible and ultraviolet (UV) light, and are commonly packaged in light-tight envelopes.
- *Other factors affecting the response*: The temperature of the chemicals strongly affects the response of radiographic film (Bogucki et al., 1997), but this is a minor problem because most commonly available developers keep the chemicals at a constant temperature. The type of reader used may also affect the response (Bos et al., 2002).

### 4.2.6.1.3. Typical Applications

Since they are not tissue equivalent, film dosimeters are particularly suited for electron dosimetry. Their use in quality assurance of radiotherapy machines (congruence of light and radiation fields, determination of collimators position, etc.) is well established.

They are also used in IMRT (Esthappan et al., 2002; Martens et al., 2002) and in interventional radiology (Morrell & Rogers, 2004; Vano et al., 1997).

A common application is in personal dosimeters and film badges; these are equipped with filters of different materials (typically aluminum and copper) and thicknesses. Comparison of readouts in all regions makes possible not only calculation of the absorbed dose, but also determination of the source that produced the exposure.

### 4.2.6.2. Radiochromic Film

#### 4.2.6.2.1. General Principles

Radiochromic films (the most typical being GAFCHROMIC® films) are a more recent alternative to radiographic films as dosimeters. A radiochromic film is a colorless film containing a dye that polymerizes when exposed to radiation, changing the color of the film different shades of blue. The resulting optical density can be read using a laser and photodiode system or a digitizer.

#### 4.2.6.2.2. Characteristics of Radiochromic Film Dosimeters

The typical range of use of radiochromic films is broader and shifted toward high doses in comparison with radiographic films. Radiochromic films have shown a good response from about 10 Gy to $10^4$ Gy (McLaughlin et al., 1991). Their main advantages are the following:

- Good tissue equivalence
- Independent of the dose rate (Butson et al., 2003; Dini, Koona, Ahbourn, & Meigooni, 2005)
- High spatial resolution (about 1200 lp/mm; McLaughlin et al., 1991) because of their grainless nature
- Nearly flat angular response
- Limited dependence on ambient parameters within a reasonable range of temperature and humidity (Abdel-Fattah & Miller, 1996)
- Insensitivity to visible light, which implies less stringent requirements in terms of packaging

The sensitometric curve of radiochromic films depends strongly on the color spectrum of the densitometer in terms of both linearity and sensitivity (Butson, Cheung, & Yu, 2004; Kellermann, Ertl, & Gornik, 1998; Lee, Fung, & Kwok, 2005).

Probably the biggest disadvantage of radiochromic films is their continuous darkening after irradiation. Since this process stabilizes after a few hours (Ali et al., 2003; Meigooni et al., 1996; McLaughlin et al., 1991), it is a common practice to read radiochromic films 24 hours after exposure. This, of course, limits their clinical use.

#### 4.2.6.2.3. Typical Applications

Because of their high spatial resolution and independence of dose rate, radiochromic films are particularly suited for measurements of high dose gradients, for instance, near brachytherapy sources and in stereotactic fields (Chiu-Tsao, de la Zerda, Lin, & Kim, 1994; Sharma, Bianchi, Conte, Novario, & Bhatt, 2004). Their use is also documented at tissue interfaces (Niromaand-Rav et al., 1996; Reinstein, Gluckman, & Meek 1998).

## 4.2.7. DIAMOND DOSIMETRY

### 4.2.7.1. General Principles

The potential of diamond detectors was investigated as early as the 1940s, although research in this field was not pursued because of the limited availability and the variability of natural diamonds. Only a very small fraction of natural diamonds—those with very low impurity levels—can be used as radiation detectors, and they need individual calibration and characterization. Research into using diamonds began again after techniques for growing synthetic diamonds, such as chemical vapor deposition (CVD), became established.

Irradiated diamonds show a linear current-voltage characteristic, the resistivity decreasing with the dose rate. This effect is due to the creation of electron-ion pairs using ionizing radiation that drift toward the electrodes when a voltage is applied.

The presence of impurities strongly influences the lifetime of charge carriers in diamond. Thus, in order to ensure full charge collection, it has been calculated that the optimal thickness of a diamond detector is about 0.1 mm to 0.3 mm (Altukhov et al., 2004).

### 4.2.7.2. Characteristics of Diamond Dosimeters

A typical diamond detector is a few cubic millimeters in volume and is sealed in a resin or polystyrene case. The bias voltage is applied by means of metal contacts. Due to the presence of defects in the diamond lattice, a space charge can be accumulated inside the crystal. This effect is known to stabilize after a certain dose, so diamond dosimeters need to be preirradiated with a dose that may vary from 0.1 Gy to 10 Gy (Cirrone et al., 2003; Prosvirin et al., 2004). The following are some of the characteristics of diamond dosimeters:

- *Tissue equivalence:* One of the main advantages of diamond dosimeters is their near-tissue equivalence ($Z = 6$), deviations from which are due mainly to the geometry and the composition of the electrodes. However, the energy response is nearly flat for photons above about 200 keV, and for lower energies the energy dependence is weaker than in other detectors (Yin et al., 2004).
- *Radiation damage*: One major advantage of diamond dosimeters is their radiation hardness: they show no change in response for photon doses up to 100 kGy (Bauer et al., 1995) and electron doses up to 1 MGy (Mainwood, 2000).
- *Dose rate dependence*: The current as a function of dose rate shows a small deviation from linearity (Burgermeister, 1981; Planskoy, 1980).
- *Dependence on ambient parameters*: Diamond detectors show a small change in sensitivity related to an increase in temperature (Nakano et al., 2003).
- *Angular dependence*: Angular dependence is negligible (Nakano et al., 2003).
- Sensitivity: Because of its smaller atomic number, wider band gap (5.5 eV compared to 3.6 eV for Si), and constraints on thickness, the efficiency of a typical diamond detector is lower than that of a typical Si detector, as shown in Figure 4.2.20. On the other hand, the wider band gap implies a lower leakage current.

### 4.2.7.3. Typical Applications

The main limitation to the widespread use of diamond dosimeters is their high cost. They are typically used for online dose rate measurements, but can also be used as TL dosimeters for offline integrated dose measurement (Borchi et al., 1998; Cuttone et al., 1999; Mobit & Sandison, 1999).

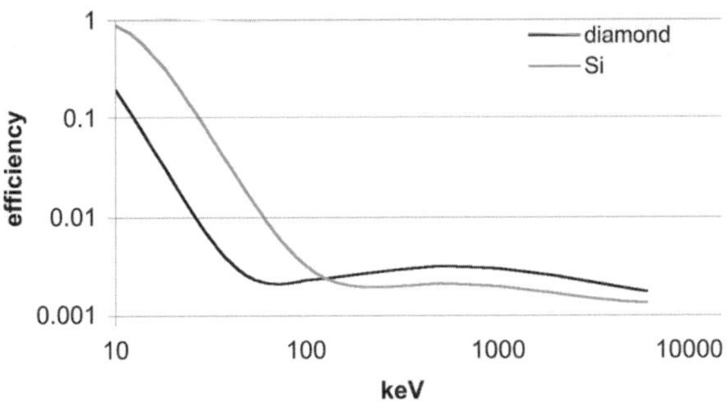


**Figure 4.2.20.** Photon absorption efficiency for a Si detector and a diamond detector, both 300 μm in thickness (data from Nowotny, 1998).

Because of their small size, diamond dosimeters are particularly suitable for measuring strong dose gradients, such as in stereotactic radiosurgery (Heydarian, Hoban, & Beddoe, 1996). They have also provided good results for less conventional uses, such as proton dosimetry (Cuttone et al., 1999; Onori et al., 2000) or α-particle dosimetry (Keddy, Nam, & Burns, 1987).

## 4.2.8. CHEMICAL DOSIMETRY

Chemical dosimetry is based on measurements of chemical changes produced by radiation. As will be discussed, some chemical dosimeters can be used as absolute dosimeters.

The use of gel-based chemical dosimeters represents the only dosimetric technique capable of providing 3-D information in solid phantoms. Gels can be shaped in any form, acting concurrently as dosimeters and phantoms, and are nearly tissue equivalent.

Three types of chemical dosimeters are used: Fricke dosimeters, polymer gels, and alanine dosimeters.

### 4.2.8.1. Fricke Dosimetry

#### 4.2.8.1.1. General Principles

A Fricke dosimeter is based on the measurement of the fraction of ferrous ions ($Fe^{2+}$) that have been oxidized to ferric ions ($Fe^{3+}$) through a series of chemical reactions triggered by radiation. More details about these reactions can be found in Greening (1985).

The original dosimeter, proposed by Fricke and coworkers in 1927, consists of a solution of ferrous sulfate in air-saturated dilute sulfuric acid. The yield of ferric ions is measured by spectrophotometry of the solution, which has absorption peaks in the UV region at 224 nm and 304 nm.

In principle, a Fricke dosimeter can be used as an absolute dosimeter, the absorbed dose in the solution being calculated as follows (Greening, 1985):

$$D = \frac{A - A_0}{\rho G\left(Fe^{3+}\right) l \varepsilon_m},$$

(4.2.5)

where $A$ and $A_0$ are the optical densities of the solution after the irradiation and before it, respectively; $\rho$ is the density of the solution; $G(Fe^{3+})$ is the radiation chemical yield of $Fe^{3+}$, that is, the amount of substance that is produced by radiation per unit energy deposited; $l$ is the length of the light path of the spectrometer; and $\varepsilon_m$ is the molar absorption coefficient of $Fe^{3+}$ solution: $\varepsilon_m = A/lc$, where $c$ is the concentration of the solute.

However, as the parameters affecting the dose response of a Fricke dosimeter vary greatly depending on the preparation, it is more common to use a Fricke dosimeter after a calibration against an absolute dosimeter rather than as an absolute dosimeter itself. Three-dimensional dose distributions can be calculated by means of optical tomography (Kelly, Jordan, & Battista, 1998).

In the 1980s, an alternative technique for measuring the amount of $Fe^{2+}$ ions was proposed by Gore, Kang, and Schulz (1984). It consists of measuring the spin relaxation times of the dosimetric solution before and after the irradiation by means of magnetic resonance, based on the linear increase of the relaxation times $T_2$ and $T_1$ as a function of the concentration of $Fe^{2+}$.

Usually the ferrous sulfate solution is dispersed in a gel matrix, typically gelatin or agarose (Schreiner, 2004). This strongly limits the diffusion of ions that causes a blur in the dose distribution when using an aqueous solution and allows 3-D dosimetry. The gel acts as a phantom and as a dosimeter at the same time, removing any problems related to discontinuity in the medium.

### 4.2.8.1.2. Characteristics of Fricke Dosimeters

As previously mentioned, the main advantage of Fricke gels is the ability to perform 3-D dosimetry. In addition, there are other advantages:

- *Tissue equivalence*: Fricke dosimeters are nearly tissue equivalent (Klassen et al., 1999; Kron, Metcalfe, & Pope, 1993).
- *Linearity*: Fricke dosimeters show good linearity up to a certain dose, depending on the concentration of iron ions. Saturation occurs when all $Fe^{2+}$ ions have been converted into $Fe^{3+}$. For typical Fricke dosimeters, saturation occurs at about 500 Gy for aqueous dosimeters (Podgorsak & Schreiner, 1992) and at about 50 Gy or less for gel dosimeters (Gambarini et al., 1994; Hazle et al., 1991; Schulz, Venkataramanan, & Huq, 1990). The minimum detectable dose is on the order of 1 Gy for magnetic resonance imaging (MRI) measurements (Olsson, Petersson, Ahlgren, & Mattsson, 1989) and can be decreased by about one order of magnitude for spectrophotometric readouts (Mattsson, Johansson, & Svensson, 1982).
- *Dose rate dependence*: Fricke dosimeters are not dose rate dependent (Olsson et al., 1989; Schulz et al., 1990).
- *Reproducibility*: Reproducibility is reported to be within a few percent (Chu et al., 1998; Johansson Bäck et al., 1998).

The main limiting factor to the spatial resolution of a Fricke dosimeter is the diffusion of ferric ions after irradiation (Olsson, Westrin, Fransson, & Nordell, 1992; Schulz et al., 1990). This factor is dependent on the time interval between the irradiation and the readout and on the dose delivered. However, gels with a low diffusion of $Fe^{3+}$ have recently been proposed (Chu, Jordan, Battista, Van Dyk, & Rutt, 2000).

### 4.2.8.1.3. Typical Applications

Fricke dosimeters are only used in beam calibration and for validating Monte Carlo algorithms in radiotherapy. They have proven valuable for both megavoltage and kilovoltage beams (Kron & Pope, 1994). Brachytherapy sources have been characterized (Schreiner et al., 1994) and less conventional uses, such as proton beam dosimetry (Bäck et al., 1999) and neutron dosimetry (Gambarini, Birattari, Colombi, Pirola, & Rosi, 2002), have been reported.

### 4.2.8.2. Polymer Gels

#### 4.2.8.2.1. General Principles

The use of polymer gel dosimeters was first proposed by Maryanski, Gore, Kennan, and Sculz (1993) in order to overcome some of the main limitations of Fricke dosimeters, the most important being the loss of spatial resolution due to ferric ion diffusion.

In a polymer gel dosimeter, monomers such as acrylamide are dispersed in a gel matrix (gelatin or agarose). Upon irradiation, the monomer polymerizes. The degree of polymerization can be determined by MRI (Maryanski et al., 1993), optical computed tomography (CT) (Xu, Wuu, & Maryanski, 2004), X-ray CT (Hilts, Jirasek, & Duzenli, 2005; Jenneson et al., 2004), ultrasound tomography (Mather & Baldock, 2003), proton spectroscopy (Murphy et al., 2000). There is a relation of proportionality between the degree of polymerization and the absorbed dose.

After the development of monomer-polymer gels known as BANG-type (bis-acrylamide, nitrogen, and gelatin) (Maryanski et al., 1996) and PAG-type (polyacrylamide gel), other gels were developed in order to overcome their main limitation, that is, their sensitivity to oxygen, which inhibits polymerization, causing a threshold effect (De Deene, Reynaert, & De Wagter, 2001; Hepworth, Leach, & Doran, 1999). In particular, in the so-called MAGIC gel (methacrylic and ascorbic acid in gelatin initiated by copper), oxygen is necessary for polymerization to take place (Fong et al., 2001).

#### 4.2.8.2.2. Characteristics of Polymer Gel Dosimeters

Polymer gels share many advantages with Fricke gels. In particular good tissue equivalence makes polymer gels suitable for low energies (Pantelis et al., 2004) and for building phantoms of any shape for the calibration of radiotherapy beams and the validation of Monte Carlo protocols.

The main advantages of polymer gels are good tissue equivalence, independence of dose rate (Maryanski et al., 1996; McJury et al., 2000; Novotny et al., 2001), and relatively high sensitivity. Ibbott et al. (1997) reported that doses as small as 0.1 Gy can be detected, while greater sensitivity has been reported by MacDougall, Miquel, Wilson, Keevil, and Smith (2005).

Although the dose values above which linear behavior is lost depend strongly on the composition of the gel (Fong et al., 2001), it can be said that, in general, saturation occurs at higher doses for MAGIC-type gels than for BANG-type gels, the first being able to work at up to several tens of grays (De Deene et al., 2002; Fong et al., 2001; Trapp et al., 2004), while the latter are suitable for dose levels within 10 Gy (Hilts et al., 2005; Maryanski et al., 1996). Gels with added ascorbic acid have a much wider range of linearity (De Deene et al., 2002).

On the other hand, the main limitation to the use of polymer gel dosimeters is a variability in response that can be as large as 15% from one dosimeter to another (MacDougall et al., 2005). Another serious limitation to widespread use is their toxicity.

Also, polymerization occurs after irradiation, causing a change in response that eventually reaches a plateau as much as several days later (MacDougall et al., 2005; McJury et al., 1999a). Postirradiation polymerization depends on several factors, including light, heat, and impurities (McJury et al., 2000). Some diffusion of monomers may also introduce errors in measurements of steep dose gradients (Vergote et al., 2004).

#### 4.2.8.2.3. Typical Applications

The application of polymer gels for the calibration of several types of radiotherapy sources has been evaluated. In particular, their use has been proposed for brachytherapy sources (Kipouros et al., 2003;

McJury et al., 1999b), for IMRT (Wuu et al., 2004), and for stereotactic radiosurgery (McJury et al., 2000; Novotny et al., 2002). Moreover, the use of polymer gels for neutron dosimetry appears promising (Uusi-Simola et al., 2003).

### 4.2.8.3. Alanine/Electron Spin Resonance Dosimetry

#### 4.2.8.3.1. General Principles

Alanine is an amino acid that can be used for high dose dosimetry in the form of pellets, films, or gels. Radiation causes the formation of alanine radicals, the concentration of which can be measured by means of electron spin resonance (ESR) or electron paramagnetic resonance (EPR) (Pilbrow, 1996).

#### 4.2.8.3.2. Characteristics of Alanine Dosimeters

Alanine dosimeters are nearly tissue equivalent (Olsson, Bergstrand, Carlsson, Hole, & Lund, 2002) and have a fairly flat energy response over the typical energy range for radiotherapy (Zeng et al., 2004, 2005). They have a linear response over a wide range up to above 40 kGy (Olsson, Lund, & Erickson, 1996; Wieser & Girzikowsky 1996).

The main limitation of alanine/ESR dosimetry is its low sensitivity; high doses are necessary to obtain good reproducibility (De Angelis et al., 1999). However, it has been reported that preirradiation with about 50 Gy allows for subsequent detection of doses as low as 2 Gy (Olsson et al., 1996).

The response depends on both temperature and humidity (Arber & Sharpe, 1993; Bugay et al., 2000; Olsson et al., 2002), thus the calibration must take into account environmental conditions. Although some fading has been reported (Arber & Sharpe, 1993; Olsson et al., 1996), alanine dosimeters are suitable for long-term information storage.

Because of the necessity of using a minimum volume of about 0.05 cm$^3$ in order to achieve an acceptable SNR ratio (Olsson et al., 2002), the spatial resolution of alanine dosimeters is not as good as that of other solid-state dosimeters. However, it is acceptable for most typical radiotherapy applications.

#### 4.2.8.3.3. Typical Applications

Because of their characteristic of long-term stability after irradiation, the use of alanine dosimeters appears promising for dosimetry comparisons among different centers (Bartolotta et al., 1993; Gall et al., 1996). Also, because of their low sensitivity, they are suitable for high dose applications, and in particular, high dose rate brachytherapy (De Angelis et al., 1999; Guzman Calcina, et al., 2005; Olsson et al., 2002), proton beam therapy (Gall et al., 1996; Onori et al., 1997), and dose monitoring in radiation-harsh environments such as particle accelerators.

## 4.2.9. SCINTILLATION DOSIMETERS

### 4.2.9.1. General Principles

Scintillation dosimetry has been proposed relatively recently and is not yet a well-established technique. Scintillation detectors are based on the conversion of the kinetic energy of charged particles into detectable light and are optically coupled to a photomultiplier. A typical scintillation material must exhibit a high light yield proportional to the energy deposited, and should be transparent to the wavelength of its own emission (Knoll, 2000). Moreover, the decay time of the induced luminescence must be short enough to allow fast signal pulses. This is particularly relevant when a fast response is needed (e.g., in IMRT). For a complete discussion of the characteristics of scintillation detectors, see Knoll (2000).

### 4.2.9.2. Characteristics of Scintillation Dosimeters

A typical scintillation dosimeter consists of a scintillation detector, a fiber-optic bundle, and a photo-multiplier tube optically coupled to each other. The detectors are usually manufactured in small sizes (a few cubic millimeters) in order to perform dose measurements with high spatial resolution. Plastic scintillators are nearly tissue equivalent (Beddar, Mackie, & Attix, 1992a).

The background light and the Cherenkov light contribution can be removed by using two light guides, one coupled to the scintillator for the signal, and an entirely separate one for measuring the background. The response from the latter can be subtracted from the total signal arising from the scintillator (Beddar et al., 2003).

Scintillation dosimeters are linear with dose and are able to detect doses in the tens of grays (Beddar, Mackie, & Attix, 1992b; Letourneau, Pouliot, & Roy, 1999). They also have good reproducibility and their response is independent of dose rate (Beddar et al., 1992b).

### 4.2.9.3. Typical Applications

The use of scintillator dosimeters has been proposed for those cases in which fast response or high spatial resolution is required, such as in IMRT and stereotactic radiosurgery (Letourneau, Pouliot, & Roy, 1999). The use of plastic scintillators for a 2-D dosimeter was proposed by Kirov et al. (1999), and recently a system for 3-D dosimetry based on a liquid scintillator for eye plaque applicators has been developed (Kirov et al. 2005).

### 4.2.10. CALORIMETRY

In this section a brief description is given of the working principle and the use of calorimeters as absolute dosimeters. In principle, measuring the increase in temperature of a material after irradiation is the most direct way of measuring the energy deposited in that material. However, an apparatus based on this method has low sensitivity (temperature increases on the order of fractions of millikelvin have to be measured [Seuntjens & Palmans, 1999]), is not easily portable, requires a long time in order to reach thermal equilibrium, and requires high precision. Thus calorimetry is limited to primary standard laboratories or to a research environments, and calorimeters are not usually commercially available for clinical measurements, although some portable devices have recently been proposed (McEwen & Duane, 2000; Palmans et al., 2004).

A calorimeter consists of a known mass of material (usually water or graphite) equipped with a high precision thermometer probe. Upon irradiation, the increase in temperature $\Delta T$ is measured and the total energy deposited is calculated according to the following equation:

$$E = \Delta Tcm, \tag{4.2.6}$$

where $E$ is the energy deposited, $c$ is the specific heat of the material, and $m$ is the mass of the material. The dose deposited in the calorimeter is equal to $E/m$, and thus is given by

$$D = \Delta Tc. \tag{4.2.7}$$

These equations are, of course, extremely simplified and hold if no chemical reactions take place upon irradiation and if the calorimetric material is thermally insulated from the environment. In order to achieve the latter condition, calorimeters are surrounded by insulating materials.

Originally calorimeters were based on graphite, because of the good tissue equivalence of that material, its ease of handling, and its high heat conductivity, which limits the time necessary to reach thermal equilibrium. More recently, water-based calorimeters have been built. The main reason for the increasing interest in water calorimetry is that dose in water is obtained directly, with no corrections being needed for the different weight of interaction mechanisms or for different energy absorption coefficients (Nutbrown et al., 2002).

Many issues with water calorimeters remain however. First, water has a higher heat capacity than graphite, so the same dose causes a smaller increase in temperature in water than in graphite. Second, the heating of other calorimeter components, having a lower heat capacity than water, can significantly affect the measurement if these components are too close to the point of measurement (Ross & Klassen, 1996). These include the thermometer probe, which must be as small as possible.

A more relevant issue is the chemical complexity of water. When water is irradiated, up to fifty reactions may take place, and the so-called heat defect (i.e., a correction for radiation-induced chemical changes) must be taken into account (Klassen & Ross, 1997). In order to limit the number of factors contributing to this heat defect, the purity of the water must be very high, or it can be saturated with nitrogen, hydrogen, or a mixture of oxygen and nitrogen (Seuntjens & Palmans, 1999).

Other physical factors that may affect the performance of a water calorimeter are convection, which can be a nonnegligible problem when measuring beams directed horizontally (Ross & Klassen, 1996), and thermal expansion. In order to limit the relative importance of the latter, the operating temperature of the calorimeter must be kept between 1°C and 4°C (Ross & Klassen, 1996).

A major technical issue that must be taken into account is the design of the temperature probe, which, as mentioned previously, must be small enough to avoid introducing errors in the measurement due to radiation-induced heating of the probe. It must also be electrically insulated from the water (Ross & Klassen, 1996; Schulz, Wuu, & Weinhous, 1987).

### 4.2.11. HOW TO CHOOSE A DOSIMETER

A dosimeter must be chosen according to the characteristics that make it suitable for a specific application. Table 4.2.2 summarizes the advantages and disadvantages of the dosimeters described in the previous sections.

## 4.3. SENSORS FOR RADIATION IMAGING

### 4.3.1. BACKGROUND

Wilhelm Conrad Röntgen discovered X-rays more than a century ago (November 8, 1895), and X-ray imaging dates back to December 22, 1895, when the world-famous radiograph of his wife's hand was taken. From the very beginning, the primary detector for imaging has been film. The most important subsequent development was the introduction of the intensifier screen. The intensifier screen absorbs incoming X-rays and reemits the absorbed energy in the form of visible light, to which the film is sensitive. Thus, at the cost of diminished spatial resolution (the lateral spread of the visible light being

**Table 4.2.2.** Advantages and disadvantages of the various dosimeters

| Device | Advantages | Disadvantages | Main uses | Typical precision achievable (95% confidence level) |
|---|---|---|---|---|
| Ionization chamber | Can be tissue equivalent<br>Absolute dosimetry possible<br>Very limited radiation damage<br>Online response | High voltage needed<br>Temperature dependent<br>Recombination at high pulse rates | Parallel plate: diagnostic beams, electron beams below 10 MeV<br>Free air: calibration of photon beams below 300 keV<br>Farmer: electron beams above 10 MeV | ±0.5% |
| TL dosimeter | Portability<br>Reusability<br>Low cost | Sensitive to ambient parameters and handling<br>Limited range of linearity (depending on TL material) | In vivo measurements<br>Depth dose measurements (both for diagnostic and radiotherapy beams depending on TL material) | ±2%–3% discs, ±1%–2% powder (Horowitz, 1981; Johns & Cunningham, 1983) |
| Si diode | Almost independent of dose rate<br>Good linearity<br>High sensitivity<br>Online response<br>Small size | Not tissue equivalent<br>Subject to radiation damage<br>Angular dependence<br>Temperature dependence | In vivo entrance and exit dose measurements<br>Intracavity measurements | ±1% (Loncol, Greffe, Vynckier, & Scalliet, 1996) |
| Radiographic film | Portable<br>2-D dosimetry possible<br>Low energy dependence for electrons<br>Small angular dependence<br>Dose rate independent | Not tissue equivalent<br>Limited range of linearity<br>Variation from batch to batch<br>Nonreusable<br>Dependence on the conditions of the development process | 2-D mapping of radiotherapy beams | ±2%–3% (Zhu et al., 2002) |
| MOSFET | Portability<br>Implantable<br>High sensitivity<br>Online response<br>Wide range of linearity | Subject to radiation damage<br>Not tissue equivalent<br>Not radiation transparent<br>Directional dependence | In vivo, online measurements<br>Intracavity measurements | ±1.5% (Jornet et al., 2004) |

*continued on next page*

**Table 4.2.2.** Advantages and disadvantages of the various dosimeters (*continued*)

| Device | Advantages | Disadvantages | Main uses | Typical precision achievable (95% confidence level) |
|---|---|---|---|---|
| OSL dosimeters | Wide range of linearity<br>Near-real-time information | Not well-established technique | In vivo diagnostic and radiotherapy dosimetry | ±0.2%–0.6% OSL; ±0.6%–1% RL (Aznar et al., 2004) |
| Radiochromic film | Tissue equivalence<br>Portability<br>2-D dosimetry<br>Wide range of linearity | Low sensitivity<br>Nonimmediate readout<br>Dependence on readout light spectrum | 2-D mapping of radiotherapy beams | ±5% (McLaughlin et al., 1991) |
| Diamond | Radiation hardness<br>Tissue equivalence<br>Small size<br>Negligible directional dependence | High cost<br>Need for preirradiation<br>Need for high voltage | Strong gradient radiotherapy beams | ±1% (Fidanzio et al., 2000) |
| Fricke dosimeters | Absolute dosimetry possible<br>Tissue equivalence<br>3-D dosimetry<br>Good linearity<br>Dose rate independent | Dependence on preparation<br>Nonreusable<br>Low sensitivity<br>Diffusion | 3-D beam calibration | ±1.5% (MacDougall et al., 2002) |
| Polymer gels | Tissue equivalence<br>3-D dosimetry<br>Good linearity<br>Non-dependence of dose rate | Toxicity<br>Strong dependence on preparation<br>Sensitivity to oxygen (BANG gels) | 3-D beam calibration | ± 1.2–3.5% within the same batch (MacDougall et al., 2005) |
| Alanine | Wide range of linearity<br>Long-term information storage<br>Dose rate independent | Low sensitivity<br>Poor spatial resolution<br>Dependence on ambient parameters | Comparison between centers<br>Harsh radiation environment | ±8%–2% for 2–10 Gy (Onori et al., 1997) |
| Scintillation detectors | Tissue equivalence<br>Online response<br>Radiation hardness | Not well-established technique | IMRT, stereotactic radiosurgery | ±3% (Bambynek et al., 2000; Petric, Robar, & Clark, 2006) |

roughly comparable to the screen thickness), the intensifier screen allows a dramatic dose reduction because the X-ray stopping power of plain film is only 1% to 3% that of a modern intensifier screen (Sabel & Aichinger, 1996).

There are many different reasons why film has survived for so long in X-ray imaging. An incomplete list would include the facts that film is extremely practical, easy to manufacture and use, reliable, and cost effective. In addition, its good spatial resolution makes it competitive for specific applications.

However, film does have a range of weaknesses. Among these, the most important is probably its poor dynamic range, which is intrinsically connected with the specific working principles of film and is thus inescapable. Basically a film consists of grains of silver bromide suspended in a gelatin. These grains offer a much larger cross section to the incoming radiation than does the gelatin, hence most interactions take place in the grains. To oversimplify somewhat, the resulting photoelectrons can be trapped in the grains, and when this happens the grains become "sensitized." Film processing removes the nonsensitized grains and converts the sensitized ones into silver, thus forming the image (Mees & James, 1966). It is therefore clear that the range of the film is strictly bracketed between sensitizing almost no grains at all ("white" image) and nearly all of them ("black" image), with no physical possibility of reaching beyond these limits. The phenomenon is effectively expressed by the film "characteristic" or "HD curve" (from Hurter and Driffield, who described it in 1890). Figure 4.2.19 (see section 4.2.6.1.1) gives the optical density of film as a function of exposure (Johns & Cunningham, 1983). The maximum contrast achievable in film imaging is thus limited, making it difficult to visualize different details on the same image. This is a problem relevant to those fields where large absorption differences are encountered. For example, exposure differences of two orders of magnitude can be encountered in the field of mammography, according to Maidment, Fahrig, and Yaffe (1993). Moreover, an unavoidable amount of image noise is caused by the intrinsic granularity of film (Barnes, 1982), and the detection efficiency is not optimized.

Further relevant limitations of analog film imaging become clear when the advantages of digital imaging are described. Basically, when digital sensors are employed, the different processes of acquisition, display, analysis, and archiving of the image are physically separated and can thus be optimized individually (Brody, 1984). This makes possible a series of improvements, as follows. First, digital imaging detectors provide much wider dynamic ranges that can become virtually infinite in the case of photon counting devices. Second, the possibility of image manipulation allows for an impressive range of operations, from the use of different gray and color scales to enhance detail visibility and stretch the contrast, to the use of sophisticated analysis tools via many kinds of image filtration. Third, digital images can be stored and archived, and can be transmitted over communication networks for remote diagnoses. Furthermore, they enable the implementation of computer-aided diagnosis techniques, which are capable of providing excellent results (see, for instance, Ikeda et al., 2004) and may be crucially important in reducing the costs of screening surveys. In order to apply the same procedures to a film image, it must be digitized by means of a scanner, which, in addition to the time needed, can introduce further sources of noise and distortion.

The use of digital detectors was boosted by the introduction of computed tomography (CT) in the early 1970s (Ambrose, 1973; Ambrose & Hounsfield, 1973; Hounsfield, 1973). In CT, the use of digital detectors is mandatory, and the advantages of having access to 3-D information prevailed over all the disadvantages imposed by the limited detector and computer technology available at the time. For planar imaging, however, these limitations prevented an immediate acceptance of digital methods, because the digital methods were not considered competitive with the high resolution and large area coverage provided by films and screen-film systems. The increasing use of CT images helped make clear the advantages of digital imaging, thus fostering their further development. The subsequent huge expansion of computer and detector technology eventually made today's systems possible.

## 4.3.2. DETECTORS FOR MEDICAL AND BIOLOGICAL IMAGING

In this section, some of the main types of detectors available for medical and biological imaging will be individually reviewed. Some recent developments and experimental prototypes of interest will also be briefly discussed within each appropriate subsection.

In general, detectors for X-ray imaging are subdivided into direct and indirect detection devices. In the direct mode, the X-ray is directly converted into electric charge in the detector material, while in the indirect mode the photon is first converted into visible light by a luminescent material, after which the visible photons are converted into charge in the detector material. Luminescent materials are usually called "phosphors" when they are coupled to detectors operating in the integration mode (e.g., charge-coupled devices [CCDs]) and "scintillators" when they are coupled to photon counting devices, as occurs for example in most nuclear medicine applications. However, it should be noted that there is no neat distinction between phosphors and scintillators, and the two terms are often used as synonyms. An overview of the most commonly used luminescent materials and their properties is presented in section 4.3.2.4.1.

There are basically three optical coupling methods employed in the indirect detection mode: proximity, lens, and fiber-optic coupling. Proximity coupling simply involves keeping the phosphor as close as possible to the detector's active surface, and provides the best results when that surface is directly coated with the phosphor material (although this can result in direct interaction of X-rays in the sensor material). However, because many devices (CCDs in particular) have limited sensitive areas, active surface magnification is often achieved by coupling a small detector area with a larger phosphor layer. In this case, relying on lens or fiber-optic coupling is mandatory. Lens coupling is simple and convenient, but often inefficient. Moreover, its use can result in geometric distortions (see, e.g., Liu et al., 2000). Thus more efficient and reliable coupling by fiber-optic bundles is often preferred. Although their use results in fixed pattern noise artifacts, as the boundaries of the individual bundles are usually discernible in the acquired image, these are easily removed by simple correction algorithms.

The basic operating principles of each detector device will be briefly reviewed and it will be made clear whether each specific device operates in the direct or indirect detection mode (or in both modalities).

## 4.3.2.1. COMPUTED RADIOLOGY: STORAGE PHOSPHOR SYSTEMS

"A new system of computed radiography that is based on new concepts and the latest computer technologies has been developed. This system eliminates the drawbacks of conventional screen-film radiography. The basic principle of the system is the conversion of the X-ray energy pattern into digital signals utilizing scanning laser stimulated luminescence (SLSL)." In this way, Sonoda, Takano, Miyahara, and Kato introduced the photostimulable phosphor (or storage phosphor, or image plate, or sometimes simply "computed radiography" [CR]) system in 1983 (Sonoda et al., 1983). This was one of the first attempts at film substitution, and time has proved it to be a very successful one: the system rapidly found extensive acceptance and is still widely used.

Different from conventional phosphors, photostimulable phosphors intentionally contain traps that capture the charges generated by X-ray interactions, so that exposure and readout phases are separated and the image is actually "stored" in the plate. The trapped charge is then released by external stimulation with a (red) laser, and its subsequent decay generates luminescent (blue) light that is collected by a light guide and detected by a photomultiplier tube (Fig. 4.3.1).

The critical parameter is the energy separation between the traps and the conduction band in the phosphor: this has to be small in order to facilitate laser stimulation, but cannot be too small because random charge release due to thermal excitation might affect image storage. Furthermore, during X-ray irradiation, part of the released charge is captured in the traps while part of it emits prompt light (which is usually discarded). This might seem to favor a design with increased trapping efficiency. However, such an increase would also imply that during laser stimulation, a large fraction of the released charge falls back into the traps instead of producing luminescence. It is easy to conclude that optimum balance can be achieved with a trapping efficiency of 50%, which means that, with respect to a conventional phosphor, only 25% of the generated charge actually results in luminescent light output. Although the basic working principle of the system is explained rather easily, some specific details of the photoluminescence mechanism have not yet been completely clarified (Blasse & Grabmaier, 1994; Seibert, 1997).

One of the technological challenges that had to be solved in CR system development was to prevent laser photons from contaminating the luminescent light readout. Although in principle it is not difficult to separate the laser red photons from the luminescence blue ones, it should be noted that when a low X-ray exposure has to be read, the ratio between blue and red photons can be as small as $10^{-8}$. This problem is solved by adding proper light filters to the readout chain and by selecting photomultiplier photocathodes with much higher efficiencies in the blue than in the red wavelengths. For commonly used bialkali photocathodes, this is typically 25% in the blue and 0.1% in the red wavelengths.

Originally CR systems were based on $BaFBr:Eu^{2+}$ (the dopant material is indicated after the colon). Basically, any $BaFX:Eu^{2+}$ compound can be used where X is bromine (Br), chlorine (Cl), iodine (I), or any mixture of these. In recent years, $BaFBr_{1-x}I_x:Eu^{2+}$ (where $x \leq 0.2$, usually 0.15) has found widespread acceptance, mainly because of the good match of its optimal stimulation wavelength with that emitted by conventional diode lasers.

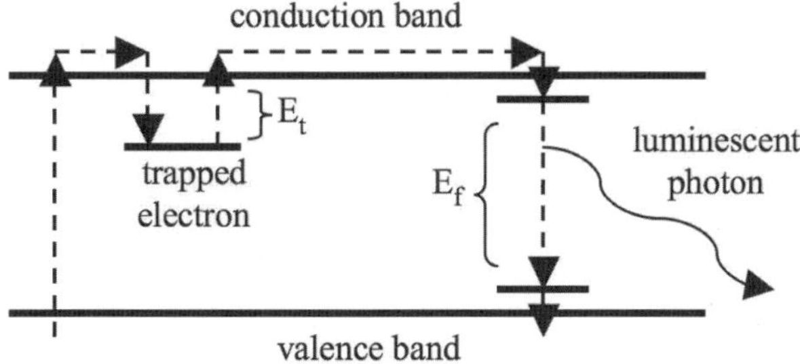


**Figure 4.3.1.** Basic principle of the storage phosphor system. The excited electron is stored in a trap located at an energy $E_t$ below the conduction band. During the readout, it is released via laser stimulation and decays, emitting a luminescent photon of energy $E_f$.

Regarding the spatial resolution of the system, the equivalent of the aperture is the cross section of the laser spot, while the spacing is determined by the scanning raster. Aside from the fact that it is not a real-time system, spatial resolution probably represents its main limitation because of the unavoidable process of light scattering inside the phosphor. Basically, since a flying laser spot is usually employed to scan the plate, this limitation arises from the scattering of laser light rather than luminescent light. The problem is also made more severe because of flare (i.e., multiple reflections from the plate to the face of the light guide and then back to the plate, resulting in luminescent light emitted from other, randomly located points) and halation (i.e., laser light reflected back and forth inside the protective layer deposited above the phosphor), which will eventually stimulate luminescent emissions from a ring of positions around the original point targeted by the laser.

Another limit is encountered in the noise performance of the system because it has a secondary quantum sink. To give an example, an absorbed 50 keV X-ray produces approximately 2000 hole-pairs in the phosphor plate; of these, about 7% are actually trapped. Fifty percent of the trapped electrons are released by the laser scan, and only 33% of the produced luminescent light is transported to the photomultiplier tube by the light guide. Here, only 25% of the photons are converted into photoelectrons, because of photocathode efficiency limitations. The system gain is thus $G \approx 2000 \times 0.07 \times 0.5 \times 0.33 \times 0.25 \approx 5.8$ (Rowlands, 2002). On a scale in which a photon counting detector represents the "optimum," because the only source of noise arises from the statistical nature of X-ray absorption and emission, the smaller the gain, the worse the noise performance (e.g., a flat-panel systems has $G \approx 1000$). However, the nonideal behavior encountered in the different stages outlined previously indicates that there is still room for possible developments (improved charge detrapping by laser stimulation on both sides of the plate, improved collection of the photostimulated luminescence, etc.). A comprehensive discussion of these can be found in Rowlands (2002).

Despite the extremely wide range of different detector systems developed during recent years, in terms of everyday practice, CR systems might be superseded only as a result of the greater acceptance of (much more expensive) flat-panel technology, and probably only to a limited extent. In some applications, such as emergency and bedside radiology, the CR system is still the most practical because of its ease of handling and portability, along with a wide dynamic range that largely solves the problem of over- or underexposure in conditions where it is very difficult, if not impossible, to rely on automatic exposure control.

### 4.3.2.2. Image Intensifiers

An image intensifier is a fast, reliable, and widely used real-time device that for many years has been the only tool for fluoroscopy. In the mid-1980s it was also used for CT applications in which high image quality was not the primary issue (e.g., radiotherapy planning; see, for instance, Arnot et al., 1984).

An image intensifier consists basically of an evacuated tube with an intensifier screen at either end and appropriate electron optics in between (Fig. 4.3.2). The input intensifier screen (typically CsI:Na because it can be deposited with a packing efficiency of nearly 100% with no binder and can be grown in columnar structures) is coupled to a photocathode (e.g., $Cs_3Sb$). X-rays impinging on the intensifier screen generate visible light photons that are converted into photoelectrons by the photocathode. These electrons then travel the whole length of the tube driven by the electric field shaped by the electrodes of the electron optical system. The electrons are accelerated along their path by an applied voltage (20 kV–35 kV), striking the output phosphor (ZnS:Cu, CdS:Cu, ZnS:Ag, CdS:Ag), which reconverts them into visible light with a high gain. The output screen is then optically coupled to a video system, originally a TV camera, but now in most cases a CCD or a CMOS sensor.

All the components have nonunity efficiency. To give an example, for a 50 keV X-ray absorbed by the input screen, approximately 2000 light photons will be generated, and typically slightly less than half of these will reach the photocathode. Typical photocathode efficiencies are in the range of 10% to 15%, which means that slightly more than one hundred electrons will be released. Electron optical coupling is usually very efficient, possibly greater than 90%. A typical applied voltage is 25 kV, and a 25 kV electron produces approximately 2000 light photons when hitting the output phosphor, so, given the previous approximations, the result is the emission of approximately 200,000 light photons. Finally, the efficiency of the output phosphor has to be taken into account, resulting in an output of $1 \times 10^5$ to $1.5 \times 10^5$ visible photons per incident 50 keV X-ray.

In addition is the fact that in order to preserve the vacuum, an entrance window is always present, which means that a certain fraction (5%–10%, depending very much on the incident X-ray spectrum) of the incoming photons will not reach the input phosphor. Originally this entrance window was made of glass; currently aluminum is the preferred material. Actually beryllium is the optimum choice because of its low atomic number, but its use is restricted to nondestructive testing because of its extremely high toxicity.

The main advantages of the image intensifier can be summarized as follows:

- Almost aberration-free electron-optic coupling
- High gain achievable by electron coupling, which overcompensates for subsequent losses in the imaging system
- Large area coverage (up to 60 cm in diameter)
- Low delivered dose

The main disadvantage is the relatively low spatial resolution: in general, the lack of sharpness increases with size minimization; the resolution is lower than in most other imaging techniques. Image contrast is also perceptibly lower compared to that obtainable with other imaging devices.

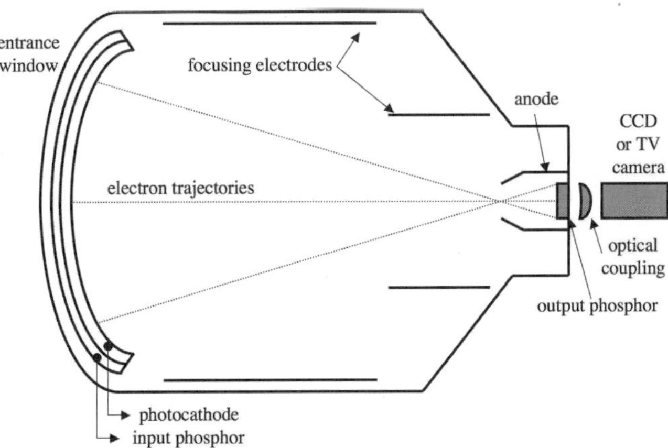


**Figure 4 3.2.** Schematic of an image intensifier.

Furthermore, in practically all cases, although to a degree that can vary from one system to another, images suffer from spatial distortion and spatial nonuniformity (the "vignetting" effect, i.e., the image is brighter in the center than on the periphery).

### 4.3.2.3. Pixel Detectors

An impressive range of pixel detectors have been (and are being) developed for a variety of different applications. Of these, CCDs and the so-called flat-panel systems are currently the most widely used in a range of medical and biological imaging applications, thus they will be treated separately in the following subsections. Their widespread acceptance was mainly due to their compactness, cost-effectiveness, and simplicity of use. Recently, however, CMOS sensor technology has proven to be competitive, especially along with CCD methods. Thus some developments based on CMOS sensors will also be briefly discussed in a dedicated subsection.

Apart from these "dominating" technologies, several other techniques have been developed or are under development. A considerable number of the relevant prototypes are based on the single photon counting mode rather than on the integration method, which means that they are affected only by the Poisson noise due to X-ray interactions and are thus capable of providing optimized image contrast. Most of them are basically spinoffs from research carried out in the field of high-energy physics, primarily regarding the design of vertex detectors (i.e., the inner part of the "barrel" of detectors surrounding the interaction region in collider experiments).

In this field, the dominating material is silicon, the relevant technology of which is well established: its charge collection properties are known in detail and it allows for excellent shaping of the electric field by tailored impurity doping. Silicon detectors are made from crystalline silicon wafers, with thicknesses usually on the order of hundreds of micrometers. Structures are formed on one of the large surfaces in the shape of rectangular pixels or strips. In the former, each individual pixel on the silicon wafer can be connected to its own electronic readout channel by bump-bonding the wafer to a readout chip: in this way, a pixel detector is obtained. This arrangement is often referred to as the "hybrid pixel technique" (Wermes, 2004), because the sensor and the front-end chip are physically separated parts of the detector module (see Fig. 4.3.3). However, the limited thickness of the wafer and

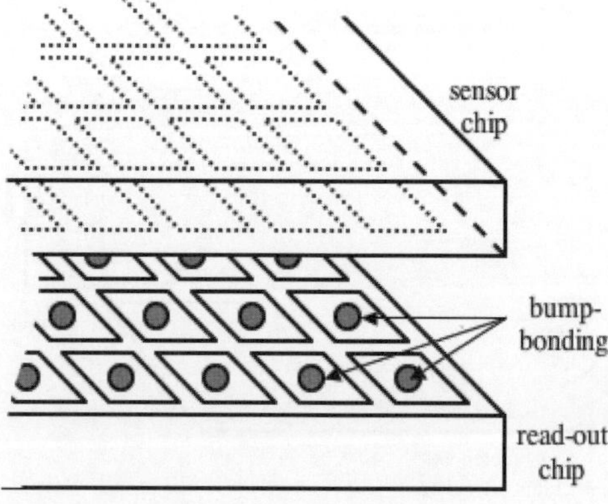


**Figure 4.3.3.** Schematic of a hybrid pixel technique detector.

the low stopping power of silicon result in low detection efficiency, thus preventing, to a large extent, the utilization of such a device in medical imaging unless indirect detection methods are employed. Thus its use is limited to biological applications (see, for instance, Datte et al., 1999), while research on other, higher-$Z$ materials is carried out to make this device usable in medical applications.

Regarding silicon, other solutions have been proposed involving the use of strip detectors (see Fig. 4.3.4). In order to improve detection efficiency, the use of such devices in edge-on geometry has been investigated (Arfelli et al., 1998). In this modality, the radiation impinges on the side rather than on the surface of the chip, with the direction of the incoming photons parallel to the implanted strips. Thus a much greater thickness (a few centimeters instead of a few hundred micrometers) is available for photon conversion. This solution is well suited to scanned acquisition systems, in which it provides a range of additional advantages. In fact, the first mammography system based on this concept has recently been commercialized by Sectra, SE (http://www.sectra.com).

Another solution implies the use of wafers with strips implanted on both surfaces, in orthogonal directions, in order to retrieve 2-D information (Alfano et al., 1993). In this case the chips are read from the sides, rather than from below as occurs in the hybrid pixel geometry. In principle it is possible to increase the detection efficiency by stacking several devices one top of another. The same detector has also been used in the somewhat less demanding field of autoradiography (Bertolucci et al., 1996).

As already mentioned, another solution consists of implementing the hybrid pixel technique with higher stopping power sensor materials; the CERN-based MEDIPIX collaboration is an outstanding reference point for the research carried out in this field (http://medipix.web.cern.ch). For instance, the use of GaAs was investigated for potential applications in mammography (Amendolia et al., 2001) and in autoradiography (Abate et al., 2001). More recently, the use of CdTe has been suggested for a range of possible applications (Chmeissani et al., 2004). Another approach to the use of GaAs detectors, based on the integration readout mode rather than on photon counting, was proposed by Sellin et al., (2001).

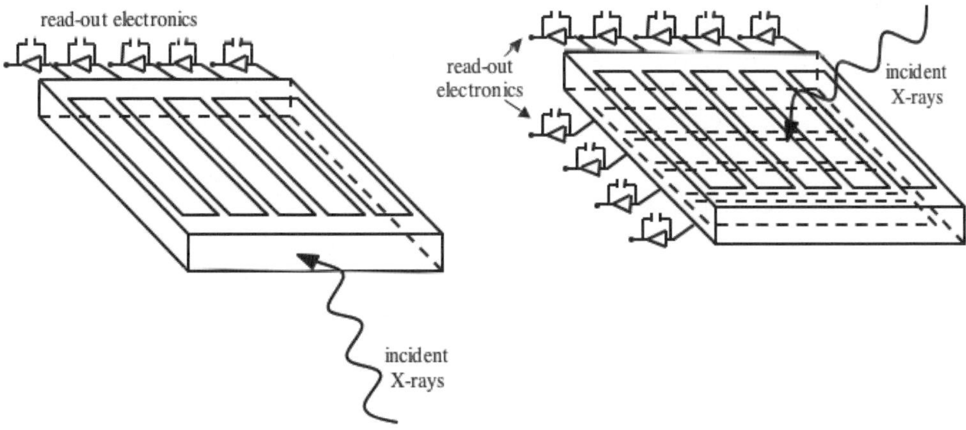


**Figure 4.3.4.** Schematic of a microstrip detector used in edge-on geometry (left) and a double-sided microstrip detector (right).

The use of CdZnTe has also been proposed for mammography applications because of its high stopping power (Mainprize et al., 2002a). In this specific case, a CCD was used as the readout device by bump-bonding it to the CdZnTe sensor.

The reported examples provide a coarse sampling of the wide range of research that is being carried out on innovative imaging devices. The subject was touched upon mainly to show that this is a huge, continuously growing field.

For the sake of completeness, photodiode arrays must be mentioned here because they were one of the first solid-state pixel devices and are still widely used (an exhaustive description can be found in Knoll, 2000). Developments based on gas detectors will also be discussed.

Gas detectors are an offspring of research carried out in high-energy physics and have been used in a range of medical and biological applications. X-ray absorption results in the creation of an electron-ion pair (instead of an electron-hole pair), and the created charge is driven to the readout electrodes by an electric field applied to the gas. The main problem with gas detectors in medical and biological imaging is their low X-ray stopping power, requiring the use of gases with the highest $Z$, xenon in particular. This is especially relevant in medical imaging, where the detection efficiency is a primary issue affecting the delivered dose, but it is a limiting factor in biological imaging as well. Nevertheless, several approaches using gas detection have been explored, especially those based on multiwire proportional chambers (MWPCs), because of their spatial resolution. These were invented by 1992 Nobel Prize Laureate G. Charpak (Charpak & Sauli, 1979). Some examples of autoradiography applications based on these detectors can be found in Angelini, Bellazzini, Brez, Massaia, and Torquati (1988) and in Dominik et al. (1989).

In medical applications, gas detectors have been mainly arranged in a geometry resembling an edge-on strip detector in such a way that a relevant gas depth is made available for photon conversion. For example, the NIKOS project for synchrotron radiation (SR) coronary angiography, historically the first SR-based program that carried out a relevant number of investigations on human patients, employed this kind of detector design (Dill et al., 1998). Much more recently, Despres et al. (2005) proposed a similar design for orthopedic X-ray imaging. In some cases, implementation of the time delay integration (TDI) readout mode has been proposed for gas detectors in a way substantially corresponding to that employed with CCDs. This approach was proposed by DiBianca and Barker (1985) and further developed by Wagenaar and Terwilliger (1995).

Some further examples of promising developmental detectors for radiation imaging will be discussed at the end of the following subsection because they are substantially upgrades of the basic CCD architecture.

### 4.3.2.3.1. Charge-Coupled Devices

Charge-coupled devices developed at Bell Laboratories in 1969 (Boyle & Smith, 1970) are probably the most compact and practical detectors currently on the market. They prevailed over competing technologies because a smaller pixel size was achievable and because they proved to be much less affected by fixed pattern noise, which was considered at the time to be the most limiting constraint associated with the use of MOS-based devices (Fry, Noble, & Rycroft, 1970). Subsequently, impressive improvements in terms of quantum efficiency, fill factor, dark current, charge transfer efficiency, smear and lag suppression, readout rate, full well capacity, and noise performance were achieved for CCDs.

A CCD is basically a monolithic silicon chip subdivided into columns by implanted potential barriers (channel stops). The surface of the chip is covered with an insulating layer (silicon dioxide or nitride) on top of which is arranged an array of metallic electrodes (gates). The voltage applied to the electrodes subdivides each column into pixels by creating a regular array of potential wells in which the charge created by radiation interaction is stored. By properly clocking the gates, it is possible to shift the stored charge down the columns, physically separating the different charge packets from one another. This is done simultaneously for all columns in such a way that an entire row is shifted downward by one position. The bottom row of the device is an analog output shift register having the input of an amplifier on one side, usually integrated into the chip itself. The charge packets are then shifted horizontally and individually clocked out. Once this stage is terminated, the vertical shift procedure outlined previously is repeated and the successive row of charge packets is horizontally shifted, and so on, until the entire device is read out (see Fig. 4.3.5).

This "full-frame" readout mechanism has the clear advantage that the entire surface of the CCD is available for X-ray exposure. But it also has a severe drawback in that the pixels have to be processed one at a time, which dramatically affects the readout time. Although in principle clock-out frequencies of several megahertz can be used, this adversely affects the noise performance of the device—optimum results are obtained with frequencies below 500 kHz. Moreover, the smear effect (i.e., irradiation during the readout phase resulting in extra charge created in the wrong position) has to be taken into account, which in some cases makes the use of shutters necessary to prevent detector exposure during the readout phase.

A possible way of reducing the readout time is segmentation of the CCD into halves or quadrants, each one with its own amplifier, or the realization of interline or frame transfer readout configurations, in which part of the CCD area is shielded from radiation and used to store the collected charge. In this way it is possible to read out the shielded area while the unshielded area collects the successive frame. In the interline configuration, CCD columns are alternately shielded, while in the frame transfer method, half of the area is shielded and used for charge storage. Since these configurations dramatically reduce the fill factor, their use is discouraged in X-ray medical and biological imaging, although in frame transfer it is possible to expose only the unshielded area, and the system is (at least partly) buttable.

When scanned acquisition procedures are used, the problem is effectively solved by reading out the device in the TDI mode. While the beam and the detector assembly are scanned across the sample in one direction, the charge in the CCD is shifted with the same speed, but in the opposite direction.

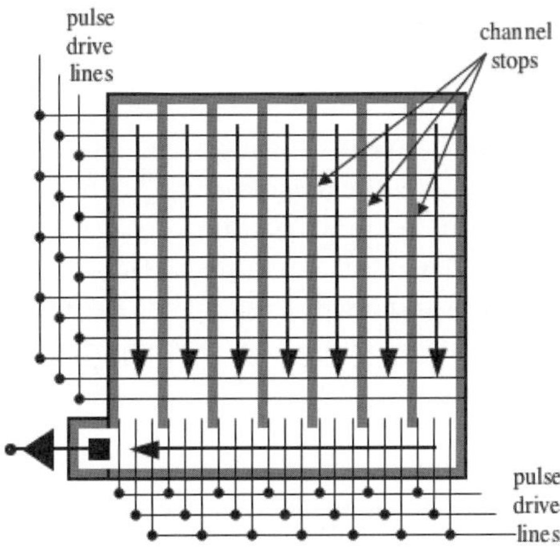


**Figure 4.3.5.** Schematic of the basic CCD architecture.

In this way the collected charge is kept stationary with respect to a given projection path in the sample and is continuously accumulated until it reaches the readout region. A complementary advantage of the TDI modality is that all detector pixels in a column contribute to the final image element, thus the effect of defective detector pixels (if any) on the final image is minimized. To give an example, the SenoScan mammography system, by Fischer Imaging (http://www.fischerimaging.com), based on the pioneering work of Maidment, Fahrig, and Yaffe (1993), works in the TDI mode.

Modern CCD architectures rely on the "buried channel" arrangement, which means that the depleted region is created within the silicon bulk, well below the silicon–insulator interface (Gruner, Tate, & Eikenberry, 2002). This avoids charge trapping at the interface above, thus making the charge lifetime much longer. This is of primary importance because the charge stored in the individual pixel has to be shifted many times along the chip before being actually read out. The buried channel arrangement, together with the well capacity of modern CCDs, which can be as large as several hundred thousand electrons, makes the development of devices with outstandingly high noise performances possible (in some cases, less than 10 electrons root-mean-square [rms]).

However, it is important to stress that, because of the extremely thin depleted region resulting in an extremely small detection efficiency, CCDs are used to detect X-rays only in the indirect conversion configuration at low X-ray energies. This implies a trade-off between resolution and efficiency, as often occurs in indirect detection techniques, which might to some extent negate one of the main advantages of CCD cameras, that is, the high spatial resolution. Some possible implementations based on deep depletion devices realized in high-resistivity silicon or, even better, higher stopping power alternative semiconductors have been devised. In such cases, however, one of the primary benefits of CCD realization is lost, namely the possibility of relying on well-established fabrication schemes, because the device has to be custom designed and fabricated. Thus alternative solutions (diode arrays, pixel arrays, etc.) are often preferred.

Alternative architectures have also been explored. In pn-CCDs, for example, the MOS structures are replaced with reverse-biased pn-diode architectures. This allows for the achievement of relatively large (hundreds of cubic micrometers) depleted volumes, consequently increasing the detection efficiency for direct X-rays. Moreover, excellent noise and speed performances have been obtained (Soltau et al., 1996).

Another innovative device arising from pn-CCD technology is the controlled-drift detector (CDD), the working principle of which is somewhere between a drift chamber and a CCD. During the irradiation phase, potential wells are established in the device by superimposing a periodic perturbation on the classic linear slope of the drift potential. Thus the charge created by irradiation is stored locally in these wells. During the readout, the perturbation is removed and the collected charge packets can drift out of the active surface one after the other (see Fig. 4.3.6). Particular care must be taken in the design of the potentials in order to keep the charge packets separated from one another, including during the readout (drift) phase, but an excellent time resolution can be achieved (Castoldi et al., 2002). In some cases, CCDs have also been used as readout devices by bump-bonding them to other, higher stopping power devices such as photodiode arrays (Mainprize et al., 2002b).

### 4.3.2.3.2. CMOS Image Sensors

For many years considered markedly inferior to CCDs, CMOS sensors are currently experiencing a resurgence in development work, and several companies have commercialized devices for X-ray imaging applications based on this technology (see, e.g., http://www.cmosxray.com, http://www.rad-icon.com, http://www.exxim-cc.com). This work has been triggered mainly by two factors where CMOS

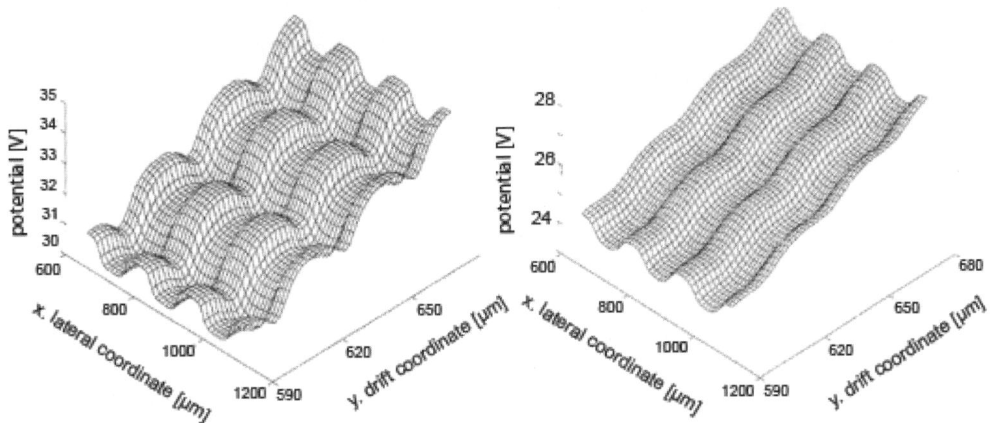

**Figure 4.3.6.** The potentials in the CDD during the acquisition (left) and readout phase (right) (from Castoldi et al., 1997).

technology is distinctly superior to CCD technology, namely low cost and low power consumption, the latter being especially important in the framework of deep space exploration experiments. Although, initially, smaller pixel dimensions were more easily achievable with CCD technology, current developments in CMOS pixel sensors have overcome this limitation. Moreover, in the design of CMOS pixel sensors, additional functions such as analog-to-digital (A/D) conversion can be integrated on the chip. And finally, as each pixel is, in practice, read out individually, there is no signal degradation due to charge transfer.

Although substantially reduced, both readout and fixed pattern noise are still perceptibly higher than in CCDs. Furthermore, it should be noted that in CMOS sensors the fill factor is always less than 100%, although this can also be the case in some CCD designs.

Pixel implementation in CMOS technology is achieved through two approaches: the passive and active schemes. The passive scheme is based on the pioneering work of Weckler (1967) in which the charge created by X-ray interactions in a photodiode (the individual pixel) is read out when the "access" transistor connecting the pixel to a bus is activated (see Fig. 4.3.7). The bus is kept at a constant voltage by a charge integrating amplifier. When the photodiode is accessed, this charge is converted into a voltage signal on the bus. This is the simplest implementation, and the one allowing the largest fill factor, but also the one with the lower noise performance, being of the order of 250 electrons rms compared with the typical 20 electrons rms of modern CCD cameras (Fossum, 1997).

This low noise performance suggested the insertion of an amplifier directly within each pixel, opening the way to active CMOS sensors. The amplifier is activated only during the readout phase, and thus it does not substantially affect the low power consumption characteristics of the device. This enhances the system performance (an overall noise level of 75 to 100 electrons rms is achievable); on the other hand, it also reduces the maximum achievable fill factor, which in some cases can be as small as 30%, as shown in Figure 4.3.8. A detailed description of a possible design of such a device can be found in, for instance, Kleinfelder et al. (2002).

Further improvements in noise performance can be achieved by moving from the active photodiode style to an active "photogate" style. With this device, noise performances comparable to those of

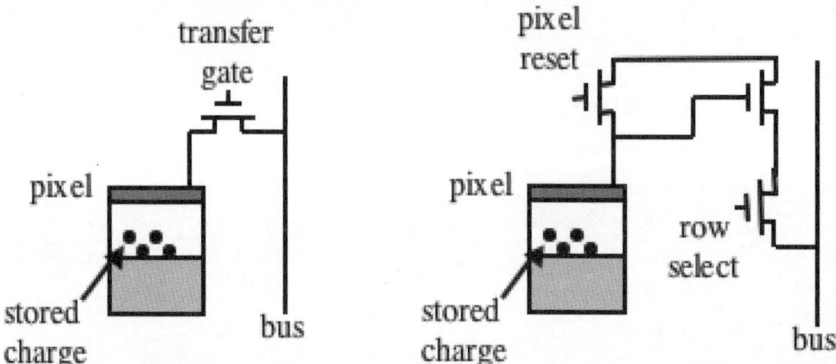


**Figure 4.3.7.** Schematic of the pixel readout structure of a CMOS sensor in the passive (left) and one of the possible active (right) configurations (a photodiode-type example is shown in this case). Since the transistors shown in the figure have to be integrated on the pixel, the active configuration provides improved noise performance but reduced fill factor (see also Figure 4.3.8).

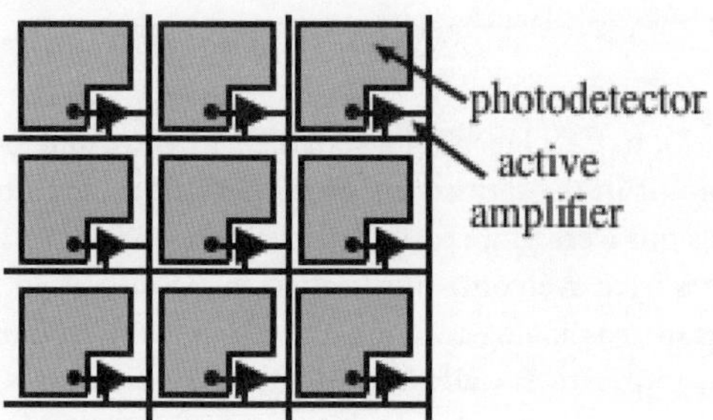


**Figure 4.3.8.** Reduced fill factor in active CMOS sensors.

CCDs are obtained. A detailed description of this device is beyond the scope of this chapter, but can be found in Mendis et al. (1997).

### 4.3.2.3.3. Flat-Panel Detectors

Progress achieved in the field of large-area active matrix arrays, basically related to the development of liquid crystal displays, has made flat-panel detector technology available at affordable costs. This technology has the capability of providing large area, high quantum efficiency, fast readout, reliable detectors applicable to almost all radiological modalities (radiology, fluorography, fluoroscopy). Thus flat-panel detectors have rapidly become the new standard in radiology.

Basically, two strategies have been followed in the development of flat-panel detectors: indirect, mostly based on amorphous silicon (a-Si; Antonuk et al., 1991; Fujieda et al., 1991); and direct (Zhao & Rowlands, 1995), mainly employing amorphous selenium (a-Se).

Indirect detection systems take advantage of the possibility provided by a-Si of realizing large area devices. Competing technologies (e.g., CCDs) are based on crystalline silicon (c-Si), in which silicon wafers, obtained by the proper cutting of c-Si grown in cylindrical shapes, are severely limited in their maximum achievable area.

Large matrices of imaging pixels arranged in regular arrays, each one consisting of a sensor (photodiode) coupled to a thin-film transistor (TFT), can be realized in a-Si. Each pixel element is connected vertically and horizontally to the electronics located on the edges of the matrix via data/control/bias lines and can thus be individually addressed and read out (see Fig. 4.3.9). In order to be used for X-ray imaging, the a-Si matrix is coated with a scintillating material to convert X-rays into visible light, which is then converted into electrons by the individual photodiodes. This coating can be realized in conventional phosphor screens such as $Gd_2O_2S$ or in columnar CsI phosphors for improved spatial resolution (see the following section for scintillating material descriptions). For use in megavoltage (portal) imaging, a metal plate can be added to improve the detection efficiency.

It should be noted that because each individual pixel must contain both the actual sensor and the transistor(s), the fill factor is always less than one, and the problem becomes more acute as the pixel size is made smaller (e.g., in mammography applications).

The same active matrix described previously (or a simplified version of it in which the photodiodes are replaced by simple electrodes with integrated storage capacitance) can be used in direct-detection flat-panel systems. In this case a photoconductor, typically a-Se, is directly evaporated onto the matrix array. The active matrix can also be realized in other materials, for example, polycrystalline silicon or CdSe, that have higher carrier mobilities (Zhao & Rowlands, 1995). The incoming radiation is then directly converted into charge in the a-Se layer without the intermediate conversion into visible light, thus providing significant advantages. A common electrode is applied on top of the photoconductor layer to produce the electric field necessary to drift the created charge toward the electrodes.

The excellent photoconductor properties of a-Se were already well known in X-ray imaging, as, for example, xeroradiography was mainly based on this material (Boag, 1973). In that case, the latent image on the photoconductor layer was read out by means of fine toner particles, resulting in an "edge enhancement" effect on the obtained images. Lately other readout schemes based, for example, on electrometer probes (Neitzel, Maack, & Gunther-Kohfahl, 1994) have been employed.

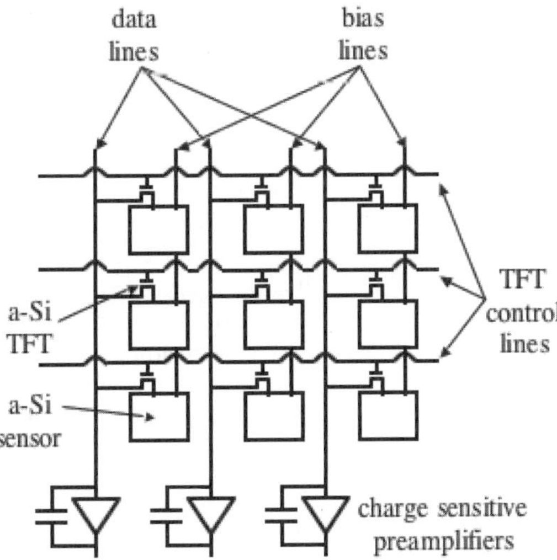


**Figure 4.3.9.** Schematic of an a-Si active matrix array. As in CMOS sensors, the transistor is integrated in each single pixel and, as a consequence, the fill factor is less than 100%.

Currently these non-real-time readout schemes have been superseded by the active matrix technology described earlier.

Both direct and indirect flat-panel detectors have proven capable of providing good performances in nearly all radiological fields, such as chest radiography (Liu & Shaw, 2004), angiography (Granfors et al., 2003), and fluoroscopy (Hunt, Tounsignant, & Rowlands, 2004). However, some open issues are still encountered in the highly demanding field of mammography. Although both indirect (Senographe 2000D; http://www.gehealthcare.com) and direct (Selenia Digital Mammography System; http://www.hologic.com) systems have already completed the U.S. Food and Drug Administration (FDA) approval process and are currently commercially available, most clinical trials have reported a reduced sensitivity compared to screen-film mammography (Pisano & Yaffe, 2005). However, these reported differences are small and in most cases have not been considered statistically significant by the researchers. Moreover, they are usually accompanied by a slight increase in specificity. It is hoped that a much larger survey, under way at the time of writing, will be capable of providing definitive answers (Galen, Staab, & Pisano, 2002). Meanwhile, research is currently in progress to evaluate and improve the performances of flat-panel detectors in this field (Jee et al., 2003; Saunders et al., 2005).

### 4.3.2.4. Scintillators and Scintillation Light Readout

Strictly speaking, a scintillator is not a "complete" detector by itself: it converts X-rays, gamma rays, or charged particles into light that must then be detected by a successive device. However, there is such a wide range of different scintillating materials with different properties and for different purposes that the subject deserves to be treated in dedicated sections. Thus this section is split in two subsections, the first dealing with specific scintillator materials, and the second dealing with the devices used to read out the scintillating light. In practice, a range of possible detectors results from combining an item taken from the first subsection with one taken from the second.

The scintillator/readout combination is widespread in biomedical imaging with ionizing radiation. It is the basis of most nuclear imaging techniques, although direct detection techniques have been proposed (e.g., by Kastis et al., 2002), where a CdZnTl pixel detector is involved. Because of the relatively high-energy X-rays usually employed, a range of CT and micro-CT techniques are also based on this detection scheme. Moreover, scintillators are the basis for all X-ray imaging techniques based on indirect detection.

Specific examples related to all these applications will be given later. Here, a general overview of the most commonly used scintillating material/readout devices is provided.

### 4.3.2.4.1. Scintillators

The basic requirements for a scintillating material in biomedical imaging are the following:

- It must have a high density and atomic number in order to achieve the maximum detection efficiency.
- It must efficiently transmit the scintillating light in order to avoid signal losses. This is achieved by using ionic crystals, or by partly covalent crystals with a band gap.
- It must provide high light yield, because the generation of a large number of scintillation photons means maximizing the information and minimizing the noise. Thus the band gap must be small.
- In most applications, speed takes primary importance. Therefore, short decay time and reduced afterglow are also fundamental parameters.

In indirect detection X-ray imaging, and especially in screen-film imaging, the green-light emitting $Gd_2O_2S$:Tb (again, the dopant material is after the colon) is widely used. Another material, blue-emitting $CaWO_4$, has also been used. For some applications, $YTaO_4$ is used in an undoped form, emitting at 350 nm, while doping with Nb shifts the emission to longer wavelengths. Although $Z$ and $\rho$ are the key parameters in detection efficiency evaluation, in X-ray imaging it is of primary importance to take into account the K-edge energy of the different materials.

Obviously, the thicker the scintillating screen, the higher the detection efficiency, but this severely affects the spatial resolution because of the lateral spread of light in the scintillator. In fact, a trade-off between the two is needed, and usually a broadening of the point spread function (PSF) on the order of the scintillator thickness is encountered.

This limitation was to a large extent removed by growing the scintillating material in columns, which act almost like individual fiber optics, thus strongly limiting the lateral light spread. This is basically achievable with CsI:Tl and CsI:Na. Currently the former is more widely used because it is less hygroscopic and matches the efficiency curve of a-Si better than the latter. A typical individual CsI:Tl column is 3 µm in diameter and can be up to approximately 5 mm in height, which allows a high detection efficiency (approximately 83% at 60 keV). Current problems with CsI:Tl are its afterglow and the phenomenon of hysteresis, which is an increase in the light yield with radiation damage. Moreover, separation between the columns is obtained by cracking, and as a consequence, light channeling may not be optimized (Spekowius et al., 1995).

In nuclear imaging the most commonly used materials are NaI, $Bi_4Ge_3O_{12}$ (BGO), $Gd_2SiO_5$ (GSO), and $Lu_2SiO_5$:Ce (LSO). Almost all of these have limitations: NaI in speed and sensitivity; BGO in speed, resolution, and brightness; and GSO in brightness. Also, because of intellectual property restrictions, LSO is currently used by only one manufacturer.

Recently a new crystal called LYSO ($Lu_{2(1-x)}Y_{2x}SiO_5$:Ce), which has characteristics very close to those of LSO, was developed and tested by a company in collaboration with the European Organization for Nuclear Research (CERN)-based collaboration CrystalClear (http://crystalclear.web.cern.ch). LYSO was also used in combination with $LuAlO_3$:Ce (LuAP) in the development of an innovative positron emission tomography (PET) scanner for small animals. Furthermore, the CrystalClear collaboration is carrying out considerable work on $PbWO_4$ (PWO), which is a very attractive material because of its relatively low production cost. However, its use is currently restricted to scientific applications because of its low light yield.

Other materials, such as $YalO_3$:Ce (YAP:Ce), are mainly used in systems for small animal examinations. These materials have lower densities, resulting in reduced detection efficiency.

Finally, easy-to-machine ceramic scintillators such as $Y_2O_3$:$Eu^{3+}$, $Gd_2O_3$:$Eu^{3+}$ codoped with Pr, and especially $Gd_2O_2S$:Pr codoped with Ce and F (GOS) have recently become common, particularly in CT, where they appear to be the optimal scintillating material. Because they are translucent, they are subject to resolution reduction due to lateral light scattering. However, this problem is kept under control with the use of rather thin devices, without an excessive detection efficiency reduction, as they are characterized by relatively high $\rho$ and $Z$ values. Moreover, the emitted light matches well the sensitivity curves of the photodiodes. Their main problem—the afterglow—is strongly reduced by the codoping procedure, although this also affects the scintillation efficiency. Research is also in progress on other ceramic materials such as ($Lu_2O_3$:Eu,Tb and $SrHfO_3$:Ce).

The main properties of the most commonly used scintillating materials are summarized in Table 4.3.1.

**Table 4.3.1.** Physical characteristics of some scintillator materials

| Material | Density (g/cm$^3$) | $\rho Z_{eff}$ ($10^6$) | Attenuation length at 511 keV (mm/prob. phot. eff.) | Hygroscopicity | Light yield (photons/MeV) | Decay time (ns) | Afterglow (% after 3 ms/100 ms) | Emission $\lambda$ max. (nm) | $DE/E$ (FWHM) at 662 keV (%), PMT readout |
|---|---|---|---|---|---|---|---|---|---|
| CsI:Na | 4.51 | 38 | 22.9/21 | Yes | 40,000 | 630 | | 420 | 7.4 |
| CsI:Tl | 4.51 | 38 | 22.9/21 | Slightly | 66,000 | 800– >6 × 10$^{-3}$ | >2/03 | 550 | 6.6 (PMT) / 4.3 (SDD)[a] |
| CaWO$_4$ | 6.1 | 89 | 13.6/32 | No | 20,000[b] | | | 420 | IM |
| YTaO$_4$:Nb | 7.5 | 96 | 11.8/29 | No | 40,000[b] | | | 410 | IM |
| Gd$_2$O$_2$S:Tb | 7.3 | 103 | 12.7/27 | No | 60,000[b] | 1 × 10$^{-6}$ | | 545 | IM |
| Gd$_2$O$_2$S:Pr,Ce,F | 7.3 | 103 | 12.7/27 | No | 35,000[b] | 4 × 10$^3$ | <0.1/<0.01 | 510 | IM |
| Gd$_2$O$_2$S:Pr(UFC) | 7.3 | 103 | 12.7/27 | No | 50,000[b] | 3 × 10$^3$ | 0.02/0.002 | 510 | IM |
| Y$_{1.34}$,Gd$_{0.60}$O$_3$: (Eu,Pr)$_{0.60}$[c] | 5.9 | 44 | 17.8/16 | No | 42,000[b] | 1 × 10$^6$ | 4.9/<0.01 | 610 | IM |
| Gd$_3$Ga$_5$O$_{12}$:Cr,Ce | 7.1 | 58 | 14.8/18 | No | 40,000[b] | 140 × 10$^3$ | <0.1/0.01 | 730 | IM |
| CdWO$_4$ | 7.9 | 134 | 11.1/29 | No | 20,000[b] | 5 × 10$^3$ | <0.1/0.02 | 495 | 6.8 |
| Lu$_2$O$_3$:Eu,Tb | 9.4 | 211 | 8.7/35 | No | 30,000[b] | >10$^6$ | >1/0.3 | 611 | IM |
| CaHfO$_3$:Ce | 7.5 | 139 | 11.6/30 | No | ≈10,000[b] | 40 | | 390 | IM |
| SrHfO$_3$:Ce | 7.7 | 122 | 11.5/28 | No | ≈20,000[b] | 40 | | 390 | IM |
| BaHfO$_3$:Ce | 8.4 | 142 | 10.6/30 | No | ≈10,000[b] | 25 | | 400 | IM |
| NaI:Tl | 3.67 | 24.5 | 29.1/17 | Yes | 41,000 | 230 | | 410 | 5.6 |
| LaCl$_3$:Ce | 3.86 | 23.2 | 27.8/14 | Yes | 46,000 | 25 (65%) | | 330 | 3.3 |
| LaBr$_3$:Ce | 5.3 | 25.6 | 21.3/13 | Yes | 61,000 | 35 (90%) | | 358 | 2.9 |

*continued on next page*

**Table 4.3.1.** Physical characteristics of some scintillator materials (*continued*)

| Material | Density (g/cm$^3$) | $\rho Z_{eff}$ (10$^6$) | Attenuation length at 511 keV (mm/prob. phot. eff.) | Hygroscopicity | Light yield (photons/ MeV) | Decay time (ns) | Afterglow (% after 3 ms/100 ms) | Emission $\lambda$ max. (nm) | *DE/E* (FWHM) at 662 keV (%), PMT readout |
|---|---|---|---|---|---|---|---|---|---|
| Bi$_4$Ge$_3$O$_{12}$ (BGO) | 7.1 | 227 | 10.4/40 | No | 9000 | 300 | | 480 | 9.0 |
| Lu$_2$SiO$_5$:Ce (LSO) | 7.4 | 143 | 11.4/32 | No | 26,000 | 40 | | 420 | 7.9 |
| Gd$_2$SiO$_5$:Ce (GSO) | 6.7 | 84 | 14.1/25 | No | 8000 | 60 | | 440 | 7.8 |
| YAlO$_3$:Ce (YAP) | 5.5 | 7 | 21.3/4.2 | No | 21,000 | 30 | | 350 | 4.3 |
| LuAlO$_3$:Ce (LuAP) | 8.3 | 148 | 10.5/30 | No | 12,000 | 18 | | 365 | ≈15 |
| Lu$_2$Si$_2$O$_7$:Ce (LPS) | 6.2 | 103 | 14.1/29 | No | 30,000 | 30 | | 380 | ≈10 |

[a] Measured with a PMT and silicon drift detector (SDD).

[b] Measured at approximately 60 keV to 80 keV; all others 6Є2 keV.

[c] Proprietary codopant.

IM, integrating mode.

van Eijk, 2002.

### 4.3.2.4.2. Scintillator Output Readout

The most common device used to convert the feeble light pulse produced by a scintillator into an easily detectable signal is the photomultiplier tube. This is basically an evacuated tube with a photo-cathode at the top. This converts the light produced by the scintillator into photoelectrons (typically a few hundred). Focusing electrodes drive these electrons to a series of dynodes that provide the actual multiplying stages. Usually the interdynode potential is on the order of a few hundred volts and the multiplication factor (the number of secondary electrons emitted per primary incident electron) of each dynode ranges from between 4 and 6 to about 10 in optimal conditions. In this way, the few hundred electrons are converted into approximately $10^7$ to $10^{10}$ charge carriers, which are then collected at the anode (see Fig. 4.3.10).

One of the main characteristics of photomultiplier tubes is their speed. If illuminated by an appropriately short light pulse, they produce an electron pulse a few nanoseconds long within a delay time of a few tens of nanoseconds. This time interval can be made one order of magnitude smaller when continuous channels, rather than multiplying structures based on dynodes, are used (De Vries & van Eijk, 1985). In this device, the multiplication effect is caused by the electrons hitting the wall of the tube rather than a series of discrete dynodes.

The classic design of a photomultiplier tube, in which all electrons generated by the photocathode are driven to the same chain of dynodes by the focusing electrodes, prevents any possible return to the original position in which the light hit the photocathode surface (and thus the position in which the original X-ray or gamma ray hit the scintillator, creating that light). On the other hand, many applications, and nuclear medicine in particular, need this information. For this reason, position sensitive photomultipliers have been developed, in which a multiplying structure capable of preserving the spatial separation of charge clouds generated by different regions of the photocathode is introduced.

The simplest solution is achieved by using continuous channels with very small diameters (tens of micrometers), arranging them in clusters to form what is called a multichannel plate (see Fig. 4.3.11). More sophisticated solutions involve the development of fine mesh structures in which each layer of horizontally displaced multiple dynodes is followed by a layer in which multiple holes are arranged to

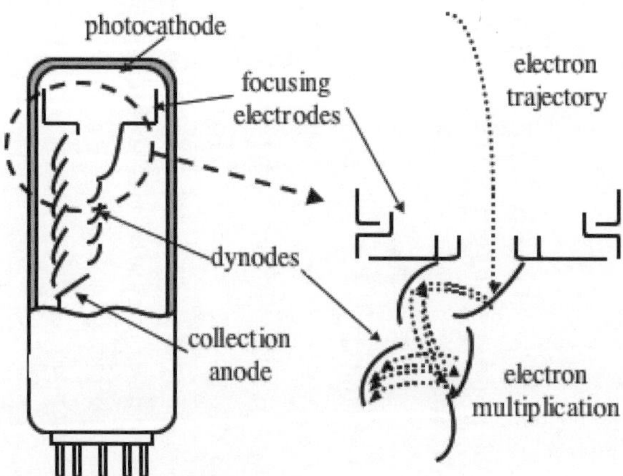


**Figure 4.3.10.** Schematic of a photomultiplier tube.

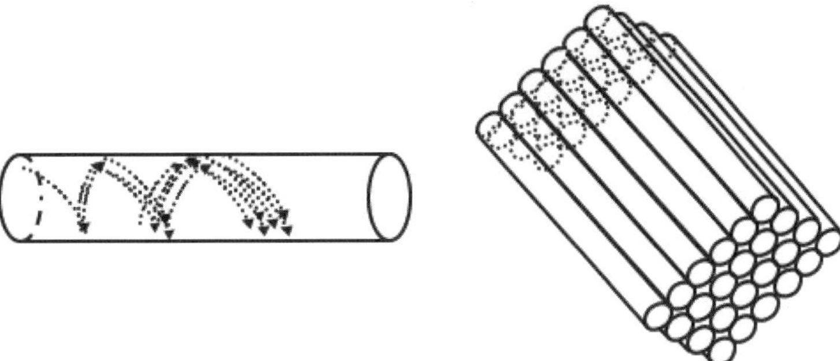

**Figure 4.3.11.** Electron multiplication via continuous channels (left) and the construction principle of the multichannel plate (right).

prevent the different charge clouds from mixing, or arrangement of the dynodes themselves in channel structures. Although in most cases these structures are capable of confining the electron avalanches properly, a nonuniform response is often observed with respect to light hitting different positions on the photocathode surface. This type of device has been successfully implemented in a range of nuclear imaging applications (Cherry et al., 1997; Meikle et al., 2002; Miyaoka, Kohlmyer, & Lewellen, 2001; Weisenberger et al., 1998).

A possible replacement for photomultiplier tubes is provided by silicon photodiodes. In general these are cheaper, more compact, and consume less power than photomultiplier tubes. Moreover, they have a broader spectral response extending to longer wavelengths, which can be important when scintillators with a significant yield at long wavelengths (CsI:Tl, BGO) are used.

Because they have no inherent multiplying effect, the number of electron-hole pairs created is at maximum equal to the number of impinging scintillation photons. Thus their use in pulse mode usually results in lower energy resolution compared to that provided by photomultiplier tubes. On the other hand, their use in current mode is much more reliable, especially for high-rate applications. This has made them the light detector of choice in many CT applications based on the use of scintillators.

In order to operate silicon photodiodes in pulsed mode, the system can be cooled to reduce the leakage current, consequently increasing the SNR. Another possibility for reducing the leakage current consists of employing materials with a wider band gap, such as $HgI_2$ (Wang, Patt, & Iwanczyk, 1996).

Alternatively, it is possible to increase the collected charge rather than to reduce the leakage current. This may be achieved by using avalanche photodiodes. In these devices, a high applied voltage accelerates the charges to energies large enough to produce additional electron-hole pairs. However, good temperature and voltage stability is required because the gain factor is strongly dependent on these parameters.

The most common configuration is known as "reach-through," where the electric field is shaped in such a way that it increases slowly along the drift region (a large fraction of the silicon bulk) and then suddenly jumps to a much higher value in the region immediately adjacent to the collection electrode (see Fig. 4.3.12). In this way, the multiplication takes place in the last part of the device, as far as possible from the entrance window. This reduces the lateral spread of the charge and makes the system more controllable. Several nuclear imaging instruments employing these devices have been devised (Lecomte et al., 1996; Ziegler et al., 2001).

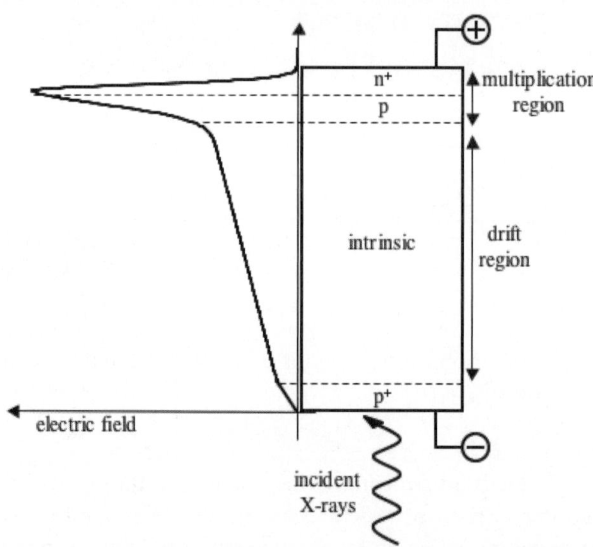


**Figure 4.3.12.** Schematic layout and electric field (not to scale) of an avalanche photodiode in the reach-through configuration.

A form of intermediate solution between those outlined previously is provided by hybrid photomultiplier tubes (sometimes called hybrid photodiodes). In these devices, a silicon detector instead of a dynode structure is used to multiply the electrons. Its construction is rather delicate: the silicon device has to be inserted into the vacuum tube, with consequent risk of contaminating the photocathode (making it inefficient) or the surface of the silicon chip itself (thus increasing the surface leakage current). Nevertheless, the number of produced charge carriers per incident electron is much higher (approximately 3000) than in conventional photomultiplier tube dynodes (typically 5, maximum 25 for specific high-gain, negative electron affinity dynode materials), and this results in increased spectral resolution. Moreover, a position-sensitive silicon detector can be used, in which case a position-sensitive hybrid photomultiplier tube results.

Gas detectors, like multiwire proportional chambers (MWPCs) have also been proposed for possible coupling with scintillators. They can actually provide a much cheaper solution (about one-third of the cost) with respect to photomultiplier tubes. Usually they have to be coupled to a crystal that produces short wavelength photons (BaF, for instance, where $\lambda = 200$ nm) and filled with a specific gas mixture capable of converting the short wavelength photon into a photoelectron. Another advantage is that large MWPCs can be easily constructed to cover remarkably large areas.

## 4.3.3. SPECIFIC APPLICATIONS

This section provides a brief and necessarily incomplete overview of a range of applications with the main goal of stressing in each case the specific detector performance requirements and providing a few examples of the most commonly used devices.

### 4.3.3.1. Computed Tomography

In CT, relatively high (80 kVp to 140 kVp) X-ray energies are used. Consequently X-ray detection is largely based on inorganic scintillators, classically $CdWO_4$, BGO, and CsI:Tl. The most common scintillating light readout scheme is based on arrays of photodiodes operated in the integration mode.

However, these scintillators have several disadvantages: relatively low light yields, imperfect matching with the sensitivity curve of the photodiodes, relatively long afterglow, sensitivity to radiation damage, and toxicity ($CdWO_4$). Therefore alternative solutions have been found. For example, one of the Siemens (SOMATON) CT scanners employed high-$Z$ gas (xenon) kept at high pressure (van Eijk, 2002), but a loss in detection efficiency was encountered. Another development was provided by innovative ceramic technologies involving the introduction of codopants to reduce the afterglow: $Y_2O_3$:$Eu^{3+}$ and $Gd_2O_3$:$Eu^{3+}$ codoped with Pr, $Gd_2O_2$S:Pr codoped with Ce and F (Grabmaier & Rossner, 1993; Greskovich & Duclos, 1997). As a consequence, ultrafast ceramic scintillating detectors rapidly became the standard in CT. Moreover, some direct detection methods have also been proposed, in some cases relying on the photon counting readout mode (Pani et al., 2004; Shikhaliev, Xu, & Molloi, 2005).

### 4.3.3.2. Mammography

Mammography is probably one of the most challenging radiological fields, as both high spatial resolution and high detection efficiency—two classically counteracting issues—are of primary importance. Although classic screen-film mammography is a precise and reliable technique, it has some shortcomings in terms of sensitivity and specificity. These might be overcome by higher image contrast (which provided the first incentive toward digital radiology) and higher resolution. However, increased spatial resolution often implies reduced detection efficiency, which is a major problem in this field because of the high radiosensitivity of the breast. Several asymmetric double-screen–double-emulsion combinations have been tested (Haus, 1990) and were proven to provide a dose reduction of up to 50%, but at the price of a reduced spatial resolution.

A further major incentive toward digital mammography arises from dynamic range requirements: according to Maidment, Fahrig, and Yaffe (1993), the optimal latitude should be 1:100, while the screen-film system is capable of providing a range of only 1:25.

The optimal pixel size for mammography is a rather controversial issue (Chan et al., 1994); at present, 50 µm is the usually chosen compromise. The first step into digital mammography was provided by photostimulable phosphor systems (Hillen, Schiebel, & Zaengel, 1987). Some of the advantages were immediately clear, including dynamic range, windowing and contrast enhancement, and image manipulation, in addition to some of the limitations, such as spatial resolution.

Flat-panel detectors are rapidly becoming the new standard. However, as mentioned previously, they show reduced sensitivity (although often accompanied by improved specificity) with respect to the classic screen-film technique (Pisano & Yaffe, 2005).

Charge-coupled device detectors are good candidates because of their high spatial resolution, but their relatively small area requires the use of tiling techniques. Because it is not easy to arrange tiled CCDs to cover the required area of 18 cm × 24 cm, slot systems are usually preferred (the Fisher system, based on CCDs operated in the TDI mode, has already been mentioned; a description can be found in Tesic, Fisher Piccaro, & Munier, 1999). Smaller systems can be used for stereotactic breast biopsy (Karellas et al., 1992; Roehrig, Fajardo, & Yu, 1993). A completely different solution, based on single photon counting edge-on microstrip detectors, has more recently been made commercially available (see section 4.3.2.3 regarding the SECTRA system).

### 4.3.3.3. Chest Radiography

The classic screen-film combination, with $Gd_2O_2S$:Tb as the typical scintillator material (Blasse & Grabmaier, 1994) and standard dimension of 35 cm × 43 cm, is still used in this application. The first digital approach to chest radiography was provided by storage phosphor systems, usually based on $BaFBr_{1-x}I_x$:Eu ($x \leq 0.2$) as the active material (Sonoda et al., 1983). In the early 1990s, a solution based on the electrostatic readout of a drum covered with amorphous selenium was introduced by Neitzel, Maack, and Gunther-Kohfahl (1994), which may be regarded as anticipatory of current flat-panel technologies.

More recently, flat-panel technology has received widespread acceptance in this field, employing direct conversion in an a-Se readout by thin-film transistor arrays (Eastman Kodak) as well as indirect conversion obtained by depositing a scintillating layer of $Gd_2O_2S$:Tb on top of an array of a-Si photodiodes, again with readout by thin-film transistors (Agfa). The typical pixel size of these devices is about 150 µm, which is considered sufficient for this kind of imaging. Other companies (Canon, GE, Varian, Trixell) rely on the use of CsI:Tl as the scintillating material because, as already mentioned, it can be grown in columnar structures providing reduced lateral light spread and thus increased spatial resolution (Jing et al., 1994; Zhao, Ristic, & Rowlands, 2004). Experimentation based on scanned systems, in some cases employing the TDI principle, has also been carried out.

### 4.3.3.4. Dental Imaging

Although dental imaging is not one of the most demanding fields in radiology, significant research has been carried out in this field. Here, small (2 cm × 3 cm or 3 cm × 4 cm) active area detectors are required. Originally the task was easily accomplished using the classic intraoral film package. A small intraoral storage phosphor system (van der Stelt, 2001) may be used, as well as direct X-ray detection in small CCDs.

### 4.3.3.5. Fluoroscopy

The X-ray image intensifier has for many years been the workhorse in fluoroscopy, and is still widely used (Hell, Knupfer, & Mattern, 2000). Its main advantages and limitations have already been discussed, but in the context of its everyday use, a further drawback is its rather bulky nature, which can make it quite impractical in some cases. Flat-panel technology is currently encountering wide acceptance in this field, and large (40 cm × 40 cm) systems based on the CsI:Tl/a-Si indirect detection modality have recently been developed.

### 4.3.3.6. Single Photon Emission Computed Tomography

Single photon emission computed tomography (SPECT) is a technique completely different from the ones discussed up to this point. It is based on the detection of radiation emitted from the human body in the form of high-energy gamma rays rather than X-rays. Its nontomographic version, often called scintigraphy, is based on a simplified version of the instrumentation discussed in the following paragraphs, and hence it will not be treated separately.

The first important factor in SPECT is that resolution and SNR are mostly driven by a collimator system rather than by the detection device itself. Planar collimators are used in scintigraphy, and conical diverging ones are the standard for SPECT. In the latter, multiple camera heads are often used to increase the sensitivity, and their rotation around the patient provides the 3-D information. As in almost all other imaging fields, the sensitivity and resolution are counteracting issues. Pinhole collimators provide maximum resolution, but minimum sensitivity and field of view, and a range of solutions has been proposed, including multiple and coded-aperture pinholes. The problem is less dramatic when lower energy X-ray photons (for instance, 27 keV to 35 keV as emitted by [125]I) are used. In this case, reabsorption within the human body becomes a limiting issue; in practice, good results are obtained only in small animal systems.

In the classical arrangement, monolithic NaI:Tl crystal plates are read out by photomultipliers arranged in hexagonal packing schemes (Jasczak, Coleman, & Lim, 1980; Short, 1984). More recent systems are arranged in rectangular packing with thicker (25 mm versus 6 mm to 12 mm) NaI:Tl crystals.

Recently, new materials have been introduced, notably $LaCl_3$:Ce and $LaBr_3$:Ce. These are capable of providing high light yield, fast response, good time resolution, excellent energy resolution (because of the small nonproportionality of the emitted light to the absorbed gamma-ray energy), while maintaining a detection efficiency comparable to that of NaI:Tl.

### 4.3.3.7. Positron Emission Tomography (PET)

PET differs from SPECT in that positron ($\beta$)-emitting radioactive tracers are inserted into the patient. After a short distance in the tissue, the emitted positron is annihilated with an electron and two 511 keV, back-to-back gamma rays are emitted.

The back-to-back nature of the emission is advantageous in that collimation is not required because position information is retrieved by the coincident detection of the two photons. The system has a high sensitivity ($10^2$ to $10^3$ higher than SPECT), but a series of key technical challenges have to be faced. Depth of interaction encoding (i.e., implementing systems capable of detecting at which depth within the scintillator crystal the gamma-ray interaction has taken place) is highly desirable in order to avoid parallax errors limiting the spatial resolution. Furthermore, with high-density materials, 511 keV photons have a high likelihood of being Compton scattered inside the detector, and being absorbed in a neighboring detector element, thus affecting the resolution.

Unlike SPECT, PET has at least two unavoidable intrinsic limits. The first is the range of the positron before annihilation (the image is actually a map of the $\beta$ annihilation positions rather than the emission centers). The second is a small noncollinearity ($\pm 0.25°$) in the back-to-back emission due to the residual momentum of the positron or the electron. These limits can only be partially compensated by means of correction algorithms.

$Bi_4Ge_3O_{12}$ is the most commonly used scintillator because of the relatively high probability (40%) of photoelectric absorption of 511 keV photons. NaI:Tl is also used because it allows large, curved crystals to be produced. However, the detection efficiency is lower than for BGO.

Considerable research has been carried out on new scintillating materials because BGO has nonoptimal light yield, speed, and energy resolution. The introduction of LSO removed some of these limitations, but as previously mentioned, its use is currently limited to only one manufacturer because of intellectual property rights. GSO is also a good candidate for solving these problems but suffers from low light yield. Further solutions based on scintillating crystals are mentioned in section 4.3.4.1. It is worth noting that alternative detection methods have also been proposed, employing, for example, liquid xenon as a scintillator and gas chambers to read the signal (Chepel et al., 1997; Collot, Jan,

& Tournefier, 2000). Finally, in small animal examinations, the use of lower density materials like $YalO_3$:Ce (YAP:Ce) is often proposed (Del Guerra et al., 2000; Weber et al., 2000).

### 4.3.3.8. Multimodal Imaging

The term *multimodal* refers to the combined use of at least two different imaging modalities. The main aim is to provide functional and morphological information at the same time. Originally this was achieved by PET/SPECT (functional) examination, quickly followed and perhaps anticipated by NMR scans (morphological). However, this approach works only in an extremely limited number of cases (mainly some applications in brain imaging), because for most other organs the results are affected by physiological motion (heartbeat, respiratory cycle, bladder filling/emptying, etc.). In this framework, optimal results are achieved by combined SPECT/CT or PET/CT scans, although problems arise from the relevant differences in the acquisition time of the two approaches. When the SPECT/CT combination is used, further complications arise because of the smaller difference in energy between the X-rays employed by the two techniques.

### 4.3.3.9. Molecular Imaging

Molecular imaging is quickly gaining predominance because of our increasing knowledge of the roles of specific genes and proteins in the development of various diseases. The adjective *molecular,* however, does not imply new kinds of imaging techniques: it arises principally from a shift in the emphasis given to the information extracted from the examination (Cherry, 2004). For ionizing radiation, the techniques employed are in fact principally PET and SPECT. Since it provides solely morphological information, CT can play only a "supporting" role in terms of providing high-resolution structural information for the interpretation and correction of data provided by other techniques (which can be SPECT and PET, but also other imaging techniques not based on ionizing radiation). Actually, in some cases, a further role of CT can be the assessment of changes in vascularization associated with or caused by a specific drug. However, the approach is to a large extent limited to the imaging of small animals, because in practice it requires very high resolution, in vivo micro-CT. In this framework, some high-efficiency detectors based on PbI and $HgI^2$ have been devised (Street et al., 2002). The problem of detection efficiency for small-animal micro-CT is not trivial, as the dose levels associated with current micro-CT techniques can kill a mouse after about ten scans, while in many cases the primary aim is to follow up the effects of a specific drug on the same animal over a relatively long time span.

The main requirements of molecular imaging can be summarized as high resolution, high sensitivity, and high accuracy in the extraction of quantitative information. The current goal is to be able to image approximately $10^9$ cells, something about the size of a grain of rice. Since it is a technique that is used to a large extent in small animal research, trade-offs can be achieved in resolution and sensitivity, which are the two classically counteracting issues in nuclear imaging.

### 4.3.3.10. Portal Imaging

Portal imaging refers to the acquisition of images during radiotherapy treatments, making use of the treatment beam itself. Because of the high energies employed, the conditions are far from optimal for imaging because image contrast is strongly suppressed. Nevertheless, this technique is absolutely essential to the quality of the treatment.

Two modalities must be distinguished: localization and verification imaging. In localization, a small portion (5% to 10%) of the total dose is delivered to the patient. This allows the checking of patient positioning as well as possible corrections before the main dose is delivered. Verification imaging, on the other hand, provides a way to assess the treatment itself.

Like practically all imaging methods, portal imaging has been based on films. Originally the film was sandwiched between two metal plates in which the high-energy, high-power treatment beam created a number of electrons that impinged upon the film. The back plate, sometimes made of plastic, was used to take advantage of the backscattered electrons. A first improvement was achieved with the so-called enhanced contrast localization system, in which a low-speed, fine-grain film was sandwiched between two phosphor screens, with a thin copper plate on top.

Such systems provide an image quality basically fulfilling the requirements of the technique. In this case, rather than being driven by image quality issues, the quest for digital devices was mainly driven by other factors, notably the necessity of processing the film, which means that several minutes are required before the image is actually accessible (Antonuk, 2002). In some cases this can make the localization image useless due to patient motion. Furthermore, a real-time imaging technique would make online adjustments of the patient position feasible during the verification stage. Finally, the overall amount of time required by film imaging techniques reduces the overall number of treatments per day, imposing a limit on the maximum number of verification images taken of the same patient during the treatment. In addition, there are the usual advantages associated with digital imaging (i.e., dynamic range, image processing, etc.). Specifically designed flat-panel detectors for megavoltage imaging can essentially fulfill all these requirements (see, for instance, Antonuk et al., 1998).

### 4.3.3.11. Autoradiography

Autoradiography allows the visualization of the radioactivity distribution within a (thin) sample. This is the only example discussed in this chapter in which not only electromagnetic radiation, but also charged particles ($\beta$) are detected. In the classical scheme, a high-sensitivity film and an intensifier screen are placed on top of the sample; sometimes a second screen is placed below the sample to increase the sensitivity, although at the price of reduced spatial resolution. The film is then read via microdensitometers (although alternative readout solutions, usually based on CCD cameras, have been proposed, as for instance by Lear, Plotnick, & Rumley, 1987). In the early 1960s, the use of the electron microscope was also proposed to achieve an extremely high resolution on particularly small and thin samples (Caro & Van Tubergen, 1962).

However, it is clear that in this application the use of intrinsically digital detector devices can result in considerable benefits, especially in terms of sensitivity (and consequently reduced exposure times). A range of possible solutions has been proposed, beginning with storage phosphor systems (Johnson, Pickett, & Barker, 1990) and including a number of different devices. For instance, the use of MWPC (Angelini et al., 1988), double-sided microstrip detectors (Bertolucci et al., 1996), detectors based on microchannel plates (Lees, Fraser, & Dinsdale, 1997), and CCDs (Ott, MacDonald, & Wells, 2000) have all been proposed. More recently, use of the MEDIPIX hybrid pixel detector has also been proposed for autoradiography (Mettivier, Montesi, & Russo, 2003). Georges Charpak developed and commercialized an autoradiography system based on a parallel plate avalanche chamber (Biospace Instruments, http://www.biospace.fr). The same company commercialized the "Micro-Imager," based on a scintillating foil connected to a CCD via an image intensifier, still widely used in the screening of gene expression (see, for instance, Salin et al., 2002).

The limited number of examples presented is probably sufficient to illustrate that devices suited for specific autoradiography applications can be obtained from many of the existing detector technologies.

The fact that inanimate samples are being imaged makes this application somewhat less demanding than most radiological ones, although a number of technical problems, especially regarding sensitivity and resolution, still have to be addressed.

## 4.4. SENSORS FOR SPECTROSCOPY

### 4.4.1. SPECIAL REQUIREMENTS FOR SPECTROSCOPY

Accurate spectral measurement requires a high degree of accuracy in the measurement of the charge deposited. For a radiation sensor, the degree of accuracy for spectral measurements is typically quoted in terms of the energy resolution, which is defined as the ability of the sensor to resolve two proximal energies. Consider a detector irradiated with a monoenergetic radiation beam and in which all interactions deposit the full amount of energy. In a perfect system, all charge pulses generated will produce the same pulse height, but in practice this is not the case, and a distribution of events is observed, as shown in Figure 4.4.1. As a general rule, a detector can resolve two energies if they are separated by more than one value of full width at half maximum (FWHM).

A variety of factors can limit the achievable accuracy, including random noise within the detector or electronics, but typically radiation detectors are quantum limited, meaning that the dominant cause of error is the statistical variation in the amount of charge generated for different events. The energy required for ionization is not a constant amount for every interaction; the ionization potential quoted earlier is the *mean* amount of energy to create an ion pair. Therefore a Gaussian distribution of pulse heights will be observed. The random nature of radiation means that Poisson statistics govern these interactions. This means that the degree of variation observed in the charge generated is proportional to the square root of the mean number of the charge, and therefore is inversely proportional to the energy resolution component due purely to statistical fluctuations. Therefore, for a given energy of radiation, the most accurate sensor for spectroscopy in a quantum-limited environment will be the one with the smallest ionization potential, as this generates the greatest amount of charge per kiloelectronvolt of energy deposited.

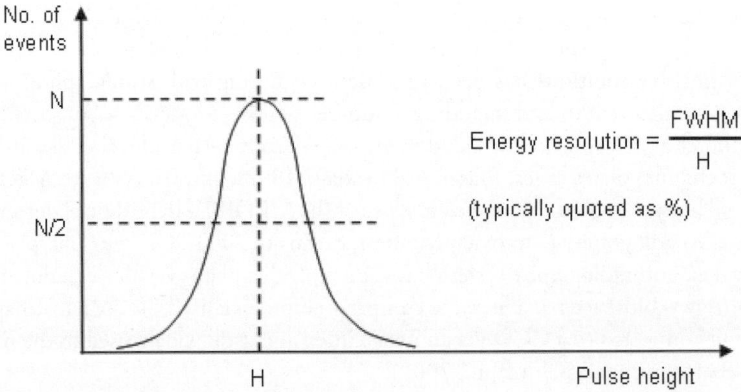


**Figure 4.4.1.** Definition of energy resolution.

In practice, the observed energy distribution is not quite Gaussian because other factors contribute to imperfections in the system. Common examples are impurities in the detector material restricting charge flow or random noise from slight defects in detector construction or from the controlling electronics (see Knoll, 2000, for further details). The FWHM of the individual sources of error add in quadrature. This departure of the measured fluctuations in the detector from Poisson statistics is quantified by the Fano factor, $F$. This is defined as

$$F = \text{observed variance in } N/\text{Poisson variance}$$

and leads to an increase in the observed energy resolution $R$ as follows:

$$R \propto \sqrt{\frac{F}{N}}.$$

In a scintillation detector, the mechanism for achieving good energy resolution is slightly more complicated than in a gas or a semiconductor, there being a two-stage procedure: (1) the conversion of ionizing radiation to light, and (2) the conversion of light to an electrical signal. The efficiency of both of these stages dictates spectroscopic performance. The conversion efficiency is typically quantified by the *light yield*, that is, the number of light photons produced per kiloelectronvolt of energy. On the other hand, the conversion of light to an electrical signal depends upon a number of factors (discussed in section 4.3.2.4). A further key point for spectroscopic work using scintillators is the linearity of light production in the scintillator. Ideally the light yield should be proportional to the deposited energy for a wide energy range. In practice, some degree of nonlinearity is observed, which is more marked in some crystals than others. For further details see Moszynski (2003).

## 4.4.2. SELECTING A DETECTOR FOR SPECTROSCOPIC MEASUREMENTS

When selecting an appropriate detector system for spectroscopy the following questions should be considered:

- What energy and type of radiation will be measured?
- What level of energy resolution is acceptable?
- What fluence rate will be encountered at the detector?
- What other detector properties are also required, such as ability to form an image, high detection efficiency, coincidence/timing information, etc.?
- What are the practical considerations; for example, are there any size restrictions or cost limitations?

Generally, all but the first question have conflicting answers, so some compromise must be reached. No detector system is perfect in all aspects, thus it is important to quantify the required parameters and assign an order of priority. For example, the following sections will show that detectors with the best energy resolution require a cooling system (electronic or cryogenic) and thus can be quite bulky. In addition, achieving the highest energy resolution with such a system imposes constraints on the pulse processing electronics, which in turn limits the count rate that can be accurately measured. Also, requirements such as high imaging spatial resolution only further complicate matters. Thus compromise is necessary.

### 4.4.2.1. Practical Requirements for Accurate Spectral Measurement

Once a detector has been selected it is important to ensure that it is operated in a way that achieves optimal spectroscopic performance. This is largely governed by the pulse processing electronics. A summary of the relevant details is presented here; for further details, see Knoll (2000).

The overall purpose of the pulse processing electronics is to accurately measure the voltage pulse produced by an event in the detector. Figure 4.4.2 shows a typical spectroscopic system configuration.

#### 4.4.2.1.1. Amplification

The purpose of the amplification stage is threefold: (1) to amplify the detector pulse so that its amplitude can be accurately measured (usually from a few millivolts to within the 0.1 V to 10 V range); (2) to shape the pulse in order to broaden the peak and thus facilitate pulse height analysis; and (3) to shape the pulse in order to eliminate slow exponential decay of the pulse to the baseline. Point 3 is necessary to ease constraints on the event rate within the detector. Many pulse-shaping amplifiers include baseline restorer circuitry to ensure that each pulse starts at a fixed level.

In many cases, such as germanium detectors, the detector pulse has a very small amplitude and thus some preamplification of the generated pulse is required. However, in detectors such as NaI(Tl)–PMT scintillation detectors, the pulse is sufficiently large due to intrinsic amplification.

For optimal energy resolution, a linear pulse-shaping amplifier is required. A user-defined gain setting allows the amplifier to be used for a range of source energies. A variety of pulse shapes are employed; for spectroscopic work, a semi-Gaussian pulse shape is often encountered (Fig. 4.4.3). If event timing information is also required, a bipolar output is useful, with accurate timing information obtained from the baseline crossover point, although some compromise in the energy resolution is observed.

A pulse-shaping amplifier integrates the detector pulse for a given duration, set by the pulse-shaping time (often user defined). For an accurate energy measurement this time should be long enough to ensure collection of the entire pulse. Too short a time will be detrimental to the energy resolution; for example, sodium iodide was measured as having an energy resolution of 3.8% at 662 keV with a long shaping time of 50 μs, compared to only 5.9% at a much shorter time of 1.2 μs (Moszynski, 2003). Shaping time requirements are detector dependent and are determined by either the charge collection time at the electrodes or the speed of the preamplifier. A germanium detector, for example, achieves the best spectroscopic performance with a shaping time of approximately 6 μs, whereas a NaI(Tl)–PMT combination requires approximately 2 μs.

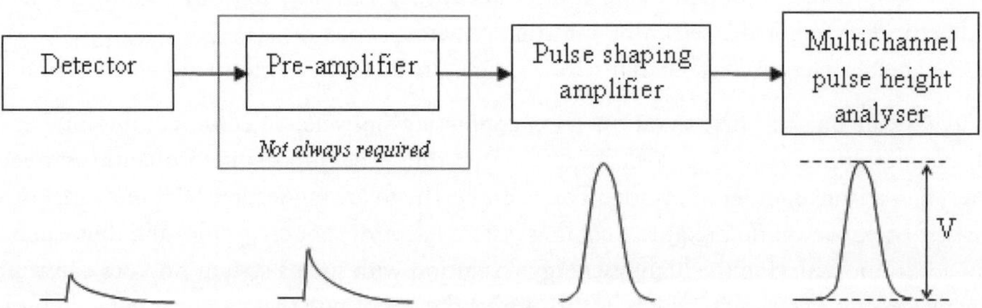


**Figure 4.4.2.** A typical spectroscopic system configuration with a demonstration of the pulses at each stage.

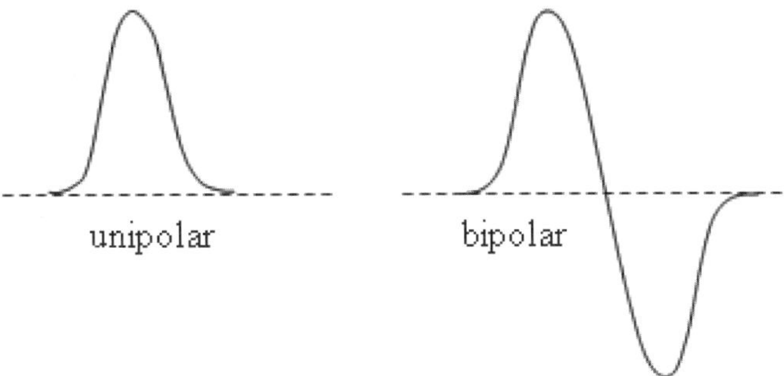



**Figure 4 4.3.** A semi-Gaussian pulse shape for good energy resolution (unipolar) and timing applications (bipolar).

### 4.4.2.1.2. Multichannel Pulse Height Analysis

The analog-shaped pulse from the amplifier is passed through an analog-to-digital (A/D) converter, sampled, and digitized. The sampling frequency of the A/D converter needs to be sufficiently high to ensure an accurate representation of the analog trace is obtained. From the digital trace, pulse height information can be measured, histogrammed into multiple channels (energy bins), and stored to a memory buffer.

### 4.4.2.1.3. Digital Signal Processing Units

Digital signal processing (DSP) units are available (e.g., the DSPEC from ORTEC) that can replace the analog approach described. The preamplified signal is sampled and digitized. The digitized trace can then be processed and analyzed. Such systems tend to offer greater flexibility in terms of signal processing than is generally available with an analog unit.

### 4.4.2.1.4. Dead Time and Pulse Pile-up

A direct relationship between the measured pulse height and the energy deposited in the detector relies on the voltage across the electrodes being at zero immediately prior to the pulse. This is not the case if the tail of a previous pulse has not yet decayed to the baseline, as illustrated in Figure 4.4.4. This situation, known as pulse pile-up, causes the measured energy to appear greater than the true value and occurs when the event rate in the detector is too high. The outcome is to effectively impose a maximum usable count rate for a detector.

The time required to process the pulse is quantified by the *dead time* and is usually quoted as a percentage of the real time. Real time is composed of detector live time, during which the detector can actively process a pulse, plus the dead time. Charge drift times in gas or semiconductor detectors are generally negligible compared to electronics effects. However, afterglow effects in certain scintillators can be significant. It is generally recommended that the dead time be less than 10% for optimal energy resolution. This corresponds to a maximum count rate of approximately 33,000 counts per second, for a pulse-shaping time of 3 μs. The maximum count rate decreases proportionately for longer pulse-shaping times.

Pulse pile-up rejection circuitry, in which two amplifiers are employed, is available to help minimize this problem. A fast pulse-shaping amplifier with a short shaping time allows adjacent pulses

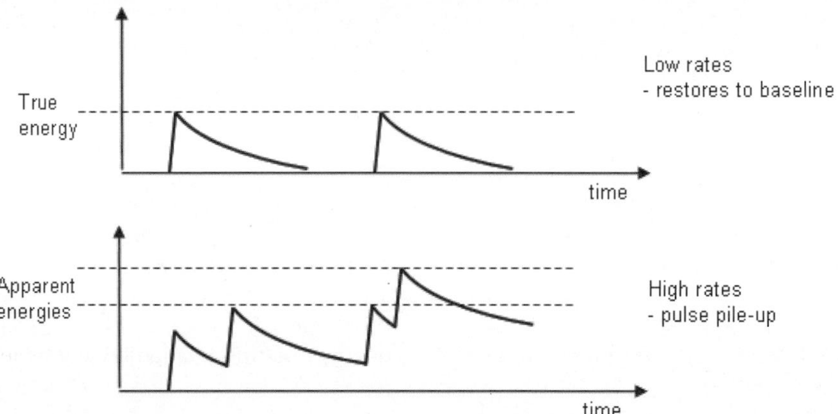


**Figure 4.4.4.** Effect of high event rates on energy measurement for paralyzable detector systems.

to be identified, but this will provide a relatively poor energy measurement, so a slower spectroscopy amplifier is used for accuracy. Alternatively, deconvolution techniques can be implemented in real time to preserve energy resolution at higher count rates (Guo, Gardner, & Mayo, 2005).

### 4.4.3. DETECTOR TYPES AND MATERIALS FOR SPECTROSCOPY

#### 4.4.3.1. X- and Gamma-ray Spectroscopy

Table 4.4.1 lists a range of common detector materials with their reported energy resolution values for photon interactions. The second column of the table shows the statistical component of the energy resolution quantified for each material. For semiconductors and gas detectors, a small ionization potential (in common terminology the *band gap* and the *w-value*, respectively) provides better energy resolution. For scintillators, a more representative parameter is the *light yield*, defined as the number of light photons generated per unit energy deposited. A high light yield generally infers that it should be (theoretically) possible to achieve good energy resolution.

A generalized summary of the table may be made by stating that semiconductor detectors typically show the best spectroscopic performance, followed by scintillators and then gas detectors. Some overlap occurs between detector types, but it is a reasonably well-followed rule. The best energy resolution of any commercially available detector is provided by high-purity germanium detectors, although their appeal is offset by their cost and bulky cooling systems. The intense commercial development of silicon over many years means that costs are low and they are widely available in a variety of forms. However, low-$Z$ and limited thickness (<1 mm is common) restrict their usefulness for direct X- and gamma-ray detection to low energies (<20 keV for good detection efficiency). Consequently, silicon devices for X- and gamma-ray detection are generally coupled to scintillators and thus suffer a reduction in spectroscopic performance. Of the room-temperature semiconductors, CdZnTe appears the most promising in terms of spectroscopic performance, and considerable effort is being expended to improve production quality (eV products; Verger et al., 2004).

The high-light-yield scintillators, in particular NaI(Tl) and CsI(Tl), demonstrate reasonable energy resolution, and their low cost and high $Z$ make them advantageous in certain applications. Sodium iodide was for many years the scintillator with the highest light yield, and so has long been

**Table 4.4.1.** Energy resolution values of common detector materials

| Detector material | Statistical parameter | Energy resolution | Comments |
|---|---|---|---|
| *Semiconductor* | *Band gap (eV per electron-hole pair)* | *All values quoted at 122 keV* | |
| Silicon | 1.12 | 150–300 eV at 5.9 keV (ORTEC products) | Value quoted for lithium drifted silicon detectors |
| Germanium | 0.67 | ≈0.5 keV (ORTEC products) | Resolution quoted is for thin, planar configurations. Poorer resolution would be expected for thicker crystals and coaxial configurations. Detector must be cooled. |
| Cadmium telluride | 1.5 | 1.8 keV (Niraula et al., 2002) | |
| Cadmium zinc telluride | 1.57 | 1.2 keV (Verger et al., 2004) | This performance is achieved with processing and correction; 3% to 10% can be expected for unprocessed signals (Feichtinger et al., 2004). |
| Mercuric iodide | 2.15 | 1.2 keV FWHM for 59.5 keV | |
| Gallium arsenide | 1.42 | 8.8 keV (Zat'ko et al., 2004) | These measurements were taken at room temperature; resolution improved to 5.65 keV at 59.5 keV at 273 K. |
| Thallium bromide | 2.68 | 6.0 keV (Onodera et al., 2004) | |
| *Scintillator* | *Light yield (photons/MeV)* | *All values quoted at 662 keV* | |
| NaI(Tl) | 38,000 | 5.9% (≈39 keV) (Moszynski, 2003) | Arguably the most commonly used scintillator for spectrometry since its discovery in 1948 (Hofstadter, 1948). Hygroscopic. |
| CsI(Tl) | 52,000 | 4.9% (≈32 keV) (Ikagawa et al., 2005) | Less hygroscopic than sodium iodide. |
| BGO | 8200 | 12% (≈79 keV) (Hu et al., 2004) | A dense, high-$Z$ scintillator optimized for detection efficiency. |

*continued on next page*

**Table 4.4.1.** Energy resolution values of common detector materials (*continued*)

| Detector material | Statistical parameter | Energy resolution | Comments |
|---|---|---|---|
| *Scintillator* | *Light yield (photons/MeV)* | *All values quoted at 662 keV* | |
| YAP:Ce | 24,000 | 4.36% ($\approx$29 keV) (Kapusta et al., 1999) | Light output shows a very linear response with energy. |
| LaBr$_3$ | 61,000 | 2.9% ($\approx$19 keV) (van Loef, Dorenbos, & van Eijk, 2001) | Both this material and the one below are new materials showing very promising spectroscopic performance. |
| CeBr$_3$ | 68,000 | 3.4% ($\approx$22 keV) (Shah et al., 2004) | |
| *Gas* | *w-value (eV/ electron-ion pair)* | *All values quoted at 662 keV* | |
| Xenon | 21.5 | 14.4 keV at 662 keV (Dmitrenko et al., 2000) | Theoretical limit of 1.3% FWHM at 140 keV and 0.6% at 662 keV (Bolotnikov & Ramsey, 1998) |

widely used. Its hygroscopic nature requires encapsulation, thus for low-energy photons or particles, cesium iodide is often the scintillator of choice. Some new chloride and bromide scintillators, namely LaCl$_3$, LaBr$_3$, and CeBr$_3$, look particularly promising for spectroscopy. Reported energy resolutions at 662 keV of 2.9% and 3.4% for LaBr$_3$ and CeBr$_3$, respectively (Shah et al., 2004; van Loef et al., 2001), indicate that they could rival the spectroscopic performance of many semiconductors.

If high count rate is a requirement, there are a number of scintillators with very short decay times that are capable of high-speed operation. Plastic organic scintillators are notable for their short decay times, although their low-$Z$/density tends to limit their application to particles or low-energy photons. For higher energy photons, BaF$_2$ and YAP:Ce offer some useful properties (Kerek et al., 1998).

Gas proportional counters or ionization chambers operated in pulse mode can provide reasonable energy resolution, often better than a scintillator, but rarely competitive with a semiconductor. The main drawback of gas detectors for photon work is the low detection efficiency compared with the other materials, which tends to limit their application to energies less than 20 keV if sensitivity is a factor, although the useful range can be extended using high pressures (for further details, see Grey, Sood, & Manchanda, 2004). Despite this, gas detectors have other advantages and provide large area coverage at relatively low cost.

### 4.4.3.2. Charged Particle Spectroscopy

Both silicon and scintillation detectors are commonly employed for charged particle detection. For spectroscopic work there is much commonality between photon and charged particle studies, but there are a few important differences. First, low-$Z$ materials tend to be preferable for electron studies, which is opposite to the situation for photons. The reason for this is that the probabilities of bremsstrahlung production and backscatter increase significantly with the atomic number of the absorber, both of which affect the spectral shape. Consequently, common detectors for electron studies are silicon—either diodes or lithium drifted devices—low-$Z$ organic scintillators such as anthracene or plastics, or liquid scintillators. Second, the detector entrance window needs careful consideration. Alpha- and beta-particle ranges are considerably shorter than equivalent energy X- or gamma rays, so detector encapsulation or surface layers become important issues. This requirement makes hygroscopic scintillators such as NaI(Tl) less suitable. Third, an advantage of the short range of the particles is that the detector can be thin or low $Z$ and still achieve good detection efficiency. Consequently, silicon detectors, which have a typical thickness of less than 1 mm, exhibit good particle absorption across a normal energy range. A final point concerns high-resolution measurements of low-energy particles. A particle interaction can deposit such small amounts of energy in the detector that they are comparable with the detector noise. Thus particle detectors for high-resolution spectroscopy are operated to provide the lowest possible noise, and a minimum energy threshold is specified. Silicon detectors, for example, are commonly cooled to minimize thermal noise.

Tables 4.4.2 and 4.4.3 provide typical energy resolution values that can be expected for common detector materials for alpha and beta detection. Similar trends are seen in X- and gamma-ray detectors, with the semiconductors demonstrating superior spectroscopic performance. Of the scintillators, anthracene is possibly the most common for beta detection because of its high light output, although requirements for other properties mean that a whole range of detector materials is encountered.

**Table 4.4.2.** Reported energy resolutions of alpha particles from [241]Am, a common source for calibrating alpha detectors

| Detector material | Energy resolution (using [241]Am at 5.48 MeV) | Reference |
|---|---|---|
| CVD diamond | 0.4% | Manfredotti (2005) |
| CsI(Tl) | 6.0% | Bhattacharjee et al. (2002) |
| YAG(Ce) | 8.4% | Bhattacharjee et al. (2002) |
| Silicon (surface barrier) | 0.4% | Rahab et al. (2001) |
| Cadmium zinc telluride | 1.8% | Pearson, Regan, & Divoli (2001) |

Note: ZnS is a common material for alpha-particle detection, but is only available as a polycrystalline powder. Consequently it is usually in the form of a thin sheet held together by a binding material. It is generally unsuitable for accurate energy measurement.

**Table 4.4.3.** Reported energy resolutions of beta particles

| Detector material | Energy resolution | Reference |
|---|---|---|
| Silicon CCD | 3 keV at 219 keV ([111]In) | Hofsäss et al. (2003) |
| Si (Li) | 2 keV at 0.976 MeV | ORTEC |
| ZnSe(Te) | ≈30 keV (3%–6%) at 0.976 MeV | Ryzhikov et al. (2005) |
| Anthracene (organic scintillator) | <10% | |
| Plastic scintillator | ≈5% | Sanchez, Ono, & Miyata (2002) |

Note: A wide range of plastic scintillators exists, each exhibiting different light yield properties. Consequently the energy resolution varies according to the material chosen.

There is some interest in developing detectors that are sensitive to different forms of radiation (e.g., simultaneous measurement of both beta and gamma interactions). For such applications it is possible to use either two separate detectors on either side of the sample, or a single detector such as silicon that can provide a good signal from both particles and low-energy gammas, or composite detectors if higher energy gamma rays are used. A composite detector consists of two detector materials, each one optimized for radiation of a particular type and energy. A recent example of this is the CsI(Tl)/ZnSe(Te) composite of Ryzhikov et al. (2005).

### 4.4.3.3. Considerations for Achieving Optimal Energy Resolution

The values provided in Tables 4.4.2 and 4.4.3 are indicative of the optimal energy resolutions that can be achieved with those materials. The following sections discuss the various factors to be considered to achieve optimal energy resolution.

### 4.4.3.4. Charge/Light Collection

Section 4.4.1 describes the dependence of energy resolution on the number of charge carriers (or light photons in the case of scintillators). In order to approach the statistical limit, charge (light) collection should be maximized. This corresponds to the shaping time of the pulse-shaping amplifier.

### 4.4.3.5. Semiconductor/Gas Detectors

For the case of semiconductor detectors or gas detectors, the electrode structure and charge transport within the material effect energy resolution. The spectroscopic performance can be considerably restricted by electrode design (Baciak & He, 2003; Lacy et al., 2004). Pixellating the electrodes reduces the energy resolution of the detector. This is largely due to spread of charge over an area greater than the pixel. Summing the charge across the struck pixel and all neighboring pixels can help recover the energy resolution (He et al., 2000). However, for each detector type and geometry, certain pixel arrangements will provide better energy resolution than others (Gros d'Aillon et al., 2005).

Poor charge transport prevents the full amount of charge from contributing to the pulse, and therefore the energy measurement. This can lead to ionic recombination caused by the interaction of mobile charge carriers with the detector material, especially at low bias voltages or large detector volumes. A possible cause of poor charge transport is impurities in the detector material, leading to charge trapping and an apparent low energy measurement. Crystal growth methods ultimately dictate the charge transport properties of a semiconductor crystal, and hence the spectroscopic performance. High-purity germanium crystals can now be produced with excellent quality, but for newer materials such as CdZnTe, the quality of crystal growth is still being explored by a variety of methods (Funaki et al., 1999; Schlesinger et al., 1999; Szeles & Eissler, 1998; Verger et al., 2004).

Charge trapping effects are frequently seen in room-temperature semiconductors, for example, cadmium telluride. This is because these materials tend to exhibit poor charge mobility (usually holes). The reader is directed to Knoll (2000) for further details. Such spectra where this is evident show a characteristic charge trapping "tail" on the low-energy side of the peak.

Various authors have reported methods for correcting for the charge trapping effect. One such technique is to use a capacitive Frisch grid, which is a modified electrode structure that minimizes the effect of hole motion such that the signal is primarily due to electrons, thus overcoming the problem of poor hole mobility (McNeill & McGregor, 2004; Montemont et al., 2001). Other suggested methods include a biparametric approach that corrects the measured pulse height using pulse rise time information (Verger et al., 2001) and pulse shape discrimination (Ho et al., 1998).

### 4.4.3.6. Scintillation Detectors

Efficient light collection in scintillation counters, and therefore good spectroscopic performance, is governed by the following factors:

1. Matching the emission spectrum of the scintillator to the absorption spectrum of the light counter
2. An efficient light counter
3. Transparency of the scintillator to its own emissions
4. A refractive index closely matched to the entrance window of the light counter to minimize reflections
5. Maximizing the amount of light that passes through the exit window of the scintillator

Points 1 and 2 are key to the spectroscopic performance of a scintillation detector. A light counter exhibiting poor quantum efficiency at the wavelength emitted by the scintillator will produce poor energy resolution. Some improvements in energy resolution can be expected using recently developed photodetectors, such as avalanche silicon photodiodes (Moszynski et al., 2002), $HgI_2$ photodetectors (Wang, Iwanczyk, & Patt, 1994), and TlBr (Hitomi et al., 2000) because of the high quantum efficiencies of these materials. However, for low-energy photons or particles, electronic noise in photodiodes tends to dominate energy resolution.

For spectroscopic work, the choice of a bright scintillator largely dictates the light counter selection according to the required spectral response. For example, the emission spectrum of NaI(Tl) (a blue–violet emitter) is commonly matched with a bialkali photocathode on a photomultiplier tube, although for other applications it is often the case that the application warrants a particular light detector which in turn governs scintillator choice. Again, for example, high-resolution imaging applications could require a CCD, which has a broad absorption spectrum typically peaking at around 600 nm to 700 nm, at the red end of the visible spectrum. CCDs are typically coupled with $Gd_2O_2S:Eu$ (commonly known as gadox–europium doped) or CsI(Tl), both of which emit some of their light at these wavelengths.

Point 5 can be achieved by applying a reflective coating to all surfaces of the scintillator other than the exit window and by choosing a suitable scintillator geometry (Naydenov, 2005). Figure 4.4.5 shows two scintillator configurations. For the one on the left, the majority of interactions occur just above the exit window. The light traveling in other directions is reflected from coated surfaces to contribute to the signal. In contrast, the scintillator on the right is required for an imaging device with good detection efficiency. A columnar scintillator structure with no reflective coatings ensures that light spread is minimized to maintain a good spatial resolution in the image, whereas good detection efficiency is ensured by a thick scintillator. However, only a small fraction of the light will reach the exit window by either direct transmission or total internal reflection, and thus the energy resolution will be poor. For example, a 3 mm thick CsI(Tl) matrix consisting of orthogonal arrays of crystal pillars with 0.6 mm × 0.6 mm cross sections showed an energy resolution of 22% FWHM at 122 keV, whereas 6% to 8% can be expected in optimal conditions (Vittori, Malatesta, & de Notaristefani, 1998).

### 4.4.3.7. Noise Reduction

Although radiation measurements are often quantum limited, section 4.4.1 showed that other noise sources are detrimental to the spectroscopic performance and should be minimized. This is particularly

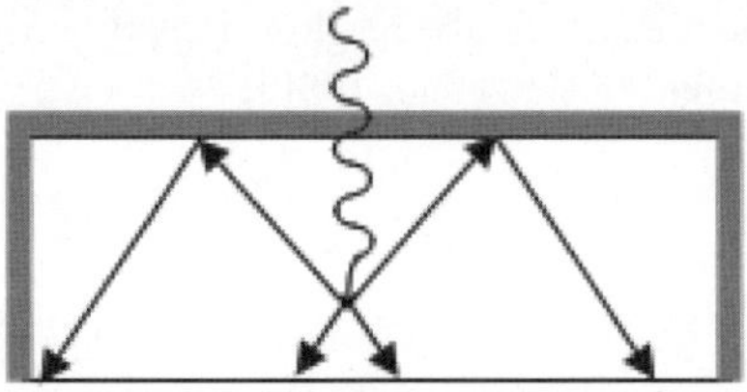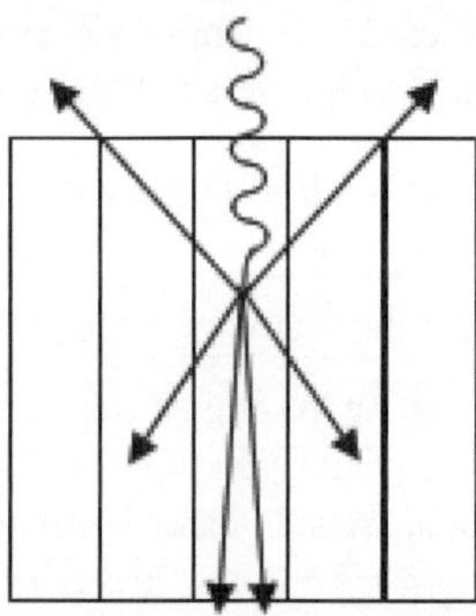

**Figure 4.4.5 Light collection efficiency in a scintillator according to geometry and reflective coatings.**

relevant for low-energy measurements where small signals are encountered. Electronic noise in the readout of the detector signal will appear as random, low voltage pulses and can dominate the lower end of the measured spectrum. Often these pulses can be removed from the spectrum using a low-level discriminator on the multichannel analyzer; however, for low-energy depositions, the pulses generated can be of comparable amplitude to the noise. This is sometimes seen in the measurement of low-energy radiation using a photodiode coupled to a scintillator. Low-energy measurements require the careful selection of a low-noise system.

While many noise sources are caused by detector design and production quality, certain noise sources depend on operation. While the band gap of germanium is sufficiently low that it must be operated at low temperatures, all semiconductor detectors show significant improvement in spectroscopic performance if cooled. For example, a GaAs detector was reported to show an FWHM of 6.8 keV at 59.5 keV at 20°C compared to 5.65 keV at 0°C (Zat'ko et al., 2004). In the case of scintillation detectors, light leakage into the crystal can add a significant background noise source to worsen performance. And in all cases, environmental effects such as electric or magnetic fields or vibration can also have detrimental effects on performance.

## 4.4.4. CORRECTION TECHNIQUES TO IMPROVE SPECTRAL MEASUREMENT

Providing the response of the system and any experimental factors that can distort the spectrum are well known, some attempt can be made at extracting a "pure" spectrum from noisy experimental data that have been distorted by the detector system. The measured spectrum is effectively the convolution of the pure spectrum with the response of the system. Provided the system response can be well described, deconvolution techniques can be applied, often following data smoothing to reduce statistical noise. Potential problems with this approach are that the system response is not accurately known across the entire measurement range and that there are differences in experimental conditions between measuring the system response and the spectral measurements that are to be corrected. Consequently, maximum likelihood techniques can be used to estimate system response. The reader is directed to Gelfgat, Kosarev, and Podolyak (1993) and Penttilä et al. (2005) for further details. However, in all cases the ability to apply corrections does not detract from the need for good quality raw data.

### 4.4.4.1. Highest Achievable Energy Resolution

The best energy resolution of any detector type is provided by cryogenic microcalorimeters. These devices operate at very low temperatures (typically less than 100 mK) and measure the elevation of temperature generated by a radiation interaction in an absorber. An energy resolution of 160 eV (FWHM) at the 59.5 keV gamma line of $^{241}$Am has been reported (Loidl et al., 2004), which compares very favorably to a value of approximately 450 eV that can be expected from the best semiconductor. The energy resolution is so superior because the excitation energies required to cause a temperature elevation in an absorber are in the microelectronvolt to millielectronvolt range: this causes considerably less statistical fluctuation than the electronvolts required for ionization in other detector types. The low-temperature operation is necessary to minimize the heat capacity of the absorber and to limit the effect of thermal fluctuations, but it creates certain practical difficulties. Such systems are not currently commercially available; details can be found in Loidl et al. (2004) and Booth, Cabrera, and Fiorini (1996).

### 4.4.4.2. Energy Measurement Using Integrating Detectors

Discussion so far has focused on detectors operating in pulse mode, which is the conventional approach. However, spectroscopy is possible with an integrating imaging sensor. CCDs and CDDs are integrating sensors that have both achieved good energy resolution (Castoldi et al., 2004; Harris et al., 2001). The technique sums the charge deposited in a pixel cluster on a calibrated image to create an energy value. It relies on the event rate in the sensor being sufficiently low compared to the integrating frame rate so that no overlap occurs between pixel clusters from separate events. A CDD operating at a frame rate of 100 kHz can achieve an energy resolution at room temperature better than 300 eV FWHM at 5.9 keV. A value of approximately 150 eV is expected with moderate (Peltier) cooling (Castoldi et al., 2004).

### 4.4.4.3. Detector Selection for Spectroscopy: Case Studies

#### 4.4.4.3.1. Case 1: High-Resolution Spectral Measurements in an X-ray Scatter Experiment

A collimated beam from a W-anode X-ray source irradiates a thin crystalline sample. We wish to accurately measure the energy spectrum diffracted to a small scatter angle, with an energy resolution better than 1 keV. The X-ray source is operated at 60 kV, emitting a continuous polyenergetic X-ray beam between 10 keV and 60 keV. The X ray fluence rate at the detector is known to be approximately 10 kcounts s$^{-1}$ mm$^{-2}$.

*Detector selection.* The main priority for this work is high energy resolution. The spectroscopic requirements effectively restrict the choice to a germanium detector. X-ray energy is relatively low, so there are no special demands on germanium crystal thickness, therefore a planar geometry would be the preferred choice. However, it is important to consider the X-ray fluence rate. Germanium detectors require a shaping time of approximately 6 μs for optimum energy resolution. This corresponds to a maximum event rate in the detector of approximately 15 kcounts s$^{-1}$, for a dead time of less than 10%. Therefore it is necessary to collimate the scattered beam at the detector to an area of 1.5 mm$^2$ in order to keep the event rate within the preferred limit and maximize spectroscopic performance.

#### 4.4.4.3.2. Case 2: Measuring a Radioisotope Distribution in a Biological Sample

A radiolabeled tracer is injected into a thick biological tissue section. We wish to dynamically image the distribution of the radiotracer through the tissue section. The radioisotope Tc99m emits gamma rays at an energy of 140 keV. The area to be imaged is 3 cm × 3 cm and a pixel size of 4 mm × 4 mm is required. In order to reduce the image contrast degradation effects of scattered radiation, an energy resolution of 10% is preferred.

*Detector selection.* An energy resolution of 10% opens up the detector choice to most semiconductor detectors, some high-light-yield scintillators, and even some gas detectors. The need to image dynamically imposes a strict demand on high detection efficiency, which at 140 keV effectively eliminates gas detectors and low-$Z$ materials such as silicon. The imaging requirement of 4 mm × 4 mm is not overly demanding, but will cause some degradation of energy resolution and restrict scintillator choice to those with the highest light yields, such as NaI(Tl) or CsI(Tl).

Thus the choices are the high-$Z$, high-light-yield scintillators and high-$Z$ semiconductors, all of which are capable of meeting the required specifications. In this situation it would be wise to consider the practical issues, which are usually dominated by cost. The most cost-effective solution would be a scintillator backed by photomultiplier tubes in an Anger gamma camera arrangement. However, if a key practical consideration is compactness, then a room-temperature semiconductor such as CdZnTe may be a good solution.

## ACKNOWLEDGEMENT

The authors are grateful to Dr. Beate Planskoy for her valuable comments and fruitful discussions on the theoretical and technical aspects of dosimetry.

## REFERENCES

Abate, L., Bertolucci, E., Conti, M., Mettivier, G., Montesi, M. C., & Russo, P. (2001). GaAs pixel arrays for β imaging in medicine and biology. *Nuclear Instruments and Methods in Physics Research Section A, 460*(1), 97–106.

Abdel-Fattah, A. A., & Miller, A. (1996). *Radiation Physics and Chemistry, 47*(4), 611–621.

Aird, E. G. A., & Farmer, F. T. (1972). The design of a thimble chamber for the Farmer dosemeter. *Physics in Medicine and Biology, 17*(2), 169–174.

Alfano, B., Bandettini, A., Bencivelli, W., Bertolucci, E., Bottigli, U., Conti, M., . . . & Stefanini, A. (1993). Digital imaging in radiology: Preliminary results obtained with a high spatial resolution 2D silicon detector. *IEEE Transactions on Nuclear Science, 40*(4), 987–991.

Ali, I., Costescu, C., Vicic, M., Dempsey, J. F., & Williamson, J. F. (2003). Dependence of radiochromic film optical density post-exposure kinetics on dose and dose fractionation. *Medical Physics, 30*(8), 1958–1967.

Almond, P. R., Biggs, P. J., Coursey, B. M., Hanson, W. F., Huq, M. S., Nath, R., & Rogers, D. W. (1999). AAPM's TG-51 protocol for clinical reference dosimetry of high-energy photon and electron beams. *Medical Physics, 26*(9), 1847–1870.

Altukhov, A. A., Afanas'ev, M. S., Kraskov, V. B., Lyubchenko, V. E., Mityagin, A. Y., Murav'ev, E. N., . . . & Spitsyn, B. V. (2004). Application of diamond in high technology. *Inorganic Materials, 40*(suppl. 1), S50–S70.

Ambrose, J. (1973). Computerized transverse axial scanning (tomography): Part 2. Clinical application. *British Journal of Radiology, 46*, 1023–1047.

Ambrose, J., & Hounsfield, G. (1973). New techniques for diagnostic radiology. *British Journal of Radiology, 46*, 148–149.

Amendolia, S. R., Bisogni, M. G., Bottigli, U., Ciocci, M. A., Delogu, P., Dipasquale, G., . . . & Stumbo, S. (2001). Test of a GaAs-based pixel device for digital mammography. *Nuclear Instruments and Methods in Physics Research Section A, 460*(1) 50–54.

American Association of Physicists in Medicine. (2004). *Tissue inhomogeneity corrections for megavoltage photon beams* (AAPM Rep. No. 85). Madison, WI: Medical Physics Publishing.

Angelini, F., Bellazzini, R., Brez, A., Massaia, M. M., & Torquati, M. R. (1988). Digital imaging with advanced gaseous detectors developed at Pisa University. *Nuclear Instruments and Methods in Physics Research Section A, 269*(2), 430–435.

Antonuk, L. E. (2002). *Physics in Medicine and Biology, 47*, R31–R65.

Antonuk, L. E., Boudry, J. M., Kim, C. W., Longo, M., Morton, E. J., Yorkston, J., & Street, R. A. (1991). Signal, noise, and readout considerations in the development of amorphous silicon photodiode arrays for radiotherapy and diagnostic X-ray imaging. *Proceedings of SPIE, 1443*, 108–119.

Antonuk, L. E., El-Mohri, Y., Huang, W., Jee, K. W., Siewerdsen, J. H., Maolinbay, M., . . . & Yorkston J. (1998). Initial performance evaluation of an indirect-detection, active matrix flat-panel imager (AMFPI) prototype for megavoltage imaging. *International Journal of Radiation Oncology, Biology, Physics, 42*(2), 437–454.

Arber, J. M., & Sharpe, P. H. G. (1993). *Applied Radiation and Isotopes, 44*(1–2), 19–22.

Arfelli, F., Bonvicini, V., Bravin, A., Cantatore, G., Castelli, E., Dalla Palma, L., . . . & Vacchi A. (1998). Mammographic phantom and breast tissue images with synchrotron radiation using a linear array silicon detector. *Radiology, 208*, 709–715.

Arnot, R. N., Willetts, R. J., Batten, J. R., & Orr, J. S. (1984). Investigations using an X-ray image intensifier and a TV camera for imaging transverse sections in humans. *British Journal of Radiology, 57*, 47–55.

Aznar, M. C., Andersen, C. E., Bøtter-Jensen, L., Bäck, S. Å. J., Mattsson, S., Kjær-Kristoffersen, F., & Medin, J. (2004). Real-time optical-fibre luminescence dosimetry for radiotherapy: Physical characteristics and applications in photon beams. *Physics in Medicine and Biology, 49*, 1655–1669.

Aznar, M. C., Hemdal, B., Medin, J., Marckmann, C. J., Andersen, C. E., Bøtter-Jensen, L., . . . & Mattsson, S. (2005). In vivo absorbed dose measurements in mammography using a new real-time luminescence technique. *British Journal of Radiology, 78*(928), 328–334.

Baciak, J., & He, Z. (2003). Comparison of 5 and 10 mm thick $HgI_2$ pixelated γ-ray spectrometers. *Nuclear Instruments and Methods in Physics Research Section A, 505*, 191–194.

Bäck, S. A., Medim, J., Magnusson, P., Olsson, P., Grusell, E., & Olsson, L. E. (1999). Ferrous sulphate gel dosimetry and MRI for proton beam dose measurements. *Physics in Medicine and Biology, 44*, 1983–1996.

Bambynek, M., Flühs, D., Quast, U., Wegeener, D., & Soares, C. G. (2000). A high-precision, high-resolution and fast dosimetry system for beta sources applied in cardiovascular brachytherapy. *Medical Physics, 27*(4), 662–667.

Barnes, G. T. (1982). *Medical Physics, 9*, 656–667.

Bartolotta, A., Fattibene, P., Onori, S., Pantaloni, M., & Petetti, E. (1993). Sources of uncertainty in therapy level alanine dosimetry. *Applied Radiation and Isotopes, 44*(1–2), 13–17.

Bauer, C., Baumann, I., Colledani, C., Conway, J. Delpierre, P., Djama, F., . . . & Zoeller, M. (1995). Radiation hardness studies of CVD diamond detectors. *Nuclear Instruments and Methods in Physics Research Section A, 367*(1–3), 207–211.

Beddar, A. S., Law, S., Suchowerska, N., & Mackie, T. R. (2003). Plastic scintillation dosimetry: Optimization of light collection efficiency. *Physics in Medicine and Biology, 48*(9), 1141–1152.

Beddar, A. S., Mackie, T. R., & Attix, F. H. (1992a). *Physics in Medicine and Biology, 37*(10), 1883–1900.

Beddar, A. S., Mackie, T. R., & Attix, F. H. (1992b). *Physics in Medicine and Biology, 37*(10), 1901–1913.

Beddar, A. S., Salehpour, M., Briere, T. M., Hamidian, H., & Gillin, M. T. (2005). Preliminary evaluation of implantable MOSFET radiation dosimeters. *Physics in Medicine and Biology, 50*(1), 141–149.

Berger, M. J., Coursey, J. S., & Zucker, M. A. (2000). *ESTAR, PSTAR, and ASTAR: Computer programs for calculating stopping-power and range tables for electrons, protons, and helium ions* (version 1.2.2). Available at http://physics .nist.gov/Star; accessed June 28, 2005. Gaithersburg, MD: National Institute of Standards and Technology.

Bertolucci, E., Conti, M., Grossi, G., Madonna, G., Mancini, E., Russo, P., . . . & Amendolia, S. R. (1996). Autoradiography with silicon strip detectors. *Nuclear Instruments and Methods in Physics Research Section A, 381*(2), 527–530.

Beutel, J., Kundel, H. L., & Van Metter, R. L. (Eds.). (2000). *Handbook of medical imaging: Vol. 1. Physics and psychophysics*. Bellingham, WA: SPIE Press.

Bhattacharjee, T., Basu, S. K., Dey, C. C., & Chatterjee, M. B. (2002). Comparative studies of YAG(Ce) and CsI(Tl) scintillators. *Nuclear Instruments and Methods in Physics Research Section A, 484*, 364–368.

Blackman, R. B., & Tukey, J. W. (1958). *The measurement of power spectra.* New York, NY: Dover.

Blasse, G., & Grabmaier, B. C. (1994). *Luminescent materials.* Berlin, Germany: Springer.

Boag, J. W. (1973). *Physics in Medicine and Biology, 18,* 3–37.

Bogucki, T. M., Murphy, W. R., Baker, C. W., Piazza, S. S., & Haus, A. G. (1997). Processor quality control in laser imaging systems. *Medical Physics, 24*(4), 581–584.

Bolotnikov, A., & Ramsey, B. (1998). Development of high-pressure xenon detectors. *Proceedings of SPIE, 3446,* 64–75.

Booth, N., Cabrera, B., & Fiorini, E. (1996). Low-temperature particle detectors. *Annual Review of Nuclear and Particle Science, 46,* 471–532.

Borchi, E., Bruzzi, M., Leroy, C., & Sciortino, S. J. (1998). *Journal of Physics D: Applied Physics, 31,* 609–616.

Bos, L. J., Danciu, C., Cheng, C. W., Brugmans, M. J., van der Horst, A., Minken, A., Mijnheer, B. J. (2002). Inter-institutional variations of sensitometric curves of radiographic dosimetric films. *Medical Physics, 29*(8), 1772–1780.

Bøtter-Jensen, L., Agersnap Larsen, N., Markey, B. G., & McKeever, S. W. S. (1997). *Radiation Measurements, 27*(2), 295–298.

Boutillon, M. (1998). *Physics in Medicine and Biology, 43,* 2061–2072.

Boyle, W. S., & Smith, G. E. (1970). *Bell Labs Technical Journal, 49,* 587–593.

Bracewell, R. N. (1986). *The Fourier transform and its applications.* New York, NY: McGraw-Hill.

Brigham, E. O. (1974). *The fast Fourier transform.* Englewood Cliffs, NJ: Prentice Hall.

Brody, W. R. (1984). *Digital radiography.* New York, NY: Raven Press.

Bugay, A., Kolesnik, S., Mehta, K., Nagy, V., & Desrosiers, M. (2000). Temperature stabilization of alanine dosimeters used for food processing and sterilization. *Applied Radiation and Isotopes, 52*(5), 1371–1373.

Burgermeister, E. A. (1981). *Physics in Medicine and Biology, 26*(2), 269–275.

Butson, M. J., Cheung, T., & Yu, P. K. N. (2004). *Physics in Medicine and Biology, 49,* N377–N381.

Butson, M. J., Yu, P. K. N., Cheung, T., & Metcalfe, P. (2003). Radiochromic film for medical radiation dosimetry. *Materials Science and Engineering: R, 41,* 61–120.

Cameron, J. R., Suntharalingam, N., & Kenney, G. N. (1968). *Thermoluminescent dosimetry.* Madison, WI: University of Wisconsin Press.

Caro, L. G., & Van Tubergen, R. P. J. (1962). *Cell Biology, 15,* 173–188.

Castoldi, A., Cattaneo, G., Galimberti, A., Guazzoni, C., Rehak, P., & Strüder, L. (2002). Room-temperature 2-D X-ray imaging with the controlled-drift detector. *IEEE Transactions on Nuclear Science, 49*(3), 989–994.

Castoldi, A., Galimberti, A., Guazzoni, C., Rehak, P., & Strüder, L. (2004). Towards large area X- and gamma-ray imagers based on controlled drift detectors. *Nuclear Instruments and Methods in Physics Research Section A, 518,* 426–428.

Castoldi, A., Guazzoni, C., Longoni, A., Gatti, E., Rehak, P., & Struder, L. (1997). Conception and design criteria of a novel silicon device for the measurement of position and energy of X-rays. *IEEE Transactions on Nuclear Science, 44*(5), 1724–1732.

Chan, H. P., Niklason, L. T., Ikeda, D. M., Lam, K. L., & Adler, D. D. (1994). Digitization requirements in mammography: Effects on computer-aided detection of microcalcifications. *Medical Physics, 21,* 1203–1211.

Charpak, G., & Sauli, F. (1979). *Nuclear Instruments and Methods in Physics Research, 162,* 405–428.

Cheng, C. W., & Das, I. J. (1996). Dosimetry of high energy photon and electron beams with CEA films. *Medical Physics, 23*(7) 1225–1232.

Chepel, V., Lopes, M. I., Kuchenkov, A., Ferreira Marques, R., & Policarpo, A. J. P. L. (1997). Performance study of liquid xenon detector for PET. *Nuclear Instruments and Methods in Physics Research Section A, 392,* 427–432.

Cherry, S. R. (2004). *Physics in Medicine and Biology, 49,* R13–R48.

Cherry, S. R., Shao, Y., Silverman, R. W., Meadors, K., Siegel, S., Chatziioannou, A., . . . & Phelps, M. E. (1997). MicroPET: A high resolution PET scanner for imaging small animals. *IEEE Transactions on Nuclear Science, 44,* 1161–1166.

Childress, N. L., Dong, L., & Rosen, I. I. (2002). *Medical Physics, 29*(10), 2384–2390.

Chiu-Tsao, S. T., de la Zerda, A., Lin, J., & Kim, J. H. (1994). *Medical Physics, 21*(5), 651–657.

Chmeissani, M., Frojdh, C., Gal, O., Llopart, X., Ludwig, J., Maiorino, M., . . . & Zwerger, A. (2004). First experimental tests with a CdTe photon counting pixel detector hybridized with a Medipix2 readout chip. *IEEE Transactions on Nuclear Science, 51*(5), 2379–2385.

Chu, K. C., Jordan, K. J., Battista, J. J., Van Dyk, J., & Rutt, B. K. (2000). Polyvinyl alcohol-Fricke hydrogel and cryogel: Two new gel dosimetry systems with low $Fe^{3+}$ diffusion. *Physics in Medicine and Biology, 45*(4), 955–969.

Chu, W. C., Guo, W. Y., Wu, M. C., Chung, W. Y., & Pan, D. H. C. (1998). The radiation induced magnetic resonance image intensity change provides a more efficient three-dimensional dose measurement in MRI-Fricke-agarose gel dosimetry. *Medical Physics, 25*(12), 2326–2332.

Chuang, C. F., Verhey, L. J., & Xia, P. (2002). *Medical Physics, 29*(6), 1109–1115.

Cirrone, G. A. P., Cuttone, G., Rafaele, L., Sabini, M. G., De Angelis, C., Onori, S., . . . & Sciortino, S. (2003). Natural and CVD type diamond detectors as dosimeters in hadron therapy applications. *Nuclear Physics B: Proceedings Supplement, 125*, 179–183.

Collot, J., Jan, S., & Tournefier, E. (2000). In: B. Aubert, J. Colas, P. Nedelec, & L. Poggioli (Eds.), *Proceedings of the IX International Conference on Calorimetry in High Energy Physics*, Annecy, France, October 9–14 (pp. 305–313). Frascati, Italy: INFN Laboratori Nazionali di Frascati.

Cunningham, I. A., & Fenster, A. (1987). *Medical Physics, 14*, 533–537.

Cunningham, I. A., Westmore, M. S., & Fenster, A. (1994). *Medical Physics, 21*, 417–427.

Cuttone, G., Azario, L., Barone-Tonghi, L., Borchi, E., Boscarino, D., Bruzzi, M., . . . & Zatelli, G. (1999). The CANDIDO project: Development of a CVD diamond dosimeter for applications in radiotherapy. *Nuclear Physics B: Proceedings Supplement, 78*, 587–591.

Dainty, J. C., & Shaw, R. (1974). *Image science*. London, England: Academic Press.

Datte, P., Birkbeck, A., Beuville, E., Endres, N., Druillole, F., Luo, L., . . . & Xuong, N.-H. (1999). Status of the digital pixel array detector for protein crystallography. *Nuclear Instruments and Methods in Physics Research Section A, 421*(3), 576–590.

De Angelis, C., Onori, S., Petetti, E., Piermattei, A., & Azario, L. (1999). Alanine/EPR dosimetry in brachytherapy. (1999). *Physics in Medicine and Biology, 44*, 1181–1191.

De Deene, Y., Hurley, C., Venning, A., Vergote, K., Mather, M., Healy, B. J., & Baldock, C. (2002). A basic study of some normoxic polymer gel dosimeters. *Physics in Medicine and Biology, 47*(19), 3441–3463.

De Deene, Y., Reynaert, N., & De Wagter, C. (2001). *Physics in Medicine and Biology, 46*, 2801–2825.

Del Guerra, A., Damiani, C., Di Domenico, G., Motta, A., Giganti, M., Marchesini, R., . . . & Zavattini, G. (2000). An integrated PET-SPECT small animal imager: Preliminary results. (2000). *IEEE Transactions on Nuclear Science, 47*, 1537–1540.

Despres, P., Beaudoin, G., Gravel, G., & de Guise, J. A. (2005). Physical characteristics of a low-dose gas microstrip detector for orthopedic X-ray imaging. *Medical Physics, 32*, 1193–1204.

De Vries, J., & van Eijk, C. W. E. (1985). *Nuclear Instruments and Methods in Physics Research Section A, 239*, 243–250.

DiBianca, F. A., & Barker, M. D. (1985). *Medical Physics, 12*, 339–343.

Dill, T., Dix, W. R., Hamm, W., Jung, M., Kupper, W., Lohman, M., . . . & Ventura, R. (1998). Intravenous coronary angiography with synchrotron radiation. *European Journal of Physics, 19*, 499–511.

Dini, S. A., Koona, R. A., Ahbourn, J. R., & Meigooni, A. S. (2005). *Journal of Applied Clinical Medical Physics, 6*(1), 114–134.

Dmitrenko, V. V., Gratchev, V. M., Ulin, S. E., Uteshev, Z. M., & Vlasik, K. F. (2000). High-pressure xenon detectors for gamma-ray spectrometry. *Applied Radiation and Isotopes, 52*, 739–743.

Dobbins, J. T., III. (2000). Image quality metrics for digital systems. In: J. Beutel, H. L. Kundel, & R. L. Van Metter (Eds.), *Handbook of medical imaging: Vol. 1. Physics and psychophysics* (pp. 161–222). Bellingham, WA: SPIE Press.

Dobbins, J. T., III, Ergun, D. L., Rutz, L., Blume, H., Hinshaw, D. A., & Clark, D. C. (1995). DQE(f) of four generations of computed radiography acquisition devices. *Medical Physics, 22*, 1581–1593.

Dominik, W., Zaganidis, N., Astier, P., Charpak, G., Santiard, J. C., Sauli, F., . . . & Townsend, D. (1989). A gaseous detector for high-accuracy autoradiography of radioactive compounds with optical readout of avalanche positions. *Nuclear Instruments and Methods in Physics Research Section A, 278*(3), 779–787.

Duggan, L., Sathiakumar, C., Warren-Forward, H., Symonds, M., McConnell, P., Smith, T., & Kron, A. T. (1999). Suitability of LiF:Mg, Cu, P and $Al_2O_3$:C for low dose measurements in medical imaging. *Radiation Protection Dosimetry, 85*, 425–428.

Ehringfeld, C., Schmid, S., Poljanc, K., Kirisits, C., Aiginger, H., & Georg, D. (2005). Application of commercial MOSFET detectors for in vivo dosimetry in the therapeutic X-ray range from 80 kV to 250 kV. *Physics in Medicine and Biology, 50*(2), 289–303.

Esthappan, J., Mutic, S., Harms, W. B., Dempsey, J. F., & Low, D. A. (2002). Dosimetry of therapeutic photon beams using an extended dose range film. *Medical Physics, 29*(10), 2438–2445.

Eveling, J. N., Morgan, A. M., & Pitchford, W. G. (1999). *Medical Physics, 26*(1), 100–107.

Feichtinger, J., Schrottner, T., Schwaiger, M., & Kindl, P. (2004). Characterisation of selected cadmium-zinc-telluride detectors. *Applied Radiation and Isotopes, 61*, 113–115.

Fidanzio, A., Azario, L., Miceli, R., Russo, A., & Piermattei, A. (2000). PTW-diamond detector: Dose rate and particle type dependence. *Medical Physics, 27*(11), 2589–2593.

Fjeld, R. A., Montague, K. J., & Haapala, M. H., Kotrappa, P. (1994). Field test of electret ion chambers for environmental monitoring. *Health Physics, 66*(2), 147–154.

Fong, P. M., Keil, D. C., Does, M. D., & Gore, J. C. (2001). Polymer gels for magnetic resonance imaging of radiation dose distributions at normal room atmosphere. *Physics in Medicine and Biology, 46*, 3105–3113.

Fossum, E. R. (1997). *IEEE Transactions on Nuclear Science, 44*, 1689–1698.

Fry, P., Noble, P., & Rycroft, R. (1970). *IEEE J. Solid-State Circuits, SC-5*, 250–254.

Fujieda, I., Cho, G., Drewery, J., Gee, T., Jing, T., Kaplan, S. N., . . . & Wildermuth, D. (1991). X-ray and charged particle detection with CsI(Tl) layer coupled to a a-Si:H photodiodes layers. *IEEE Transactions on Nuclear Science, 38*, 255–262.

Fujita, H., Tsai, D., Itoh, T., Doi, K., Morishita, J., Ueda, K., & Ohtzuka, A. (1992). A simple method for determining the modulation transfer function in digital radiography. *IEEE Trans Med Imaging, 11*, 34–39.

Funaki, M., Ozaki, T., Satoh, K., & Ohno, R. (1999). Growth and characterization of CdTe single crystals for radiation detectors. *Nuclear Instruments and Methods in Physics Research Section A, 436*, 120–126.

Galen, B., Staab, E., & Pisano, E. D. (2002). *Academic Radiology, 9*, 374–375.

Gall, K., Derosiers, M., Bensen, D., & Serago, C. (1996). *Applied Radiation and Isotopes, 47*(11/12), 1197–1199.

Gambarini, G., Arrigoni, S., Cantone, M. C., Molho, N., Facchielli, L., & Sichirollo, A. E. (1994). Dose-response curve slope improvement and result reproducibility of ferrous sulphate doped gels analysed by NMR imaging. *Physics in Medicine and Biology, 39*, 703–717.

Gambarini, G., Birattari, C., Colombi, C., Pirola, L., & Rosi, G. (2002). Fricke-gel dosimetry in boron neutron capture therapy. *Radiation Protection Dosimetry, 101*, 419–422.

Gaza, R., McKeever, S. W. S., & Akselrod, M. S. (2005). *Medical Physics, 32*(4), 1094–1002.

Gelfgat, V. I., Kosarev, E. L., & Podolyak, E. R. (1993). Programs for signal recovery from noisy data using the maximum likelihood principle. *Computer Physics Communications, 74*, 335–348.

Giger, M. L., Doi, K., & Metz, C. E. (1984). *Medical Physics, 11*, 797–805.

Gore, J. C., Kang, Y. S., & Schulz, R. J. (1984). *Physics in Medicine and Biology, 29*(10), 1189–1197.

Grabmaier, B. C., & Rossner, W. (1993). *Nuclear Tracks and Radiation Measurements, 21*, 43–45.

Granfors, P. R., Aufrichtig, R., Possin, G. E., Giambattista, B. W., Huang, Z. S., Liu, J., & Ma, B. (2003). Performance of a 41 × 41 cm² amorphous silicon flat panel X-ray detector designed for angiographic and R&F imaging applications. *Medical Physics, 30*(10), 2715–2726.

Greening, J. R. (1985). *Fundamentals of radiation dosimetry* (2nd ed.). Bristol, England: Adam Hilger.

Greskovich, C., & Duclos, S. (1997). *Annual Review of Materials Science, 27*, 69–88.

Grey, D., Sood, R., & Manchanda, R. (2004). Resolution and spectral characteristics of ultra high pressure proportional counters using various quench gases. *Nuclear Instruments and Methods in Physics Research Section A, 527*, 483–511.

Gros d'Aillon, E., Gentet, M. C., Montémont, G., Rustique, J., & Verger, L. (2005). Simulation and experimental results on monolithic CdZnTe gamma-ray detectors. *IEEE Transactions on Nuclear Science, 52*(6), 3096–3102.

Gruner, S. M., Tate, M. W., & Eikenberry, E. F. (2002). *Review of Scientific Instruments, 73*, 2815–2842.

Grusell, E., & Rikner, G. (1985). *Acta Radiologica: Therapy, Physics, Biology, 23*, 465–469.

Grusell, E., & Rikner, G. (1986). *Physics in Medicine and Biology, 31*, 527–534.

Grusell, E., & Rikner, G. (1993). *Physics in Medicine and Biology, 38*, 785–792.

Guo, W., Gardner, R., & Mayo, C. (2005). A study of the real-time deconvolution of digitized waveforms with pulse pile up for digital radiation spectroscopy. *Nuclear Instruments and Methods in Physics Research Section A, 544*, 668–678.

Guzman Calcina, C. S., de Almeida, A., Oliveira Roche, J. R., Abrego, F. C., & Baffa, O. (2005). Ir-192 HDR transit dose and radial dose function determination using alanine/EPR dosimetry. *Physics in Medicine and Biology, 50*, 1109–1117.

Harris, E., Royle, G., Speller, R., & Mooney, M. (2001). A CCD based gamma-ray dosimeter. *Nuclear Instruments and Methods in Physics Research Section A, 458*, 227–232.

Haus, A. G. (1990). *Radiology, 174*, 628–637.

Hazle, J. D., Hefner, J., Nyerick, C. E., Wilson, L., & Boyer, A. (1991). Dose-response characteristics of a ferrous-sulphate-doped gelatin system for determining radiation absorbed dose distributions by magnetic resonance imaging (Fe MRI). *Physics in Medicine and Biology, 36*(8), 1117–1125.

He, Z., Li, W., Knoll, G. F., Wehe, D. K., & Du, Y. F. (2000). Effects of charge sharing in 3-D position sensitive CdZnTe gamma-ray spectrometers. *Nuclear Instruments and Methods in Physics Research Section A, 439*, 619–624.

Heitler, W. (1954). *The quantum theory of radiation*. Oxford, England: Clarendon Press.

Hell, E., Knupfer, W., & Mattern, D. (2000). *Nuclear Instruments and Methods in Physics Research Section A, 454*, 40–48.

Hepworth, S. J., Leach, M. O., & Doran, S. J. (1999). *Physics in Medicine and Biology, 44*(8), 1875–1884.

Heydarian, M., Hoban, P. W., & Beddoe, A. H. (1996). *Physics in Medicine and Biology, 41*(1), 93–110.

Hillen, W., Schiebel, U., & Zaengel, T. (1987). *Medical Physics, 14*, 744–751.

Hilts, M., Jirasek, A., & Duzenli, C. (2005). *Physics in Medicine and Biology, 50*(8), 1727–1745.

Hitomi, K., Muroi, O., Shoji, T., Hiratate, Y., Ishibashi, H., & Ishii, M. (2000). Thallium bromide photodetectors for scintillation detection. *Nuclear Instruments and Methods in Physics Research Section A, 448*, 571–575.

Ho, W. C. G., Boggs, S. E., Lin, R. P., Slassi-Sennou, S., Madden, N. W., Pehl, R. H., & Hull, E. L. (1998). Pulse-shape discrimination techniques for correcting the effects of radiation damage in germanium coaxial detectors. *Nuclear Instruments and Methods in Physics Research Section A, 412*, 507–514.

Hofsäss, H., Vetter, U., Ronning, C., Uhrmacher, M., Bharuth-Ram, K., Hartmann, R., & Strüder, L. (2003). Electron emission channeling spectroscopy using X-ray CCD detectors. *Nuclear Instruments and Methods in Physics Research Section A, 512*, 378–385.

Hofstadter, R. (1948). *Physics Review, 74*, 100.

Holmes-Siedl, A. (1974). *Nuclear Instruments and Methods in Physics Research Section A, 121*, 169–179.

Horowitz, Y. S. (1981). *Physics in Medicine and Biology, 26*(4), 765–824.

Hounsfield, G. (1973). *British Journal of Radiology, 46*, 1016–1022.

Hu, G., Wang, S., Li, Y., Xu, L., & Li, P. (2004). The influence of temperature gradient on energy resolution of $Bi_4Ge_3O_{12}$ (BGO) crystal. *Ceramics International, 30*, 1665–1668.

Hunt, D. C., Tounsignant, O., & Rowlands, J. A. (2004). *Medical Physics, 31*, 1166–1175.

IAEA. (1997). *The use of plane parallel ionization chambers in high energy electron and photon beams—An international code of practice for dosimetry* (Technical reports series 381). Vienna, Austria: International Atomic Energy Agency.

IAEA. (2000). *Absorbed dose determination in external beam radiotherapy—An international code of practice for dosimetry based on standards of absorbed dose to water* (Technical reports series 398). Vienna, Austria: International Atomic Energy Agency.

Ibbott, G. S., Maryanski, M. J., Eastman, P., Holcomb, S. D., Zhang, Y., Avison, R. G., . . . & Gore, J. C. (1997). Three-dimensional visualization and measurement of conformal dose distributions using magnetic resonance imaging of BANG polymer gel dosimeters. *International Journal of Radiation Oncology, Biology, Physics, 38*(5), 1097–1103.

ICRU. (1979). *Average energy required to produce an ion pair* (Report no. 31). Washington, DC: International Commission on Radiation Units and Measurements.

ICRU. (1980). *Radiation quantities and units* (Report no. 33). Washington, DC: International Commission on Radiation Units and Measurements.

ICRU. (1984). *Stopping powers for electrons and positrons* (Report no. 37). Washington, DC: International Commission on Radiation Units and Measurements.

ICRU. (1992). *Photon, electron, proton and neutron interaction data for body tissues* (Report no. 46). Washington, DC: International Commission on Radiation Units and Measurements.

Ikagawa, T., Kataoka, J., Yatsu, Y., Saito, T., Kuramoto, Y., Kawai, N., . . . & Kawabata, N. (2005). Study of large area Hamamatsu avalanche photodiode in a γ-ray scintillation detector. *Nuclear Instruments and Methods in Physics Research Section A, 538,* 640–650.

Ikeda, D. M., Birdwell, R. L., O'Shaughnessy, K. F., Sickles, E. A., & Brenner, R. J. (2004). Computer-aided detection output on 172 subtle findings on normal mammograms previously obtained in women with breast cancer detected at follow-up screening mammography. *Radiology, 230,* 811–819.

Jasczak, R. J., Coleman, R. E., & Lim, C. B. (1980). *IEEE Transactions on Nuclear Science, 27,* 1137–1153.

Jee, K. W., Antonuk, L. E., El-Mohri, Y., & Zhao, Q. (2003). System performance of a prototype flat-panel imager operated under mammographic conditions. *Medical Physics, 30*(7), 1874–1890.

Jenneson, P. M., Atkinson, E. C., Wai, P., & Doran, S. J. (2004). *Journal of Physics: Conference Series, 3,* 257–260.

Jing, T., Goodman, C. A., Drewery, J., Cho, G., Hong, W. S., Lee, H., . . . & Wildermuth, D. (1994). Amorphous silicon pixel layers with cesium iodide converters for medical radiograph. *IEEE Transactions on Nuclear Science, 41*(4), 903–909.

Johansson Bäck, S. Å., Magnusson, P., Franson, A., Olsson, L. E., Montelius, A., Holmberg, O., . . . & Mattsson, S. (1998). Improvements in absorbed dose measurements for external radiation therapy using ferrous dosimeter gel and MR imaging (FeMRI). *Physics in Medicine and Biology, 43*(2), 261–276.

Johns, H. E., & Cunningham, J. R. (1983). *The physics of radiology* (4th ed.). Springfield, IL: Charles C. Thomas.

Johnson, R. F., Pickett, S. C., & Barker, D. L. (1990). *Electrophoresis, 11,* 355–360.

Jornet, N., Carrasco, P., Jurado, D., Ruiz, A., Edualdo, T., & Ribas, M. (2004). Comparison study of MOSFET detectors and diodes for in vivo dosimetry in 18 MV beams. *Medical Physics, 31*(9), 2534–2542.

Jornet, N., Ribas, M., & Eudaldo, T. (2000). *Medical Physics, 27*(6), 1287–1293.

Jursinic, P. A., & Nelms, W. E. (2003). *Medical Physics, 30*(5), 870–879.

Kapusta, M., Balcerzyk, M., Moszynski, M., & Pawelke, J. (1999). *Nuclear Instruments and Methods in Physics Research Section A, 421,* 610.

Karellas, A., Harris, L. J., Liu, H., Davis, M., & D'Orsi, C. (1992). Charge-coupled device detector: Performance considerations and potential for small-field mammographic imaging applications. *Medical Physics, 19,* 1015–1023.

Kastis, G. A., Wu, M. C., Balzer, S. J., Wilson, D. W., Furenlid, L. R., Stevenson, G., . . . & Appleby, M. (2002). Tomographic small-animal imaging using a high-resolution semiconductor detector. *IEEE Transactions on Nuclear Science, 49,* 172–175.

Keddy, R. J., Nam, T. L., & Burns, R. C. (1987). *Physics in Medicine and Biology, 32*(6), 751–759.

Kellermann, P. O., Ertl, A., & Gornik, E. (1998). *Physics in Medicine and Biology, 43*(8), 2251–2263.

Kelly, R. G., Jordan, K. J., & Battista, J. J. (1998). *Medical Physics, 25*(9), 1741–1750.

Kember, N. F. (1994). *Medical radiation detectors—Fundamental and applied aspects.* Bristol, England: Institute of Physics Publishing.

Kerek, A., Klamra, W., Norlin, L.-O., Novák, D., Westman, S., Lidberg, J., . . . & the CRYRING staff. (1998). Fast inorganic scintillators for beam diagnostics at extreme high vacuum. *Sixth European Particle Accelerator Conference (EPAC 98), June 22–26, Stockholm, Sweden* (pp. 1577–1579). Bristol, England: Institute of Physics Publishing.

Kipouros, P., Papagiannis, P., Sakelliou, L., Karaiskos, P., Sandilos, P., Baras, P., . . . & Baltas, D. (2003). 3D dose verification in $^{192}$Ir HDR prostate monotherapy using polymer gels and MRI. *Medical Physics, 30*(8), 2031–2039.

Kirov, A. S., Hurlbut, C., Dempsey, J. F., Shrinivas, S. B., Epstein, J. W., Binns, W. R., . . . & Williamson, J. F. (1999). Towards two dimensional brachytherapy dosimetry using plastic scintillator: New highly efficient water equivalent plastic scintillator materials. *Medical Physics, 26*(8), 1515–1523.

Kirov, A. S., Piao, J. Z., Mathur, N. K., Miller, T. R., Devic, S., Trichter, S., . . . & LoSasso, T. (2005). The three dimensional scintillation dosimetry method: Test for a [106]Ru eye plaque applicator. *Physics in Medicine and Biology, 50*(13), 3061–3081.

Klassen, N. V., & Ross, C. K. (1997). *Journal of Research of the National Institute of Standards and Technology, 102,* 63–74.

Klassen, N. V., Shortt, K. R., Seuntjens, J., & Ross, C. K. (1999). *Physics in Medicine and Biology, 44*(7), 1609–1624.

Klein, O., & Nishina, Y. (1929). *Zeits fur Physics, 52,* 853–862.

Kleinfelder, S., Bichsel, H., Bieser, F., Matis, H. S., Rai, G., Retiere, F., . . . & Yamamoto, E. (2002). Integrated X-ray and charged particle active pixel CMOS sensor arrays using an epitaxial silicon sensitive region. *Proceedings of SPIE, 4784,* 208–217.

Knoll, G. F. (2000). *Radiation detection and measurement* (3rd ed.). New York, NY: Wiley.

Kron, T., Metcalfe, P., & Pope, J. M. (1993). *Physics in Medicine and Biology, 38*(1), 139–150.

Kron, T., & Pope, J. M. (1994). *Physics in Medicine and Biology, 39*(9), 1337–1349.

Lacy, J., Athanasiades, A., Shehad, N., Sun, L., Lyons, T., Martin, C., & Bu, L. (2004). Cylindrical high pressure xenon spectrometer using scintillation light pulse correction. In: *IEEE Nuclear Science Symposium Conference Record* (vol. 1), October 16–22, Rome, Italy (pp. 16–20). New York, NY: IEEE.

Lear, J. L., Plotnick, J., & Rumley, S. (1987). *Journal of Nuclear Medicine, 28,* 218–222.

Lecomte, R., Cadorette, J., Rodrigue, S., Rouleau, D., Bentourkia, M., Yao, R., & Msaki, P. (1996). Initial results from the Sherbrooke avalanche photodiode PET scanner. *IEEE Transactions on Nuclear Science, 43,* 1952–1957.

Lee, K. Y., Fung, K. K. L., & Kwok, C. S. (2005). *Medical Physics, 32*(6), 1485–1490.

Lees, J. E., Fraser, G. W., & Dinsdale, D. (1997). *Nuclear Instruments and Methods in Physics Research Section A, 392,* 349–353.

Letourneau, D., Pouliot, J., & Roy, R. (1999). *Medical Physics, 26*(12), 2555–2561.

Liu, H., Jiang, H., Fajardo, L. L., Karellas, A., & Chen, W. R. (2000). Lens distortion in optically coupled digital X-ray imaging. *Medical Physics, 27*(5), 906–912.

Liu, X., & Shaw, C. C. (2004). *Medical Physics, 31,* 98–110.

Loidl, M., Leblanc, E., Bouchard, J., Branger, T., Coron, N., Leblanc, J., . . . & Enss, C. (2004). High-energy resolution X-ray, gamma and electron spectroscopy with cryogenic detectors. *Applied Radiation and Isotopes, 60,* 363–368.

Loncol, T., Greffe, J. L., Vynckier, S., & Scalliet, P. (1996). *Radiation Oncology, 41*(2), 179–187.

MacDougall, N. D., Miquel, M. E., Wilson, D. J., Keevil, S. F., & Smith, M. A. (2005). Evaluation of the dosimetric performance of BANG3 polymer gel. *Physics in Medicine and Biology, 50*(8), 1717–1726.

MacDougall, N. D., Pitchford, W. G., & Smith, M. A. (2002). *Physics in Medicine and Biology, 47,* R107–R121.

Maidment, A. D., Fahrig, R., & Yaffe, M. J. (1993). *Medical Physics, 20,* 1621–1633.

Maidment, A. D., Yaffe, M. J., Plewes, D. B., Mawdsley, G. E., Soutar, I. C., & Starkowski, B. G. (1993). Imaging performance of a prototype scanned-slot digital mammography system. *Proceedings of SPIE, 1896,* 93–103.

Mainprize, J. G., Ford, N. L., Yin, S., Gordon, E. E., Hamilton, W. J., Tumer, T. O., & Yaffe, M. J. (2002a). A CdZnTe slot-scanned detector for digital mammography. *Medical Physics, 29,* 2767–2781.

Mainprize, J. G., Ford, N. L., Yin, S., Tumer, T., & Yaffe, M. J. (2002b). A slot-scanned photodiode-array/CCD hybrid detector for digital mammography. *Medical Physics, 29,* 214–225.

Mainwood, A. (2000). *Semiconductor Science and Technology, 15,* R55–R63.

Manfredotti, C. (2005). CVD diamond detectors for nuclear and dosimetric applications. *Diamond and Related Materials, 14,* 531–540.

Marre, D., & Marinello, G. (2004). *Medical Physics, 31*(1), 50–56.

Martens, P., Claeys, I., Wagter, C. D., & Neve, W. D. (2002). The value of radiographic film for the characterization of intensity-modulated beams. *Physics in Medicine and Biology, 47*(13), 2221–2234.

Maryanski, M. J., Gore, J. C., Kennan, P., & Schulz, R. J. (1993). NMR relaxation enhancement in gels polymerized and cross-linked by ionizing radiation: A new approach to 3D dosimetry by MRI. *Magnetic Resonance Imaging, 11*(2), 253–258.

Maryanski, M. J., Ibbott, G. S., Eastman, P., Schulz, R. J., & Gore, J. C. (1996). Radiation therapy dosimetry using magnetic resonance imaging of polymer gels. *Medical Physics, 23*, 699–705.

Mather, M. L., & Baldock, C. (2003). *Medical Physics, 30*(8), 2140–2148.

Mattsson, L. O., Johansson, K. A., & Svensson, H. (1982). *Acta Radiologica: Oncology, 21*, 139–144.

McEwen, M. R., & Duane, S. C. (2000). *Physics in Medicine and Biology, 45*, 3675–3691.

McJury, M., Oldham, M., Cosgrove, V. P., Murphy, P. S., Doran, S., Leach, M. O., & Webb, S. (2000). Radiation dosimetry using polymer gels: Methods and applications. *British Journal of Radiology, 73*(873), 919–929.

McJury, M., Oldham, M., Leach, M. O., & Webb, S. (1999a). *Physics in Medicine and Biology, 44*(8), 1863–1873.

McJury, M., Tapper, P. D., Cosgrove, V. P., Murphy, P. S., Griffin, S., Leach, M. O., . . . & Oldham, M. (1999b). Experimental 3D dosimetry around a high-dose-rate clinical $^{192}$Ir source using a polyacrylamide gel (PAG) dosimeter. *Physics in Medicine and Biology, 44*(10), 2431–2444.

McKinlay, A. F. (1981). *Thermoluminesence dosimetry*. Bristol, England: Adam Hilger.

McLaughlin, W. L., Yun-Dong, C., Soares, C. G., Miller, A., Van Dyk, G., & Lewis, D. F. (1991). Sensitometry of the response of a new radiochromic film dosimeter to gamma radiation and electron beams. *Nuclear Instruments and Methods in Physics Research Section A, 302*, 165–176.

McNeil, W. J., & McGregor, D. S. (2004). Single-charge-carrier-type sensing with an insulated Frisch ring CdZnTe semiconductor radiation detector. *Applied Physics Letters, 84*, 1988–1990.

Mees, C. E., & James, T. H. (1966). *The theory of the photographic process* (3rd ed.). New York, NY: Macmillan.

Meigooni, A. S., Sanders, M. F., Ibbott, G. S., & Szeglin, S. R. (1996). *Medical Physics, 23*(11), 1883–1888.

Meikle, S. R., Kench, P., Weisenberger, A. G., Wojcik, R., Smith, M. F., Majewski, S., . . . & Fulham, M. J. (2002). A prototype coded aperture detector for small animal SPECT. *IEEE Transactions on Nuclear Science, 49*, 2167–2171.

Mendis, S. K., Kemeny, S. E., Gee, R. C., Pain, B., Staller, C. O., Kim, Q., & Fossum, E. R. (1997). CMOS active pixel image sensors for highly integrated imaging Systems. *IEEE Journal of Solid-State Circuits, 32*(2), 187–197.

Mettivier, G., Montesi, M. C., & Russo, P. (2003). *Physics in Medicine and Biology, 48*, N173–N181.

Miyaoka, R. S., Kohlmyer, S. G., & Lewellen, T. K. (2001). *IEEE Transactions on Nuclear Science, 48*, 1403–1407.

Mobit, P. N., & Sandison, G. A. (1999). *Medical Physics, 26*(11), 2503–2507.

Montemont, G., Arques, M., Verger, L., & Rustique, J. (2001). A capacitive Frisch grid structure for CdZnTe detectors. *IEEE Transactions of Nuclear Science, 48*, 278–281.

Morrell, R. E., & Rogers, A. (2004). *Physics in Medicine and Biology, 49*(24), 5559–5570.

Moszynski, M. (2003). Inorganic scintillators in gamma-ray spectrometry. *Nuclear Instruments and Methods in Physics Research Section A, 505*, 101–110.

Moszynski, M., Szawlowski, M., Kapusta, M., & Balcerzyk, M. (2002). *Nuclear Instruments and Methods in Physics Research Section A, 485*, 504.

Muench, P. J., Meigooni, A. S., Nath, R., & McLaughlin, W. L. (1991). *Medical Physics, 18*(4), 769–775.

Murphy, P. S., Cosgrove, V. P., Schwarz, A. J., Webb, S., & Leach, M. O. (2000). Proton spectroscopic imaging of polyacrylamide gel dosimeters for absolute radiation dosimetry. *Physics in Medicine and Biology, 45*(4), 835–845.

Nakano, T., Suchowerska, N., Bilek, M., McKenzie, D. R., Ng, N., & Kron, T. (2003). High dose-rate brachytherapy source localization: Positional resolution using a diamond detector. *Physics in Medicine and Biology, 48*(14), 2133–2146.

Naydenov, S. (2005). Spectrometric properties of detectors with regular and chaotic light collection and improvement of the intrinsic energy resolution. *Nuclear Instruments and Methods in Physics Research Section A, 537*, 397–401.

Neitzel, U., Maack, I., & Gunther-Kohfahl, S. (1994). *Medical Physics, 21*, 509–516.

Niraula, M., Nakamura, A., Aoki, T., Tomita, Y., & Hatanaka, Y. (2002). Stability issues of high-energy resolution diode type CdTe nuclear radiation detectors in a long-term operation. *Nuclear Instruments and Methods in Physics Research Section A, 491*, 168–175.

Niromaand-Rav, A., Razavi, R., Thobejane, S., & Hartner, K. W. (1996). *International Journal of Radiation Oncology, Biology, and Physics, 34*(2), 475–480.

Novotny, J., Jr., Novotny, J., Spevacek, V., Dvorak, P., Cechak, T., Liscak, R., . . . & Vymazal, J. (2002). Application of polymer gel dosimetry in gamma knife radiosurgery. *Journal of Neurosurgery, 97*(suppl. 5), 556–562.

Novotny, J., Jr., Spevacek, V., Dvorak, P., Novotny, J., & Cechak, T. (2001). Energy and dose rate dependence of BANG-2 polymer-gel dosimeter. *Medical Physics, 28*(11), 2379–2386.

Nowotny, R. (1998). *XmuDat: Photon attenuation data on PC* (IAEA-NDS 195). Vienna, Austria: International Atomic Energy Agency.

Nutbrown, R. F., Duane, S., Shipley, D. R., & Thomas, R. A. S. (2002). *Physics in Medicine and Biology, 47*(3), 441–454.

Olivo, A., Rigon, L., Arfelli, F., Cantatore, G., Longo, R., Menk, R. H., . . . & Castelli, E. (2000). Experimental evaluation of a simple algorithm to enhance the spatial resolution in scanned radiographic systems. *Medical Physics, 27*(11), 2609–2616.

Olsson, L. E., Petersson, S., Ahlgren, L., & Mattsson, S. (1989). *Physics in Medicine and Biology, 34*(1), 43–52.

Olsson, L. E., Westrin, B. A., Fransson, A., & Nordell, B. (1992). *Physics in Medicine and Biology, 37*(12), 2243–2252.

Olsson, S., Bergstrand, E. S., Carlsson, A. K., Hole, E. O., & Lund, E. (2002). Radiation dose measurements with alanine/agarose gel and thin alanine films around a $^{192}$Ir brachytherapy source, using ESR spectroscopy. *Physics in Medicine and Biology, 47*, 1333–1356.

Olsson, S., Lund, E., & Erickson, R. (1996). Dose response and fading characteristics of an alanine-agarose gel. *Applied Radiation and Isotopes, 47*(11/12), 1211–1217.

Onodera, T., Hitomi, K., Shoji, T., & Hiratate, Y. (2004). Pixellated thallium bromide detectors for gamma-ray spectroscopy and imaging. *Nuclear Instruments and Methods in Physics Research Section A, 525*, 199–204.

Onori, S., De Angelis, C., Fattibene, P., Pacilio, M., Petetti, E., Azario, L., . . . & Lo Nigro, S. (2000). Dosimetric characterization of silicon and diamond detectors in low-energy proton beams. *Physics in Medicine and Biology, 45*(10), 3045–3058.

Onori, S., d'Errico, F., De Angelis, C., Egger, E., Fattibene, P., & Janovsky, I. (1997). Alanine dosimetry of proton therapy beams. *Medical Physics, 24*(3), 447–453.

Ott, R. J., MacDonald, J., & Wells, K. (2000). *Physics in Medicine and Biology, 45*, 2011–2027.

Palmans, H., Thomas, R., Simon, M., Duane, S., Kacperek, A., Dusautoy, A., & Verhaegen, F. (2004). A small-body portable graphite calorimeter for dosimetry in low-energy clinical proton beams. *Physics in Medicine and Biology, 49*(16), 3737–3749.

Pani, S., Longo, R., Dreossi, D., Montanari, F., Olivo, A., Arfelli, F., . . . & Castelli, E. (2004). Breast tomography with synchrotron radiation: Preliminary results. *Physics in Medicine and Biology, 49*, 1739–1754.

Pantelis, E., Karlis, A. K., Kozicki, M., Papagiannis, P., Sakelliou, L., & Rosiak, J. M. (2004). Polymer gel water equivalence and relative energy response with emphasis on low photon energy dosimetry in brachytherapy. *Physics in Medicine and Biology, 49*, 3495–3514.

Pearson, C. J., Regan, P. H., & Divoli, A. (2001). The application of CdZnTe detectors for coincident α-γ spectroscopy. *Nuclear Instruments and Methods in Physics Research Section A, 462*, 393–396.

Penttilä, A., Heinäsmäki, S., Sankari, R., Aksela, S., & Aksela, H. (2005). Resolution enhancement by deconvolution. *Journal of Electron Spectroscopy and Related Phenomena, 144*, 979–981.

Petric, M. P., Robar, J. L., & Clark, B. G. (2006). *Medical Physics, 33*(1), 96–105.

Pilbrow, J. R. (1996). *Applied Radiation and Isotopes, 47*(11/12), 1465–1470.

Pisano, E. D., & Yaffe, M. J. (2005). *Radiology, 354*, 353–362.

Planskoy, B. (1980). *Physics in Medicine and Biology, 25*(3), 519–532.

Planskoy, B. (1983). Dose measurement. In: N. M. Bleehen, E. Glatstein, & J. L. Haybittle (Eds.), *Radiation therapy planning*. New York, NY: Marcel Dekker.

Podgorsak, M. B., & Schreiner, L. J. (1992). *Medical Physics, 19*(1), 87–95.

Prosvirin, D. V., Amosov, V. N., Krasil'nikov, A. V., & Gvozdeva, N. M. (2004). A dosimeter for on-line dose rate monitoring based on a natural diamond detector. *Instruments and Experimental Techniques, 47*(5), 675–677.

Rabbani, M., Shaw, R., & Van Metter, R. J. (1987). *Journal of the Optical Society of America A, 4*, 895–901.

Rahab, H., Keffous, A., Menari, H., Chergui, W., Boussaa, N., & Siad, M. (2001). Surface barrier detectors using aluminum on n- and p-type silicon for alpha-spectroscopy. *Nuclear Instruments and Methods in Physics Research Section A, 459*, 200–205.

Ramani, R., Russell, S., & O'Brien, P. (1997). *International Journal of Radiation Oncology, Biology, and Physics, 37*(4), 959–964.

Reinstein, L. E., Gluckman, G. R., & Meek, A. G. (1998). *Physics in Medicine and Biology, 43*(10), 2703–2708.

Rikner, G., & Grusell, E. (1983). *Physics in Medicine and Biology, 28*(11), 1261–1267.

Roehrig, H., Fajardo, L., & Yu, T. (1993). *Proceedings of SPIE, 1896*, 213–220.

Rose, A. (1973). *Vision: Human and electronic (Optical physics and engineering)*. New York, NY: Plenum.

Ross, C. K., & Klassen, N. V. (1996). *Physics in Medicine and Biology, 41*, 1–29.

Rowlands, J. A. (2002). *Physics in Medicine and Biology, 47*, R123–R166.

Ryzhikov, V., Gal'chinetskii, L., Katrunov, K., Lisetskaya, E., Gavriluk, V., Zelenskaya, O., . . . & Chernikov, V. (2005). Composite detector for mixed radiations based on CsI(Tl) and dispersions of small ZnSe(Te) crystals. *Nuclear Instruments and Methods in Physics Research Section A, 540*, 395–402.

Sabel, M., & Aichinger, H. (1996). *Physics in Medicine and Biology, 41*, 315–368.

Saez-Vergara, J. C., Romero, A. M., Ginjaume, M., Ortega, X., & Miralles, H. (1999). Photon energy response matrix for environmental monitoring systems based on LiF:Mg, Ti and hypersensitive phosphors (Lif:Mg, Cu, P and $\alpha$-Al$_2$O$_3$:C). *Radiation Protection Dosimetry, 85*, 207–211.

Saini, A. S., & Zhu, T. C. (2002). *Medical Physics, 29*(4), 622–630.

Salin, H., Vujasinovic, T., Mazurie, A., Maitrejean, S., Menini, C., Mallet, J., & Dumas, S. (2002). A novel sensitive microarray approach for differential screening using probes labelled with two different radioelements. *Nucleic Acids Research, 30*, e17.

Sanchez, A. L. C., Ono, H., & Miyata, H. (2002). Bench test of small plastic scintillator tiles for the JLC EM calorimeter. Presented at the Accelerator and Particle Physics Institute, Iwate, Japan, February 13–16, 2002.

Saunders, R. S., Jr., Samei, E., Jesneck, J. L., & Lo, J. Y. (2005). Physical characterization of a prototype selenium-based full field digital mammography detector. *Medical Physics, 32*(2), 588–599.

Scalchi, P., & Francescon, P. (1998). *International Journal of Radiation Oncology, Biology, and Physics, 40*(4), 987–993.

Schlesinger, T. E., Greaves, M., Ross, S., Brunett, B. A., Van Scyoc, J. M., & James, R. B. (1999). Role of uniformity and geometry in Imarad-type gamma-ray spectrometers. *Proceedings SPIE, 3768*, 16.

Schreiner, L. J. (2004). *Journal of Physics: Conference Series, 3*, 9–21.

Schreiner, L. J., Crooks, I., Evans, M. D. C., Keller, B. M., & Parker, W. A. (1994). Imaging of HDR brachytherapy dose distributions using NRM Fricke-gelatin dosimetry. *Magnetic Resonance Imaging, 12*, 901–907.

Schulz, R. J., Venkataramanan, N., & Huq, M. S. (1990). *Physics in Medicine and Biology, 35*(12), 1611–1622.

Schulz, R. J., Wuu, C. S., & Weinhous, M. S. (1987). *Medical Physics, 14*(5), 790–796.

Seibert, J. A. (1997). Computed radiography: Technology and quality assurance. In: G. D. Frey & P. Sprawls, Jr. (Eds.), *Proceedings of the 1997 AAPM Summer School: The expanding role of medical physics in diagnostic imaging*. Madison, WI: Advanced Medical Publishing.

Sellin, P. J., Rossi, G., Renzi, M. J., Knights, A. P., Eikenberry, E. F., Tate, M. W., . . . Gruner, S. M. (2001). Performance of semi-insulating gallium arsenide X-ray pixel detectors with current-integrating readout. *Nuclear Instruments and Methods in Physics Research Section A, 460*(1), 207–212.

Seuntjens, J., & Palmans, H. (1999). *Physics in Medicine and Biology, 44*, 627–646.

Shah, K., Glodo, J., Higgins, W., van Loef, E., Moses, W., Derenzo, S., & Weber, M. (2004). CeBr$_3$ scintillators for gamma-ray spectroscopy. In: *IEEE Nuclear Science Symposium Conference Record*, October 16–22, Rome, Italy. New York, NY: IEEE.

Sharma, S. D., Bianchi, C., Conte, L., Novario, R., & Bhatt, B. C. (2004). Radiochromic film measurement of anisotropy function for high-dose-rate Ir-192 brachytherapy source. *Physics in Medicine and Biology, 49*(17), 4065–4072.

Shikhaliev, P. M., Xu, T., & Molloi, S. (2005). *Medical Physics, 32*, 427–436.

Short, M. D. (1984). *Nuclear Instruments and Methods in Physics Research Section A, 221*, 142–149.

Smith, F. A. (2000). *A primer in applied radiation physics*. London, England: World Scientific Publishing.

Soltau, H., Holl, P., Kemmer, J., Krisch, S., Zanthier, C. V., Hauff, D., . . . Krämer, J. (1996). Performance of the pn-CCD X-ray detector system designed for the XMM satellite mission. *Nuclear Instruments and Methods in Physics Research Section A, 377*, 340–345.

Sonoda, M., Takano, M., Miyahara, J., & Kato, H. (1983). Computed radiography utilizing scanning laser stimulated luminescence. *Radiology, 148*(3), 833–838.

Spekowius, G., Boerner, H., Eckenbach, W., Quadflieg, P., & Laurenssen, G. J. (1995). Simulation of the imaging performance of X-ray image intensifier/TV camera chains. *Proceedings of SPIE, 2432,* 12–23.

Sprawls, P. (1997). Computed radiography: Technology and quality assurance. In: G. D. Frey & P. Sprawls, Jr. (Eds.), *Proceedings of the 1997 AAPM Summer School: The expanding role of medical physics in diagnostic imaging.* Madison, WI: Advanced Medical Publishing.

Street, R. A., Ready, S. E., Van Schuylenbergh, K., Ho, J., Boyce, J. B., Nylen, P., . . . & Hermon, H. (2002). Comparison of PbI$_2$ and HgI$_2$ for direct detection active matrix X-ray image sensors. *Journal of Applied Physics, 91,* 3345–3355.

Szeles, C. S., & Eissler, E. E. (1998). Current issues of high-pressure Bridgman growth of semi-insulating CdZnTe. *Materials Research Society, 487,* 3–12.

Tesic, M. M., Fisher Piccaro, M., & Munier, B. (1999). *European Journal of Radiology, 31,* 2–17.

Toivonen, M., Chernov, V., Jungner, H., Aschan, C., & Toivonen, A. (1998). The abilities of LiF thermoluminescent detectors for dosimetry at boron neutron capture therapy beams. *Radiation Measurements, 29*(3–4), 373–377.

Trapp, J. V., Michael, G., Evans, P. M., Baldock, C., Leach, M. O., & Webb, S. (2004). Dose resolution in gel dosimetry: Effect of uncertainty in the calibration function. *Physics in Medicine and Biology, 49*(10), N139–N146.

Uusi-Simola, J., Savolainen, S., Kangasmaki, A., Heikkinen, S., Perkiö, J., Abo Ramadan, U., . . . & Auterinen, I. (2003). Study of the relative dose-response of BANG-3 polymer gel dosimeters in epithermal neutron irradiation. *Physics in Medicine and Biology, 48*(17), 2895–2096.

van der Stelt, P. F. (2001). *Nuclear Instruments and Methods in Physics Research Section A, 460,* 45–49.

van Eijk, C. W. E. (2002). Inorganic scintillators in medical imaging. *Physics in Medicine and Biology, 47,* R85–R106.

van Loef, E., Dorenbos, P., & van Eijk, C. (2001). *Applied Physics Letters, 77,* 1467.

Vano, E., Guibelalde, E., Fernandez, M. J., Gonzalez, L., & Ten, J. I. (1997). Patient dosimetry in interventional radiology using slow films. *British Journal of Radiology, 70*(830), 195–200.

Verger, L., Boitel, M., Gentet, M. C., Hamelin, R., Mestais, C., Mongellaz, F., . . . & Sanchez, G. (2001). Characterization of CdTe and CdZnTe detectors for gamma-ray imaging applications. *Nuclear Instruments and Methods in Physics Research Section A, 458,* 297–309.

Verger, L., Drezet, A., Gros d'Aillon, E., Mestais, C., Monnet, O., Montémont, G., . . . & Peyret, O. (2004). New perspectives in gamma-ray imaging with CdZnTe/CdTe. In: *IEEE Nuclear Science Symposium Conference Record,* October 16–22, Rome, Italy. New York, NY: IEEE.

Vergote, K., De Deene, Y., Vanden Bussche, E., & De Wagter, C. (2004). *Physics in Medicine and Biology, 49*(19), 4507–4522.

Vittori, F., Malatesta, T., & de Notaristefani, F. (1998). Comparison between YAP:Ce and CsI(Tl) multipillar matrices. *Nuclear Instruments and Methods in Physics Research Section A, 418,* 497–506.

Wang, Y. J., Iwanczyk, J. S., & Patt, B. E. (1994). *IEEE Transactions on Nuclear Science, NS-41,* 910.

Wang, Y. J., Patt, B. E., & Iwanczyk, J. S. (1996). Detector optimization for hand-held CsI(Tl)/HgI gamma-ray scintillation spectrometer applications. *IEEE Transactions on Nuclear Science, 43,* 1277–1281.

Weber, S., Bauer, A., Herzog, H., Kehren, H., Mühlensiepen, J., Vogelbruch, H., . . . & Halling, H. (2000). Recent results of the TierPET scanner. *IEEE Transactions on Nuclear Science, 47,* 1665–1669.

Weckler, G. P. (1967). *IEEE Journal of Solid-State Circuits, SC-2,* 65–73.

Weisenberger, A. G., Kross, B., Majevsky, S., Wojick, R., Bradley, E. L., & Saha, M. S. (1998). Design features and performance of a CsI(Na) array based gamma camera for small animal gene research. *IEEE Transactions on Nuclear Science, 45,* 3053–3058.

Welsh, K. T., & Reinstein, L. E. (2001). *Medical Physics, 28*(5), 844–849.

Wermes, N. (2004). *IEEE Transactions on Nuclear Science, 51,* 1006–1015.

White, D. R. (1977). *Physics in Medicine and Biology, 22,* 219–230.

Wieser, A., & Girzikowsky, R. (1996). *Applied Radiation and Isotopes, 47*(11/12), 1269–1275.

Wuu, C. S., Xu, U., & Maryanski, M. J. (2004). *Journal of Physics: Conference Series, 3,* 297–300.

XCOM. Computer program available from the National Institute Standards & Technology. See http://www.nist.gov

Xu, Y., Wuu, C. S., & Maryanski, M. J. (2004). *Medical Physics, 31*(11), 3024–3032.

Yaffe, M. J., & Rowlands, J. A. (1997). *Physics in Medicine and Biology, 42,* 1–39.

Yin, Z., Hugtenurg, R. P., Green, S., & Beddoe, A. H. (2004). *Nuclear Instruments and Methods in Physics Research Section B, 213*, 646–649.

Yukihara, E. G., Yoshimura, E. M., Lindstrom, T. D., Ahmad, S., Taylor, K. K., Mardirossian, G. (2005). High-precision dosimetry for radiotherapy using the optically stimulated luminescence technique and thin $Al_2O_3$:C dosimeters. *Physics in Medicine and Biology, 50*(23), 5619–5628.

Zat'ko, B., Dubecký, F., Boháček, P., Gombia, E., Frigeri, P., Mosca, R., . . . Kordoš, P. (2004). On the spectrometric performance limit of radiation detectors based on semi-insulating GaAs. *Nuclear Instruments and Methods in Physics Research Section A, 531*, 111–120.

Zeng, G. G., McEwen, M. R., Rogers, D. W. O., & Klassen, N. V. (2004). An experimental and Monte Carlo investigation of the energy dependence of alanine/EPR dosimetry: I. Clinical X-ray beams. *Physics in Medicine and Biology, 49*(2), 257–270.

Zeng, G. G., McEwen, M. R., Rogers, D. W. O., & Klassen, N. V. (2005). An experimental and Monte Carlo investigation of the energy dependence of alanine/EPR dosimetry: II. Clinical electron beams. *Physics in Medicine and Biology, 50*(6), 1119–1129.

Zhao, W., Ristic, G., & Rowlands, J. A. (2004). *Medical Physics, 31*, 2594–2605.

Zhao, W., & Rowlands, J. A. (1995). *Medical Physics, 22*, 1595–1604.

Zhu, X. R., Jursinic, P. A., Grimm, D. F., Lopez, F, Rownd, J. J., & Gillin, M. T. (2002). Evaluation of Kodak EDR2 film for dose verification of intensity modulated radiation therapy delivered by a static multileaf collimator. *Medical Physics, 29*(8), 1687–1692.

Ziegler, S. I., Pichler, B. J., Boening, G., Rafecas, M., Pimpl, W., Lorenz, E., . . . & Schwaiger, M. (2001). A prototype high-resolution animal positron tomograph with avalanche photodiode arrays and LSO crystals. *European Journal of Nuclear Medicine, 28*(2), 136–143.

## ABOUT THE AUTHORS

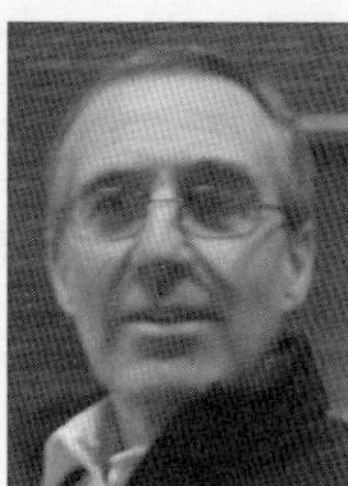

**Professor Robert Speller** obtained his first degree and PhD in physics from Imperial College London. He has over 40 years experience in radiation physics and currently holds a chair in the Department of Physics Applied to Medicine at University College London (UCL) and is head of the Radiation Physics Research Group. He has particular interests in scattered radiation fields and sensors and has published widely in these fields.

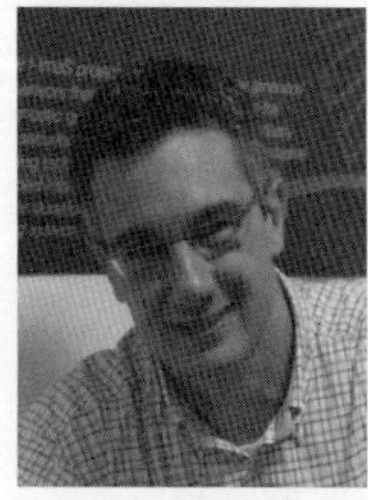

**Dr. Alessandro Olivo** did both his undergraduate and postgraduate studies in Trieste, Italy, obtaining his "Laurea" in physics *summa cum laude* in 1995 and his PhD in 2000. Following his PhD award he spent five years at ELETTRA, the synchrotron facility in Trieste, developing new X-ray imaging techniques and collaborating in the design of the first station for in vivo mammography with synchrotron radiation. Having been awarded a Marie Curie Fellowship, he moved to UCL in 2005, where he invented a new method to produce X-ray phase contrast images with conventional sources. Thanks to these results, he was awarded a Career Acceleration Fellowship by EPSRC to build a research group, which is currently developing the new methods in areas such as medical imaging, homeland security, material science, and others. In 2010 he was appointed senior lecturer in X-ray imaging.

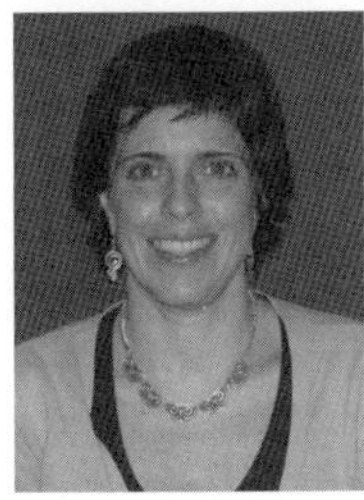

**Dr. Silvia Pani** obtained her "Laurea" degree (MPhys) and her PhD in physics from the University of Trieste (Italy) in 1996 and 2001, respectively. She then worked on the design and commissioning of the first synchrotron beamline dedicated to in vivo breast imaging at the synchrotron facility, ELETTRA. From 2004 to 2007 she worked at UCL as a Marie Curie Fellow and at St. Bartholomew's and the London NHS trust on the development of novel X-ray techniques for tissue analysis, breast and dental imaging, and the identification of illegal substances in parcels. In 2008 she became a lecturer in applied radiation physics at the University of Surrey, Guildford, UK.

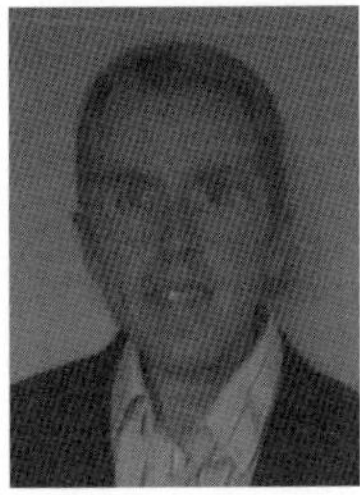

**Dr. Gary Royle** is currently senior lecturer at the Department of Medical Physics and Bioengineering at UCL. He obtained a physics degree from Imperial College London before completing a PhD in medical physics at UCL. He has over twenty years of experience in the field of medical radiation physics, primarily devoted to the detection and analysis of ionizing radiation for medical applications. This work has lead to one hundred and fifty publications and three patents. He has also taught extensively in this field and for many years ran a masters degree program in medical radiation physics.

# CHAPTER 5

# Nonionizing Electromagnetic Radiation

## Sensors for Radiometric and Photometric Measurements

E. Theocharous

*Optical Measurement Group*
*National Physical Laboratory, Teddington, TW11 0LW, UK*

## 5.1. INTRODUCTION

Radiometry is defined as the science and technology of the measurement of optical radiation, which is in turn defined as electromagnetic radiation of wavelengths between 1 nm and 1000 μm. Photometry is the science and technology of the measurement of optical radiation as it is perceived by the human eye, and can be considered as a special case of radiometry. The eye is sensitive only to wavelengths in the 360 nm to 830 nm range (CIE, 1983), which is often referred to as "light."

This chapter deals with radiometric, photometric, and spectroradiometric sensors. Radiometric sensors, or "radiometers," are defined as instruments that are designed to measure one or more of the radiometric quantities or parameters used to quantify the characteristics of a source, beam, or field of optical radiation. The term *radiometer* is usually associated with instruments that respond over a relatively wide but well-defined range of wavelengths of optical radiation. This range of wavelengths should be included in the specification of each radiometer.

Photometric sensors or "photometers" are defined as instruments designed to measure one or more of the photometric quantities or parameters used to quantify the characteristics of a source, beam, or field of optical radiation. All photometric measurements are weighted by the spectral response of the human eye. When measurements are made using the eye as the detector, this is referred to as visual photometry. More generally, however, photometric measurements are carried out using photodetectors whose spectral responsivity has been engineered to simulate the spectral response of the average human eye. This is referred to as physical photometry. Physical photometry also includes measurements made using mathematical calculations to correct spectroradiometric measurements for the spectral response of the human eye. In the case of photometers, there is no need to specify a wavelength range of response since the response of a photometer will, by definition, follow the internationally agreed relative spectral responsivity of the average human eye, which is known as the *spectral luminous efficiency function* (CIE, 1983) or the $V(\lambda)$ function.[1]

The optical radiation emission of all sources varies with wavelength, so it is important to know the wavelength distribution of their radiometric parameters. Another class of radiometric sensors has been developed to address this task by dispersing the optical radiation being evaluated into its spectral components. These instruments are known as spectroradiometers. Their design is usually more complex than broadband radiometers and photometers because they employ a component such as a diffraction grating, prism, or Fourier transform (FT) spectrometer that disperses the incident radiation into its component wavelengths.

This chapter will begin by defining the most important radiometric and photometric parameters because it is these parameters that radiometric and photometric sensors are intended to measure. The relation between the various radiometric and photometric parameters will be highlighted because every radiometer and photometer employs a photodetector to convert the total radiant power incident on its active area into an electrical signal. This is convenient if the aim is to measure radiant power, but to measure another radiometric or photometric quantity, the relationship between that quantity and the radiant or luminous power incident on the detector is required for the former to be measured. This is relatively straightforward because the relationship between the various radiometric or photometric parameters is purely geometrical, as will be shown in the next two sections.

## 5.1.1. DEFINITIONS OF THE MAJOR RADIOMETRIC ENTITIES AND UNITS

Radiant power, sometimes referred to as radiant flux, is defined as the time derivative of radiant energy and represents the rate of flow of that radiant energy. It is denoted by the symbol $\Phi$ and has units of watts. Radiant power is used, for example, to quantify the power of a laser beam. Total radiant power or flux is frequently encountered in radiometry, and this is the total radiant power emitted by a source in all directions. Note that radiant energy or "exposure" can be calculated by integrating the radiant power over a period of time. Radiant intensity[2] is the radiant power radiated from a source into a unit solid angle[3] in a defined direction and is expressed in units of watts per steradian (W sr$^{-1}$). Radiant intensity is denoted by the symbol $I$ and is associated with point, isotropic[4] sources and sources whose dimensions are small compared to the distance between the source being characterized and the observer. Irradiance is the radiant power incident on a surface per unit surface area from a hemisphere. It is denoted by the symbol $E$ and has units of watts per square meter (W m$^{-2}$). Radiant exitance refers

---

1   $V(\lambda)$ corresponds to photopic vision. For scotopic vision, an alternative $V'(\lambda)$ is defined (CIE, 1983).

2   The term intensity has different meanings when it is used in different fields. In radiometry it is defined as radiant power per unit solid angle and has units of watts per steradian (W sr$^{-1}$). The same term is (wrongly) used to mean irradiance or radiant power and it is even used to denote radiance in atmospheric physics (Palmer, 1993).

3   Solid angle is the three-dimensional (3-D) equivalent of the plane angle. The solid angle of a cone is defined as the ratio of the area cut out on a spherical surface with its center at the apex of that cone divided by the square of the radius of the sphere. It has units of steradians (sr). A hemisphere has a solid angle of $2\pi$ sr.

4   An isotropic source is a spherical source that radiates uniformly in all directions, that is, its radiant intensity is the same in all directions.

to the radiant power radiated into a hemisphere from a surface of unit area. It is denoted by the symbol $M$ and also has units of watts per square meter. Finally, radiance, denoted by the symbol $L$, is defined as the radiant power per unit solid angle per unit projected area (Datla & Parr, 2005) and is expressed in units of watts per square meter per steradian ($W\ m^{-2}\ sr^{-1}$). Radiance is considered a fundamental radiometric parameter (Nicodemus, 1963) because all other radiometric entities can be derived from radiance by integrating over area (to get radiant intensity), solid angle (to get irradiance or radiant exitance), or area and solid angle (to get radiant power).

The purpose of this chapter is to describe the design, calibration, and operation of instruments that measure these radiometric (as well as photometric) quantities. It is important to stress that there are a host of instruments wrongly referred to as radiometers. For example, a radiation thermometer or pyrometer consists of a photodetector, a band-pass filter, and an assembly that defines the solid angle over which the photodetector detects radiation. This means that a radiation thermometer measures the spectral radiance of the source or scene in its field of view (FOV) integrated over the bandwidth of the instrument. However, these instruments are not calibrated in terms of radiometric units. Instead, they use Planck's law to relate the spectral radiance of the source to its radiant temperature and are calibrated in units of temperature. For this reason they cannot be considered as radiometers. The definition of radiometric sensors should be restricted to instruments measuring radiometric parameters. Some instruments have exotic names such as pyranometers, pyrheliometers, and pyrgeometers. Since these instruments measure irradiance, they are by definition radiometers, despite their colorful names, and they are addressed in section 5.5.9.

## 5.1.2. DEFINITIONS OF THE MAJOR PHOTOMETRIC QUANTITIES AND UNITS

For each radiometric parameter there is a corresponding photometric or luminous parameter. The corresponding photometric parameters are represented by the same symbol but are differentiated by the use of a subscript. The absence of a subscript or the use of the subscript $e$ denotes a radiometric parameter, while the corresponding photometric parameter is denoted by the subscript $v$.

Luminous power, or flux, is the photometric equivalent of radiant flux. It is denoted by $\Phi_v$ and has units of lumens (lm). The total luminous power or flux is defined as the total luminous power emitted by a source. Luminous intensity is defined as the luminous flux radiated from a point source into a unit solid angle in a defined direction and is denoted by $I_v$. Luminous intensity is measured in candela (cd), which is equal to $1\ lm\ sr^{-1}$. The candela is of particular importance because it is one of the seven SI base units (BIPM, 1998). The photometric unit corresponding to irradiance is the illuminance ($E_v$), and it is defined as the luminous flux from a complete hemisphere incident on a unit surface area. It is measured in lux, which is equal to an illuminance of $1\ lm\ m^{-2}$. Luminance is the photometric quantity corresponding to radiance and is defined as the luminous flux per unit solid angle per unit projected area. It is denoted by $L_v$ and has units of lumens per steradian per square meter or candela per square meter. There are a host of other photometric units that can make the field of photometry confusing to a newcomer to the field. The reader is referred elsewhere for further information on these units (Palmer, 2001).

## 5.1.3. DEFINITIONS OF THE SPECTRORADIOMETRIC QUANTITIES AND UNITS

Radiometric sensors quantify optical radiation covering wide spectral ranges. Spectroradiometers measure the "spectral concentration" of radiometric parameters. Spectroradiometric parameters are defined as the derivatives of the corresponding radiometric quantities with respect to wavelength. They are denoted with the prefix *spectral,* covering parameters such as spectral irradiance, spectral radiant power, and so on. They represent the ratio of a parameter over a narrow wavelength range divided by the wavelength range. Spectroradiometric units refer to the parameter per unit wavelength interval, so they include a $\lambda^{-1}$ factor. For example, the units of spectral irradiance will be watts per square meter per micrometer (W m$^{-2}$ $\mu$m$^{-1}$). The total radiometric value of a parameter can be calculated by integrating the spectroradiometric (spectral) parameter over the wavelength range of interest. Spectroradiometric parameters are denoted by using a subscript $\lambda$, so $L_\lambda$ and $E_\lambda$ denote spectral radiance and spectral irradiance, respectively.

The definition of the spectral luminous efficiency function, or $V(\lambda)$ function, allows a photometric parameter $X_v$ to be determined from its corresponding spectroradiometric parameter $X_\lambda$ by the following relationship (CIE, 1983):

$$X_v = K_m \int_{360}^{830} X_\lambda(\lambda)\, V(\lambda)\, d\lambda, \tag{5.1}$$

where $K_m$ is the proportionality constant in the definition of the candela[5] whose value is taken as 683 lm W$^{-1}$. Note that it is considerably more difficult to convert a photometric parameter to the corresponding radiometric parameter and can only be done when the relative spectral emission of the source is known (Palmer, 2001).

## 5.1.4. LAMBERTIAN SOURCES AND THEIR IMPORTANCE TO RADIOMETRIC AND PHOTOMETRIC SENSORS

Prior to embarking on the treatment of different types of radiometric and photometric sensors, the properties of a Lambertian source must be summarized. This is a special type of source. The emission characteristics of blackbodies (Hollandt et al., 2005) and the exit ports of integrating spheres[6] (McCluney, 1994) are excellent approximations to those of a Lambertian source. The emissions of many objects that are encountered in everyday life also represent adequate approximations. Furthermore, radiometric and photometric theory and calculations simplify considerably when a Lambertian source is considered. For example, the radiant exitance $M$ of a Lambertian source is related to its radiance $L$ by the relationship[7] $M = \pi L$, allowing calculations for this type of source to be significantly simplified.

A Lambertian source is defined as the source whose radiance appears the same when viewed from any direction. The radiant intensity is estimated by integrating the radiance over the area of the source.

---

5    The candela is defined as the luminous intensity, in a given direction, of a source that emits monochromatic radiation at a frequency of $540 \times 10^{12}$ Hz and has a radiant intensity in that direction of 1/683 W sr$^{-1}$.

6    An integrating sphere (also known as an Ulbricht sphere) is a hollow sphere whose interior walls are coated with a material of very high diffuse reflectance. Radiation entering through a small port (the entrance port) is scattered off the sphere walls many times (see Figure 5.8). The total radiant power leaving through another port (the exit port) will be a constant fraction of the total radiant power entering the sphere regardless of the spatial and angular distribution with which it is incident on the entrance port. This makes integrating spheres ideal candidates for cosine collectors (see section 5.5.7.1.2). Furthermore, radiation entering the sphere will be "thoroughly mixed" after numerous diffuse reflections off the sphere walls, so the exit port of the sphere will have a spatially uniform radiance, which is the fundamental characteristic of a Lambertian source.

7    Note that the factor relating $M$ and $L$ is not $2\pi$, but $\pi$. This is because of the definition of radiance in terms of the "projected area," which introduces a factor of $\cos(\theta)$. The factor of $\pi$ (rather than the expected $2\pi$) appears when the radiance is integrated over a hemisphere to estimate the radiant exitance.

It is easy to show that for a Lambertian source, the apparent radiant intensity of the source is proportional to the cosine of the angle between the direction from which the source is being observed and the normal to that surface. In fact, this is Lambert's law. Examples of Lambertian sources include (apart from blackbody radiators and integrating spheres) flat radiating surfaces as well as passive, reflective surfaces such as surfaces painted with a good matte white paint. If such surfaces are uniformly illuminated, they will appear equally bright from whatever direction they are being viewed.

## 5.2. RADIOMETRIC AND PHOTOMETRIC SENSORS

All radiometric and photometric sensors consist of three main components:

- A photodetector that converts the radiant power incident on it into an electrical signal that is amplified further using some support electronics
- A spectral filter that defines the spectral response profile of the radiometer (with contributions from other parts such as the imaging components and the photodetector)
- A system of apertures or imaging optics that define the area and range of angles over which the radiometer receives optical radiation, as the only differences between the various radiometric entities are purely geometrical

Sections 5.2.1 through 5.2.4 deal with sensors measuring radiant and luminous power, irradiance and illuminance, radiant and luminous intensity, and radiance and luminance, respectively. The only difference between radiometric and photometric sensors is that the latter incorporates band-pass filters that modify the spectral responsivity to follow the $V(\lambda)$ profile. It is therefore sensible to deal with radiometric and photometric quantities together. For the purposes of clarity, radiometric terms will be used whenever possible, but the reader can change the text to the corresponding photometric quantities, with obvious changes to the meaning.

### 5.2.1. RADIANT POWER AND LUMINOUS POWER SENSORS

The most straightforward radiometric quantity to measure is radiant power. The familiar laser power meters measure the radiant power of the output beams from lasers. The main requirement is that the diameter of the active area of the photodetector being used should be larger than the diameter of the cross section of the beam of optical radiation being measured (see Fig. 5.1). This ensures that all radiant power within the beam is incident within the active area of the detector. In this case, the photodetector output will be proportional to the radiant power incident on the detector, assuming that

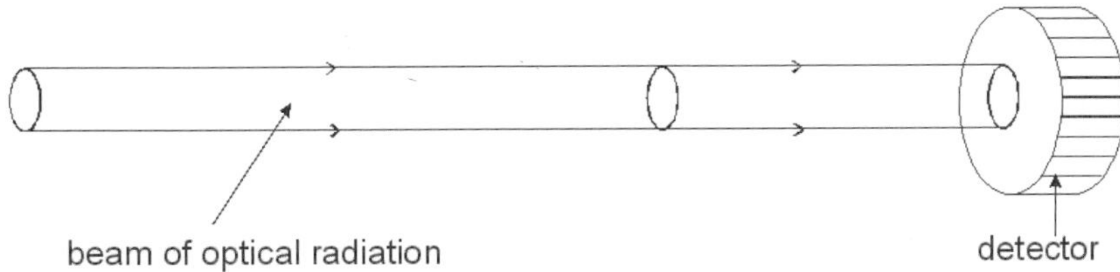


**Figure 5.1.** In a radiant power sensor, the optical beam has to underfill the active area of the photodetector.

the value of the radiant power being measured is within the linear range of the detector response. Care should be exercised when dealing with Gaussian beams because their beam diameter is often defined by the position where the beam irradiance drops to $1/e^2$ of the value of the peak irradiance. This, however, includes only 86% of the total power in the beam (Boivin, 1981; Day, 2005).

Radiometers measuring radiant power are available with photon detectors as well as thermal detectors. Photon detectors have lower noise equivalent power (NEP) values (see sections 5.2.5 and 5.3.8; Limperis & Mudar, 1989; Theocharous & Birch, 2002) and are used to measure relatively low values of radiant power (typically less than 1 mW) unless an attenuator is used in the beam of optical radiation before it reaches the photodetector. The best form of attenuation is provided by integrating spheres (McCluney, 1994), which offer significant benefits when used in high-power laser power meters. This is because, apart from introducing attenuation values of many orders of magnitude, the attenuation they introduce is independent of the direction of the incident beam as well as its state of polarization. The latter is of particular interest to laser power meters. Commercially available radiant power meters, combining a photon detector with an integrating sphere attenuator, are capable of measuring radiant power values up to 10 W. Some have a silicon and an InGaAs detector mounted on the sphere that extends the measurement range from the ultraviolet (UV) to approximately 1.6 μm.

In contrast to photon detectors, thermal detectors rely on the temperature increase caused by the incident radiation. Despite their relatively poor NEP values (Limperis & Mudar, 1989; Theocharous & Birch, 2002), thermal detectors can be engineered to have a linear range of response extending to very high radiant powers (e.g., hundreds of watts; Day, 2005). Another advantage of thermal detectors is that they have a relatively flat (constant) spectral responsivity, which means that they can be used over wide wavelength ranges.

Detectors of optical radiation exhibit various degrees of spatial nonuniformity[8] in their response; that is, the same beam illuminating different parts of the active area of the detector will give different readings (Theocharous, Fox, & Prior, 1996). Whereas some silicon detectors have spatial nonuniformities less than 0.1%, thermal detectors as well as thin-film photoconductor photon detectors (e.g., PbS, PbSe, and HgCdTe) exhibit spatial nonuniformities greater than 10% (Theocharous, 2006; Theocharous, Ishi, & Fox, 2004). Even when photodetectors with good spatial uniformities are used, it is important to illuminate the same part of the photodetector active area during the power meter calibration as during subsequent use. While centering a beam of visible radiation on a detector is relatively straightforward, it is difficult to accomplish the same task with beams of UV radiation,[9] and is particularly difficult with infrared (IR). One established technique used to aid the alignment of a beam of IR radiation is to arrange for a visible beam to overlap the IR beam (Theocharous et al., 1998b).

Other issues that contribute to the combined uncertainty of a measurement of radiant power will be discussed in section 5.3.

### 5.2.1.1. Total Radiant Power and Total Luminous Power Sensors

In contrast to radiant power meters that monitor the radiant power of beams, luminous power measurements mostly address the total luminous power emitted by a source in all directions. Two methods

---

8   Spatial nonuniformity of response is defined as the maximum percent deviation of the detector response relative to the maximum response. The nonuniformity should be measured with a probe beam diameter that is at least ten times smaller than the active area of the detector being evaluated.

9   A number of targets, including white paper, fluoresce when illuminated with UV radiation, and this is used routinely for the alignment of UV beams.

have been developed for measuring the total luminous power of sources. The first method places the test source inside an integrating sphere whose diameter is large compared to the source being characterized. A detection system located at the exit port of the integrating sphere provides a reading of $V_{test}$. The test source is then replaced by a reference source whose total luminous power is known. If the output of the detection system corresponding to the reference source is given by $V_{ref}$, then the total luminous power of the test source is given by equation 5.2 (CIE, 1989):

$$\Phi_{test} = \frac{V_{test}}{V_{ref}} \, \Phi_{ref} ,$$

5.2

where $\Phi_{test}$ and $\Phi_{ref}$ are the total luminous power of the test and reference sources, respectively. The integrating sphere method is a quick and simple method that captures the entire output of the source being investigated. The biggest drawback of this method is that it requires a source whose total luminous power is known (see equation 5.2). There are further drawbacks due to the nonideal characteristics of integrating spheres. A method for measuring the total luminous power of sources using an integrating sphere that does not require a reference source has been developed (Ohno, 1994). However, this method is difficult to execute because it requires the detailed characterization of the spatial reflectance characteristics of the integrating sphere being used. The adoption of this method has been limited (Ohno, 2005).

The second method for measuring total radiant/luminous power utilizes a goniophotometer. In this instrument, a detector is allowed to move on the surface of an imaginary sphere while it is always pointing toward the center of that sphere (see Fig. 5.2). The source whose total luminous power is being sought is placed at the center of the imaginary sphere so that the detector measures its luminous intensity at different points on the surface of this imaginary sphere. The total luminous power can then be calculated by integrating the luminous intensity over a $4\pi$ solid angle. The length of the goniophotometer arms can vary from less than 1 m to more than 10 m. The longer arms are needed to ensure that the goniophotometer arm is much longer than the largest dimension of the source being measured so that the inverse square law approximation remains valid (McCluney, 1994). Longer arm lengths are

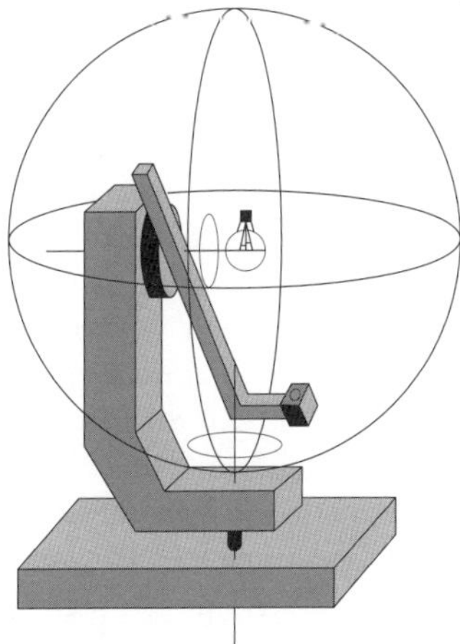

**Figure 5.2.** Schematic of a goniophotometer with the test source at the center and the photometer moving on the surface of an imaginary sphere.

often achieved by folding the path of the radiation emitted by the source using plane mirrors (CIE, 1987a). However, care is needed when using a mirror goniophotometer, because polarization effects may be introduced by the mirror reflection.

The goniospectroradiometer is a variation of the goniophotometer and is able to measure the wavelength-resolved, angle-dependent emission characteristics of sources. Goniospectroradiometers are particularly useful when dealing with light-emitting diode (LED) sources and displays whose emission characteristics in different angular orientations are wavelength dependent.

### 5.2.2. IRRADIANCE AND ILLUMINANCE SENSORS

Irradiance is the most widely measured radiometric parameter because it describes the spatial concentration of radiant power. For example, the irradiance from a UV lamp illuminating a UV-cured epoxy determines the time required for the epoxy to receive the required exposure. Radiometers measuring irradiance should accept radiation from a hemispherical solid angle, hence they require a cosine response (see section 5.2.2.1). However, a number of applications require the measurement of irradiance (illuminance) from a particular source, which may be relatively small in size and located at some distance from the sensor. This means that the source illuminates the radiometer within a relatively small range of angles. In this case, there is no need for the irradiance (illuminance) meter to have a cosine response, provided its narrow angular acceptance is greater than the range of angles over which the source illuminates the radiometer. Indeed, it is beneficial for an irradiance (illuminance) sensor not to have a cosine response, because absence of the cosine corrector increases the radiant power reaching the photodetector and reduces the stray light contribution from other sources.

There are two types of irradiance (illuminance) sensors, one without a diffuser, shown schematically in Figure 5.3(a), which can be used to measure the irradiance due to individual small sources, and one with a diffuser (cosine corrector), shown in Figure 5.3(b), which can be used to measure irradiance from a complete hemisphere, as, for example, in the measurement of global solar irradiance (see section 5.5.9). Both types of irradiance sensor include a photodetector and a band-pass filter, which in the case of an illuminance meter, modifies the relative spectral responsivity of the sensor to the $V(\lambda)$ function. The irradiance sensor with a diffuser has that diffuser mounted immediately behind the aperture. Here, it is imperative that the irradiance (illuminance) sensor has an aperture at the front, so that the sensor has a well-defined area. The same aperture can act as the plane of reference for the sensor from which the distance to the source being characterized is measured. This distance is important when the irradiance sensor is used as a radiant (luminous) intensity sensor (see section 5.2.3) and as a radiance (luminance) sensor (see section 5.2.4). Furthermore, the aperture (and aperture body) must be as thin as possible to ensure that radiation, at very large angles of incidence, strikes the diffuser. The thickness of the aperture wall has been identified as one of the reasons why the contribution of radiation incident at large angles is underestimated (Martin, Currie, & Pye, 1999). The shape of plate diffusers is designed to protrude slightly from the aperture in order to ensure that incident grazing radiation contributes equally to the response of the radiometer.

The type of diffuser (cosine corrector) used by irradiance (illuminance) sensors depends on the cost of the instrument as well as the performance being sought. Low-cost, commercially available devices use plastic diffusers that have a very limited performance and are strongly dependent on wavelength. Quartz and sapphire plates as well as polytetrafluoroethylene (PTFE) discs and opal glass diffusers offer better performance. Opal glass diffusers in particular exhibit good stability and

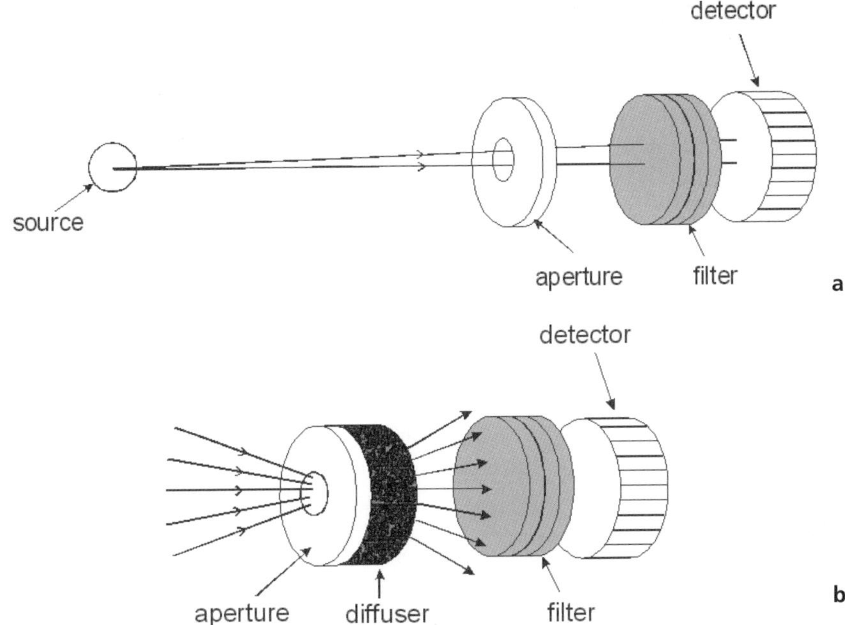


**Figure 5.3.** (a) Irradiance (illuminance) sensor without a diffuser. (b) Irradiance (illuminance) sensor with a diffuser.

resistance to UV radiation, but in some cases can exhibit fluorescence. Integrating spheres should offer the best cosine response characteristics if designed properly (Budde, 1983), but their use is limited to the highest performance applications because of high cost, poor "photon utilization," and relatively large physical size.

### 5.2.2.1. The Importance of Cosine Response in Radiometric and Photometric Sensors

Consider a ray of optical radiation incident within the active area of a photodetector. If the detector response to this ray is independent of the direction of the incident ray, then the detector is said to have a cosine response, because the response of the same detector to a beam of radiation whose cross-sectional area overfills the active area of the detector, $A_{det}$, is proportional to the cosine of the angle of incidence, $\theta$. This is because it is the projected area of the detector in the direction of the incident beam that is relevant and is given by $A_{det} \cos \theta$. A sensor with a cosine response is able to measure correctly the irradiance of a field incident on the sensor, irrespective of the angular distribution of the incident field. If the angular response of an irradiance (illuminance) sensor differs from the ideal cosine response, then large errors can be expected when the angular distribution of the irradiance field being measured differs substantially from the field used during the calibration of the sensor.

A characterization of the angular response of several commercially available radiometers and photometers demonstrated that their angular response differed significantly from the ideal cosine response (Michalsky, Harrison, & Berkheiser, 1995). The angular response characteristics of radiometers are discussed in section 5.5.7.1.2.

## 5.2.3. RADIANT INTENSITY AND LUMINOUS INTENSITY SENSORS

Measurement of the radiant (luminous) intensity requires measurement of the radiant (luminous) power emitted by a source in a well-defined solid angle. Since the solid angle over which radiation is collected is defined as the area of the sensor aperture divided by the square of the distance between the source and that aperture, the radiant intensity is measured using an irradiance meter such as the silicon trap detector with a calibrated aperture described in section 5.5.3. If the distance between the source and the aperture is $d$, then the radiant intensity $I$ can be calculated from equation 5.3:

$$I = Ed^2, \tag{5.3}$$

where $E$ is the irradiance measured by the irradiance sensor (see Fig. 5.4).

This technique is also applied by the National Standards Laboratories for the realization of the candela using photometers whose absolute spectral responsivity has been calibrated and is traceable to a primary standard detector (such as a cryogenic radiometer) through a series of calibration steps (Goodman & Key, 1988). Some industrial organizations are also beginning to adopt detector-based photometric measurements, mainly because photometers have good long-term stability, are much more robust in terms of resistance to mechanical shock than transfer standard lamps, and their response is linear over a very wide range of inputs.

## 5.2.4. RADIANCE AND LUMINANCE SENSORS

### 5.2.4.1. The Simple Radiance Sensor or Gershun Tube Radiometer

From the definition of radiance, it is clear that a radiance sensor measures the radiant power emitted by a unit surface area of a source in a unit solid angle. Therefore the minimum components of a radiance meter are a photodetector and a means of defining both the solid angle and source area. The simplest form of a radiance sensor consists of two apertures of area $A_1$ and $A_2$ separated by a distance $d$, as shown in Figure 5.5. The planes of the two apertures are perpendicular to the axis joining their centers. The first aperture, $A_1$, defines the area of the source from which radiant power is being collected, whereas the second aperture, $A_2$, and the distance, $d$, define the solid angle over which radiation is being gathered. If the absolute value of the radiant power $\Phi$ going through both apertures is measured, then the radiance of the source in the FOV of this simple radiometer can be estimated from equation 5.4:

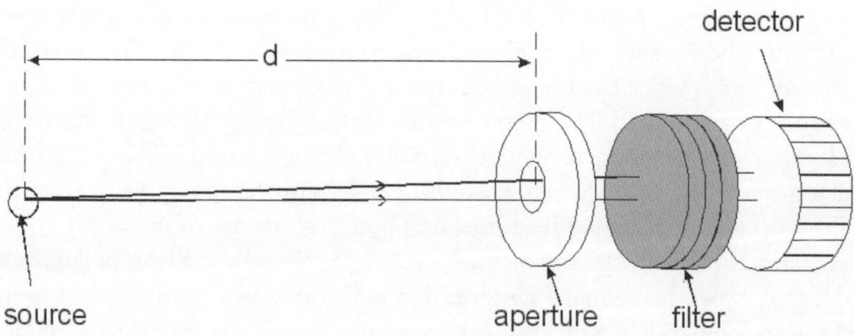


**Figure 5.4.** A radiant intensity sensor based on an irradiance sensor.

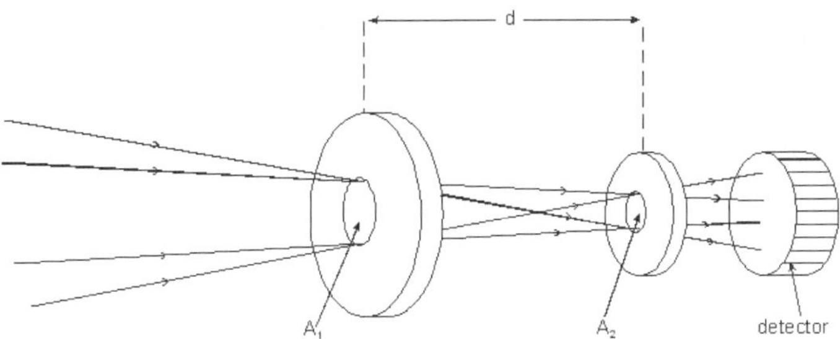


**Figure 5.5.** A simple radiance/luminance sensor.

$$L = \frac{\Phi d^2}{A_1 A_2}.$$

(5.4)

Note that equation 5.4 is only valid when $d$ is much larger than the diameters of $A_1$ and $A_2$. The reader is referred elsewhere for the full equation relating these parameters (Datla & Parr, 2005; Wyatt, 1987).

Despite its simplicity, this type of radiometer (also known as a Gershun tube radiometer) is being used to measure the radiance of extended sources because it does not involve any imaging components. Imaging optics introduce attenuation and ghost images due to Fresnel reflections from the surfaces, in addition to scattering that contributes to the size-of-source effect (Ohtsuka & Bedford, 1989). This method is frequently used by the National Standards Laboratories to measure the spectral radiance of blackbody sources from which the radiant temperature is estimated using Planck's formula (Harrison et al., 1998). Usually aperture $A_2$ is combined with a photodetector to form an irradiance sensor or, if a band-pass filter is included, a filter radiometer calibrated as an entity in units of output per unit spectral irradiance.

This simple radiometer has a significant drawback. It requires that the source have a relatively large area in order to overfill the FOV of the radiometer. The diameters of the areas of some of the high-temperature blackbodies used by the National Standards Laboratories can be as small as 3 mm. This means that the diameters of the two apertures have to be kept small, while the distance $d$ between the two apertures has to be large in order to ensure that the emission area of the blackbody overfills the FOV of the radiometer.

### 5.2.4.2. The Lensed Radiance and Luminance Sensor

The addition of an imaging component such as a lens in the vicinity of the first aperture $A_1$ (see Fig. 5.5), as shown in Figure 5.6, offers very clear benefits, particularly when it is being used to characterize small-area sources. The focal length of this lens and the distance between the radiometer and the source are chosen so that the image of the source is formed in the plane of the second aperture, also known as the field stop. Due to the principle of conservation of radiance (McCluney, 1994), the radiance of the image formed in the plane of the field stop is equal to the product of the radiance of the source multiplied by the transmittance of the lens. The area of the field stop determines the area over which radiance is integrated, while the area of the entrance aperture (aperture stop in Fig. 5.6) and the distance between the two apertures define the solid angle over which radiation is collected. The

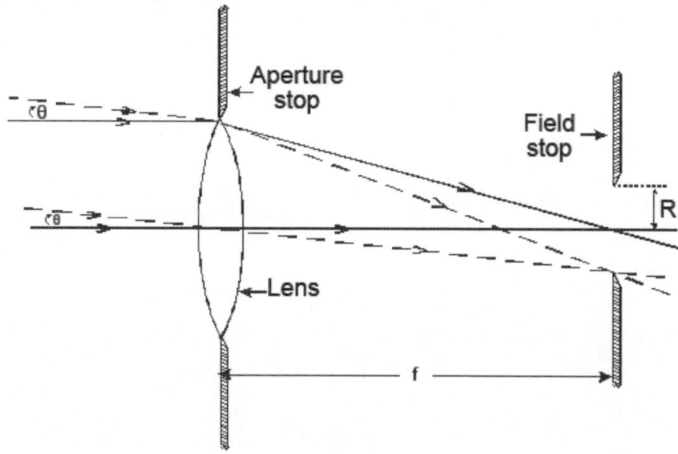


**Figure 5.6.** A radiance meter using an imaging component (photodetector not shown).

radiance of the source can be calculated in the same way as in the Gershun tube radiometer, except that in the case of the lensed radiometer, another factor has to be introduced into equation 5.4 to account for the transmission of the lens. When the distance between the two apertures is equal to the focal length of the lens (i.e., the instrument is imaged at infinity), then the diameter of the second aperture defines the FOV (half angle $\theta$, given by $R/f$, where $R$ is the radius of the second aperture), thus the reason for calling this aperture the "field stop."

Some manufacturers of radiance (luminance) sensors offer viewing aids that are part of, or can be attached to, these instruments so that the operator can view the source being characterized. This is particularly useful when the source has a small physical size. Figure 5.7 shows an example of such a viewing aid available from Bentham Instruments, Reading, UK. It consists of a plane mirror with a hole at its center mounted at an angle to the optical axis. The lens forms an image of the object in the plane of this hole and the part of the image that coincides with the aperture passes through and is relayed onto the photodetector using another lens. The observer sees the image of the object through the eyepiece, with a black spot on it corresponding to the part of the image being measured. This ensures that only radiation from the part of the object that appears "black" is measured. These viewing attachments are available with a number of interchangeable lenses, ranging from a microscope objective that can image objects at a distance of a few millimeters, to lenses that image objects located at infinity. A number of different mirrors (with apertures) are also available. Each mirror has a different aperture diameter so that a range of areas of the object can be selected and analyzed.

Filters can be mounted between the aperture and the photodetector. The addition of a $V(\lambda)$ filter turns this instrument into a luminance meter. In some instruments, a filter wheel is incorporated that allows spectral radiance measurements of the source, integrated over the bandwidth of each filter.

### 5.2.4.3. Imaging Radiometers and Photometers

The field stop and photodetector of a radiance (luminance) sensor can be replaced by a two-dimensional (2-D) detector array (also known as a detector matrix). In this case each pixel, in combination with the lens and the entrance aperture, constitutes a radiance sensor. This means that, with a 2-D

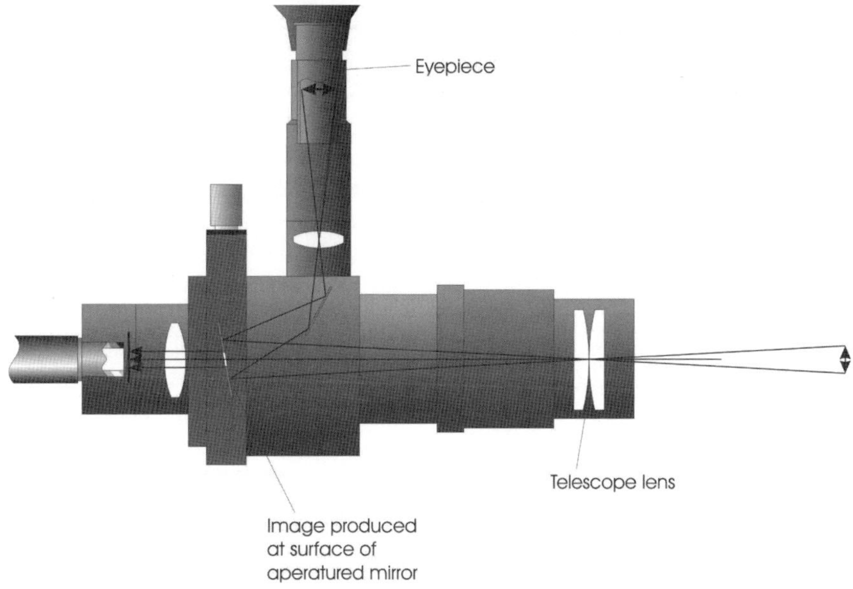


**Figure 5.7.** Schematic of a viewing aid for radiance and luminance meters (courtesy of Bentham Instruments, Reading, UK)

detector array installed, the imaging radiometer provides an image of the object that is a map of the spatial distribution of the radiance (luminance). Since it is difficult to determine the active area of each pixel, the responsivity of an imaging radiometer has to be calibrated. This is done by pointing the radiometer at an extended source whose emission area overfills the FOV of the imaging radiometer and whose radiance (luminance) is known. Imaging radiometers are becoming more widely accepted because of the extra information they can provide. The output of an imaging luminance sensor based on a 512 × 512 pixel detector matrix is equivalent to one-quarter million luminance sensors. Detector arrays have already been adopted for a number of radiometers used for Earth observation (Butcher et al., 1997; Butler, Johnson, & Barnes, 2005). In other applications they are used to provide hyperspectral imaging by giving spatial information in one direction, while the other dimension is used to provide spectral information (Barnsley et al., 2004).

## 5.2.5. SPECTRORADIOMETRIC SENSORS

Spectroradiometers are used in radiometric measurements requiring spectral resolution. These instruments include an entrance aperture that defines an area over which optical radiation is collected. Immediately behind this aperture is a diffuser that provides the spectroradiometer with a cosine response. Radiation enters a wavelength-selecting mechanism that usually takes the form of a grating monochromator (Grum & Becherer, 1979). In this case, the grating monochromator sequentially isolates the radiant power at different wavelengths and this is converted to an electrical signal by the photodetector–amplifier combination mounted after the exit slit of the monochromator. The type of photodetector used is determined by the wavelength of radiation being detected. Grating monochromators are relatively bulky and slow, but they are very well characterized. However, both grating and prism monochromators have low "throughput" or "entendue" (McCluney, 1994) because of the small size of their slits.

The most important photodetector parameter in spectroradiometry is the NEP (Limperis & Mutar 1989; Theocharous & Birch, 2002). The NEP of a photodetector is equal to the radiant power required to illuminate the photodetector in order to generate an output equal to the root-mean-square (rms) electrical noise present at the detector output. The NEP of radiometric sensors defines their ability to measure small optical signals and is discussed further in section 5.3.8. Examination of detector brochures shows that photomultipliers offer the lowest (i.e., best) NEP values in the visible and particularly in the UV spectrum because they offer high internal gain values combined with very low noise (Budde, 1983). However, care should be taken when using photomultipliers because they can exhibit nonlinear responses. Silicon detectors are excellent for detecting wavelengths in the 400 nm to approximately 1 μm range. InGaAs detectors are the obvious choices for wavelengths in the 950 nm to 1.6 μm range, whereas extended InGaAs detectors respond to up to 2.5 μm, but they have relatively small active areas. InSb detectors offer the best performance for wavelengths in the 2.5 μm to 5.3 μm range, and the addition of a cold filter improves their performance in the 1.6 μm to 2.5 μm wavelength region (Theocharous & Birch, 2002). For wavelengths longer than 5.3 μm, HgCdTe detectors are extensively used. However, at these long wavelengths, the advantages of photon (quantum) detectors over thermal detectors are not as pronounced compared to those at the short wavelengths. Indeed, thermal detectors are being used in a significant number of IR radiometric sensors (Theocharous & Birch, 2002). Some near-IR spectroradiometers use PbS detectors to detect radiation with wavelengths in the 1 μm to 2.5 μm region (Corredera et al., 1991). It was recently shown that the response of PbS detectors suffers from serious nonlinearity issues, even for low values of incident spectral irradiance (Theocharous, 2006). This makes the use of this type of detector in most radiometric measurements unacceptable unless nonlinearity correction algorithms are adopted (Sanders, 1972).

Fourier transform (FT) spectrometers offer some advantages when used as spectroradiometers compared to scanning monochromators (Chunnilall, Fox, & Theocharous, 1997). However, FT spectrometers are more complicated instruments and are considerably more expensive. They have been applied to a few IR radiometers, where the long wavelengths make the mechanical tolerance requirements less severe. However, they have had little impact in UV or visible spectroradiometry. Care should be exercised when using FT spectrometers in IR spectroradiometry because the detector simultaneously "sees" the entire output of the source being monitored. It was recently shown that IR detectors such as HgCdTe (CMT) detectors have relatively low thresholds of nonlinear response that can easily be exceeded in spectroradiometric applications involving FT spectrometers (Theocharous et al., 2004).

Some spectroradiometers utilize circular variable filters (Ivanov et al., 2000) or a filter wheel with a number of band-pass filters mounted on it (Biggar, 1998). These filtering methods result in low-cost, compact spectroradiometers. The signal-to-noise ratio (SNR) at the output of these radiometers is high because of the significant throughput of circular variable and band-pass filters. However, the spectral resolution with which the source emission can be characterized is very poor compared to diffraction grating and FT-based spectroradiometers. Very few spectroradiometers are based on prisms because the dispersion of prisms is less than that produced by diffraction gratings. Moreover, the bandwidth of a prism monochromator depends on its wavelength setting (Grum & Becherer, 1979).

## 5.2.5.1. Spectroradiometers Based on Diode Array Spectrometers

A widely adopted development in low-cost, low-performance spectroradiometers is the detector array spectrometer (Stark, 2002). In a conventional scanning monochromator, a single wavelength is sequentially generated and detected by a single detector. In a diode array spectrometer, multiple detectors are used to accomplish the simultaneous measurement of a large number of spectral detection bands. Each pixel in the array acts as an exit slit for a particular wavelength. Figure 5.8 shows the schematic of a spectroradiometer based on a diode array spectrometer for measuring spectral irradiance. The earliest systems were restricted to silicon detector arrays covering the 300 nm to 1000 nm wavelength range. Wavelength range was extended to 1.7 µm with the development of germanium and InGaAs detector arrays. More recently, arrays based on extended InGaAs detectors and also PbS detectors have extended the long wavelength limit to 2.5 µm. Arrays based on InSb and HgCdTe detectors, whose response extends to wavelengths longer than 10 µm, are available, but they are currently prohibitively expensive and require cooling to cryogenic temperatures (Rogalski, 1995).

There are obvious advantages to be gained by using a detector array spectrometer, including speed (all wavelengths are recorded simultaneously), compactness, light weight, and more efficient use of the available photons. However, diode array spectrometers suffer from a number of drawbacks compared to double grating monochromators, the main one being the much higher levels of stray light encountered. In reporting the stray light characteristics of a spectrometer, several qualifying instrument parameters have to be considered (Arthurs, Drummond, & Kremer, 1995). The ability to suppress stray light depends on factors such as the wavelength being observed, the spectrum of the source being analyzed, the quality of the components, and the type of photodetection system used. A single grating monochromator can usually suppress stray light down to 1 part in $10^4$, whereas a double grating monochromator can suppress stray light to less than 1 part in $10^8$. Compare these values with stray light levels encountered in a diode array spectrometer, which are typically 1 part in $10^3$, but can be as high as 1 part in 10 (Zong et al., 2006).

A detector array spectrometer is inherently restricted to a single spectrometer. The higher stray light levels encountered in diode array spectrometers are to be expected. In a diode array spectrometer, the detector array is "immersed" in the spectrometer so that it receives stray light over a full hemisphere ($2\pi$ sr). The stray light depends on radiation scattered from optical components, but in a diode array spectrometer, the radiation reflected by the detector array itself has been found to make a significant contribution to the stray light (Arthurs et al., 1995). This is not an issue with a monochromator-based system because the detector is placed outside the instrument. Furthermore, one of the main attractions of diode array spectrometers is their small size, but this makes it difficult to suppress stray light by, for example, adding baffles. The spectroradiometer arrangement shown in Figure 5.8 is a particularly poor example because radiation exits the integrating sphere over a $2\pi$ solid angle, but only the radiation within the solid angle supported by the grating aperture is utilized (typically in an $F/4$ cone). The remaining radiation contributes to stray light. In some instruments, radiation is guided to the diode array spectrometer using optical fibers. This can benefit stray light, but the use of optical fibers can introduce a host of other problems.

Stray light problems are particularly serious in applications requiring the measurement of low-UV spectral irradiance levels in the presence of high irradiance of longer wavelengths. This is the type of situation encountered in the measurement of the spectral irradiance of a tungsten lamp in the UV spectral region. The problem is made worse by the fact that the detector arrays being used are based on silicon, which has a considerably higher responsivity at long wavelengths compared to UV wavelengths.

Methods have been proposed and demonstrated that quantify the stray light contribution in the output of diode array spectrometers (Brown et al., 2003; Zong et al., 2006). This implies that the stray light contribution in diode array spectrometers can potentially be taken into account. However, measurement of the stray light component in diode array spectrometers is not straightforward because it requires a suite

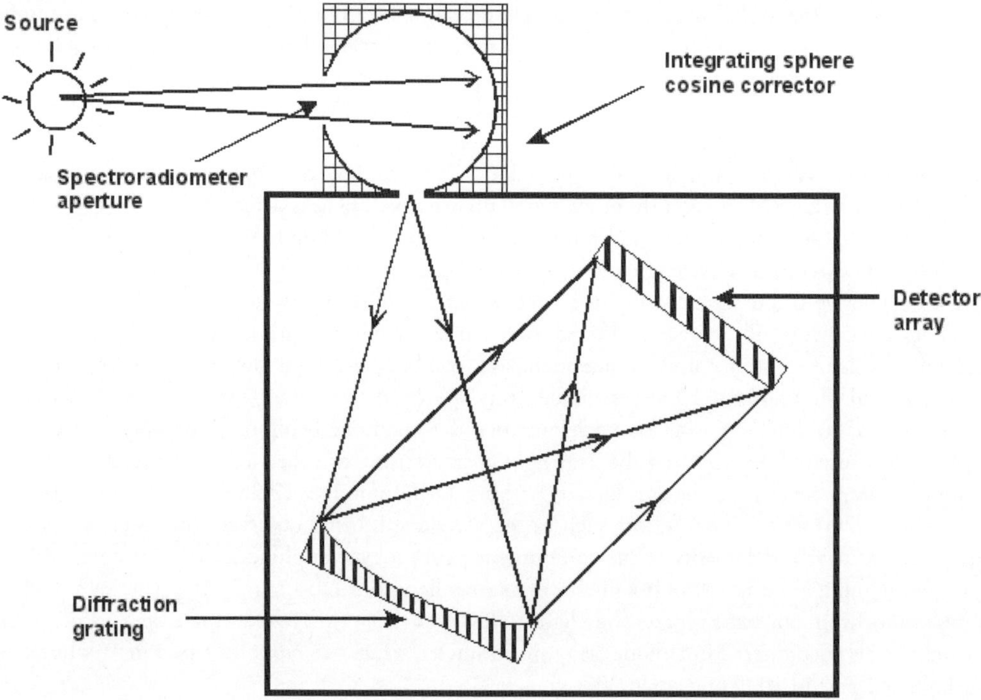


**Figure 5.8.** Schematic of a diode array spectroradiometer with an integrating sphere cosine corrector.

of tunable lasers currently found only in a few National Standards Laboratories. Furthermore, the stray light characteristics are unique to the way a diode array spectrometer is illuminated. If the illumination of the diode array spectrometer changes, then a different stray light correction is required.

## 5.3. PARAMETERS DETERMINING THE PERFORMANCE OF RADIOMETRIC AND PHOTOMETRIC SENSORS

All parameters that determine the performance of a radiometric (photometric) sensor must be fully characterized. This is essential to quantify the magnitude of their effect on the sensor output and allow the uncertainty budget associated with measurements involving that sensor to be prepared. CIE Report No. 53 provides an extensive discussion of all the parameters that can influence the performance of radiometers and photometers (CIE, 1982). The uncertainty contribution due to external influences is determined by changing the magnitude of the external influence and measuring the resulting change in the radiometer responsivity. The most important parameters that determine the performance of radiometric and photometric sensors are summarized in sections 5.3.1 through 5.3.10.

### 5.3.1. RESPONSIVITY

Responsivity is important because it is the parameter that transforms the output of the radiometer (photometer) into the corresponding value of the radiometric (photometric) unit being measured. It is the main parameter measured during calibration of the instrument (CIE, 1984a). However, for comparing the performances of different radiometric and photometric sensors, responsivity is not a particularly useful parameter because it represents the slope of the instrument output versus input plot. This can be made to have almost any value by adding appropriate electrical amplification at the output of the photodetection system incorporated in the sensor. The photodetector also produces electrical noise, and this too is amplified by any subsequent amplification stages. This means that the addition of an extra amplification stage will improve the responsivity of a radiometer significantly, yet it is unlikely to benefit the minimum resolvable change in the radiometric quantity being measured. Thus any claims relating to the responsivity of a radiometer by a manufacturer should be treated with caution.

Sometimes the term *sensitivity* is used to describe the performance of instruments including radiometers and photometers. This is a term that has two possible meanings. It is sometimes used to denote the responsivity of a radiometer, as described previously, but it is also frequently used to denote the ability of the radiometer to detect and resolve small input signals. However, the correct parameter used to describe the ability of a sensor to measure small input signals is the NEP (Theocharous & Birch, 2002). Noise equivalent irradiance (NEI) and noise equivalent radiance (NER) are used to denote the corresponding parameters for irradiance and radiance. In this chapter the term *sensitivity* is avoided to prevent this potential source of confusion.

The characterization of the responsivity of radiometric and photometric sensors should include measurement of the out-of-band response. The UV response of a photometer is generally defined as the ratio of the output when the photometer is illuminated with a specified UV source filtered with a UV-blocking filter divided by the output with the UV-blocking filter removed (CIE, 1982). A similar definition is used to specify the long-wavelength out-of-band response of photometers. Similar definitions are used to quantify the out-of-band response of radiometers. The out-of-band responsivity of filter radiometers can be suppressed to less than 0.001% of the peak response relatively easily using good quality interference filters. Blocking to 1 part in $10^7$ is possible with some effort. Filters should be selected to block radiation well beyond the edge of photodetector response. Silicon detectors are frequently assumed to respond up to 1.1 μm, yet they have measurable responsivities to wavelengths well beyond 1.3 μm.

Care should also be taken when switching the range of radiometric and photometric sensors. The range is usually altered by changing the electrical amplification at the output of the photodetector in steps of 10:1. The relationship between various ranges should be measured by comparing the readings of different ranges when a stable source is used to illuminate the instrument (Goodman, 1989).

### 5.3.2. LINEARITY AND DYNAMIC RANGE

The linearity of a radiometer (photometer) is the property whereby the output of the instrument is directly proportional to the value of the input parameter being measured. If this condition is valid, then the detector responsivity is constant over a range of inputs that must accompany any definition of linearity along with the specified tolerance in nonlinearity. Radiometrists have devised a number of methods for measuring detector nonlinearity, details of which can be found elsewhere (Budde, 1983). They have also devised methods of correcting the nonlinearity of sensors provided the linearity characteristics of an instrument are fully known (Sanders, 1972). The characterization of the nonlinearity of some radiometric and photometric sensors can be harder to determine. While the linearity of radiant power sensors can be measured using techniques identical to those used for photodetectors, the linearity of radiant intensity and luminous intensity sensors can be evaluated using the inverse square law. The linearity of irradiance (illuminance) and radiance (luminance) sensors can be evaluated using calibrated attenuators (Martin et al., 1999), but absolute linearity measurement methods such as the flux superposition method should be utilized whenever possible (Budde, 1983). These methods measure the individual responses of a sensor to two beams of radiation against the response when the two beams are acting together. The use of an integrating sphere provides the best choice for combining the output of two beams to produce a near-Lambertian source. The main drawback of using a sphere is the severe attenuation it introduces (Budde, 1983).

The linearity of radiance and irradiance sensors is sometimes evaluated by illuminating with the output of a blackbody and relying on Planck's law to predict the spectral radiance or irradiance with which the radiometer is illuminated as the blackbody temperature is varied. This method requires the spectral radiance or irradiance responsivity of the radiometer to be accurately known, and is particularly prone to errors due to any out-of-band response of the radiometer.

The dynamic range of a radiometer is defined as the ratio of the highest input signal for which the linearity specification of the radiometer is not exceeded divided by the lowest detectable signal. This is usually taken as the noise equivalent parameter, selected for a unit bandwidth. The dynamic range should not be confused with the measurement range, which is the difference between the maximum and the minimum measurable inputs.

## 5.3.3. TEMPERATURE COEFFICIENT OF RESPONSE

The temperature coefficient of response of a radiometer (photometer) defines the effect of the ambient temperature on the absolute spectral responsivity of the instrument. It is given by the percentage change in the responsivity of the instrument resulting from an increase in the ambient temperature of 1°C. It is calculated by measuring the absolute spectral responsivity of the instrument while it is sequentially maintained at two temperatures around ambient. Note that the temperature coefficient of response of radiometers can be wavelength dependent. Figure 5.9 shows the output of a UV radiometer whose response peaked at 360 nm as its temperature was increased every 20 minutes in steps of 2°C, from 20°C to 30°C. The temperature coefficient of response of this radiometer is estimated to be +0.29% °C$^{-1}$.

In a photometer, the aperture and the silicon photodiode contribute very little to its temperature coefficient of response. The temperature coefficient of response of S1337 silicon photodiodes was reported to be less than 0.01% °C$^{-1}$ between 500 nm and 800 nm (Lei & Fischer, 1993). However, the temperature coefficient of response of photometers is relatively high, primarily due to the $V(\lambda)$ filter, which utilizes colored glasses. The spectral transmission characteristics of colored glasses are known to be strongly dependent on temperature. All good quality photometers have their temperature stabilized by heating the photometer to a few degrees above ambient or by stabilizing the temperature using either a thermoelectric cooler or by placing it inside a temperature-controlled water jacket.

In the IR spectrum, some photodetectors exhibit very high temperature coefficients of response. The temperature coefficient of PbS detectors, which are a very popular choice in radiometers operating in the 1 μm to 3 μm wavelength range, was measured to be around 4% °C$^{-1}$ (Theocharous, 2006). Therefore the temperature stabilization of PbS-based radiometers is paramount.

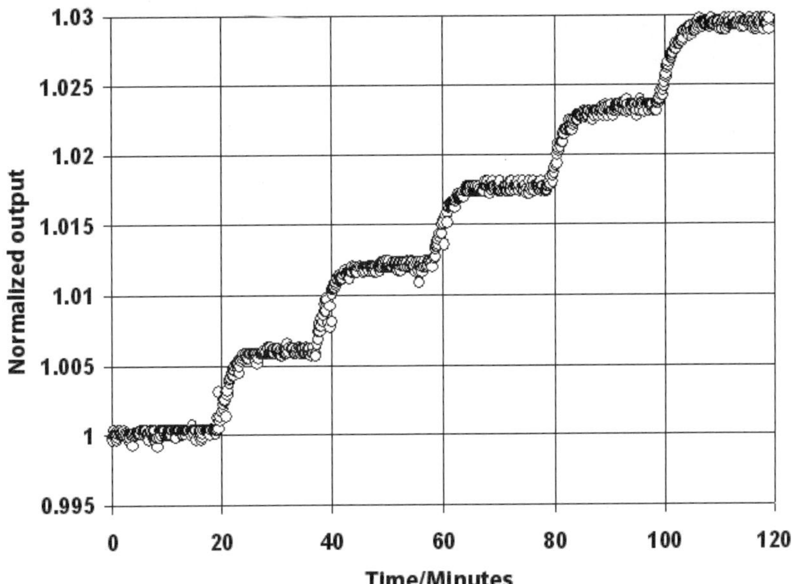

**Figure 5.9.** Normalized output of a UV radiometer as the temperature was increased every 20 minutes in steps of 2°C, from 20°C to 30°C.

## 5.3.4. SPATIAL UNIFORMITY OF RESPONSE

The spatial uniformity of response of radiometric sensors was discussed in association with radiant power meters (see section 5.2.1).

## 5.3.5. ANGULAR RESPONSE

The response of a radiometric or photometric sensor to a ray[10] of optical radiation incident on its active area should be the same irrespective of the angle of incidence. In this case the sensor is said to have an ideal cosine response. The angular response profile of radiometers is measured by mounting them on a turntable so that they are rotated about a vertical axis through their front aperture. The radiometers are illuminated with collimated radiation whose cross section overfills the entrance aperture of the radiometer under test.

Depending on the size of the source being characterized, the FOV of a radiometer (photometer) can be deliberately restricted to reduce clutter.[11] In the case of radiance (luminance) sensors, much effort is directed toward limiting the FOV of the sensors to ensure that only the output of the source being characterized contributes to the sensor response. This is accomplished by placing apertures or baffles at appropriate positions within the radiometer. In this case, radiometers are characterized by

---

10  A ray of light has an infinitely small cross section.

11  Clutter is defined as any optical signal detected by a radiometer that originates from a target other than the one being monitored by the radiometer. Clutter includes optical signals that are generated by the source being monitored but that find their way into the radiometer after being reflected/scattered by other objects in the FOV of the radiometer.

their ability to reject the output from sources that are not in their FOV. For example, a radiometer monitoring the radiance of the surface of the earth from a space platform requires a good out-of-field stray light rejection to ensure that stray radiation from the sun (which has a far higher radiance than the earth) does not contribute to the sensor output.

### 5.3.6. POLARIZATION

The absolute spectral responsivity of radiometers, photometers, and spectroradiometers generally exhibits some dependence on the state of polarization of the radiation being measured. The output of many sources, such as those based on monochromators (Palmer, 2000), some filament lamps (CIE, 1984b; Kostkowski, 1997), as well as skylight, are partially polarized. The dependence of radiometer responsivity on the state of polarization of the incident radiation must be fully characterized. Each component of a radiometer is expected to introduce some degree of polarization (CIE, 1984b), so the polarization contribution from each sensor component should be analyzed separately. This is because it can provide a better understanding of the polarization characteristics of the instrument and can aid in reduction of the polarization effects through improvements in instrument design (CIE, 1984b). Alternatively, at least the linear polarization characteristics of the complete radiometer should be quantified. This is done by measuring the instrument responsivity while the plane of polarization of the incident radiation is rotated (CIE, 1982).

### 5.3.7. TEMPORAL RESPONSE

The response time of a radiometric sensor defines how quickly the output of the sensor can follow a rapidly changing incident signal. Mathematically it specifies how quickly the output of the sensor increases in response to a step change in the incident signal. The temporal response of a radiometer is governed by the type of photodetector used and by any signal integration utilized. Thermal detectors have slower response times, and some radiometric sensors using thermal detectors can have response times in excess of 40 s (WMO, 2006). Photon detectors are inherently faster, offering response times faster than $10^{-9}$ s. However, the temporal response of radiometers is considerably slower than this in order to reduce the instrument electrical bandwidth and thus reduce the noise power at the output of the sensor (Theocharous & Birch, 2002).

### 5.3.8. THE ABILITY OF A RADIOMETRIC SENSOR TO DETECT SMALL SIGNALS

The ability of a sensor to detect small signals depends on the noise power present at the sensor output. This ability is best quantified by the NEP, NEI, and NER. These are equal to the radiant power, irradiance, and radiance, respectively, required to produce an output signal that is equal to the rms noise present at the sensor output. The NEP of a sensor is therefore the radiant power required to illuminate the sensor in order to generate an output signal with an SNR of unity. For "white" noise, the noise power is proportional to the electrical[12] detection bandwidth (Munroe, 1982). All noise equivalent parameters are normalized to a unit bandwidth and the NEP of a radiant power sensor is given in units of watts

---

12  The electrical bandwidth of a radiometer is different from its wavelength bandwidth, as the latter is governed by any wavelength-selective optical component that may be present before the radiation reaches the photodetector.

per root hertz (W Hz$^{-1/2}$). The presence of the frequency units confirms the importance of the detection bandwidth in the detection of small input signals.

### 5.3.9. STABILITY AND AGING

The responsivity of radiometric and photometric sensors changes slowly with time and is known as aging. Aging is accelerated when the sensors are operated outside the specified conditions of operation. Instruments using interference filters sometimes exhibit large sudden changes in their responsivity of up to 1%. These changes are believed to originate from the relaxation of the dielectric constituent layers of the interference filter. The effect of aging is minimized by frequent recalibration of the sensors. Another source of aging was identified in the responsivity of IR radiometers due to the deposition of a thin film of ice on cooled detectors (Theocharous, 2005b), cooled windows (Theocharous, 2005a), and cooled interference filters (Theocharous, Hawkins, & Fox, 2005). These aging effects are reversible because they can be temporarily eliminated by evacuating the detector dewars while they are baked at about 50°C.

### 5.3.10. "BACKGROUND" OR "DARK" MEASUREMENTS AND THE DEFINITION OF RADIOMETRIC ZERO

In taking measurements using radiometric and photometric sensors, it is important to include "background" or "dark" readings. The aim of these measurements is to eliminate the effects of clutter and stray light as well as any biasing due to the photodetector dark signal and the electrical amplification circuitry. Clutter was defined in section 5.3.5. Ideally clutter should be eliminated by removing its source, but where this is not possible, positioning of the optical shutter becomes critical. Note that switching the source "off" is not a good option because it removes radiation that is emitted by the source and would contribute to the radiometer output by being reflected or scattered into the radiometer under test by walls and other objects. It is usually advantageous to introduce a shutter halfway between the source and the radiometer. The aperture of the shutter when open should be just larger than necessary to allow the radiation from the source to enter the defining aperture of the radiometer.

Any body whose temperature is above absolute zero emits IR radiation, so the presence of bodies at ambient temperature in the FOV of an IR radiometer can affect the instrument reading. Measurements should include a "background measurement," that is, with the shutter closed to ensure that contributions from other sources of optical radiation are eliminated. In IR spectroradiometry the radiance of the shutter must be low compared to the radiance being measured, and that may require cooling the shutter to cryogenic temperatures (Theocharous et al., 1998a).

## 5.4. CALIBRATION OF RADIOMETRIC AND PHOTOMETRIC SENSORS

Calibration is defined as the process that establishes (under specified conditions) the relationship between the output of a measuring instrument, such as a radiometer, photometer, or spectroradiometer, and the corresponding known values of a standard. Calibration identifies the unique quantitative relationship between the output of a radiometric sensor and the radiometric parameter that the sensor is aiming to measure. For detailed discussions on recommended procedures for the calibration of sensors designed to measure the various radiometric and photometric parameters, see Boivin (2005) and Fox and Rice (2005).

The definition of a calibration should specify the conditions under which that calibration was performed. It is important to stress what is referred to by the present author as the "golden rule" of radiometry, which states that the calibration of an instrument should be performed under conditions identical to those under which the instrument is going to be operated. This is because there are many parameters that affect the performance of radiometric sensors (e.g., temperature, illumination conditions, etc.). By using the sensor under the same conditions as those under which it was calibrated, the effects of these external influences are minimized.

The preferred method for all radiometric calibrations is direct substitution. This means that a standard, reference photometer exists, so that another photometer can be calibrated against it by alternately allowing the two photometers to view the same source of optical radiation. The main advantage of direct substitution is that the effects of a number of external influences need not be known because they are common to both measurements.

It is important that the calibration of a radiometric sensor be "traceable." Traceability has a very clear definition in metrology. It is defined as the property of the result of a measurement whereby it can be related to stated references, usually national and international standards, through an unbroken chain of comparisons, all having stated uncertainties (Ehrlich & Rasberry, 1997; ISO, 1993). Unfortunately the interpretation of traceability by some instrument manufacturers and users who declare the calibration of their instruments as being traceable to National Standards Laboratories is not always as rigorous as the true definition requires.

Another important outcome of the calibration process is that it provides the combined uncertainty associated with that calibration of the instrument. This uncertainty value, often wrongly referred to as error, is necessary whenever the radiometer is being used, in order to calculate the combined uncertainty of the radiometric measurement being performed. A calibration chain may involve several steps, with each step adding an extra uncertainty contribution. This can result in a much larger final combined uncertainty in the calibration of a radiometer than would be expected from the uncertainty of the base standard. Therefore there is a need to keep the number of calibration steps as few as possible. Currently there is typically a difference of two orders of magnitude between the uncertainty in laboratory radiometric measurements compared with the uncertainty in field measurements.

Lasers are frequently used in the calibration of radiometric and photometric sensors because they offer truly monochromatic radiation of very high spectral radiance (Anderson, Fox, & Nettleton, 1992; Zalewski & Duda, 1983). The output from lasers is spatially and temporally coherent and causes interference effects when passing through windows or filters due to interreflections. This problem can be eliminated by introducing a small wedge angle, typically 0.1°, in these components (Boivin, 1981).

## 5.5. SOME EXAMPLES OF RADIOMETRIC AND PHOTOMETRIC SENSORS

The applications of radiometric and photometric sensors are numerous and varied. However, with the exception of a few areas such as photometric measurements, UVA, UVB, and solar irradiance measurements, as well as some biomedical applications, the market for these instruments is relatively small. This means that there is a vast amount of scientific literature describing custom built radiometric sensors that were developed to address specific requirements. Dedicated radiometers have been developed that are operating in space for Earth observation applications, while others have been developed to act as primary or secondary transfer standard radiometers. While the number of the former type is growing as man's efforts to quantify the effects of global warming increase (Butler et al., 2005), the total number of some radiometers of the latter type (e.g., the number of cryogenic radiometers) is limited to a few dozen, one in each of the major National Standards Laboratories, where they are used as primary radiometric standards.

Some examples of radiometric and photometric sensors were discussed in previous sections. The characteristics of some further examples of such sensors will be summarized in order to indicate the variety of applications in which these sensors are being used. Sections 5.5.1 through 5.5.5 deal with primary and secondary transfer standard radiometers. Photometers are discussed throughout this chapter, but are revisited in section 5.5.6. Section 5.5.7 deals with UV radiometers and the measurement of irradiance in UV phototherapy treatment, while sections 5.5.8 through 5.5.10 deal with solar radiation measurements.

## 5.5.1. THE CRYOGENIC RADIOMETER

The cryogenic radiometer is the most important radiometric sensor developed to date because it is used to link all radiometric measurements to the SI system of units with an uncertainty that is an order of magnitude lower than alternative methods (Fox & Rice, 2005). The cryogenic radiometer was, from a radiometric perspective, initially designed to measure the radiant power of laser beams (Martin, Fox, & Key, 1985), although it has also been used to measure the radiant power of quasi-monochromatic beams exiting from a monochromator (Boivin & Gibb, 1995/1996). The cryogenic radiometer is an electrical substitution radiometer (ESR). An ESR compares the heating effect of optical radiation with that of a substituted amount of electrical heating. ESRs have been known for more than 100 years (Fox & Rice, 2005). However, they operate at ambient temperatures, so uncertainty contributions due to incomplete absorption of the incident radiant power and the nonequivalence of the effects of electrical and radiant heating limit the combined uncertainty to greater than 0.1% (Boivin & Smith, 1978; Willson, 1979). Quinn and Martin (1985) demonstrated that operating an ESR at temperatures below 10 K reduces these uncertainty contributions significantly. At these low temperatures the specific heat capacity of copper decreases significantly, allowing the use of large, highly absorbing cavities instead of flat targets. Radiative losses (which are proportional to the fourth power of the absolute temperature) are minimized and convective losses are eliminated because the cavity is operating in a vacuum. The first cryogenic radiometer dedicated to the measurement of radiant power was assembled at the National Physical Laboratory (NPL; Teddington, UK) and measurement uncertainties of 0.005% were achieved (Martin et al., 1985).

Figure 5.10 shows the layout of the NPL mechanically cooled cryogenic radiometer (Fox et al., 1995/1996). The laser beam enters through a window positioned at Brewster's angle so the uncertainty in the measurement of its transmission is minimized. The beam is absorbed by the radiometer cavity, whose (measured) absorbance is in excess of 99.998%. The increase in the cavity temperature due to the incident beam is measured and is equated to the increase in temperature (with the laser beam interrupted) resulting from the electrical power supplied to the radiometer cavity through a resistive electric heater. In this way the radiant power of the laser beam is equated to electrical standards linked to the SI system of units. The same laser beam is used to illuminate transfer standard detectors so that their absolute radiant power responsivity can be measured and, through a chain of calibrations, every radiometric measurement can be made traceable to the SI system of units. Most major National Standards Laboratories currently operate at least one example of a cryogenic radiometer that provides the primary standard for all radiometric and photometric measurements in their respective countries.

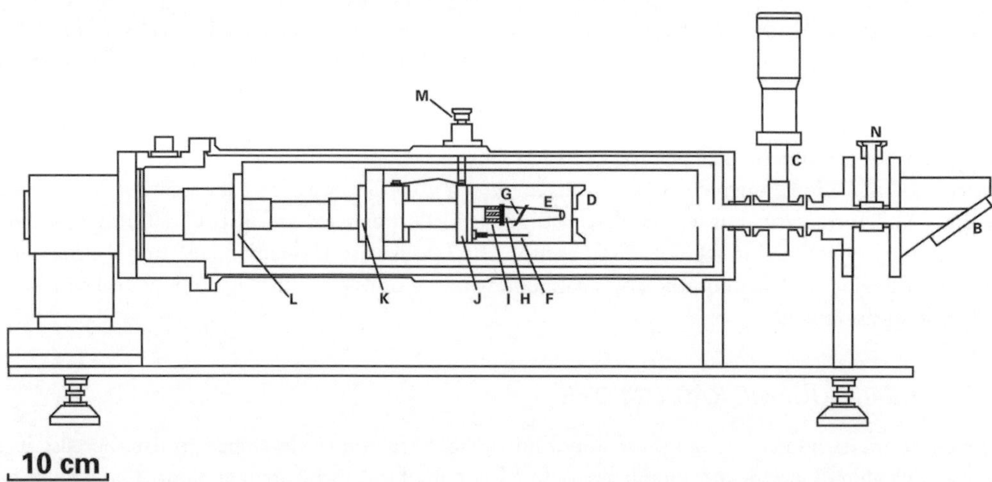



**Figure 5.10.** Schematic of a mechanically cooled cryogenic radiometer. The laser beam enters through the Brewster angle window B. C is the gate valve and D the quadrant detector used for aligning the laser beam into the cavity. E is the radiometer cavity; G the heater; H the PhFe thermometer; I the reference heat link; J the reference temperature heat sink; and K is the second-stage cooler.

## 5.5.2. TRAP DETECTORS

Arguably the second most significant development in radiometry is the silicon "trap" detector as conceived by Zalewski and Duda (1983), and in its more modern form as first described by Fox (1991). Silicon photodiodes offer very high internal quantum efficiencies in the 400 nm to 950 nm wavelength range, but their external quantum efficiency is compromised by a relatively high Fresnel reflection loss. A silicon trap detector takes advantage of the fact that the reflection from the surface of a silicon photodiode is highly specular, so a number of silicon photodiodes are arranged so that the radiation reflected by the first photodiode strikes the second photodiode, and so on, until the reflected component is small. Figure 5.11 shows a schematic of a reflection silicon trap detector consisting of four photodiodes. The silicon photodiodes are positioned so that they are optically in series, but electrically wired in parallel, so that the total generated photocurrent is available from a single output.

It is difficult to isolate and measure the reflected component of a reflection trap detector, so transmission trap detectors were devised in which the residual radiation is transmitted through the trap detector and is available to be detected and measured (Gardner, 1994).

The main advantage of trap detectors is the reduction in the uncertainty associated with the determination of the reflectance of the silicon photodiodes, and thus the reduction in the variation of their external quantum efficiency with wavelength. The predictable spectral responsivity of trap detectors allows the interpolation of their spectral responsivity with low uncertainty. Silicon trap detectors can be calibrated at laser wavelengths against the cryogenic radiometer with a $2\sigma$ uncertainty of 0.02% (Fox, 1991). The main drawback of a trap detector is the limited FOV, which depends on the number and size of the silicon photodiodes it contains. Furthermore, the shunt resistance of a silicon trap is considerably lower than the shunt resistance of a single silicon photodiode. Trap detectors based on

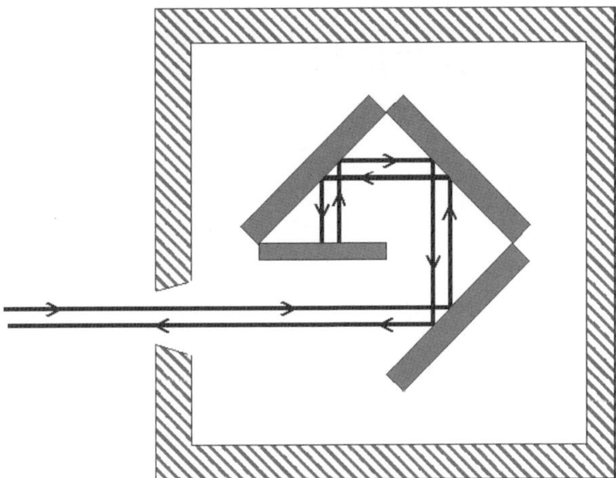

**Figure 5 11.** Schematic of a four-photodiode reflection trap detector.

InGaAs (Fox, 1993) and germanium (Stock, Heine, & Hofer, 2003) have also been reported, but their component photodiodes produce relatively poor performance.

## 5.5.3. THE ABSOLUTELY CALIBRATED IRRADIANCE SENSOR

It was pointed out in the previous section that the radiant power responsivity of a silicon trap detector can be calibrated at laser wavelengths against the cryogenic radiometer with a $2\sigma$ uncertainty of ±0.02% (Fox, 1991). If a small precision circular aperture whose diameter is measured against national length standards is mounted in front of a calibrated trap detector, the trap-aperture combination becomes an irradiance sensor whose absolute irradiance responsivity is known with a $2\sigma$ uncertainty of 0.05% (Fox, Martin, & Nettleton, 1991). This absolutely calibrated irradiance sensor is used extensively by National Standards Laboratories for absolute irradiance calibrations in the 400 nm to 950 nm wavelength range. Note that a trap detector is necessary as the detector in the absolutely calibrated irradiance sensor because the radiation reflected from it is small.[13] If the reflected component is significant, then some radiation is scattered by the aperture back onto the detector, thus introducing significant uncertainty contributions in the absolute calibration of the irradiance sensor.

The calibration of the spectral responsivity of irradiance sensors that do not use diffusers requires that the entrance aperture of the instruments be illuminated with a monochromatic, spatially uniform irradiance distribution. Leading National Standards Laboratories routinely use an integrating sphere source (Anderson et al., 1992) to accomplish this task. The output from a laser is guided to an integrating sphere using a multimode optical fiber. The output port of the integrating sphere is a good Lambertian source and the radiance of the exit port is stabilized to better than 0.1% using a technique demonstrated by Fowler, Lind, and Zalewski (1979). The real image of this port formed by a lens has an irradiance distribution that has excellent spatial uniformity. A length of the multimode fiber used to guide the laser

---

13  A transmission trap detector has no reflected component at all (Gardner, 1994).

output to the sphere is immersed in an ultrasonic bath. The speckle pattern contained within the image of the integrating sphere exit port is modulated at high frequencies due to the action of the ultrasonic bath on the multimode fiber. In this way the speckle noise is eliminated (Anderson et al., 1992).

### 5.5.4. THE FILTER RADIOMETER

Any optical sensor that consists of a photodetector, a precision aperture, and a band-pass filter that defines the spectral responsivity of the unit can be considered a "filter radiometer." For example, a photometer is a filter radiometer with a $V(\lambda)$ spectral response profile. Figure 5.12 shows a schematic of an NPL filter radiometer (Fox et al., 1991). The importance of filter radiometers is that they can be used to characterize the emission of "polychromatic" sources, provided their absolute spectral irradiance responsivity is known. National Standards Laboratories calibrate the absolute spectral irradiance responsivity of a filter radiometer against an irradiance sensor such as a trap detector and calibrated aperture combination, as described in the previous section (Anderson et al., 1992). Calibrated filter radiometers have a number of applications, including the measurement of the thermodynamic temperature of blackbodies (Fox et al., 1991) or the luminous intensity of incandescent lamps (Goodman & Key, 1988) with a less than 0.1% uncertainty (Fox, 1995/1996). The detailed design of filter radiometers varies between different research groups, with some filter radiometers utilizing narrowband interference filters, while others are based on broadband colored glass filters (Harrison et al., 1998). The temperature of the NPL filter radiometers is controlled using a water jacket (see Fig. 5.12), whereas

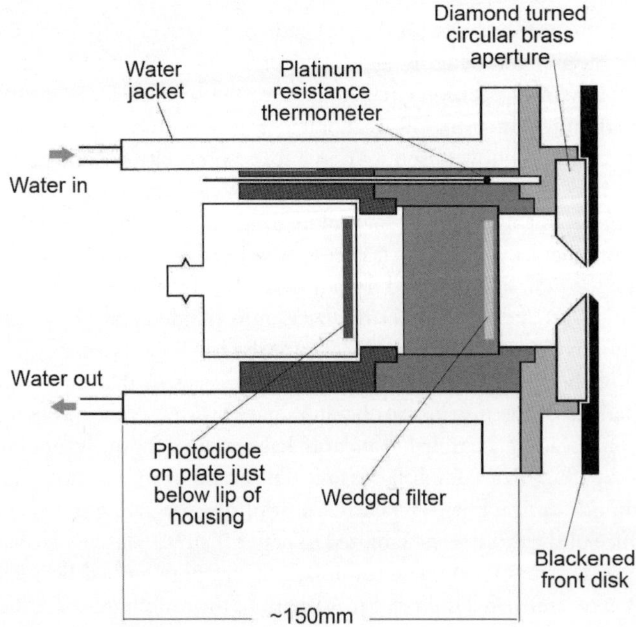


**Figure 5.12.** Schematic of the NPL filter radiometer.

other institutions use thermoelectric-based temperature control (Eppeldauer, Brown, & Lykke, 2005). The problems encountered in filter radiometers are similar to those encountered in photometers, including out-of-band response, particularly for wavelengths longer than the peak response, and aging. The out-of-band response should be measured and accounted for, while the effects of aging can be partly overcome by frequent recalibration.

Figure 5.13 shows the absolute spectral irradiance responsivity of an IR filter radiometer (includes a preamplifier) whose response peaks around 3.7 μm (Theocharous et al., 2005). This radiometer is used in association with a facility called "AMBER" (Theocharous et al., 1998a) to measure the radiance of near-ambient-temperature blackbodies.

## 5.5.5. THE ELECTRICALLY CALIBRATED PYROELECTRIC RADIOMETER

The electrically calibrated pyroelectric radiometer (ECPR) is a form of an ESR developed at the National Bureau of Standards (NBS; now the National Institute of Standards and Technology [NIST]) in the 1970s (Phelan & Cook, 1973). The ECPR is based on a pyroelectric detector that detects the modulated optical radiation incident on its active area. Electrical heating is also supplied to the pyroelectric crystal using the same detector electrodes. The electrical heating is modulated with the same wavefront as the incident optical radiation, but is applied 180° out of phase (see Fig. 5.14). By adjusting the electrical heating so that the pyroelectric detector produces a null reading, the radiant power of the optical beam can be equated to the electrical power dissipated in the detector electrodes. A version of the ECPR has been produced commercially for more than 30 years (Day, 2005). However,

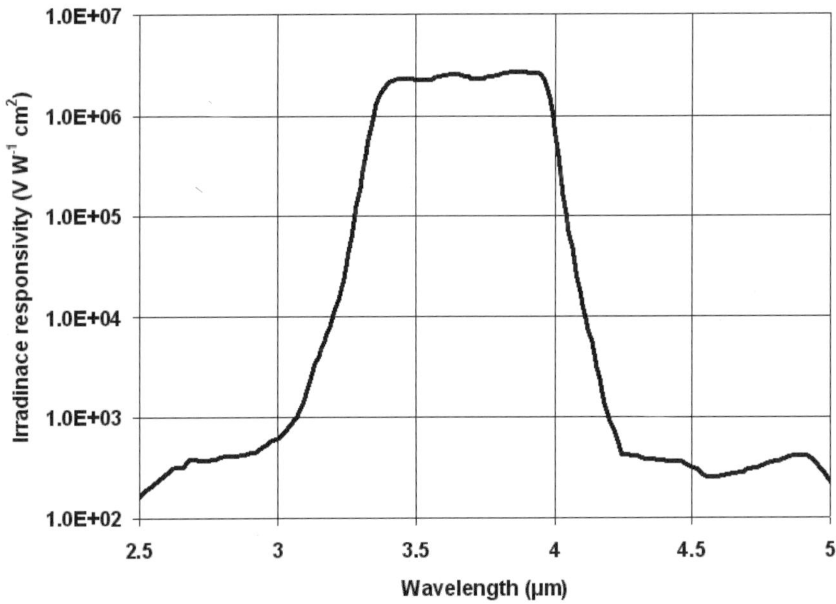


**Figure 5.13.** Spectral irradiance responsivity of the NPL 3.7 μm filter radiometer.

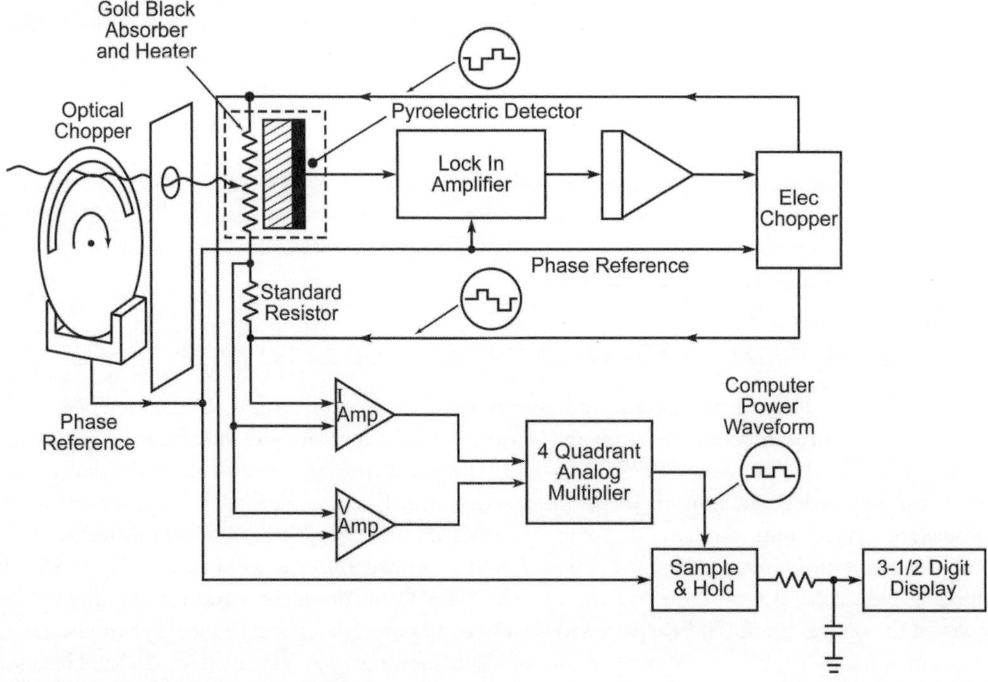


**Figure 5.14.** The ECPR radiometer layout (Day, 2005).

the measurement uncertainty when using an ECPR is much higher than the uncertainty in the measurement of the electrical power. Uncertainty contributions due to the finite reflectance of the black coating, the nonequivalence of the optical and electrical power, spatial uniformity of response of the pyroelectric detector, heating of the electrical leads, and differences in the duty cycles limit the overall uncertainty of such a measurement to about 1%. The cryogenic radiometer, which was described in section 5.5.1, also employs electrical substitution, but by operating at cryogenic temperatures, it is able to eliminate some of the uncertainty contributions that plague ECPRs. The commercially available ECPRs are coated with gold-black coatings that offer excellent absorbance combined with spectral flatness in the IR spectrum (Nelms & Dawson, 2005). ECPRs have been used by industry as well as some National Standards Laboratories as a radiant power standard for many years.

### 5.5.6. PHOTOMETRIC SENSORS

The most important design task in photometric sensors is to re-create the relative spectral responsivity of the human eye as defined by the $V(\lambda)$ function (CIE, 1983). To accomplish this task, two techniques are currently being employed: the use of band-pass filters and the use of spectroradiometers.

#### 5.5.6.1. Broadband Photometers

The first method involves the addition of a specially designed filter of the appropriate transmission so that the relative spectral responsivity of the resulting photometer (including the transmission of all imaging components and the spectral responsivity of the photodetector) matches the $V(\lambda)$ profile. A brief summary on the construction of $V(\lambda)$ filters is given in section 5.5.6.2. Silicon photodiodes are used exclusively in broadband photometers because they combine good NEP values with excellent linearity of response, long-term stability, small size, low voltage power requirements, and low cost. Indeed, certain types of silicon photodiodes have been adopted as the "detector of choice" by all major National Standards Laboratories for the most demanding radiometric and photometric applications (Boivin, 2005). Components in a photometer can be made of glass, in contrast to radiometers, which may require exotic materials such as silica, $CaF_2$, ZnSe, and even reflective imaging optics. Developing a photometer whose relative spectral responsivity exactly matches the $V(\lambda)$ profiles is a difficult task.

The degree with which the relative spectral responsivity of a photometer matches the $V(\lambda)$ function is characterized by the $f_1'$ term, defined in CIE Report No. 69 (CIE, 1987b). Values of $f_1'$ for the best available illuminance and luminance meters are typically a few percent (CIE, 1987b), although some manufacturers claim $f_1'$ values of 1%. Figure 5.15 shows the relative spectral responsivity of a photometer along with the $V(\lambda)$ function (CIE, 1983) and indicates that there are significant differences between the two. The procedure for correcting the spectral mismatch between the spectral responsivity of a photometer and the $V(\lambda)$ function requires knowledge of the "spectral mismatch correction factor." This requires knowledge of the relative spectral emission of the source whose emission characteristics are being evaluated (CIE, 1987b; Ohno, 2005). The spectral responsivity of photometers is usually found to deviate significantly from the $V(\lambda)$ function in the wings, where the contribution of incident radiation to those wavelengths is considerably smaller than near the center.

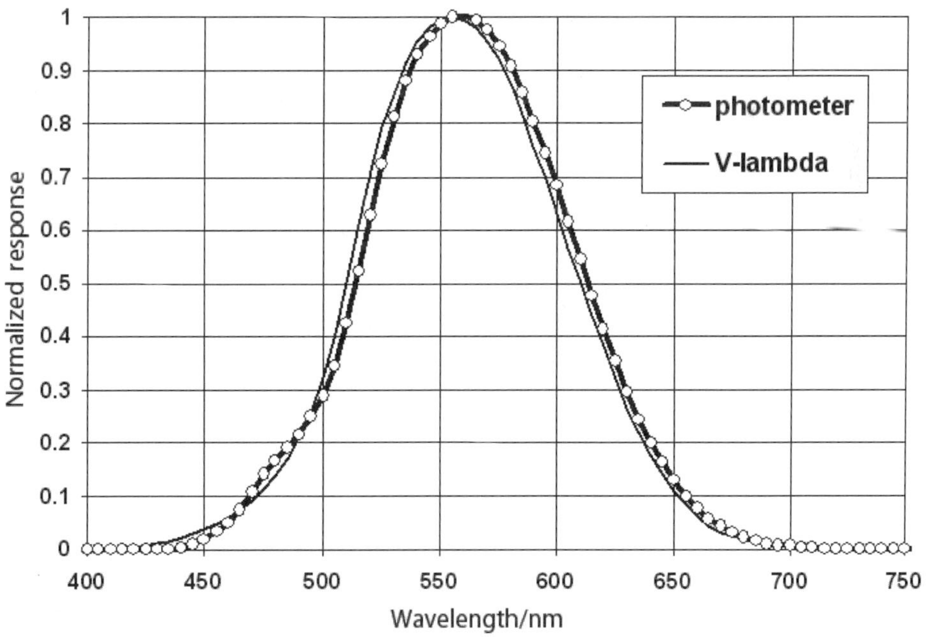



**Figure 5.15.** Relative spectral response of a photometer along with the $V(\lambda)$ function (CIE, 1983).

This is a good design compromise when the photometer is used to measure the output of a source with a broad emission spectrum, such as an incandescent source. However, this design compromise introduces significant errors when it is used to measure the output of narrowband sources such as LEDs emitting near the edges of the $V(\lambda)$ function (CIE, 1997).

An illuminance meter is required to have an angular response profile that matches the ideal cosine response. This is difficult to achieve, and an error $f_2$ is used to quantify the deviation of the angular response of an illuminance sensor from that ideal cosine response (CIE, 1987b). There is an extensive discussion on $f_2$ in the section dealing with UV radiometers used for the measurement of irradiance in phototherapy treatment cabinets (see section 5.5.7.1.2).

The spectral responsivity of silicon photodiodes changes little with temperature in the 380 nm to 780 nm wavelength region (Lei & Fischer, 1993). However, the transmissions of the component colored glass filters used in the assembly of $V(\lambda)$ filters depend greatly on temperature, so the responsivity of photometers exhibits relatively large temperature coefficients of response. For this reason active temperature stabilization is used in all high-performance photometers to ensure that drifts due to ambient temperature fluctuations are minimized. The active temperature control can be a water jacket or a thermoelectric cooler, but it can sometimes take the form of a heater that raises and maintains the temperature of the photometer by about 5°C above ambient.

Most manufacturers of low-cost photometric and radiometric sensors offer products that perform multiple measurement tasks by connecting the appropriate optical head to the control unit. Some instruments can even accept two optical heads simultaneously, which allows measurement of the photometric and radiometric output of a source at the same time.

Illuminance meters are used extensively to prove that illumination conditions conform to recommendations made by various organizations regarding the level of illuminance required for humans to complete various tasks. Requirements for illuminance levels range from 20 lux to 20,000 lux, when viewing objects of small size and low contrast (Kaufman & Christensen, 1989). In order to demonstrate compliance with these recommendations, a number of illuminance meters are commercially available from a number of vendors (McCluney, 1994). Most illuminance meters are compact, handheld instruments consisting of a diffuser that should provide the meter with a near-cosine response, a band-pass filter, a photodetector with some supporting electronics, and a display. The transmission of the filter is selected so that the relative spectral responsivity of the illuminance meter matches the $V(\lambda)$ function.

Luminance meters are arguably the most important photometric sensors simply because they measure luminance, which is the luminous quantity detected by the human eye. Some objects are self-luminous (e.g., television monitors), while others reflect or scatter radiation from other sources. The bulk of commercially available luminance meters are compact, handheld instruments of very basic construction. The optical heads of a number of these low-cost photometers are designed so they can be converted from an illuminance sensor into a luminance sensor simply by replacing the diffuser, used as a cosine corrector during illuminance measurements, with a lens of the appropriate focal length. More expensive luminance sensors rely on more sophisticated designs and often utilize bespoke components. Some are equipped with viewing optics to identify the target whose luminance is being measured (see section 5.2.4.2).

All commercially available photometric sensors, even those costing as little as $200, include a microprocessor to give these instruments improved functionality. The performance of these instruments may appear impressive to a newcomer to the field, but an experienced radiometrist knows that the performance of a radiometer is governed by the analog rather than the digital part of the instrument, and in particular the photodetector, optics (including wavelength selecting components), and in the case of irradiance meters, the quality of the cosine corrector. The performance of an instrument cannot be verified by the resolution of the digital display, or even by its repeatability—that is, its ability to give the same reading when illuminated by the same value of the radiometric parameter being measured.[14] It is accuracy that is important in the output of a radiometer rather than repeatability.[15] Accuracy is defined as the difference in the reading of an instrument and the true value of the parameter being measured. Since the true value is not known, the value measured or provided by National Standards Laboratories is the accepted "true" value, hence the importance of traceable calibrations. Understanding the performance of an instrument also requires the determination of its behavior under different environmental and illumination conditions. It is the author's opinion that a vendor's data cannot be relied upon to identify the best photometer for a particular application. It is generally acknowledged that vendors exaggerate the performance of their products, relying on the inability of the customer to verify their claims. This, unfortunately, applies in varying degrees to most radiometric sensors. Despite their drawbacks, broadband photometers offer relatively simple construction combined with low cost, small size, fast response time, and good SNRs.

## 5.5.6.2. The Construction of V(λ) Filters

The spectral responsivity of a photometric sensor should ideally follow the $V(\lambda)$ profile. Although the spectral response of all photon (as opposed to thermal) detectors varies significantly with wavelength over the visible part of the spectrum, the relative spectral responsivity of a photometer must be modified to follow the $V(\lambda)$ curve by adding optical filters of the appropriate transmission. Although multilayer dielectric (interference) filters with $V(\lambda)$ transmission have been fabricated (Dobrowolski, 1970), colored glass filters are preferred because, by comparison, they exhibit greater robustness and have smoother transmission profiles. Liquid $V(\lambda)$ filters based on solutions of chemicals in distilled water are also being used.

Two methods based on colored glasses have been developed that can provide filters with transmission profiles resembling the $V(\lambda)$ curve. The first method employs a stack of different color glasses, typically four, which are arranged together so that radiation passes through each filter sequentially (Budde, 1983). The thickness of each filter is used to fine-tune the relative spectral response profile of the photometer. The normalized product of the spectral transmittance values of the glass filters multiplied by the spectral responsivity of the detector being used results in a match to the $V(\lambda)$ curve (Wright, Sanders, & Gignac, 1969). The second method for producing $V(\lambda)$ filters involves small-size colored glass filters of different types placed side by side, like a mosaic. The overall transmission of this filter (in combination with the detector spectral responsivity) produces a photometer with a spectral responsivity that follows the $V(\lambda)$ profile. This type of $V(\lambda)$ filter is known as a Dressler or mosaic filter, and has the advantage that the spectral profile of the photometer can be fine-tuned by altering the fraction of the total aperture of the radiometer covered by each type of colored glass (Davies & Wyszecki, 1962). On the other hand, mosaic filters require that the photometer aperture always be illuminated with spatially and spectrally uniform irradiance. This is something that should ideally be the case, but is not always guaranteed in practice.

---

14  The manufacturers of some commercially available radiometers/photometers stress the excellent repeatability of their products in their brochures without any reference to their absolute accuracy.

15  In some applications, particularly in process control applications in industry, instrument repeatability may be sufficient and absolute accuracy may not be required.

Currently only one company produces mosaic $V(\lambda)$ filters, whereas photometric filters based on glass filters placed in series are available from a number of vendors. Because of the limited number of available colored glasses, neither filter design can hope to produce a photometer with a perfect $V(\lambda)$ response profile. The ability of the relative spectral responsivity of photometers to match the $V(\lambda)$ function is variable, with the more expensive photometers generally offering a better spectral match. Mosaic filters offer a better match to the $V(\lambda)$ profile because their structure (area and thickness of each component glass) allows finer tuning. However, they are more expensive and, predictably, their transmission is spatially nonuniform. This is less of a drawback when mosaic filters are used with cosine correctors or diffusers.

### 5.5.6.3. Photometers Based on Spectroradiometry

Spectroradiometers record the complete spectrum of a source from which its photometric parameters can be mathematically derived by multiplying the measurements by the $V(\lambda)$ function and then integrating as described by equation 5.1. A good example that demonstrates the usefulness of spectroradiometers is the measurement of the photometric parameters of sources with narrow emission spectra, such as LEDs. Broadband photometers are aimed at measuring the photometric parameters of broadband sources such as tungsten filament lamps, as discussed in section 5.5.6.1. Serious errors can be expected when the photometric output of an LED is being measured (CIE, 1997) because its emission is near the edges of the $V(\lambda)$ function. This should not present a problem when a spectroradiometer is being used, since the exact $V(\lambda)$ profile is stored in the software and is always available to convert the data into the appropriate photometric quantity using equation 5.1.

Spectroradiometers are relatively complex, bulky, slow, power hungry, and expensive instruments, therefore, in applications where spectral resolution is not required, broadband radiometers are used. The development of diode array spectrometers has eliminated some of these drawbacks, although some new problems have been identified (see section 5.2.5.1).

## 5.5.7. CHARACTERIZATION OF BIOLOGICAL EFFECTS USING RADIOMETRIC SENSORS

The most important parameter in characterizing the effect of optical radiation on a biological system is the "biological effective irradiance." A good example of this is the measurement of illuminance, which quantifies the effectiveness of optical radiation to produce a response when observed by the human eye. Illuminance is measured by a photometer whose relative spectral responsivity matches the response of the human eye. In the same way, the biologically effective irradiance can be measured using a radiometer whose relative spectral responsivity matches the "biological action spectrum" of the biological process being characterized. In the absence of such a radiometer, the measurement can be accomplished by measuring the spectral irradiance at the point of interest using a spectroradiometer. The spectral irradiance so measured can then be numerically combined with the "action spectrum"[16] of the biological process being measured to calculate the biologically effective irradiance, $E_{BE}$, using the very simple relationship in equation 5.5 (Diffey, 1982):

$$E_{BE} = \int_{0}^{\infty} E_{\lambda}(\lambda) \, A(\lambda) \, d\lambda, \qquad (5.5)$$

---

16  The action spectrum is defined as the effectiveness of radiation of different wavelengths to produce the biological effect being studied.

where $E_\lambda(\lambda)$ is the measured spectral irradiance due to a source at point $P$ and $A(\lambda)$ is the relative action spectrum. Note that if $A(\lambda)$ is substituted with the relative effectiveness of radiation detected by the human eye, $V(\lambda)$, then equation 5.5 can be used to calculate the illuminance at point $P$.

### 5.5.7.1. UV Radiometers for Phototherapy Treatment

Ultraviolet radiometers form the second most important subsection of radiometric sensors after photometric sensors. UV radiation is used in the treatment of a number of skin diseases. PUVA is a form of such treatment in which photoactive psoralens drugs are combined with UV radiation to treat a skin disease called psoriasis (Newing, Bullen, Davies, & Powell, 1986). The treatment includes irradiation of the patient with UV radiation in special irradiation cabinets (Green, Diffey, & Hawk, 1992). The UV exposure received by patients during such treatments must be carefully controlled in order to ensure that the benefits of the UV photochemotherapy treatment outweigh the potentially harmful effects caused by UV radiation, such as skin cancer (Currie et al., 2001; Martin & Pye, 2000). UV radiometers must be able to accurately measure the irradiance inside different phototherapy cabinets so that the potentially harmful side effects are minimized and measurements from different hospitals can be compared and reconciled. However, problems with the measurement of UV irradiance inside phototherapy cabinets were identified some time ago, when Diffey (1978) reported apparent variations in the dose required to clear psoriasis between different treatment centers, ranging from 12 J cm$^{-2}$ to 200 J cm$^{-2}$. For years, individual hospitals relied on radiometers with good stability (rather than good measurement accuracy) to offer treatment based on reproducible UV dosimetry. This ensured that the conditions inside the phototherapy cabinets were carefully controlled, even though the absolute value of irradiance inside the cabinets was not known (Newing et al., 1986). The measured differences in the doses for the treatment of psoriasis were caused by the calibration of the UV radiometers used to measure the irradiance inside the phototherapy cabinets. The different spectral response profiles of the radiometers being used were identified as one reason for the discrepancies. Deviations between the angular response profile of UV radiometers and the ideal cosine response were identified as another reason for the discrepancies (Coleman, Collins, & Sanders, 2000; Newing et al., 1986).

### 5.5.7.1.1. Spectral Responsivity Issues of UV Radiometers

The spectral response profile of UV radiometers used in phototherapy treatment must follow the action spectrum of the biological process they are designed to measure. In the case of a UVB radiometer, the sensor must have a spectral responsivity that is constant in the 280 nm to 315 nm wavelength range and zero response outside this region. No such sensor is known to exist; UV radiometers fail to meet both conditions to various degrees. The spectral responsivity of UV radiometers varies over the wavelength range over which they are designed to respond. The radiometers also exhibit some response where they should have no response—the long-wavelength out-of-band response of UV radiometers based on silicon detectors was identified as a serious issue. Figure 5.16 shows the spectral irradiance responsivity of two broadband UV radiometers used to determine the exposure of photoresist in semiconductor lithography (Larason & Cromer, 2001). Both radiometers have low but not insignificant spectral responsivity throughout the 450 nm to 680 nm wavelength range. More importantly, one of these radiometers (meter A) shows considerable out-of-band response for wavelengths in the 700 nm to 1000 nm region. This is due to some transmission by the glass filter used to define its spectral response profile, combined with the higher responsivity of the silicon photodiode at longer wavelengths (Larason & Cromer, 2001).

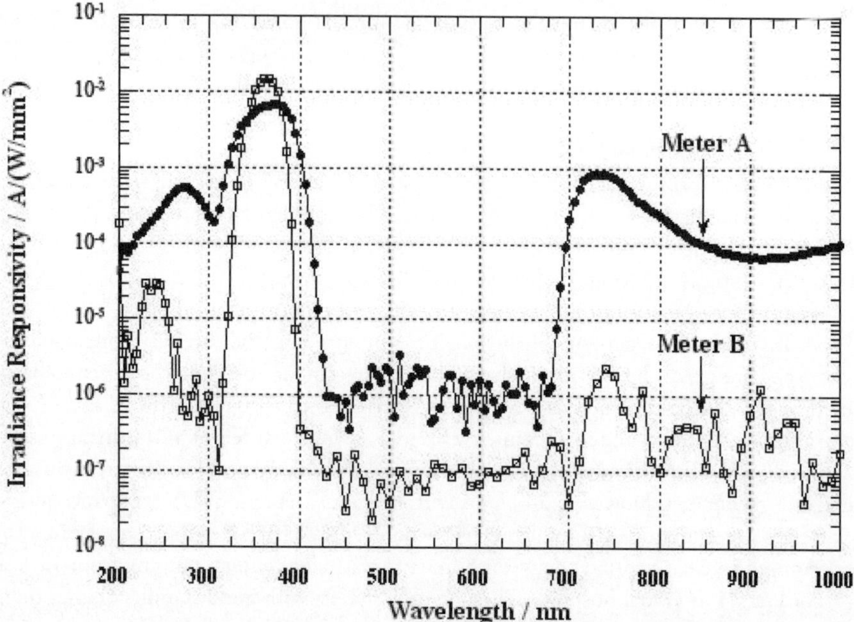



**Figure 5.16.** Spectral irradiance responsivity of two UV radiometers. Meter A suffers from significant out-of-band response (Larason & Cromer, 2001).

The presence of out-of-band responses in UV radiometers means that their output depends not only on the spectral power distribution of the source in the wavelength range of interest (315 nm to 400 nm for a UVA radiometer), but also the spectral power distribution outside this wavelength range (Diffey, 1982). If meter A, whose response is shown in Figure 5.16, is considered to be a UVA radiometer, then the out-of-band response will contribute 3.5 times more to the output of this meter when monitoring the irradiance of an FEL lamp[17] than the in-band response (Larason & Cromer, 2001). The in-band response is the product of the spectral distribution of the source and the meter responsivity integrated over the 315 nm to 400 nm wavelength range. The out-of-band response is the corresponding product integrated over all wavelengths outside the 315 nm to 400 nm range. The out-of-band contribution when the same radiometer (meter A, Fig. 5.16) measures the UVA irradiance from a deuterium lamp[18] will be only 35% of the in-band contribution. This is mainly due to the responsivity of meter A at wavelengths lower than 300 nm. The increased responsivity for wavelengths shorter than 300 nm was shown to be caused by fluorescence of the diffuser used in this radiometer (Larason & Cromer, 2001). This example demonstrates the importance of the emission spectrum of the source being measured by a radiometer with a nonideal spectral response profile.

---

17  FEL lamps are tungsten halogen lamps with double-coiled tungsten filaments. These lamps are used extensively as spectral irradiance transfer standards.

18  Deuterium lamps are discharge lamps that emit a continuous spectrum in the UV wavelengths. These lamps are used extensively as spectral irradiance transfer standards in the 200 nm to 370 nm wavelength range.

### 5.5.7.1.2. Angular Profile Issues in UV Radiometers

The angular response profile of UV radiometers should match the ideal cosine response (Coleman et al., 2000). The angular response profiles of a number of commercially available UV radiometers have been measured by mounting them on a turntable so that they can be rotated about a vertical axis through their front aperture. The radiometers are illuminated by the quasi-collimated output of a UV source (Diffey & Challoner, 1978; Mountford & Davies, 1987). The angular response profile of these radiometers was shown to differ significantly from the ideal cosine response in all cases. When these data were incorporated into mathematical models, it was predicted that the readings of these radiometers could be up to 50% in error when they were used to measure the irradiance from extended sources such as those encountered in phototherapy treatment cabinets (Martin & Pye, 2000; Pye & Martin, 2000).

A radiometer whose angular response profile differs from the ideal cosine response can still be used to measure sources having the same geometrical extent as the source standard against which the radiometer was calibrated (Gibson & Diffey, 1989). However, the UV standard sources calibrated by National Standards Laboratories such as NPL are either deuterium or tungsten lamps, which are effectively point sources when compared to the sources used in phototherapy treatment cabinets (Martin & Pye, 2000). This, in combination with the deviation of the angular response of these radiometers from the ideal cosine response, could account for the magnitude of the errors observed when the radiometers are monitoring the irradiance inside the cabinets (Martin & Pye, 2000). A figure of merit, $f_2$, exists that quantifies the deviation of the angular response of irradiance meters from the ideal cosine response (CIE, 1987b; Pye & Martin, 2000). Measurements showed that the responses of most UV radiometers examined were lower than the true cosine response for angles of incidence as small as 20° and the difference increased progressively with increasing angles of incidence (Martin & Pye, 2000). This meant that the contribution of radiation at large angles of incidence would be underestimated. Numerical modeling showed that radiometers with $f_2$ values of 20% are expected to measure the irradiance inside phototherapy cabinets by up to 50% less than the actual value (Martin & Pye, 2000). These findings have serious implications in phototherapy treatment and currently prevent the comparison of treatment regimes at different hospitals. They also prevent the measurement of cumulative UV doses for individual patients, as well as proper assessment of the risks of photochemotherapy treatments.

Unfortunately, manufacturers of UV radiometric sensors exaggerate the measuring capabilities of their products. This results in the common belief that radiometers able to measure UVA, UVB, and UVC radiation are widely available (Gibson & Diffey, 1989). Furthermore, the cosine response characteristics of UV radiometric sensors are often reported as a polar plot of the instrument response at different angles of incidence versus angle of incidence (and this is also true for photometric sensors). The corresponding plot for a sensor with an ideal cosine response is a circle. However, it is difficult to assess from this type of plot the deviation of an instrument response from the ideal cosine response (Gibson & Diffey, 1989). A plot of the percentage deviation of the instrument response from the ideal cosine response at different angles would be much more informative and revealing.

Ultraviolet radiometers with $f_2$ values down to 5% are highly desirable. This is because the angular response profile uncertainty contribution will not be the major component in the measurement accuracy of irradiance in phototherapy treatment cabinets (Pye & Martin, 2000). In theory, different types of diffusers, whether they are integrating spheres, quartz, sapphire, or PTFE plates, should be able to provide an adequate cosine response. In practice, however, diffusers exhibit significant variations from the true cosine response (Martin et al., 1999; Stobbart & Diffey, 1980), and this can only be attributed to inadequate design. In one study (Pye & Martin, 2000), the angular response profile of twenty-four UVB and UVC radiometers, each with a different cosine corrector, was evaluated using monochromatic radiation. The results of this study showed that the "raised PTFE" diffuser exhibited the smallest variation of its angular response with wavelength, while "ground quartz" diffusers exhibited the largest (Pye & Martin, 2000). However, ground quartz diffusers are more robust compared with PTFE diffusers. An alternative design combining a PTFE disc with a ground quartz diffuser was used and was shown to have $f_2$ values down to 10%, while ensuring a robust diffuser (Pye & Martin, 2000).

Although no integrating sphere diffusers have been used in combination with broadband UV radiometers, they have been evaluated with spectroradiometers. Surprisingly the angular response characteristics of these spectroradiometers were relatively poor. This was attributed to the design of the input optics, which, in spectroradiometers, requires a higher throughput to ensure an adequately high signal-to-noise output ratio (Martin et al., 1999). Another problem identified with integrating sphere diffusers is the distance between the entrance aperture of the sphere (which is also the entrance aperture of the irradiance sensor) and the actual sphere volume, that is, the sphere wall thickness. This thickness determines how closely the angular response profile follows the true cosine response at very large angles (Martin et al., 1999). A large sphere wall thickness, often encountered in Spectralon-based spheres, results in the contribution of radiation at very high angles of incidence being underestimated. Another factor causing the angular response profile of integrating spheres to deviate from the true cosine response is the presence of baffles. Baffles are used inside integrating spheres to prevent radiation from being detected after a single reflection off the sphere walls. The presence of baffles causes the contribution at certain angles to be underestimated (Martin et al., 1999). The main disadvantage of using integrating spheres as cosine correctors is their very low transmission efficiencies, that is, the ratio of the radiant power reaching the photodetector to the radiant power entering the sphere, which can be as low as 0.01% (Budde, 1983).

## 5.5.8. SOLAR RADIOMETERS

### 5.5.8.1. Solar UVB Monitoring and the Robertson–Berger Radiometer

Some components of solar radiation that are transmitted by Earth's atmosphere are harmful to human health. The requirement to quantify the amount of this radiation reaching Earth's surface has resulted in a variety of commercially available UV radiometers claiming to measure the UVA, UVB, and UVC components with impressively low uncertainties.

The discovery of the depletion of stratospheric ozone over Antarctica in the 1980s (Farman, Gardner, & Shanklin, 1985) highlighted the necessity for ground-based solar UV monitoring. Measurements of solar UVB radiation can reveal variations in stratospheric ozone, but they require the availability of stable, well-characterized radiometers (Leszczynski, 2002). Three different types of instruments are currently being used for these measurements: spectroradiometers, multichannel radiometers, and erythemally weighted broadband radiometers whose spectral response resembles that of the erythemal effective spectrum. Comparisons between spectroradiometer-based instruments show large discrepancies between their readings (Early et al., 1998). These discrepancies were attributed to nonideal cosine response, errors in wavelength calibrations, variations in bandwidth, and ambient temperature fluctuations. Errors in early measurements using broadband UV radiometers were very serious. The failure to identify stratospheric ozone depletion over Antarctica can be partly attributed to the unreliability of the measurements using these radiometers (Leszczynski, 2002).

The most widely deployed broadband radiometer for measuring solar UV radiation is based on an instrument originally developed by Robertson (1972). The design was improved by Berger (1976), and Robertson–Berger (R–B) radiometers are now used extensively, including within a global network measuring doses of sun-burning UV radiation (Diffey, 1991). A number of variations of the R–B radiometer are now commercially available. Figure 5.17 shows a schematic of the optical layout of the basic unit.

Solar radiation strikes the top of the UV-transmitting glass dome that provides environmental protection while its dome shape aids the cosine response characteristics of the instrument. Radiation is then spectrally filtered by a UV band-pass filter before it strikes the magnesium tungstate phosphor ($MgWO_4$) on the lower surface of the filter. The $MgWO_4$ phosphor absorbs the UV radiation transmitted by the UV band-pass filter and fluoresces in the green part of the spectrum. The green fluorescence is then isolated using a green band-pass filter and this filtered radiation is converted into an electrical signal using a photodetector. Older versions of R–B radiometers used a vacuum photodiode, whereas newer versions employ a GaAsP photodiode (Dichter, Beaubien, & Beaubien, 1993). The latter has its peak spectral response near the green part of the spectrum, but no response in the red part, thus aiding the suppression of solar radiation of wavelengths longer than the green that leaks through the filters.

The spectral and angular profiles of R–B radiometers differ significantly from the ideal. The spectral responsivity of a number of these sensors overestimate the UVB component of response and underestimate the response for the UVA range. The integrated response of the same radiometers over a ±70° range of angles differs from –20% to +30% from that of a radiometer with an ideal cosine response (Leszczynski, 2002).

Robertson–Berger radiometers have to operate outside the laboratory and must therefore be characterized in terms of the validity of their calibration under different ambient temperatures and humidity levels. In the early 1990s, problems due to a high temperature coefficient of response and poor angular and spectral characteristics were reported in R–B-type UV radiometers (Johnsen & Moan, 1991). Also, the temperature coefficient of response was shown to be wavelength dependent.

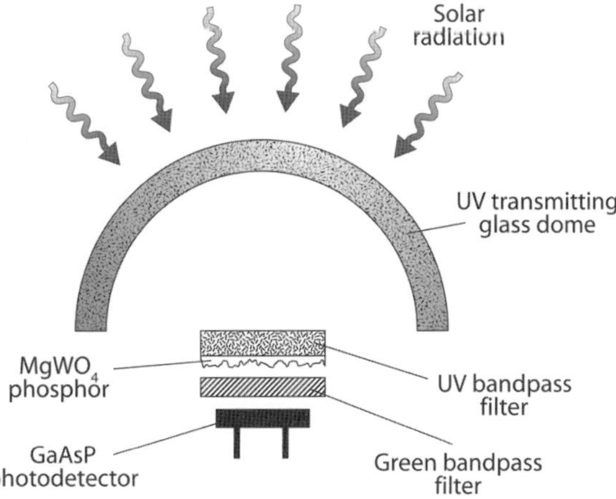


**Figure 5.17.** Schematic of the optical layout of a basic Robertson–Berger radiometer.

For a wavelength of 254 nm, the temperature coefficient of response was –0.68% °C$^{-1}$, while the corresponding values at 302 nm and 315 nm were +0.43 °C$^{-1}$ and +1.46% °C$^{-1}$, respectively. These values suggest that the spectral response profile of this radiometer was shifting to longer wavelengths with increasing temperature. This is in agreement with observations showing that the efficiency of the phosphor used by these radiometers decreases by approximately 0.5% °C$^{-1}$ and that its absorption is temperature dependent (WMO, 2006). Newer versions of the R–B radiometer have been introduced that have their internal temperature actively controlled, and their operating range is specified typically in the –40°C to +50°C range. However, variations in ambient temperature were still shown to have a significant effect on the output of new versions of these radiometers, despite their internal temperature stabilization. An increase of 20°C in the ambient temperature resulted in a reduction in the spectral responsivity of these radiometers by as much as 10% in the UVB range and by as much as a factor of 2 in the UVA range (Huber et al., 2002). The exact changes depended on the individual instrument and the relative humidity inside its housing (Huber et al., 2002). Some of the problems associated with the phosphor have been overcome with the development of UVB radiometers that do not use a phosphor, but include an interference filter to define their spectral responsivity (WMO, 2006).

## 5.5.9. MEASUREMENT OF SOLAR RADIATION ON EARTH'S SURFACE

One of the most important applications of radiometers is in the measuring of solar radiation incident on Earth and that reflected or scattered by the surface of the earth and by the clouds back to space. The difference between these measurements should equal the thermal radiation emitted by the earth into space based on its finite absolute temperature. If this equality does not hold, then changes can be expected in Earth's climate. The importance of this application has resulted in the development of a number of radiometers to perform these measurements, some of which are land-based and are commercially available, while others are unique and are viewing Earth from space.

The accepted value of the solar irradiance at the mean Earth–sun distance is approximately 1368 W m$^{-2}$ (although there is significant debate about the exact value). On the surface of the earth, the solar irradiance is lower due to the attenuation the radiation experiences in propagating through the atmosphere. Moreover, whereas outside the atmosphere the solar irradiance is simply a measure of its direct component (there is no diffuse component), on Earth's surface the measurement is considerably more difficult. This is because the radiometer is required to have a cosine response in order to measure the contribution of the diffuse component from radiation scattered by the clouds.

The sun can be approximated to a blackbody operating at a temperature of 5600 K. Approximately 97% of this radiation is confined in the 290 nm to 3 μm wavelength range. Assuming that the earth is at a temperature of 300 K, then 99.99% of the thermal radiation emitted by the earth is in wavelengths longer than 3 μm. It is clear that the spectrum of the solar radiation reaching Earth and the thermal radiation emitted by the earth do not overlap, so they can be treated separately (WMO, 2006). Currently considerable efforts are being made to measure Earth's incoming and outgoing radiation in order to determine the difference to within a few watts per square meter (Stoffel et al., 2000).

Three basic instruments are currently used to characterize the solar irradiance reaching Earth's surface. The pyranometer measures the global solar irradiance, that is, the combination of direct radiation coming from the sun as well as diffuse radiation that has been scattered while traversing Earth's atmosphere. Pyranometers measure the radiation incident on a horizontal surface from a 2π solid angle in the 300 nm to 3 μm wavelength range. Their spectral response is limited to this range by the glass domes they use. Some pyranometers use a "shading" disk to block the direct component of solar radiation and are therefore able to measure the diffuse component only. A tracking system is required to move the disk so that it always blocks direct solar radiation from reaching the instrument.

The use of thermopile detectors means that pyranometers have a very slow response time, as long as 60 s (WMO, 2006) in some cases. They also have a relatively poor NEI. Manufacturers of pyranometers based on thermopiles quote an instrument resolution of 1 W m$^{-2}$. This does not present a significant problem when measuring global solar irradiance because its value can be greater than 1000 W m$^2$, depending on weather conditions.

The pyrheliometer is another type of radiometer that measures direct solar irradiance in the 300 nm and 3 µm wavelength range. Pyrheliometers have collimator tubes that limit the angular acceptance of solar radiation to about 5° (full angle), compared to a 0.5° angle subtended by the solar disk. A pyrheliometer has to be mounted on a tracker that maintains the optical axis of the instrument in the direction of the sun during the day. The relative uncertainty of measurements using a thermopile-based pyrheliometer has been estimated to be 2%, with the dominant contribution coming from changes in the thermal environment of the instrument (Stoffel et al., 2000). Full details on the performance of pyrheliometers can be found elsewhere (WMO, 2006).

Pyrradiometers measure the total radiation in the 300 nm to 100 µm wavelength range. They are based on thermal detectors, which must have a flat spectral responsivity in this range. Because of the very wide wavelength range, total radiation is measured by splitting the range into two regions: the 0.3 µm to 3 µm region, which is covered by pyranometers, and the 3 µm to 100 µm region, which is measured using another type of radiometer called a pyrgeometer. The pyrgeometer uses a silicon dome that has an interference filter deposited on its inside surface to block radiation below 3 µm.

The glass and silicon domes used by these instruments provide some environmental protection to their thermopile detectors. When these instruments are used outdoors, they are exposed to strong sunlight, resulting in significant temperature increases. Thermopiles have relatively large temperature coefficients of response. In order to overcome problems due to ambient temperature fluctuations, pyranometers employ two thermopile sensing elements, one painted with a highly absorbing paint and a second painted with a reflective paint. By measuring the difference between the temperatures of the two elements, the dependence of the output of the pyranometer on ambient conditions can be minimized (Beaubien, Bisberg, & Beaubien, 1997). Pyranometers also have active temperature stabilization in order to minimize the effect of ambient temperature fluctuations. However, it appears that the incoming radiation raises the temperature of the thermopile element and disturbs the thermal balance within the instrument by introducing temperature gradients. These result in variable-offset systematic errors whose magnitude, in the case of a modified Eppley precision pyranometer, have been shown to be proportional to the difference between the fourth power of the radiometer dome and the thermopile detector temperatures, in accordance with the Stephan–Boltzmann radiation law (Bush et al., 1999).

Pyranometers using nonthermal detectors are also available. However, they respond only to fairly narrow wavelength ranges because of the narrow wavelength ranges of the photodetectors. A pyranometer based on a silicon detector will only respond to radiation in the 300 nm to 1 µm wavelength range. Furthermore, the spectral responsivity of nonthermal detectors, such as silicon detectors, is a strong function of wavelength. Therefore measurement of the total irradiance from the output of a pyranometer with a silicon detector requires knowledge of the absolute spectral responsivity of the radiometer as well as the relative spectral irradiance of the radiation being measured. The main advantages of silicon-based pyranometers are their fast temporal responses (faster than 1 ms), lower cost, and lower NEI because of the superior noise characteristics of silicon detectors.

### 5.5.10. MEASUREMENT OF TOTAL SOLAR IRRADIANCE FROM SPACE

Total solar irradiance (TSI) is defined as the irradiance from the sun, integrated over all wavelengths, reaching Earth at the mean Earth–sun distance. It is impossible to measure TSI on the surface of the earth because of absorption by Earth's atmosphere, so measurements of TSI have to be performed in space. A series of radiometers on different space platforms have been monitoring the TSI from space since 1978 (Butler et al., 2005). Electrical substitution radiometry is the preferred method used by these radiometers.

Measurements of TSI indicate that the output of the different radiometers is precise because they all appear capable of reproducing the 11-year-cycle fluctuations present in the TSI. However, absolute measurements from different instruments differ by much more than the reported measurement uncertainties. The spread of these measurements, coupled with gaps in measurements where no data are available, means that no conclusions can be unambiguously drawn from these data on the long-term behavior of TSI.

The discrepancies between measurements made by different instruments may be due to differences or errors in the prelaunch calibration of these instruments, or to degradation of the instruments while in orbit (Wehrli, Frohlich, & Romero, 1995/1996). Some instruments have more than two cavities that are exposed to solar radiation for different durations in order to quantify solar degradation. Both the prelaunch calibration and the degradation while in orbit are being addressed in some current instruments, but the aim of 0.01% uncertainty in the measurement of TSI is ambitious. Indeed, this value is very close to the uncertainty of the best radiometric measurements carried out using cryogenic radiometry (Martin et al., 1985). The use of cryogenic radiometers in space for the measurement of TSI has been proposed, but funding for such a project has not yet been secured (Martin & Fox, 1993). This concept continues to be developed for the future (Fox et al., 2003).

## ACKNOWLEDGMENTS

The author wishes to thank Julie Taylor, Nigel Fox, Teresa Goodman, and Gina Theocharous for reading the manuscript and suggesting improvements. He also wishes to thank Helen Kearney for the preparation of some of the figures.

## DISCLAIMER

The identification of certain commercial equipment does not imply recommendation or endorsement by NPL nor does it imply that the equipment identified is the best available for the purpose.

## REFERENCES

Anderson, V. E., Fox, N. P., & Nettleton, D. H. (1992). Highly stable, monochromatic and tuneable optical radiation source and its application to high accuracy radiometry. *Applied Optics, 31*(4), 536–545.

Arthurs, E. G., Drummond, I., & Kremer, A. (1995). Stray light performance of UV multichannel spectral measuring instruments. In: C. Burgess & D. G. Jones (Eds.), *Spectrophotometry, luminescence and colour: Science and compliance.* Amsterdam, Netherlands: Elsevier, 399–413.

Barnsley, M. J., Settle, J. J., Cutter, M. A., Lobb, D. R., & Teston, F. (2004). The PROBA/CHRIS mission: A low-cost smallsat for hyperspectral multiangle observations of the earth surface and atmosphere. *IEEE Transactions on Geoscience and Remote Sensing, 42,* 1512–1520.

Beaubien, D. J., Bisberg, A., & Beaubien, A. F. (1997). Investigations in pyranometer design. *Journal of Atmospheric and Oceanic Technology, 15*(3), 677–686.

Berger, D. S. (1976). The sunburning ultraviolet meter: Design and performance. *Photochemistry and Photobiology, 24*(6), 587–593.

Biggar, S. F. (1998). Calibration of a visible and near infrared portable transfer radiometer. *Metrologia, 35*(4), 701–706.

BIPM [Bureau International des Poids et Mesures]. (1998). *The international system of units (SI)* (7th ed.). Sèvres, France.

Boivin, L. P. (1981). Some aspects of radiometric measurement involving Gaussian laser beams. *Metrologia, 17*(1), 19–25.

Boivin, L. P. (2005). Realisation of spectral responsivity scales. In: A. C. Parr, R. U. Datla, & J. L. Gardner (Eds.), *Optical radiometry*. Amsterdam, Netherlands: Elsevier.

Boivin, L. P., & Gibb, K. (1995/1996). Monochromator-based cryogenic radiometry. *Applied Optics, 32*(6), 565–570.

Boivin, L. P., & Smith, T. C. (1978). Electrically calibrated radiometer using a thin film thermopile. *Applied Optics, 17*(19), 3067–3075.

Brown, S. W., Johnson, B. C., Feinholz, M. E., Yarbrough, M. A., Flora, S. J., Lykke. K. R., & Clark, D. K. (2003). Stray light correction algorithms for spectrographs. *Metrologia, 40*, 81–83.

Budde, W. (1983). Physical detectors of radiation. In: F. Grum & C. J. Bartleson (Eds.), *Optical radiation measurements* (vol. 4). New York, NY: Academic Press.

Bush, B. C., Valero, F. P. J., Simpson, A. S., & Bignone, L. (1999). Characterization of thermal effects in pyranometers: A data correction algorithm for improved measurement of surface insolation. *Journal of Atmospheric and Oceanic Technology, 17*, 165–175.

Butcher, G. I., Holland, A. D., Cole, R. E., Nelms, N., Wood, R. A., & Higashi, R. E. (1997). Infrared detectors for the GERB instrument on MSG. *Proceedings of SPIE, 3122*, 384–389.

Butler, J. J., Johnson, B. C., & Barnes, R. A. (2005). The calibration and characterization of earth remote sensing and environmental monitoring instruments. In: A. C. Parr, R. U. Datla, & J. L. Gardner (Eds.), *Optical radiometry*. Amsterdam, Netherlands: Elsevier.

Chunnilall, C. J., Fox, N. P., & Theocharous, E. (1997). Radiometric applications of Fourier-transform spectrometers. *Mikrochimica Acta, 14*, 175–177.

CIE [International Commission on Illumination]. (1982). Methods of characterising the performance of radiometers and photometers (Publication No. 53). Vienna, Austria.

CIE. (1983). *The basis of physical photometry* (Publication No. 18.2). Vienna, Austria.

CIE. (1984a). *Determination of the spectral responsivity of optical radiation detectors* (Publication No. 64). Vienna, Austria.

CIE. (1984b). *Polarisation: Definitions and nomenclature, instrument polarisation* (Publication No. 59). Vienna, Austria.

CIE. (1987a). *The measurement of absolute luminous intensity distributions* (Publication No. 70). Vienna, Austria.

CIE. (1987b). *Methods of characterising illuminance meters and luminance meters* (Publication No. 69). Vienna, Austria.

CIE. (1989). *The measurement of the luminous flux* (Publication No. 84). Vienna, Austria.

CIE. (1997). *Measurement of LEDs* (Publication No. 127). Vienna, Austria.

Coleman, A. J., Collins, A., & Sanders, J. E. (2000). Traceable calibration of ultraviolet meters used with broadband, extended sources. *Physics in Medicine and Biology, 45*(1), 185–196.

Corredera, P., Corrons, A., Campos, J., & Pons, A. (1991). Realization of an infrared spectroradiometer. *Applied Optics, 30*(10), 1279–1284.

Currie, D. D., Evans, A. L., Smith, D., Martin, C. J., McCalman, S., & Bilsland, D. (2001). An automated dosimetry system for testing whole body ultraviolet phototherapy cabinets. *Physics in Medicine and Biology, 46*(2), 333–346.

Datla, R. U., & Parr, A. C. (2005). Introduction to optical radiometry. In: A. C. Parr, R. U. Datla, & J. L. Gardner (Eds.), *Optical radiometry*. Amsterdam, Netherlands: Elsevier.

Davies, W. E. R., & Wyszecki, G. W. (1962). Physical approximation of colour mixture functions. *Journal of the Optical Society of America, 52*(6), 679–685.

Day, G. W. (2005). Laser radiometry. In: A. C. Parr, R. U. Datla, & J. L. Gardner (Eds.), *Optical radiometry*. Amsterdam, Netherlands: Elsevier.

Dichter, B. K., Beaubien, A. F., & Beaubien, D. J. (1993). Development and characterisation of a new solar ultraviolet-B irradiance detector. *Journal of Atmospheric and Oceanic Technology, 10*, 337–344.

Diffey, B. L. (1978). PUVA, a review of ultraviolet dosimetry. *British Journal of Dermatology, 98*(6), 703–705.

Diffey, B. L., & Challover, A. V. J. (1978). Absolute radiation dosimetry in photochemotherapy. *Physics in Medicine and Biology, 23*(6), 1124–1129.

Diffey, B. L. (1982). *Ultraviolet radiation in medicine.* Bristol, England: Adam Hilger.

Diffey, B. L. (1991). Solar ultraviolet radiation effects on biological systems. *Review in Physics in Medicine and Biology, 36*(3), 299–328.

Dobrowolski, J. A. (1970). Optical interference filters for the adjustment of spectral response and spectral power distribution. *Applied Optics, 9*(6), 1396–1402.

Early, E. A., Thompson, A., Johnson, C., DeLuisi, J., Disterholft, P., Wadle, D., . . . & Hays, D. S. (1998). The 1995 North American interagency intercomparison of ultraviolet monitoring spectroradiometers. *Journal of Research of the National Institute of Standards and Technology, 103*, 15–62.

Ehrlich, C. D., & Rasberry, S. D. (1997). Metrological timelines in traceability. *Metrologia, 34*(6), 503–514.

Eppeldauer, G. P., Brown, W. S., & Lykke, K. R. (2005). Transfer standard filter radiometers: Applications to fundamental scales. In: A. C. Parr, R. U. Datla, & J. L. Gardner (Eds.), *Optical radiometry.* Amsterdam, Netherlands: Elsevier.

Farman, J. C., Gardner, B. G., & Shanklin, J. D. (1985). Large losses of total ozone in Antarctica reveal seasonal $ClO_x$/$NO_x$ interaction. *Nature, 315*, 207–210.

Fowler, J. B., Lind, M. A., & Zalewski, E. F. (1979). *A servo-controlled electro-optical modulator for CW laser power stabilization control* (NBS Technical Note 987). Gaithersburg, MD: National Bureau of Standards.

Fox, N. P. (1991). Trap detectors and their properties. *Metrologia, 28*(3), 197–202.

Fox, N. P. (1993). Improved near-infrared detectors. *Metrologia, 30*(4), 321–325.

Fox, N. P. (1995/1996). Radiometry with cryogenic radiometers and semiconductor photodiodes. *Metrologia, 32*(6), 535–543.

Fox, N. P., Aiken, J., Barnett, J. J., Briottet, X., Carvell, R., Frohlich, C., . . . & Zalewski, E. (2003). Traceable radiometry underpinning terrestrial and helio studies (TRUTHS). *Advances in Space Research, 32*(11), 2253–2261.

Fox, N. P., Haycocks, P. R., Martin, J. E., & Ul-Haq, I. (1995/1996). A mechanically cooled portable cryogenic radiometer. *Metrologia, 32*(6), 581–584.

Fox, N. P., Martin, J. E., & Nettleton, D. H. (1991). Absolute determination of the thermodynamic temperatures of the melting points of gold, silver and aluminium. *Metrologia, 28*(5), 357–374.

Fox, N. P., & Rice, J. P. (2005). Absolute radiometers. In: A. C. Parr, R. U. Datla, & J. L. Gardner (Eds.), *Optical radiometry.* Amsterdam, Netherlands: Elsevier.

Gardner, J. L. (1994). Transmission trap detectors. *Applied Optics, 33*(25), 5914–5918.

Gibson, P., & Diffey, B. L. (1989). Broadband radiometry. In: B. L. Diffey (Ed.), *Radiation measurements in photobiology.* London, England: Academic Press.

Goodman, T. M. (1989). Calibration of light sources and detectors. In: B. L. Diffey (Ed.), *Radiation measurement in photobiology.* London, England: Academic Press.

Goodman, T. M., & Key, P. J. (1988). The NPL radiometric realisation of the candela. *Metrologia, 25*(1), 29–40.

Green, C., Diffey, B. L., & Hawk, J. L. M. (1992). Ultraviolet radiation for the treatment of skin disease. *Physics in Medicine and Biology, 37*(1), 1–20.

Grum, F., & Becherer, B. J. (1979). Radiometry. In: F. Grum & C. J. Bartleson (Eds.), *Optical radiation measurements.* New York, NY: Academic Press.

Harrison, N. J., Fox, N. P., Sperfeld, P., Metzdorf, J., Khlevnoy, B. B., Stolyarevskaya, R. I., . . . & Sapritsky, V. I. (1998). International comparison of radiation-temperature measurements with filtered detectors over the temperature range 1380 K to 3100 K. *Metrologia, 35*(4), 283–288.

Hollandt, J., Seidel, J., Kein, R., Ulm, G., Migdall, A., & Ware, M. (2005). Primary sources for use in radiometry. In: A. C. Parr, R. U. Datla, & J. L. Gardner (Eds.), *Optical radiometry.* Amsterdam, Netherlands: Elsevier.

Huber, M., Blumthaler, M., Schreder, J., Bais, A., & Topaloglou, C. (2002). Effects of ambient temperature on Robertson–Berger-type erythemal dosimeters. *Applied Optics, 41*(21), 4273–4277.

ISO [International Organisation for Standardisation]. (1993). *International vocabulary of basic terms in metrology* (2nd ed.). Geneva, Switzerland.

Ivanov, V. S., Lisiansky, B. E., Morozova, S. P., Sapritsky, V. I., Melenevsky, U. A., Xi, L. Y., & Pei, L. (2000). Medium-background radiometric facility for calibration of sources and sensors. *Metrologia, 37*(5), 599–602.

Johnsen, B., & Moan, J. (1991). The temperature sensitivity of the Robertson–Berger sunburn meter, model 500. *Journal of Photochemistry and Photobiology B: Biology, 11*(3–4), 277–284.

Kaufman, J. E., & Christensen, J. F. (1989). *IES lighting ready reference*. New York, NY: Illuminating Engineering Society of North America.

Kostkowski, H. I. (1997). Reliable spectroradiometry. La Plata, MD: Spectroradiometry Consulting.

Larason, T. C., & Cromer, C. L. (2001). Sources of error in UV radiation measurements. *Journal of Research of the National Institute of Standards and Technology, 106*, 649–656.

Lei, F., & Fischer, J. (1993). Characterisation of photodiodes in the UV and the visible spectral region based on cryogenic radiometry. *Metrologia, 30*(4), 297–303.

Leszczynski, K. (2002). *Advances in traceability of solar ultraviolet radiation measurements* (STUK-A189). Helsinki, Finland: STUK (Radiation and Nuclear Safety Authority).

Limperis, T., & Mudar, J. (1989). Detectors. In: W. L. Wolfe & G. J. Zissis (Eds.), *The infrared handbook* (3rd ed.). Washington, DC: Office of Naval Research.

Martin, C. J., Currie, G. D., & Pye, S. D. (1999). The importance of the radiometer angular response for ultraviolet phototherapy dosimetry. *Physics in Medicine and Biology, 44*(4), 843–855.

Martin, C. J., & Pye, S. D. (2000). A study of the directional response of ultraviolet radiometers: II. Implications for ultraviolet phototherapy derived from computer simulations. *Physics in Medicine and Biology, 45*(9), 2713–2729.

Martin, J. E., & Fox, N. P. (1993). Cryogenic solar absolute radiometer (CSAR). *Metrologia, 30*, 305–308.

Martin, J. E., Fox, N. P., & Key, P. J. (1985). A cryogenic radiometer for absolute radiometric measurements. *Metrologia, 21*(3), 147–155.

McCluney, W. R. (1994). *Introduction to radiometry and photometry*. Boston, MA: Artech House.

Michalsky, J. J., Harrison, L. C., & Berkheiser, W. E., III. (1995). Cosine response characteristics of some radiometric and photometric sensors. *Solar Energy, 54*(6), 397–402.

Mountford, P. J., & Davies, V. J. (1987). Ultraviolet radiometry of clinical sources with a multijunction thermopile. *Clinical Physics and Physiological Measurement, 8*(4), 325–335.

Munroe, D. M. (1982). Signal-to-noise ratio improvement. In: P. H. Sydenham (Ed.), *The handbook of measurement science* (vol. 1). New York, NY: John Wiley & Sons.

Nelms, N., & Dawson, J. (2005). Goldblack coating for thermal infrared detectors. *Sensors and Actuators A: Physical, 120*(2), 403–407.

Newing, A., Bullen, M. A., Davies, I. H., & Powell, N. L. (1986). Metrology in clinical practice. Part 1: Treatment with long wave ultraviolet radiation. *Journal of the Society for Radiological Protection, 6*(1), 33–37.

Nicodemus, F. E. (1963). Radiance. *American Journal of Physics, 31*(5), 368–377.

Ohno, Y. (1994). Integrating sphere simulation-application to total flux scale realisation. *Applied Optics, 33*(13), 2637–2647.

Ohno, Y. (2005). Photometry. In: A. C. Parr, R. U. Datla, & J. L. Gardner (Eds.), *Optical radiometry*. Amsterdam, Netherlands: Elsevier.

Ohtsuka, M., & Bedford, R. E. (1989). Measurement of size-of-source effects in an optical pyrometer. *Measurement, 7*(1), 2–6.

Palmer, C. (2000). *Diffraction grating handbook* (4th ed.). Rochester, NY: Richardson Grating Laboratory.

Palmer, J. M. (1993). Getting intense on intensity. *Metrologia, 30*, 371–372.

Palmer, J. M. (2001). Radiometry and photometry: Units and conversions. In: M. Bass (Ed.), *Handbook of optics* (vol. 3, 2nd ed.). New York, NY: McGraw-Hill.

Phelan, R. J., & Cook, A. R. (1973). Electrically calibrated pyroelectric optical radiation detector. *Applied Optics, 12*(10), 2492–2500.

Pye, S. D., & Martin, C. J. (2000). A study of the directional response of ultraviolet radiometers: I. Practical evaluation and implications for ultraviolet measurement standards. *Physics in Medicine and Biology, 45*(9), 2701–2712.

Quinn, T. J., & Martin, J. E. (1985). A radiometric determination of the Stephan-Boltzmann constant and thermodynamic temperature between –40°C and +100°C. *Philosophical Transactions of the Royal Society of London, Series A: Mathematical, Physical and Engineering Sciences, 316*, 85–189.

Robertson, D. F. (1972). *Solar ultraviolet radiation in relation to human sunburn and skin cancer.* Unpublished PhD thesis, University of Queensland, Brisbane, Queensland, Australia.

Rogalski, A. (1995). *Infrared photon detectors.* Bellingham, WA: SPIE Optical Engineering Press.

Sanders, C. L. (1972). Accurate measurements and corrections for nonlinearities in radiometers. *Journal of Research of the National Bureau of Standards, 76A*, 437–453.

Stark, E. W. (2002). Near infrared array spectrometers. In: J. M. Chalmers & P. R. Griffiths (Eds.), *The handbook of vibrational spectroscopy* (Vol. 1, pp. 393–435). New York, NY: John Wiley & Sons.

Stobbart, D., & Diffey, B. L. (1980). A comparison of some commercially available UVA meters used in photochemotherapy. *Clinical Physics and Physiological Measurement, 1*(4), 267–273.

Stock, K. D., Heine, R., & Hofer, H. (2003). Spectral characterisation of Ge trap detectors and photodiodes used as transfer standards. *Metrologia, 40*(1), S163–S166.

Stoffel, T. L., Reda, I., Myers, D. R., Renne, D., Wilcox, S., & Treadwell, J. (2000). Current issues in terrestrial solar radiation instrumentation for energy, climate and space applications. *Metrologia, 37*(5), 399–402.

Theocharous, E. (2005a). On the drifts exhibited by cryogenically cooled InSb infrared filtered detectors and their importance to the ATSR-2 and Landsat-5 earth observation missions. *Applied Optics, 44*(20), 4181–4185.

Theocharous, E. (2005b). On the stability of the spectral response of cryogenically cooled InSb infrared detectors. *Applied Optics, 44*(29), 6087–6092.

Theocharous, E. (2006). Absolute linearity measurements on a PbS detector. *Applied Optics, 45*(11), 2381–2386.

Theocharous, E., & Birch, J. (2002). Detectors for mid and far infrared spectroscopy: Selection and use. In: J. M. Chalmers & P. R. Griffiths (Eds.), *The handbook of vibrational spectroscopy* (Vol. 1, pp. 349–367). New York, NY: John Wiley & Sons.

Theocharous, E., Fox, N. P., & Prior, T. R. (1996). A comparison of the performance of infrared detectors for radiometric applications. *Proceedings of SPIE, 2815*, 56–69.

Theocharous, E., Fox, N. P., Sapritsky, V. I., Mekhontsev, S. N., & Morozova, S. P. (1998a). Absolute measurements of black-body emitted radiance. *Metrologia, 35*(4), 549–554.

Theocharous, E., Hawkins, G., & Fox, N. P. (2005). Reversible ageing effects in cryogenically-cooled infrared filter radiometers. *Infrared Physics and Technology, 46*(4), 339–349.

Theocharous, E., Ishi, J., & Fox, N. P. (2004). Absolute linearity measurements on HgCdTe detectors in the infrared. *Applied Optics, 43*(21), 4182–4188.

Theocharous, E., Prior, T. R., Haycocks, P. R., & Fox, N. P. (1998b). High-accuracy, infrared spectral responsivity scale. *Metrologia, 35*, 543–548.

Wehrli, C., Frohlich, C., & Romero, J. (1995/1996). Space degradation of SOVA sunphotometers on EURECA. *Metrologia, 32*(6), 653–656.

Willson, R. C. (1979). Active cavity radiometer type IV. *Applied Optics, 18*(2), 179–188.

WMO [World Meteorological Organisation]. (2006). *Guide to meteorological instruments and methods of observation* (7th ed., WMO No. 8). Geneva, Switzerland.

Wright, H., Sanders, C. L., & Gignac, D. (1969). Design of glass filter combinations for photometers. *Applied Optics, 8*(12), 2449–2455.

Wyatt, C. L. (1987). *Radiometric system design.* New York, NY: Macmillan.

Zalewski, E. F., & Duda, C. R. (1983). Silicon photodiode with 100% external quantum efficiency. *Applied Optics, 22*(18), 2867–2873.

Zong, Y., Brown, S., Johnson, B., Lykke, L., & Ohno, Y. (2006). Simple spectral stray light correction method for array spectroradiometers. *Applied Optics, 45*(6), 1111–1119.

## ABOUT THE AUTHOR

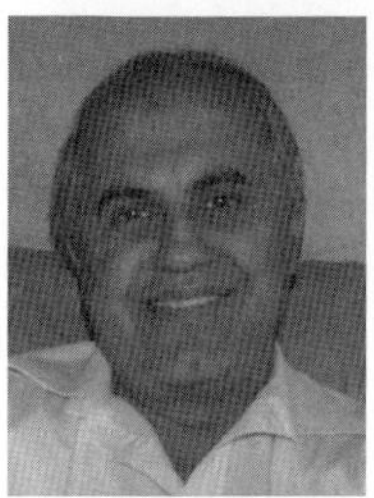

**Dr. Evangelos Theocharous** (Theo) was awarded a royal scholarship to study physics at Imperial College, London, and later a University of London studentship to complete his PhD at the same college in the field of photo-dissociation spectroscopy. He joined the Central Electricity Research Laboratory in 1981, where he developed fiber-optic sensors for the electricity supply industry. In 1986 he moved to the Instrument Development Group at BP Research Laboratories, where he worked on online process analysis using near-infrared (NIR) spectroscopy, infrared thermography, and the development of dedicated optical instruments for controlling the production of advanced materials. In 1993 he joined the Radiometry Section at NPL. His main interest is in infrared radiometry and he has published more than forty papers in this field. He is married, with two daughters and a son.

# CHAPTER 6

# MEDICAL ULTRASOUND SENSORS

## Thomas L. Szabo

*Department of Biomedical Engineering*
*Boston University, Boston, MA, USA*

## 6.1. INTRODUCTION

The transducer is the one indispensable part of a medical ultrasound system. Although much of this chapter describes the properties of piezoelectric transducers in general, emphasis will be placed on arrays for diagnostic imaging. Like many other sensors, medical ultrasound transducers perform their ordinary transduction functions of converting electrical signals to pressure (or stress) waves and vice versa, but what distinguishes them is their ability to perform imaging as well. In this chapter the physical principles of transducers, preferred piezoelectric materials for transduction, design considerations, single-element and array configurations, the characteristics needed for imaging and focusing, and new developments in transducer technology are explored.

A transducer can be considered to be a black box, as shown at the top of Figure 6.1. A short electrical pulse, $v_i(t)$, enters the left side and emerges out the other end as a pressure (or stress) wave, $p_i(t)$. This wave reflects from an object in its path and returns to the transducer, $p_r(t)$, where it is converted back to an electrical signal, $v_0(t)$, as illustrated at the bottom of Figure 6.1.

These conversions are possible because of piezoelectric material inside the transducer. Piezoelectricity was discovered by the Curie brothers in the 1880s. They found that an electric charge appeared on electrodes placed on a compressed quartz crystal: the direct piezoelectric effect. They also verified the reverse piezoelectric effect, that a displacement is caused by a voltage applied to a quartz crystal. These reciprocal piezoelectric effects enable the reception of pressure pulse echoes and the transmission of pressure waves into media such as the body.

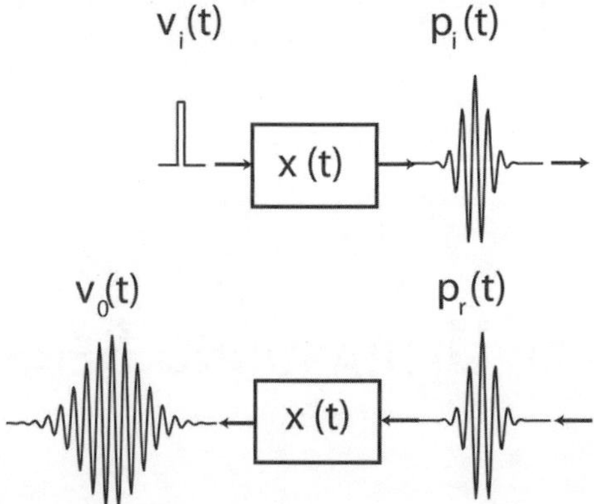



**Figure 6.1.** (top) Excitation voltage, $v_i(t)$, produces an incident pressure pulse, $p_i(t)$, through transducer, $x(t)$. (bottom) Reflected wave, $p_r(t)$, is converted back to voltage, $v_0(t)$.

When a transducer is placed in the basic echo ranging system shown in Figure 6.2, the pulse echoes from different tissue interfaces and objects can be seen in what is a called an A-mode (for amplitude) display.

If the same transducer is now moved in a controlled way in a direction transverse to the acoustic path (straight out of the transducer) and the result is displayed, an imaging system can be created as shown in Figure 6.3. Here the display indicates the increasing time dimension as straight downward. Each vertical line in the display corresponds to a different sequential position of the transducer. The length of this line is the round-trip time it takes for an acoustic pulse in a medium with a sound speed $c$ to travel to a target at a distance $z$ and return: $t = 2z/c$. The scanning function of a moving single transducer can also be accomplished by a series of inline transducers that are electronically switched on and off sequentially, as also shown in Figure 6.3. This arrangement is called a transducer array, and each individual transducer is called an array element. Arrays are not only used to switch groups of elements on to create acoustic lines in an image; they also focus and steer acoustic beams. Focusing and steering are accomplished electronically by delaying pulses sent to individual elements to form a wavefront that functions as an electronic lens. Furthermore, the focusing can be changed rapidly and automatically or modified by the imaging system user; it is described in more detail in section 6.8.2.

## 6.2. WAVE TRANSMISSION AND REFLECTION

In order to learn how a piezoelectric transducer works, it is important to understand acoustic waves. These waves are small mechanical longitudinal disturbances that propagate through materials without altering them permanently. The positive values of these pressure waveforms (such as those illustrated in Fig. 6.1) represent compression, while the negative values represent rarefaction. These instantaneous disturbances are pressure $p$ (in megapascals $10^6$ pascals) and particle velocity $v$ (in meters per second), and they are related by the acoustic characteristic impedance $Z$ (in megarayls [$10^6$ rayls or 1 Mrayl is equivalent to $10^6$ kg m$^{-2}$ s$^{-1}$]) by equation 6.1,

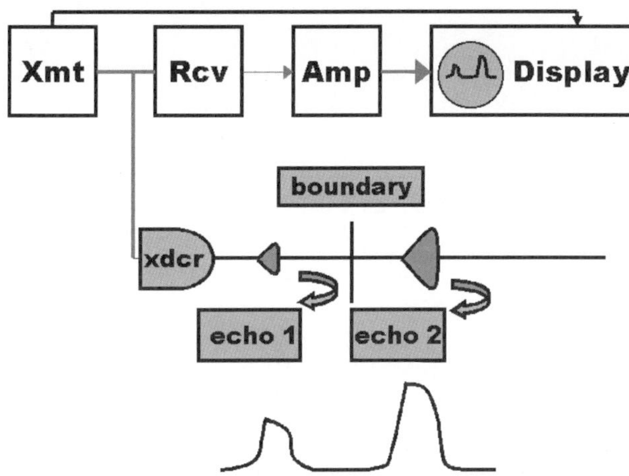


**Figure 6.2.** Basic echo ranging system consisting of a transmitter (Xmt), transducer (xdcr), receiver (Rcv), amplifier (Amp), and oscilloscope display. Pulse echoes are shown below at delays corresponding to depths of reflecting objects.

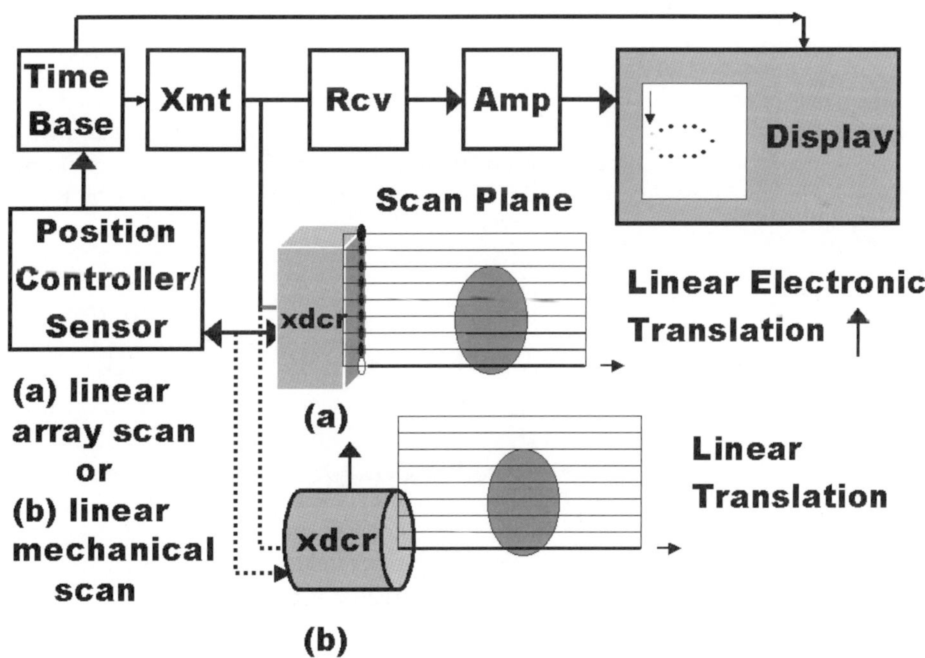


**Figure 6.3.** Basic elements of a pulse echo imaging system shown with linear scanning of two types: (a) electronic linear array scanning, which involves switching from one element to another; and (b) mechanical scanning, which involves controlled translation of a single transducer.

$$p = Zv, \tag{6.1}$$

in which pressure and particle velocity can be considered to be the mechanical analogs of the electrical variables voltage and current. If the wave is not moving forward, but backward, then

$$p = -Zv. \tag{6.1a}$$

When a pressure wave is incident on a boundary between two different acoustic media with acoustic impedances of $Z_1$ and $Z_2$, some of the pressure is reflected and the rest is transmitted into the second medium, as illustrated in Figure 6.4. The ratio of the reflected pressure to the incident pressure is given by the pressure acoustic reflection factor:

$$\mathrm{RF} = \frac{Z_2 - Z_1}{Z_2 + Z_1}. \tag{6.2}$$

Likewise, the ratio of the pressure transmitted into the second medium relative to the incident pressure is given by the pressure acoustic transmission factor:

$$\mathrm{TF} = \frac{2Z_2}{Z_2 + Z_1}. \tag{6.3}$$

In the absence of losses, these factors are related by

$$TF = RF + 1. \tag{6.4}$$

As an example of material parameters used for these factors, a typical piezoelectric ceramic has an impedance of 34 Mrayls, whereas tissue or water has an impedance of 1.5 Mrayls. A perfectly rigid material has infinite impedance and air has no resistance (0 Mrayls). Factors for how well an acoustic pressure from a ceramic with $Z_1$ = 34 Mrayls couples into different materials are summarized in Table 6.1.

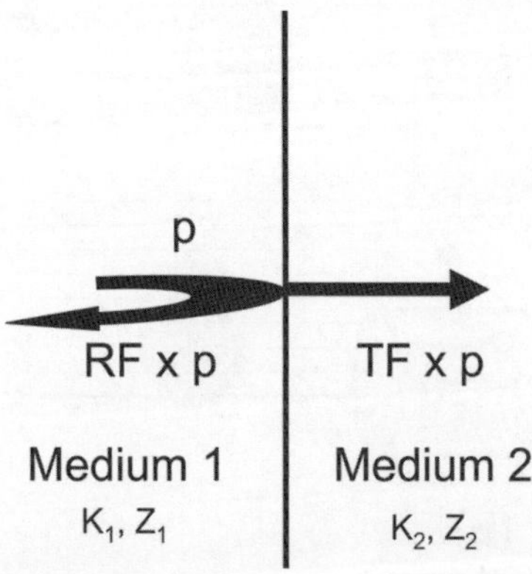


**Figure 6.4.** A pressure wave (wavenumber $K_1$) in a medium with an acoustic impedance of $Z_1$ is incident on a boundary with a semi-infinite medium. An acoustic impedance of $Z_2$ and reflected and transmitted waves (wavenumber $K_2$) result.

**Table 6.1.** Reflection (RF) and transmission (TF) factors and average power transmission coefficient (TFP) for different boundaries for $Z_1 = 34$ Mrayls

| $Z_2$ **(Mrayls)** | **RF** | **TF** | **TFP** |
|---|---|---|---|
| $Z_1$ | 0 | 1 | 1 |
| 0 | −1 | 0 | 0 |
| ∞ | 1 | 2 | 0 |
| 1.5 | −0.915 | 0.085 | 0.162 |

When the load material has an impedance equal to the ceramic, all the pressure is transmitted. For an air load, the pressure is totally reflected and inverted. For a rigid load, a curious result seems to occur: there is a reflected pressure and a transmitted pressure of twice the incident pressure. Pressure is not everything; particle displacement has not been considered. The average power transmission coefficient (TFP), which accounts for both pressure and displacement, is

$$\text{TFP} = \frac{p_2 v_2^* / 2}{p_1 v_1^* / 2} = \frac{\dfrac{|p_2|^2}{2Z_2}}{\dfrac{|p_1|^2}{2Z_1}} = \frac{4 Z_1 Z_2}{|Z_1 + Z_2|^2} \tag{6.5}$$

In terms of the TFP, the rigid and air load cases result in no power being transmitted. The final case of a ceramic with a tissue load shows that little of the power is transferred into the tissue. In order to determine how to improve this situation, it is necessary to explore the operation of a transducer.

## 6.3. TRANSDUCER TIME RESPONSE

The piezoelectric material in the form of a transducer is shown in Figure 6.5. The left and right electrode surfaces each have an area $A$ and they are separated by a thickness $d$. The electrical properties of the material are a dielectric constant or permittivity, $\varepsilon^s$ (under a condition of constant strain), and its relative form, $\varepsilon_r^s$. The transducer looks like a capacitor with a value of

$$C_0 = \varepsilon^s A/d = \varepsilon_r^s \varepsilon_0 A/d, \tag{6.6}$$

where the permittivity of free space is $\varepsilon_0 = 8.85 \times 10^{-12}$ Fm$^{-1}$. The acoustical properties are the speed of sound in the ceramic of $c_c$ (ms$^{-1}$), an acoustic impedance $Z_c$ (Mrayls), an acoustic wavenumber $k_c = 2\pi f/c_c$, and $f$ is frequency (in MHz).

Piezoelectric materials differ from ordinary elastic materials where Hooke's law prevails:

$$\sigma = C^D e, \tag{6.7a}$$

where $\sigma$ is the stress in the material, $C^D$ is the elastic stiffness constant for piezoelectrics obtained under a constant electric displacement field $D$ (shown here as a superscript notation), which is

$$D = C_0 V/A, \tag{6.7b}$$

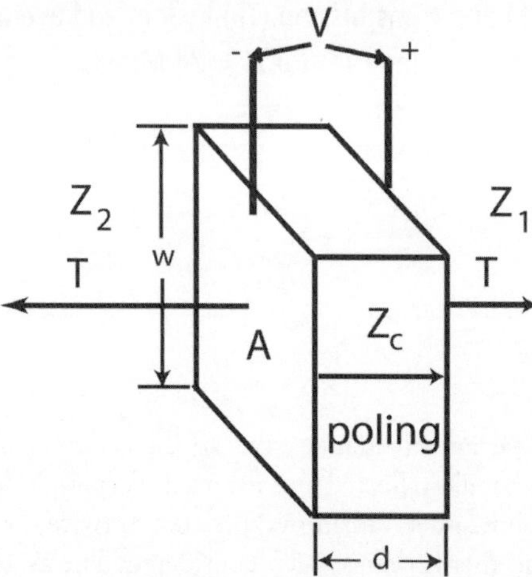



**Figure 6.5.** Voltage applied to an electroded piezoelectric slab of impedance $Z_c$ of thickness $d$, width $w$, and length $L$ creates creates stress waves $T$ into the adjacent media of impedances $Z_1$ and $Z_2$.

and $e$ is strain. The important link between the electrical and acoustical worlds is through the piezoelectric constant $h$ [force (newtons)/charge (coulombs)] of the material. A modified one-dimensional (1-D) Hooke's law for piezoelectric materials with an added piezoelectric term, $hD$, is

$$\sigma = C^D e - hD. \tag{6.8}$$

Under the condition of constant strain, forces are equal to $F = \sigma A$ and therefore, from equation 6.8, the forces as a function of time $t$ are formed at the electrodes in response to charges generated by a voltage signal $V(t)$ across the electrodes:

$$F(t) = \sigma A = hC_0 V(t)/2. \tag{6.9}$$

Redwood (1963) derived an alternative transducer model that provides insights into how a transducer response is created from an impulse excitation. This model is further simplified by neglecting secondary piezoelectric coupling and assuming a large impedance across the electrical port. If the applied voltage is an impulse, then force impulses with the magnitude described by equation 6.9 are generated at the electroded interfaces at time $t = 0$ with the polarities illustrated in Figure 6.6. The force depicted as $F_a$ propagates forward to the right with a negative magnitude is given by

$$F_a = \frac{-2Z_1}{Z_c + Z_1}(hC_0 V / 2), \tag{6.10a}$$

which can be recognized as the product of the TF (see equation 6.3) for the boundary and the magnitude (from equation 6.9):

$$F_a = -(1 + r_1)F_0, \tag{6.10b}$$

where

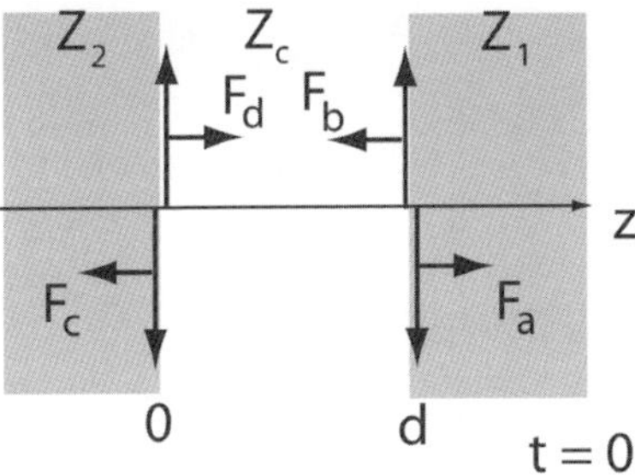


**Figure 6.6.** Force impulses excited by a voltage impulse at time $t = 0$ travel in both directions.

$$r_1 = \frac{Z_1 - Z_c}{Z_c + Z_1},\qquad(6.10\text{c})$$

and

$$F_0 = (hC_0 V/2).\qquad(6.10\text{d})$$

Simultaneously $F_b$ propagates backward into the piezoelectric as

$$F_b = (1 - r_1)F_0.\qquad(6.11)$$

Also, at $t = 0$, $F_c$ (negative force) moves backward into medium $Z_2$ as

$$F_c = -(1 + r_2)F_0,\qquad(6.12\text{a})$$

where

$$r_2 = \frac{Z_2 - Z_c}{Z_c + Z_2},\qquad(6.12\text{b})$$

and now the transmission factor for the boundary between $Z_c$ and $Z_2$ is appropriate so that $F_d$ propagates forward:

$$F_d(0) = (1 - r_2)F_0.\qquad(6.13)$$

This force propagates into the material $Z_1$ at the front or right end of the transducer. From the back of the piezoelectric, $F_d$ crosses the front boundary at a time $t = d/c_c$, as illustrated in Figure 6.7, as

$$F_d(d/c_c) = (1 + r_1)F_d(0) = (1 + r_1)(1 - r_2)F_0 = (1 - r_2)|F_d|.\qquad(6.14)$$

Also as depicted in Figure 6.7, $F_b$ bounces off the back wall and crosses the front boundary at a time $t = 2d/c_c$. Similarly, the reflected portion of $F_d$ also reflects off the back wall and crosses the front boundary at a time $t = 3d/c_c$, and so on. The series of impulses passing into $Z_1$ normalized to $F_a$ is shown on the right side of Figure 6.7.

This series of impulses can be applied to several practical examples given in Table 6.2. When the piezoelectric has air on both sides, this configuration is not useful because power is totally reflected and not transmitted. The backside material with impedance $Z_2$ is called the backing. For a front load matched to the piezoelectric and air as the backing, the time signature [–1, 2, –1] for an impulse

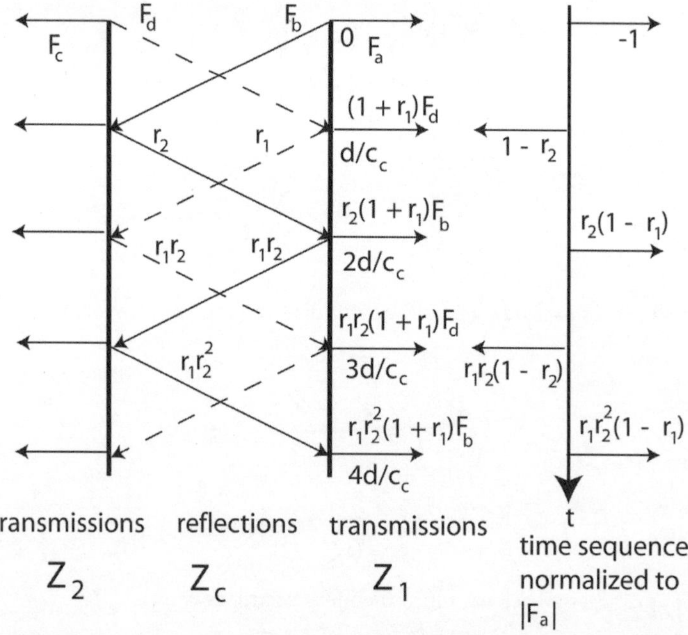



**Figure 6.7.** (left) Reflection diagram for determining time sequence of force pulses moving into medium 1. (right) Time sequence produced in medium $Z_1$ normalized to force $|F_a|$.

**Table 6.2.** Time sequences normalized to $|F_a|$ for four loading conditions

| Case | $Z_2$ | $Z_1$ | Time sequence |
| --- | --- | --- | --- |
| a | 0 | $Z_c$ | $-1, 2, -1$ |
| b | $Z_c$ | $Z_c$ | $-1, 1$ |
| c | $Z_w$ | $Z_c$ | $-1, 1.915, -0.915$ |
| d | $Z_c$ | $Z_w$ | $-1, 1$ |

excitation is given by Figure 6.8. A number of other cases of interest are also depicted in Figure 6.8. When both sides are matched to the piezoelectric, the resulting pulse is short [−1, 1]. If the backing is tissue but the front load is matched, a longer pulse results [−1, 1.915, −0.915]. For the reversal of these loads, a short pulse is again achieved [−1, 1].

Alternatively these effects can be viewed in the frequency domain. The matched case is of particular interest; it has a spectrum that is centered on the frequency $f_0$ and its odd multiples. This frequency, $f_0$, is called the resonant frequency and can be interpreted as a half-wavelength resonance:

$$f_0 = c_c/2d = c_c/[2(\lambda/2)]. \tag{6.15}$$

The speed of sound between the electrodes is given by

$$c_c = \sqrt{C^D/\rho}, \tag{6.16}$$

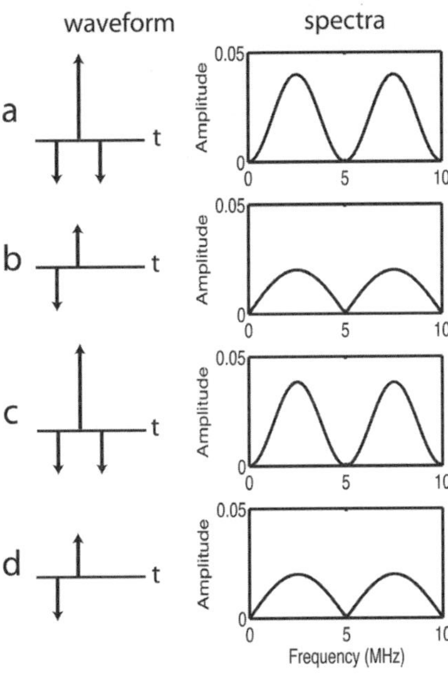


**Figure 6.8.** (left) Pressure sequences in $Z_1$ for the four cases of Table 6.2 normalized to the magnitude of $F_a$. (right) Corresponding spectra.

where $\rho$ is density (in kg/m$^3$). From the spectra in Figure 6.8, it is evident that the second and fourth cases have the widest spectra, or greatest bandwidths; these have two humps centered at $f_0$ and $3f_0$ with a null at $2f_0$. For example, if $f_0 = 2.5$ MHz, there would be a null at 5 MHz and a harmonic at 7.5 MHz.

As an example of how a spectrum is calculated, the matched case is examined. When a voltage impulse is applied across the electrodes, the piezoelectric effect creates impulsive $\delta$ forces at the electrodes, given by equation 6.17:

$$F(t) = -F_0[\delta(t) - \delta(t - d/c_c)]. \tag{6.17}$$

To obtain the spectrum of this response, take the Fourier transform of equation 6.17:

$$F(f) = -j2F_0\exp(-j\pi fd/c)\sin[\pi f/(2f_0)], \tag{6.18}$$

an expression with maxima at odd harmonics, $f = (2n + 1)f_0$ (note $n = 0, 1, 2, 3, \ldots$) of the fundamental resonance, as shown in Figure 6.8.

## 6.4. TRANSDUCER MODELS

### 6.4.1. SIMPLIFIED MODEL

Most often, transducers are designed and modeled in the frequency domain as the three-port device shown in Figure 6.9. External connections are made to the transducer through the electrical port. From here the complex transducer impedance can be measured as a function of frequency. After conversion

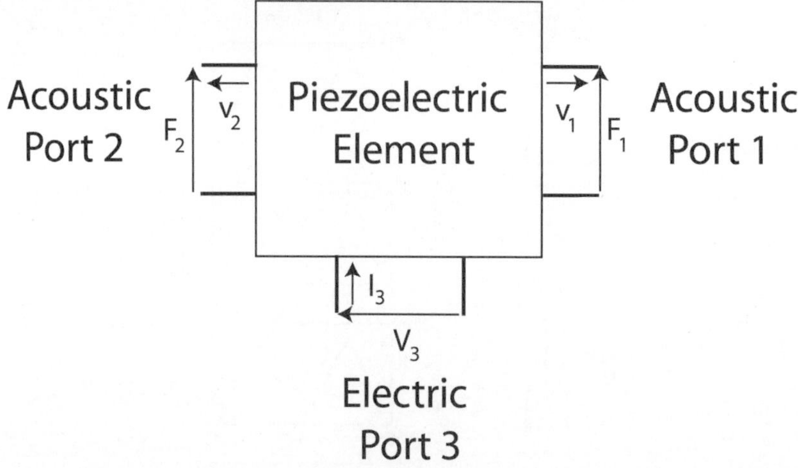


**Figure 6.9.** Representation of a three-port piezoelectric device with electric port and two acoustic ports. Here $F_1$ and $v_1$ represent the pressure and particle velocity at acoustic port 1 (usually the front of the piezoelectric); $F_2$ and $v_2$ represent the pressure and particle velocity at acoustic port 2; and $I_3$ and $V_3$ represent the current and voltage at electrical port 3.

to acoustic forces by the piezoelectric ability of the transducer, the resulting forces are split between the back and front loads, for which there are two acoustic ports.

For the matched case (Szabo, 2004), it is straightforward to develop a simple equivalent circuit model of the electrical impedance. The impedance of the transducer can be expected to have the reactance of a capacitor. However, because of strong acoustic coupling, there is an additional acoustic radiation impedance component, $Z_A(f)$, illustrated in Figure 6.10(a).

The overall electrical impedance is

$$Z_T(f) = Z_A(f) - j(1/\omega C_0) = R_A(f) + j[X_A(f) - 1/\omega C_0], \tag{6.19}$$

where $\omega = 2\pi f$. Here $Z_A$ is the acoustic radiation impedance, of which $R_A$ and $X_A$ are its real and imaginary parts. $R_A$ can be found from the total real electrical power flowing into the transducer for an applied voltage $V$ and current $I$:

$$W_E = II^* R_A/2 = |I^2| R_A/2, \tag{6.20}$$

where current is $I = j\omega q = j\omega C_0 V$, $q$ is charge, and $I^*$ denotes a complex conjugate. The total power radiated from both sides of the transducer into a surrounding medium of specific acoustic impedance, $Z_c = \rho c_c A$ (where $\rho$ is density, $c_c$ is the speed of sound in the transducer crystal, and $A$ is the cross-sectional area of the transducer) equal to that of the crystal is

$$W_A = A\sigma\sigma^*/(2Z_c/A) = A^2|F(f)/A|^2/2Z_C = |hC_0 V\sin(\pi f/2f_0)|^2/2Z_C. \tag{6.21a}$$

Setting the powers of equations 6.20 and 6.21a equal, the solution for $R_A$ is

$$R_A(f) = R_{AC}\operatorname{sinc}^2(f/2f_0), \tag{6.21b}$$

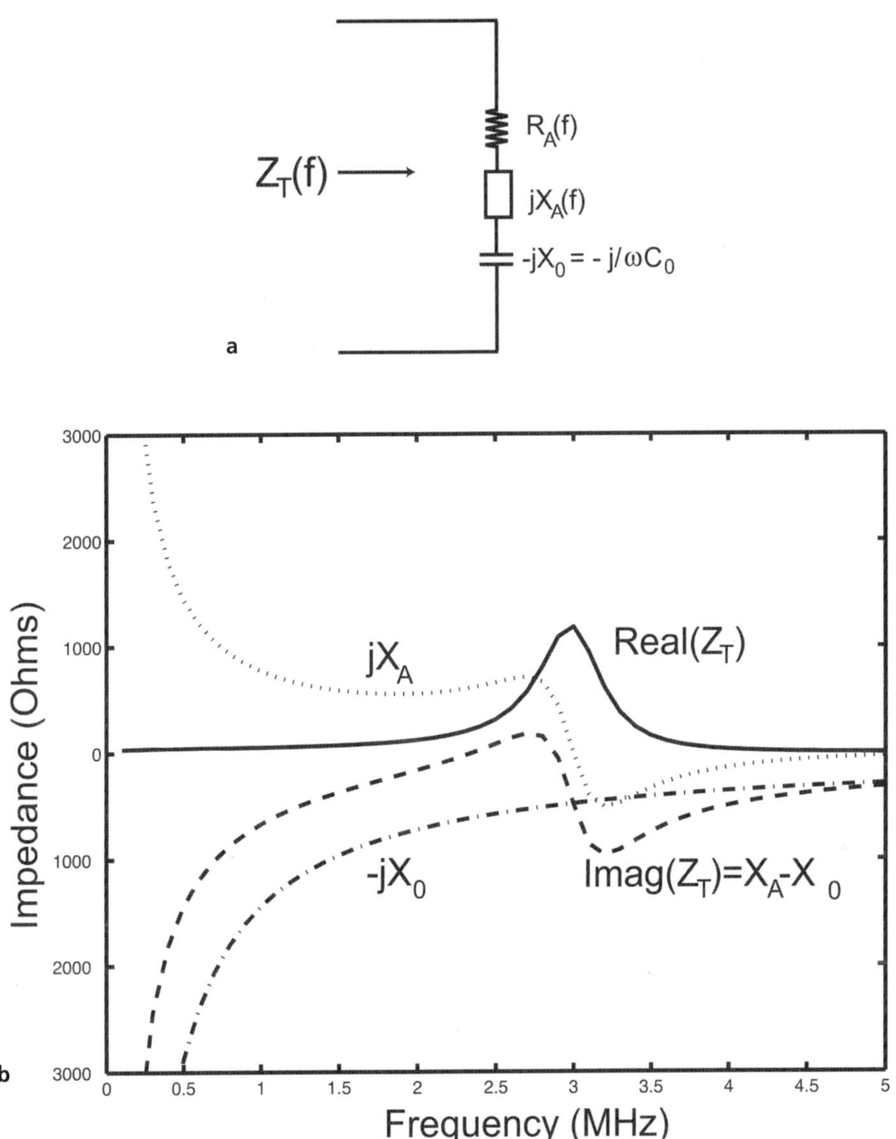


**Figure 6.10.** (a) Transducer equivalent circuit and (b) transducer impedance as a function of frequency.

where $\operatorname{sinc}(x) = \sin(\pi x)/(\pi x)$ and

$$R_{AC} = \frac{k_T^2}{4f_0 C_0} = \frac{d^2 k_T^2}{2A\varepsilon^S c_c}. \qquad (6.21c)$$

The electroacoustic coupling constant is $k_T$, a measure of mutual coupled energy to stored energy (Kino, 1987), and $k_T = h/\sqrt{C^D/\varepsilon^s}$. Alternatively, $h$ is proportional to $k_T$, which is more widely used than $h$. This coupling constant is an indicator of sensitivity; for example, the forces generated at the electrodes in equation 6.10 are proportional to $k_T$. Interesting properties of $R_{AC}$ include an inverse proportionality to the capacitance and area of the transducer, and a direct dependence on the square of the thickness $d$. Later, electrical loss, defined in equation 6.23, will be shown to be proportional to $R_{AC}$, which in turn is proportional to the coupling constant squared. Note that at resonance,

$$R_A(f_0) = \frac{k_T^2}{\pi^2 f_0 C_0}.$$

(6.21d)

Network theory requires that the imaginary part of an impedance be related to the real part, so the radiation reactance can be found as

$$X_A(f) = \frac{2R_{AC}}{\pi} \mathrm{sinc}(f/f_0).$$

(6.21e)

In this case, $R_A$ is maximum at $f = 0$ MHz and $X_A$ is zero at the resonant frequency.

## 6.4.2. GENERAL EQUIVALENT CIRCUIT MODELS

In order to simulate transducer operation for design, a more comprehensive model is required. For example, a more typical transducer impedance in which the acoustic ports have unequal loads is plotted as a function of frequency in Figure 6.10(b). Here $R_A$ is maximum near the resonant frequency and there $X_A$ is zero. This calculation was made with a transducer equivalent circuit model. Two of the most widely applied equivalent circuit models are the Mason (Berlincourt, Curran, & Jaffe, 1964) and the Krimholtz, Leedom, and Matthaei (KLM; Leedom, Krimholtz, & Matthaei, 1978). Both these approaches are based on the same piezoelectric equations and give identical numerical results. They are 1-D frequency domain models that rely on electrical analogs for acoustic variables. Even though the derivations of these models are beyond the scope of this chapter, the KLM model will be described briefly so that transducer design trade-offs can be explained.

The key advantage of the KLM model, shown in Figure 6.11, is that the piezoelectric element is simulated by a three-port architecture in which the electrical port (port number 3) is separated from the acoustic part, which is split into two opposite directions, ending up in acoustic ports 1 and 2. The electrical leg of this model starts at port 3 and includes a capacitor, an unusual electrical capacitance-like element, $C'$,

$$C' = -C_0/k_T^2 \mathrm{sinc}(f/f_0),$$

(6.22a)

and an electroacoustic transformer with a turns ratio of

$$\phi = k_T \left(\frac{1}{2f_0 C_0 Z_c}\right)^{1/2} \mathrm{sinc}(f/f_0),$$

(6.22b)

that is connected to the center point of the T junction in Figure 6.11. This center point represents the center of the piezoelectric element. The electrical equivalent circuit model of acoustic propagation is

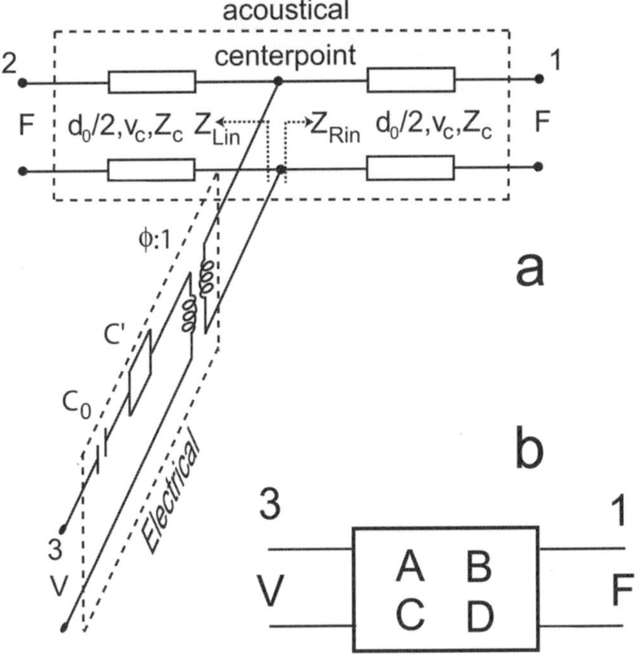


**Figure 6.11.** (a) Schematic representation of the KLM transducer three-port equivalent circuit model. (b) ABCD representation of KLM model by an ABCD matrix between electrical port 3 and acoustic port 1.

a transmission line. Thus two acoustic transmission lines extend in each direction toward ports 1 and 2 to represent acoustic wave propagation through the halves of the piezoelectric in the forward and backward directions, respectively. Each of these transmission lines represent half the piezoelectric element with a length $d_0/2 = d/2$, a sound speed $v_c = c_c$ and an impedance $Z_c$.

Outside the core KLM piezoelectric element, additional acoustic layers can be added on each acoustic port as acoustic transmission lines terminating in loads at either end, as shown in Figure 6.12 (Szabo, 2004). On the electrical port, a suitable electrical source and appropriate electrical matching elements can be attached. Since interest is focused on the transducer as an electromechanical device, for convenience the entire model can be represented as a four-element ABCD matrix with electrical attachment on the left side (port 3) and a final acoustic load on the other side (port 1), as in Figure 6.11(b). This black-box representation with applied voltage on one side and force on the other is reminiscent of the operation described in Figure 6.1.

Even though much of the current discussion is based on one-way acoustic transduction, because of the reciprocal nature of piezoelectricity, the methodology can be extended to reception as well. An example of what is called a round-trip or transmission–reception model is illustrated by Figure 6.13. On the left, a transmitter $V_1$ is connected through a matching network and source impedance $Z_1$ through an electrical cable to the overall forward transducer model represented by matrix ABCD. The transmitted force is applied to the medium represented by $Z_F$. This force serves as a source with the impedance of the medium for the return path. By reciprocity, the matrix representing the receive transduction process is

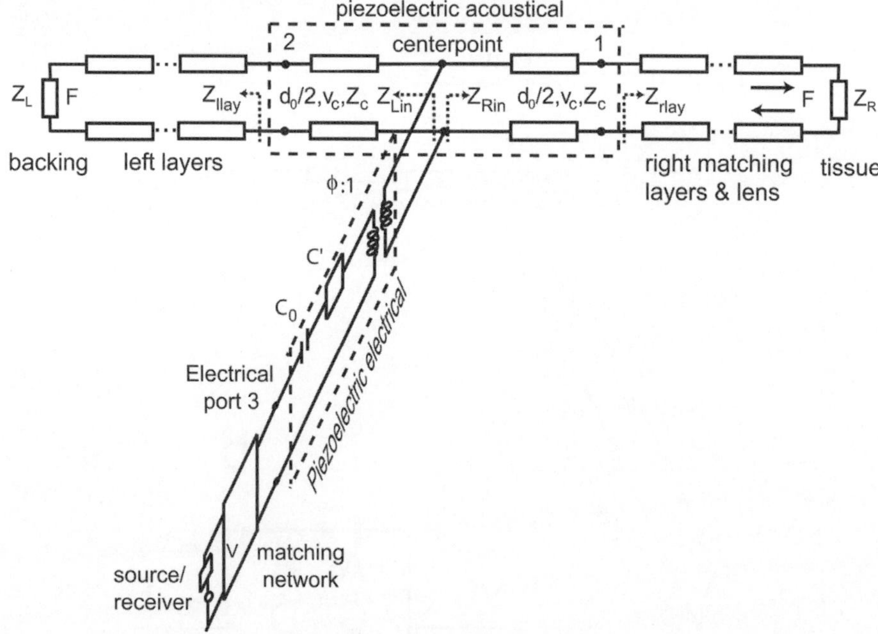



**Figure 6.12.** Overall equivalent circuit transducer model.

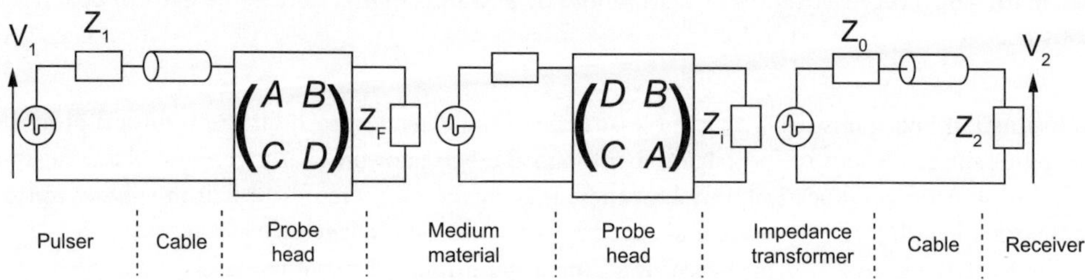



**Figure 6.13.** Equivalent circuit for the round-trip response of a transducer with cable and a lens (the properties of the lens are included in the probe head matrix; from Saitoh et al., 1999).

reversed and ends in a load. The voltage across this load is applied across an electrical impedance matching transformer through a cable back to a final electrical impedance load $Z_2$.

## 6.5. DESIGN CONSIDERATIONS

### 6.5.1. ELECTRICAL ASPECTS

The advantages of models for the simulation of transducer performance include prediction of electrical impedance, frequency characteristics, impulse response, and any variable inside the transducer structure, such as voltage and force waveforms, electrical mismatch, electroacoustic efficiency, and power transfer. Simulations allow design optimization and evaluation as well as comparison to measurements.

The KLM model can predict numerically the electrical impedance of the transducer as described in general by equation 6.19. It also provides a means of deriving a more general expression for radiation resistance at resonance. For the case where the impedance looking from the right face of the piezoelectric crystal to the right is $Z_R = Z_w$, the impedance of water or tissue, and that looking from the left face of the crystal is $Z_L = Z_B$, the backing impedance:

$$R_A(f_0) = R_{A0} = \frac{2k_T^2}{\pi^2 f_0 C_0}\left(\frac{Z_c}{Z_L + Z_R}\right) = \frac{2k_T^2}{\pi^2 f_0 C_0}\left(\frac{Z_c}{Z_B + Z_w}\right). \qquad (6.23)$$

Note that as a sanity check, if instead the loads are made equal to $Z_L = Z_R = Z_c$, the conditions under which the simpler model was derived, equation 6.23 reduces to the simple model result of equation 6.21d.

Quantitative measures of transducer efficiency as a function of a frequency are shown in Figure 6.14. Insertion loss is a measure of the round-trip or complete transmission and reception efficiency. As illustrated in Figure 6.14(a), insertion loss (IL) is defined as the ratio of the amount of electrical power from an electrical source ($R_g$) that reaches an electrical receiver load ($R_f$) as $W_f$ with the device inserted between the source and final electrical load $R_f$ over the power reaching the load with the device removed. It can be expressed as

$$IL(f) = \frac{W_f(\text{with transducer})}{W_f(\text{without transducer})} = \left[\left|\frac{V_f(f)}{V_g(f)}\right|^2\left(\frac{R_f + R_g}{R_f}\right)^2\right], \qquad (6.24)$$

where $W_f$ is the power delivered to the load. In order to provide a quantitative measure of overall one-way transducer electroacoustic efficiency, the transducer loss is useful (Szabo, 2004). In this case, as shown in Figure 6.14(b), the equivalent electrical load is $R_f = Z_R$, the right acoustic load from acoustic port 1 in Figure 6.12. Transducer loss is defined as the maximum available electrical power ($W_g$) from an electrical source ($R_g$) reaching an acoustic load ($R_f = Z_R$) with the device inserted between the source and load divided by the power reaching the load ($Z_R$) with the device removed, as shown in Figure 6.14(b).

To complete the electrical part of the transducer model, a source and matching network are added, as in Figure 6.15. The simplest form of electrical matching is a series tuning inductor, as shown on the left side of Figure 6.15. Ultimately, in terms of electrical power efficiency, what counts is the amount of time average power is transferred to the real part of the transducer impedance, $R_A$. One simple way to achieve this over a reasonable bandwidth is to tune the transducer capacitance out with a series inductor. In general, a more elaborate tuning network can be developed, as described by the $A_{ET}B_{ET}C_{ET}D_{ET}$ matrix shown on the right side of Figure 6.15.

An expression for the electrical loss (EL), which is the acoustic power reaching $R_A$ divided by the maximum power available from a source with an impedance $R_g$ as a function of frequency, can be written as

$$EL(f) = \frac{4R_A R_g}{\left|R_g + A_{ET}Z_T + B_{ET}\right|^2}, \qquad (6.25a)$$

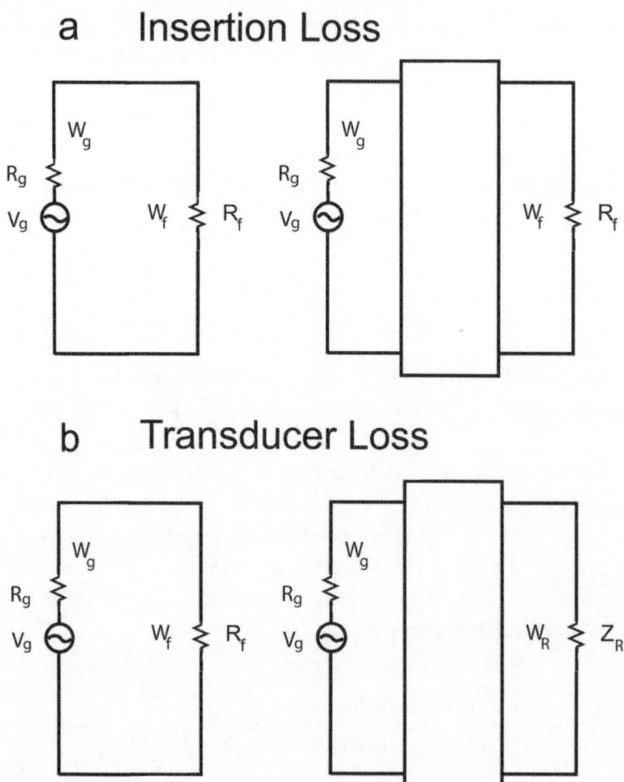



**Figure 6.14.** (a) Transducer insertion loss shown as a comparison of the source and load without and with a device in between. The device in the box is the transmit and receive transduction characteristics, similar to the representation of Figure 6.13, with correspondences between $V_1$ and $V_g$, $Z_1$ and $R_g$, and $Z_2$ and $R_f$. (b) Similar transducer loss definition for a one-way transducer, with the box representing what is between electrical port 3 and acoustic port 1 of Figure 6.12.

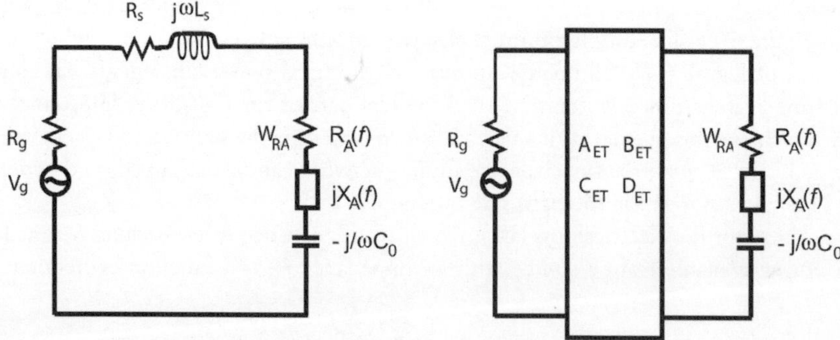



**Figure 6.15.** Electrical voltage source and electrical matching network. (a) Simple series inductor and resistor. (b) ABCD representation of a more general network.

where $R_g$ is the source impedance (often taken to be 50 ohms) and $A_{ET}$ and $B_{ET}$ are matrix elements of the general network given by Figure 6.15. In the particular implementation in which the series inductor and resistor, $L_s$ and $R_s$, are absorbed into the overall matrix, the electrical loss assumes a straightforward meaning:

$$\mathrm{EL}(f) = \frac{4R_A R_g}{\left(R_A + R_g + R_s\right)^2 + \left(X_A - \dfrac{1}{\omega C_0} + \omega L_s\right)^2} . \qquad (6.25b)$$

If at resonance, $R_A = R_g$ and $R_s$ is small, and the inductive reactance cancels the capacitive reactance, then $\mathrm{EL}(f_0) = 1.0$, or there is perfect electrical power transfer (no electrical loss). This result is an idealized result at one frequency. In general, the radiation resistance is a complicated function of frequency and the electrical loss achievable over a frequency range depends on several variables in equations 6.25a and 6.25b.

Electrical loss is only part of the story. The transfer of power from an electrical source to an acoustic load such as tissue, $Z_R$, is described by transducer loss (depicted in Fig. 6.14[b]):

$$\mathrm{TL}(f) = \mathrm{EL}(f)\mathrm{AL}(f), \qquad (6.25c)$$

where acoustical loss (AL), a measure of how much power reaches the intended acoustic load, is described next.

## 6.5.2. ACOUSTICAL ASPECTS

### 6.5.2.1. Acoustic Loading Effects

The missing piece is acoustical loss. From the KLM model, the electrical power that manages to reach the real electrical load, $R_A(f)$, is split in two directions, as shown in Figure 6.12. It is only the power reaching the tissue that is of importance. For simple real loads on each side of the piezoelectric—impedance $Z_R$ on the right and $Z_L$ on the left—the acoustical power at resonance has a simple form for typical loads:

$$\mathrm{AL}(f_0) = \frac{Z_R}{Z_L + Z_R} = \frac{Z_W}{Z_B + Z_W} . \qquad (6.26)$$

It is instructive to revisit the four cases described by Figure 6.8 and Table 6.2 at resonance. For the first case (a), in which the backing is air and the front (right) load is matched, AL = 1; however, this occurs only over a small frequency range. For case (b), in which the loads are matched to the piezoelectric, $Z_L = Z_C = Z_R$ and AL = 0.5; half the power goes in each direction. If $Z_R = Z_W$ for tissue or water and the backing is matched to the crystal, $Z_L = Z_C$, the acoustic loss is inefficient, AL = 0.042 for case (d). In case (c), the loads are reversed and AL = 0.958. This last combination looks like it has potential. A short pulse is obtained for the matched case on both sides, but half the power is lost in the process. In summary, from a combined time and frequency perspective, a reasonably short pulse and high forward efficiency can be realized in practice by acoustically matching the forward direction, as explained next, and by using a low-impedance backing. For example, with a matching layer the piezoelectric "sees" an effective forward load of $Z_C$, and with $Z_2 = 6$ Mrayls, the acoustic loss can be raised to a value of AL = 0.85.

### 6.5.2.2. Matching Layers

To alleviate the typical acoustic impedance mismatch between the high impedance of a piezoelectric material and the low impedance of tissue, one or more matching layers are employed. The concept of an acoustic transformer comes from a curious characteristic of transmission lines that are used to represent acoustic layers. The input impedance $Z_1$ of a quarter-wavelength long acoustic transmission line of characteristic impedance $Z_0$ and load $Z_2$ is

$$Z_1 = Z_0^2/Z_2. \qquad (6.27a)$$

This result explains how an acoustic layer can present an impedance of $Z_1$ while loaded with a different impedance, $Z_2$. The matching layer value, $Z_0$, needed to achieve this impedance transformation is (equation 6.27a rearranged)

$$Z_{ml} = \sqrt{Z_1 Z_2}. \qquad (6.27b)$$

As discussed previously, the use of a matching layer appeared to be most effective for combining reasonably short pulse length with minimal acoustical loss or high forward acoustic power efficiency. Note that acoustic loss (or transducer or electrical loss) is often expressed in decibels (dB) as

$$AL_{dB} = 10\log_{10}(AL), \qquad (6.28)$$

so that a desired value of loss of 1 is 0 dB (no loss). To achieve the case (d) situation, but with a low acoustic loss, the needed matched forward impedance, $Z_R$, can be realized by, for example, a matching layer (ML) value of

$$Z_{ml} = \sqrt{Z_1 Z_2} = \sqrt{34 * 1.5} = 7.14 \text{Mrayls}. \qquad (6.29)$$

Use of a matching layer has an additional benefit of widening the overall spectrum. More matching layers increase bandwidth further, while still achieving impedance matching (Szabo, 2004).

In summary, by envisioning the overall transducer loss as a product of electrical and acoustical losses, each type of loss can be evaluated and reduced by electrical or acoustical matching to optimize transducer power efficiency to the acoustic load. In practice, the two losses are interrelated so that design is more challenging and improving efficiency must be balanced between obtaining good bandwidth and short pulse length.

### 6.5.3. PERFORMANCE CRITERIA

Primary performance criteria for transducers are based on round-trip characteristics, as illustrated in Figures 6.16 and 6.17. Insertion loss measurements, as practically implemented, are performed with a load equal to the source impedance, $R_f = R_g$ in Figure 6.14(a), usually a value of 50 ohms. This condition is equivalent to referencing the measured power with the transducer inserted to the maximum power available from the source. Another often used performance measure is the overall round-trip voltage transfer function. An overall transducer simulation can be constructed from the product of a chain of ABCD matrices representing electrical matching and transduction transfer functions and an acoustic lens, as shown in Figure 6.13 (Szabo, 2004).

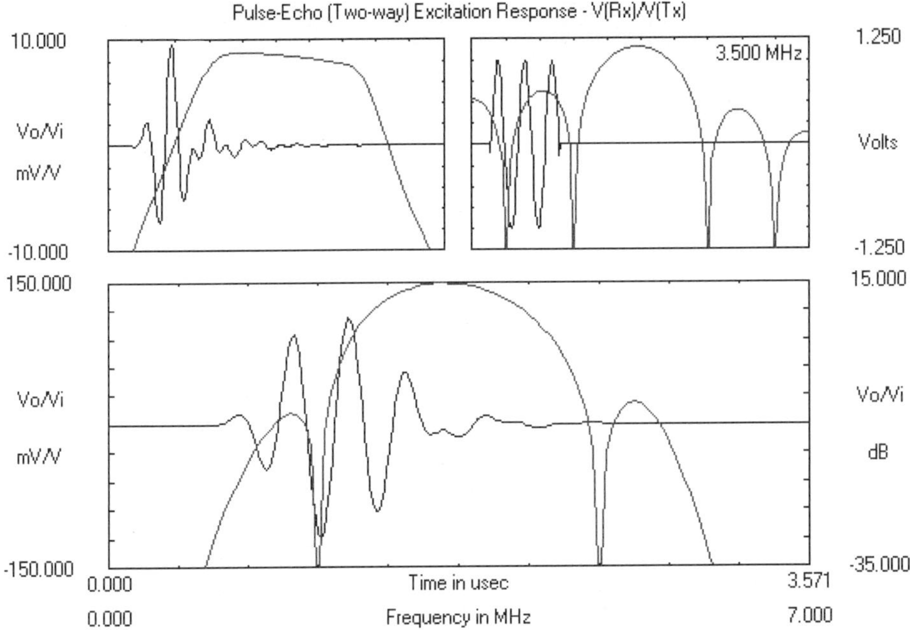


**Figure 6.16.** (top left) Pulse echo impulse response and spectrum for a 3.5 MHz linear array design. (top right) 3.5 MHz, 2.5 cycle sinusoid excitation pulse and spectrum. (bottom) Resultant output pulse and spectrum. All calculations were made using the by PiezoCAD transducer design program. (Courtesy of G. Keilman, Sonic Concepts.)

Both insertion loss and this transfer function are measured from a pulse echo signal from a known reflector (usually flat) positioned at the focal length of the transducer. Corrections may have to be made for diffraction effects, as discussed in section 6.8. Spectral data can then be compared with insertion loss predictions. A typical simulation for this case is shown in Figure 6.16. In the upper-left panel, the voltage transfer function versus frequency is simultaneously displayed with the impulse response of the transducer, the time response counterpart of the transfer function. Typically transducers are driven by a selected pulse drive such as the 2.5 cycle, 3.5 MHz pulse in the upper-right panel of Figure 6.16 and its associated spectrum. The overall responses to the 3.5 MHz driving pulse (upper-right panel) are shown in the lower panel. Note that the final spectrum is the product of the two spectra above.

The overall relation between the responses is depicted in Figure 6.16. In the frequency domain the voltage transfer functions can be multiplied as

$$V_0/V_i(f) = [V_f/V_g(f)]P(f), \qquad (6.30)$$

where the output voltage over input voltage transfer ratio $(V_0/V_i)$ is the product of the transducer transfer ratio $(V_f/V_g(f))$ and the drive pulse spectrum $(P(f))$. In the time domain counterpart of equation 6.30, the output waveform is the time convolution of the impulse response of the transducer and the drive pulse $P(t)$,

$$V_0/V_i(t) = [V_f/V_g(t)] * P(t), \qquad (6.31)$$

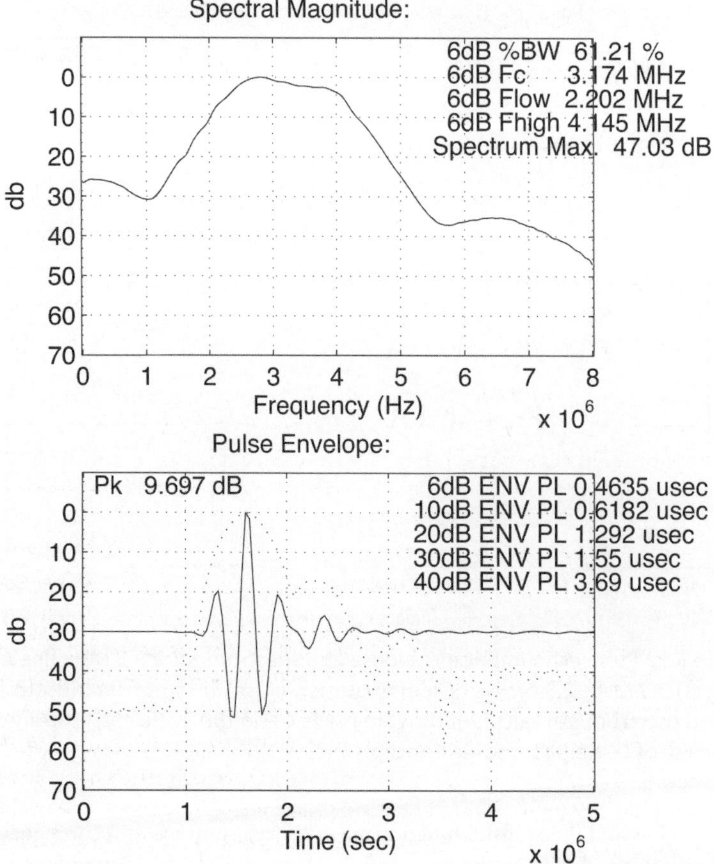



**Figure 6.17.** (top) Transducer response spectral magnitude and a –6 dB bandwidth. (bottom) Transducer impulse response and its envelope measured in pulse lengths (PLs) in dB.

in which $V_0/V_i(t)$ is the inverse Fourier transform of the overall transfer function and $V_f/V_g(t)$ is the transducer impulse function.

Measures of performance are usually given in widths on a dB scale, as depicted in Figure 6.17. For example, bandwidth is the half power or –6 dB width below the peak value of the round-trip transducer spectral magnitude (transfer function or insertion loss). A –6 dB center frequency is defined as the mean frequency value between the two frequencies at which the –6 dB points occur:

$$f_c = (f_{high} - f_{low})/2. \tag{6.32}$$

The time response can also be quantified by determining various dB widths below the peak pulse envelope value, such as –6, –10, and –20 dB PLs. The shortness of the lower dB lengths indicates a steep, well-defined, short pulse with low-amplitude trailing time sidelobes needed for unambiguous resolution of small pulse echo targets.

## 6.6. TRANSDUCER CONSTRUCTION

### 6.6.1. SINGLE-ELEMENT TRANSDUCERS

The construction of transducers falls into two major categories: single-element and arrays. The construction of a typical single-element transducer is illustrated in Figure 6.18. The piezoelectric element, backing, matching layer, and lens are identifiable. If a lens is not included, the surface of the transducer can be formed into a shape appropriate for focusing (discussed later), such as a spherical surface. Because of their relatively large area, electrical matching is much easier for single-element transducers than for array elements.

### 6.6.2. ARRAYS

An array is a configuration of individually addressable transducers (called elements) usually mounted on a common base in a geometric arrangement. A typical arrangement is depicted by Figures 6.19 and 6.20. While the individual elements contain the same stack of materials found in the bigger single-element versions, the geometry is more critical in their performance. The plane containing the cross section of the array (shown as the shaded part of the array in Fig. 6.19) is parallel to the imaging or azimuth plane. In this view, the width of each element, $w$, and its period, $p$, are shown. The elements are rectangular parallelepipeds usually mounted on a backing. The length dimension of an element, $L$ (or $L_y$ in Fig. 6.20), lies in the orthogonal plane (containing $d$ and $L$), called the elevation plane.

The resonant frequencies of a piezoelectric element are strongly dependent on the direction of poling (described in the next section) and its geometry. As the dimensions of the element along the three orthogonal directions approach each other, intercoupling among resonant modes increases. Extreme cases include those in which dimensions (usually in the plane orthogonal to the poling direction) are far different than in the intended direction of vibration, thus shifting the unwanted resonant frequencies out of band. For example, the lateral dimension of the piezoelectric of a typical single-element transducer is much greater than the thickness, so the thickness piezoelectric coupling coefficient, $k_T$, is

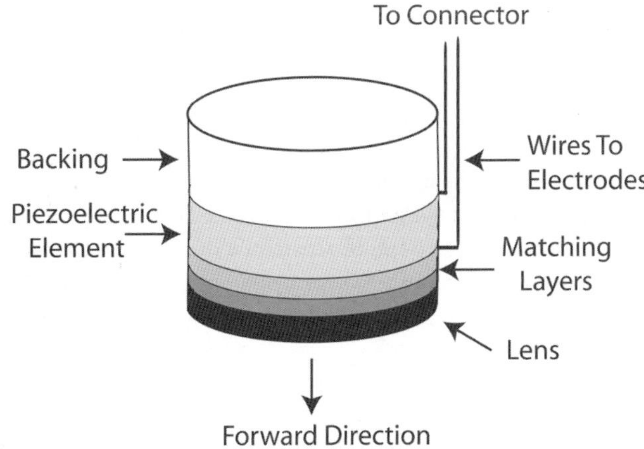



**Figure 6.18.** Construction of a single-element transducer showing layers.

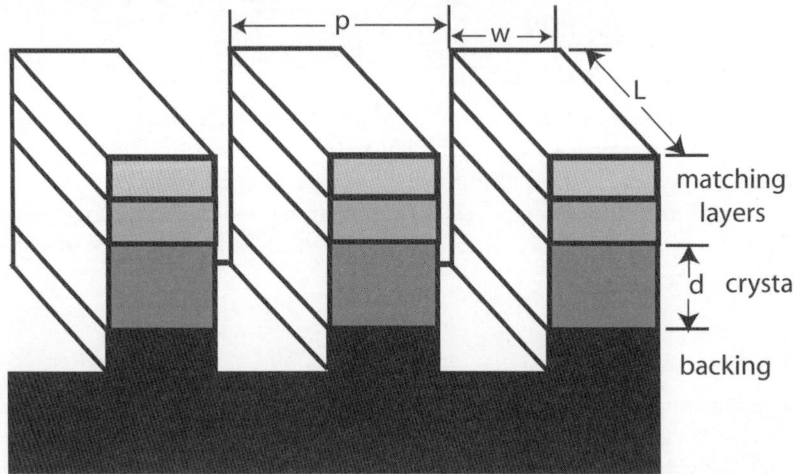

**Figure 6.19.** Construction of a 1-D array showing layers, backing, and dimensions of the elements.

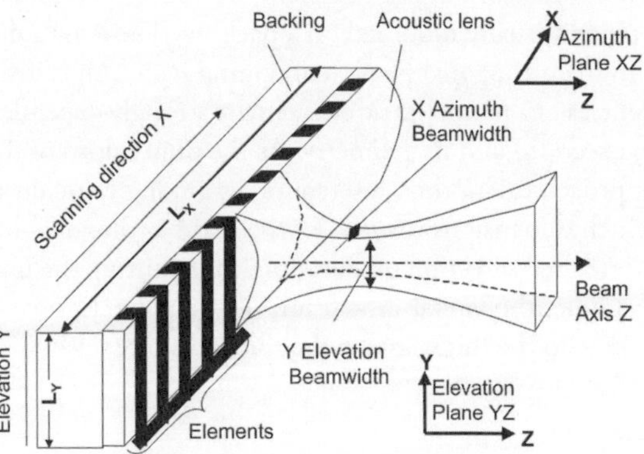


**Figure 6.20.** A 1-D phased array in both the azimuth and elevation planes showing focusing of the beam.

appropriate. Another extreme case is the bar mode where the lateral dimensions are much smaller than the resonant bar length dimension, resulting in a coupling constant, $k_{33}$.

In the case of an array element, the coupling is dependent on the geometry, especially the width-to-thickness ratio, $w/d$. As long as this ratio is kept below approximately 0.7, the beam mode and corresponding coupling constant, $k_{33}'$, provide a surprisingly larger coupling than the thickness mode. For example, for a typical piezoelectric ceramic, $k_T = 0.5$ and $k_{33}' = 0.7$. A final consideration in array design is overall array element size in terms of the area $A$ and thickness $d$ that determine the capacitance, as in equation 6.6. Recall that the radiation resistance is inversely proportional to the capacitance (see equation 6.23), which in turn determines the radiation resistance of an element. The small areas involved (a typical 5 MHz array element is 1.5 mm$^2$) result in large values of radiation resistance, and consequently, a considerable electrical mismatch (see equation 6.25b). These considerations lead to a discussion of what materials are most suitable for medical imaging arrays.

## 6.7. PIEZOELECTRIC MATERIALS

### 6.7.1. DIPOLES

Piezoelectric ferroelectric materials are full of electric dipoles in domains that, if aligned, can be manipulated either by electric fields or by the application of mechanical forces (Safari, Panda, & Janas, 1996). These dipoles, which carry opposite-sign charges on their ends, and their domains are initially randomly oriented. A special property of these piezoelectric materials is that under the application of a high electric field and elevated temperature, the process of poling occurs, where dipole domains align and stay that way semipermanently for a decade or more. Once in this polarized state, the material responds by expanding and contracting depending on the sign of the applied voltage on its electrodes, and reciprocally, produces charges on its electrodes if the material is compressed or stretched. Piezoelectric materials vary in their ability to respond to outside stimuli and in their electrical and acoustical characteristics. These characteristics are summarized in Table 6.3 and described in the following sections.

### 6.7.2. TYPES OF MATERIALS

#### 6.7.2.1. Piezoceramics

Piezoelectric ceramics are polycrystalline and have reasonably high coupling because most of their dipole domains align under poling, as indicated by the left side of Figure 6.21. These ceramics, such as lead-zirconate-titanate (PZT),[1] provide a family of options with high coupling, a high dielectric constant, low cost, and stability, as long as temperature is kept below the Curie temperature of the material. A drawback of these piezoceramics is their relatively high acoustic impedance (30 Mrayls or higher), but this impedance mismatch with soft tissues can be alleviated by intermediary matching layers. These materials and their variants and improved versions have been the most popular piezoelectric materials.

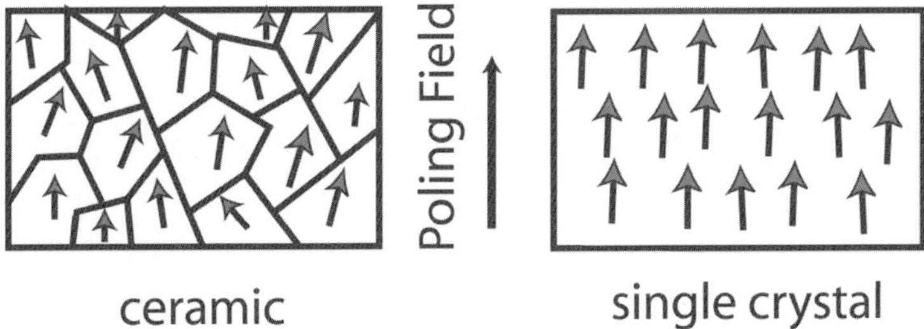


**Figure 6.21.** (left) Poled domains in a poled polycrystalline ferroelectric. (right) Highly aligned dipoles in a domain-engineered, poled single crystal ferroelectric.

---

1    Trademark, Vernitron Piezoelectric Division.

**Table 6.3.** Piezoelectric materials

| Material | $\rho$ $10^3$ kg m$^{-3}$ | $\varepsilon_{330}^{s}/\varepsilon$ | $k_T$ | $c_{TL}$ km s$^{-1}$ | $z_L$ mr | $k_{33}'$ | $c_{33L}'$ km s$^{-1}$ | $z_{33}'$ mr | $k_{33}$ | $c_{33L}$ km s$^{-1}$ | $z_{33}$ mr |
|---|---|---|---|---|---|---|---|---|---|---|---|
| PZT-5A | 7.75 | 830 | .49 | 4.350 | 33.71 | .66 | 3.227 | 25.01 | .705 | 3.693 | 28.62 |
| PZT-5H | 7.50 | 1470 | .50 | 4.560 | 34.31 | .70 | 3.800 | 29 | .75 | | |
| LiNbO$_3$ | 4.64 | 39 | .49 | 7.36 | 34.2 | | | | | | |
| Quartz | 2.65 | 4.5 | .093 | 5.0 | 13.3 | | | | | | |
| PVDF | 1.78 | 12 | .11 | 2.2 | 3.92 | | | | | | |
| PMN-PT | 8.06 | 680 | .64 | 4.646 | 37.45 | .9066 | 3.057 | 24.64 | .94 | 3.343 | 26.94 |
| PZN-PT | 8.31 | 1000 | .5 | 4.03 | 33.49 | .878 | 2.624 | 21.81 | .91 | 2.417 | 20.09 |
| Comp A | 6.01 | 376 | .80 | 3.0 | 18.03 | | | | | | |
| Comp B | 4.37 | 622 | .66 | 3.79 | 16.58 | | | | | | |

Sources: Kino, 1987; Park and Shrout, 1997; Ritter et al., 2000.

Note: Comp A is a 1-3 composite with 69% PZN-PT and 31% D-80 filler.

Comp B is a 1-3 composite with 51% Navy-type VI (equivalent to PZT-5H) and 49% D-80 filler.

MR = megarayls. The subscript L is for longitudinal wave; therefore, $c_{TL}$ represents the thickness mode longitudinal sound speed.

### 6.7.2.2. Single Crystals

Single crystal ferroelectrics have highly ordered domains, moderate coupling constants, low dielectric constants, and low losses. While they are useful for high frequencies, their low dielectric constants and need for optical-grade cutting methods make them unsuitable for arrays. Examples are lithium niobate ($LiNbO_3$), lithium tantalate ($LiTaO_3$), and quartz ($SiO_2$).

### 6.7.2.3. Organic Polymers

Piezoelectric organic polymers are soft, plastic-like materials that can be made piezoelectric. These materials have the advantages of conformability and low acoustic impedance. Drawbacks are the very low dielectric constants, high dielectric losses, and relatively weak coupling. Two popular piezo-polymers are polyvinylidene fluoride (PVDF; Kawai, 1969) and copolymer PVDF with triflouroethylene (Ohigashi et al., 1984). Extensive information on these polymers can be found in IEEE (2000).

### 6.7.2.4. Domain-Engineered Single Crystals

The most recent development in piezoelectric materials is the making of domain-engineered single crystals. Through a specialized, elaborate manufacturing process, electric domains can be made to almost perfectly align, as illustrated on the right side of Figure 6.21. The results are an extremely high coupling constant ($\approx 0.9$), moderate dielectric constants, and moderate acoustic impedances. The most common formulations include PZN-PT and PMN-PT in various percentage combinations (Gururaja et al., 1999; Park & Shrout, 1997; Saitoh et al., 1999).

### 6.7.2.5. Complex Ceramics

A new class of complex system piezoelectrics, such as PSMNZT, share similar properties with PZT in terms of bandwidth and acoustic properties. Their advantage of much higher permittivity, $\varepsilon_r^s$, provides significantly improved electrical matching for small elements (Hosono & Yamashita, 2005).

### 6.7.2.6. Composites

Finally, composite materials combine existing piezoelectric materials in a structure meant to improve on the individual properties of the constituent materials. Two common composite architectures are shown in Figure 6.22. In a 1-3–style composite, piezoelectric posts are embedded in a soft matrix material such as epoxy. The posts, because of their slender geometry, have a higher coupling constant than that for a thickness mode vibration, and the overall acoustic impedance is low because these posts make a low volume fraction of the material. Similarly the 2-2 composite combines sheets of piezoelectric with layers of a soft material such as epoxy. The main disadvantages of these composites are a more complicated manufacturing process and an overall lower dielectric constant (Gururaja et al., 1985; Newnham, Skinner, & Cross, 1978; Ritter et al., 2000).

## 6.7.3. COMPARISON OF MATERIALS

Even though for certain circumstances a particular piezoelectric material will have an advantage, is there a way to compare different materials for array applications? Two important characteristics for an array element are broad bandwidth and electrical impedance matching. An assumption is made that acoustical impedance matching with matching layers can improve the acoustic matching for most

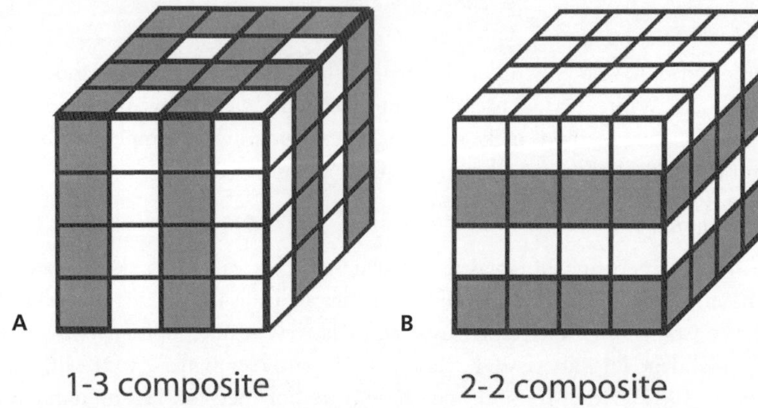



**Figure 6.22.** (a) 1-3 composite structure. (b) 2-2 composite structure. (From Safari et al., 1996.)

piezoelectric materials. For bandwidth, a first-order estimate of one-way –3 dB bandwidth (BW) is related to the electrical $Q$, such that

$$\text{BW} = 1/Q_e = \omega_0 C_0 R_{A0} = \frac{4k^2}{\pi}, \qquad (6.33)$$

in which matching layers are assumed as well as $Z_B << Z_C$ and $k = k_{33}{}'$, the appropriate coupling constant for an array geometry for most materials except $LiNbO_3$ and PVDF, for which $k_T$, the thickness coupling constant, is used. Furthermore the electrical bandwidth is assumed to be much smaller than the acoustic bandwidth from the acoustic loss factor, and therefore dominates. Acoustic radiation resistance is directly proportional to the coupling constant squared and inversely proportional to clamped capacitance or the relative dielectric constant, $\varepsilon_r^s$ according to equation 6.23; thus a figure of merit, the relative impedance factor, $\gamma$, is the relation

$$\gamma = \varepsilon_r^s/(1000k^2). \qquad (6.34)$$

In other words, the larger this figure of merit the better. It serves as a means of comparing the relative electrical impedance of a small array element of a fixed size, with the implication that the smaller the number, the greater the electrical impedance mismatch with the source, which is typically 50 ohms; therefore the electrical loss of equation 6.25 is greater (in terms of dBs). These two figures of merit are plotted in Figure 6.23 for materials with the constants appropriate for a geometry in common use. Composite A is a composite material that uses domain-engineered single crystal PZN-PT (Ritter et al., 2000); composite B is a composite using PZT-5H. Ideally, materials toward the upper-right corner of the graph would be best for array applications. The domain-engineered single crystals and their composites have the advantage based on bandwidth. The PSMNZT material is a standout because of its relative impedance factor. While no single material has high values in both criteria, the most important single criterion is bandwidth, because it affects both the image quality and functionality of the transducer, as described in section 6.10.1. Adequate sensitivity, for example, electrical loss (equation 6.25b), which in turn is proportional to $R_A$ and in turn is proportional to $k^2$ (equation 6.23),

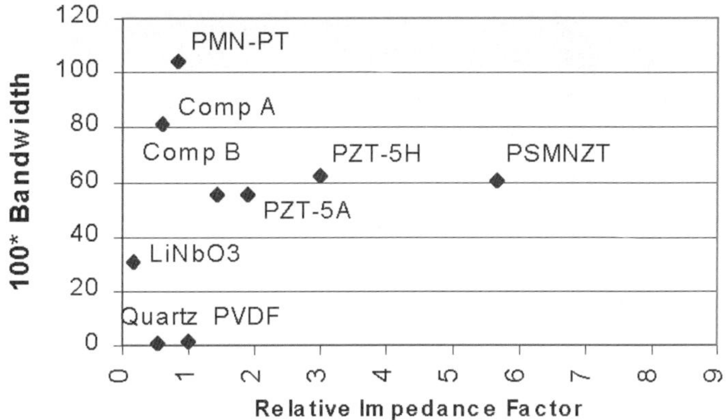


**Figure 6.23.** Estimate of fractional −3 dB bandwidth versus relative impedance factor, $\gamma$, for various piezoelectric materials.

is also a prerequisite to satisfactory performance to receive acoustic pulse echoes that have been attenuated by tissue absorption, which increases with distance and frequency. As discussed in section 6.4.2, reciprocity arguments can be invoked for receive sensitivity to be comparable to transmission efficiency if the receive load is made equal to that of the source impedance.

## 6.8. FOCUSING

### 6.8.1. DIFFRACTION

In order to improve image resolution, arrays have the ability to focus their beams electronically. Because the overall dimensions of transducers are on the order of tens of wavelengths, acoustic waves do not radiate in straight lines, but diffract instead. Diffraction is caused by the radiation of sound waves from different locations on the aperture (transducer face) and the mutual interference of these radiated waves. The result is a complicated pattern such as that shown in Figure 6.24 from a line aperture analogous to a slit in optics.

Two of the most common aperture shapes are the circle and rectangle, shown in Figure 6.25. The circular aperture is most often found in single-element transducers. A slice of the three-dimensional (3-D) beam in a plane is what is usually depicted as a beam plot or beam cross section in graphs in a plane parallel to the aperture plane. For the circular-shaped aperture, because of circular symmetry about the $z$ axis, beam plots in any plane containing the radial dimension and the beam axis, here the $z$ axis, will be identical. For example, at a fixed depth, $z$, a beam profile as a function of the $x$ axis will be the same as one that is along the $y$ axis because of circular symmetry. Most arrays have the shape of a rectangle. For the rectangular aperture, the beam formation differs in the two major planes: the azimuth or scanning plane containing the $x$ and $z$ axes, and the elevation plane, containing the $y$ and $z$ axes (see Fig. 6.20). For example, the beam amplitude described by Figure 6.24 corresponds to an $xz$ plane from a rectangular aperture. In each of these two planes, the rectangular aperture can be represented by a line aperture of length $L$.

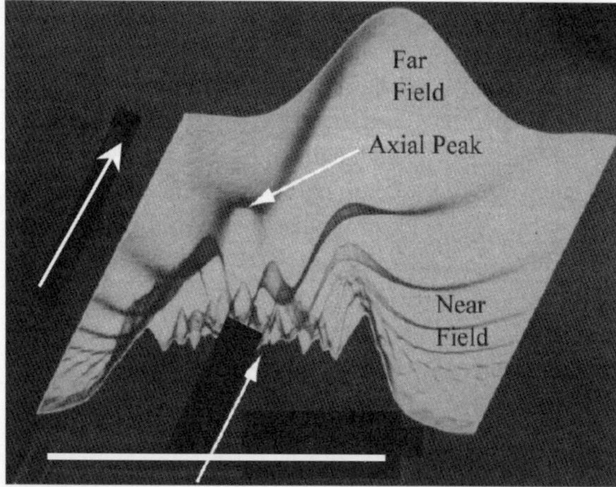



**Figure 6.24.** Diffracted field of a 40 wavelength wide line aperture. The vertical axis is intensity, shown as a gray scale (maximum equals full white). Beam axis is compressed relative to the lateral dimension, and 1920 wavelengths are shown along the propagation axis $z$.

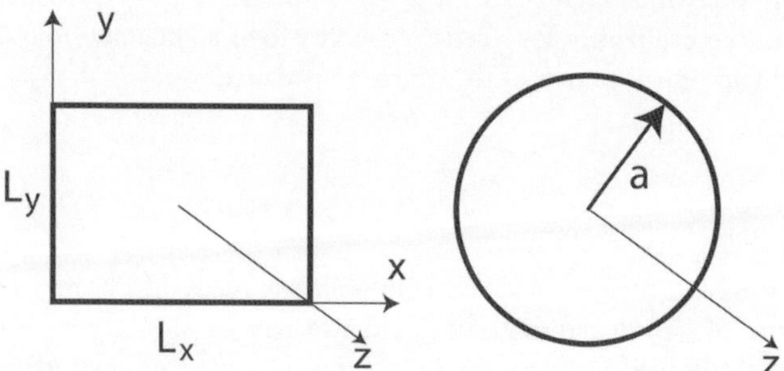



**Figure 6.25.** (left) Rectangular aperture with lengths of $L_x$ parallel to the $x$ axis and $L_y$ parallel to the $y$ axis. The $z$ axis is perpendicular to the $xy$ plane of the aperture. (right) Circular aperture of radius $a$.

Beams, under conditions of continuous wave excitation, have recognizable landmarks, such as the axial peak denoted in Figure 6.24. An unexpected outcome of the radiation from apertures is that there is a region where the beam narrows. The depth where the last axial peak occurs is called the transition distance, $z_t$, or the natural focal length, $F_N$. This transition depth demarcates two regions, one with peaks and valleys, called the near field, and one with a beam with a single peak diminishing in amplitude width and broadening with distance, called the far field, as illustrated in Figure 6.24.

The transition depth for a circular aperture of radius $a$ is

$$z_t = a^2/\lambda.$$ (6.35a)

For a rectangular aperture, the transition distance for a line aperture $L_x$ in the $xz$ plane is

$$z_t \approx L_x^2/(\pi\lambda). \tag{6.35b}$$

The natural focal length is the distance to the last axial peak and is approximately the transition distance.

A cross section of the beam perpendicular to the beam axis is called a beam plot. The –6 dB width at half of the maximum amplitude is called the "full width at half maximum" (FWHM). Beam plots are shown in Figure 6.26.

The far-field beam pattern for a rectangular aperture is the Fourier transform of the amplitude across the aperture. In the case of uniform illumination along a line aperture in the $xz$ plane,

$$A(x_0, 0, 0) = \prod \left( x_0 / L_x \right), \tag{6.36a}$$

where

$$\prod (x / L) = \begin{cases} 0 & |x| > L/2 \\ 1/2 & |x| = L/2 \\ 1 & |x| < L/2 \end{cases}, \tag{6.36b}$$

the far-field pressure pattern $p$ at a field point in the $xz$ plane is a sinc function,

$$p(x, z, f) = \frac{L_x \sqrt{P_0 f}}{\sqrt{c_0 z}} e^{i\pi/4} \frac{\sin\left(\pi L_x x f / c_0 z\right)}{\left(\pi L_x x f / c_0 z\right)} = \frac{L_x \sqrt{P_0}}{\sqrt{\lambda z}} e^{i\pi/4} \mathrm{sinc}\left(\frac{L_x x}{\lambda z}\right), \tag{6.37a}$$

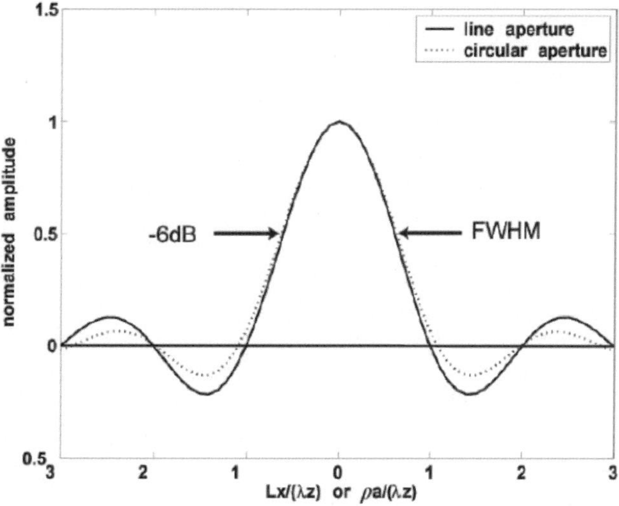


**Figure 6.26.** Far-field jinc beam shape from a circular aperture normalized to maximum value, and far-field sinc function from a square aperture with the same aperture area.

where $p_0$ is pressure on the face of the aperture and $c_0$ is the speed of sound in the propagation medium (tissue or water). A plot of this pattern is shown in Figure 6.26. This equation also applies to the elevation plane if $y$ replaces $x$ and $L_y$ replaces $L_x$. The overall pressure far-field pattern is the product of the $x$ and $y$ far-field contributions.

In the case of a uniform amplitude $p_0$ on a circular aperture of radius $a$, the far-field pressure pattern is the two-dimensional (2-D) Fourier transform of the circularly symmetric aperture function:

$$p(\bar{\rho}, z, \lambda) \approx \frac{jp_0 \pi a^2}{\lambda z} \frac{2J_1(2\pi\bar{\rho}a / (\lambda z))}{2\pi\bar{\rho}a / (\lambda z)} = jp_0 \left( \frac{\pi a^2}{\lambda z} \right) jinc \left( \frac{\bar{\rho}a}{\lambda z} \right), \qquad (6.37b)$$

where $J_1$ is the Bessel function of the first kind and $\bar{\rho}$ is the radial distance to an observation point at $(\bar{\rho}, z)$. A plot of this pattern is also given in Figure 6.26. Note from equation 6.37b that the shapes of the far-field patterns are maintained with distance as their amplitudes decrease and beams broaden with distance.

From these far-field patterns, it is easy to determine the FWHM beamwidths. For the rectangular aperture in the $xz$ or $yz$ plane,

$$\text{FWHM} = 1.206\lambda z/L, \qquad (6.38a)$$

where $L$ is the appropriate line aperture for that plane. Similarly, for a circular aperture,

$$\text{FWHM} = 0.7047\lambda z/a. \qquad (6.38b)$$

Note that the apertures for beam plots in Figure 6.26 were determined by assuming a square aperture with an area equal to that of a circular aperture of radius $a$.

## 6.8.2. FOCUSING PRINCIPLES

In order to narrow the beams even more and at different depths, geometric focusing is applied. Like focusing in optics, acoustic focusing is implemented most often with a type of lens. Unlike optics, both concave and convex converging lenses can be made because materials exist such that their sound speeds are either greater or less than that of surrounding water or tissue (refer to Fig. 6.27). In other words, the index of refraction can be less than one as well as greater than one. Under the principles of ray optics, rays converge at the geometric focal point, $F$. From the reciprocal law of lenses, the overall total focal length is the combined effect of the natural focal length and the geometrical focal length:

$$\frac{1}{F_{total}} = \frac{1}{F_N} + \frac{1}{F} \qquad (6.39)$$

in which $F_N = z_t$. This approximate relationship shows that the location of the axial peak for a focusing aperture is now moved in from the geometrical focal length. For example, if the natural focal length is 100 mm and the geometric focal length is 50 mm, the overall resulting focal length is 33.3 mm.

In the focal plane, the beam pattern is the same shape as that in the far field of an unfocused aperture, like those shown in Figure 6.26. For these shapes, equations 6.37a and 6.37b apply with the substitution $z = F$. Similarly the $-6$ dB beamwidths at the focal plane can also be found from equations 6.38a and 6.38b with $z = F$, and these are biodicated in Figure 6.26. For rectangular apertures, beam shapes are found in either the imaging or azimuth plane or the elevation plane.

These planes are shown for a linear array in Figure 6.20. So far, solid apertures have been described. Arrays can be considered to be spatially sampled apertures. The beams for both a solid and an adequately sampled aperture are similar. Element sampling along the $x$ direction is considered to be adequate when the element period $p_e \leq \lambda/2 = c_0/2f$, or equivalently, greater than or equal to the Nyquist rate; therefore the overall azimuth aperture for $N$ elements is $L_x = Np_e$, where $p_e$ is the element period. Unless the sampling rate is at or above the Nyquist rate at the highest frequency in the transducer signal bandwidth, artifacts known as grating lobes will occur at unintended spatial locations. The 1-D array actually has two types of focusing mechanisms, as depicted in Figure 6.20. The azimuth or scan plane, here the $xz$ plane, is focused electronically, whereas the elevation or $yz$ plane is focused by a fixed mechanical lens and has an aperture $L_y$.

Electronic focusing allows the transmit focal length to be selected by the system user. Note that the depth of field or the range over which resolution is narrow depends on the focal length chosen, as illustrated schematically in Figure 6.27.

On reception, diffraction and focusing principles similar to those for transmission apply. A wavefront from an object intersects a region of the finite active aperture on reception. The phase and amplitude of an incoming wave vary with the spatial location of intersection. One important difference for focusing on reception is that real-time dynamic focusing can be applied. Nearly ideal focusing is achieved by this process at all depths on reception. Real-time dynamic focusing is possible because the delay of returning signals is known, so an appropriate electronic lens can be created at each depth. Steering and focusing of the beam is only possible in the imaging plane. Because the elevation plane has a fixed focus, resolution outside the azimuth plane degrades from the elevation plane focal region. Two-dimensional arrays have recently become commercially available in which nearly 3000 active elements are used to both focus and steer the beam electronically. In this arrangement, the full focusing power of the 2-D array can be varied in both depth and angle. More details can be found in section 6.10.2.

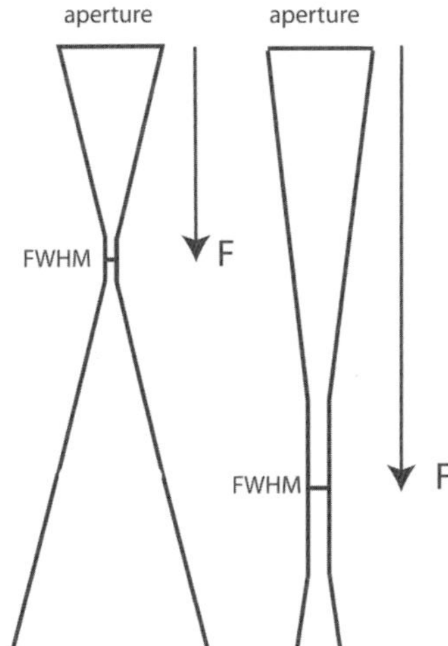


**Figure 6.27.** Schematic showing that doubling the transmit focal length alters the depth of field or the range over which adequate resolution is maintained.

## 6.9. RELATION OF IMAGE FORMATS TO TRANSDUCER TYPES

### 6.9.1. IMAGE FORMATS

In order to perform the scanning function described in the introduction, several geometric arrangements are possible. The two basic scanning movements are translation and rotation. Simple translation is shown in Figure 6.28(a). Here several elements are switched on at one time to form an active aperture. In the center of this aperture a focused beam is sent and pulse echoes are received. An element on one end of the aperture is turned off and a new one on the other end is turned on simultaneously through an electronic switch. The transmission and reception cycle is repeated to form new acoustic lines until the total number of lines required to complete an image frame are produced. Then the process begins anew for the next frame. The number of elements selected for an active aperture are chosen to maintain a consistent resolution with depth. As is apparent from equation 6.38a, this objective is attained when a constant $F$ number equal to $F/L$ is maintained.

In Figure 6.28(b), a similar process is performed on a curved or convex surface. In this approach, the scan lines, instead of pointing straight down, fan out in radial lines. The advantage of this method is that a larger angular coverage is obtained for the same electronic complexity as the linear array. Also, simpler electronics can be used for focusing without steering.

Simple rotation is depicted in Figure 6.28(c). In this configuration the active aperture remains in the center of the array, although the number of elements activated may vary with the focal depth chosen. Scanning is achieved by steering the beam through small angular increments until a sector is swept from right to left (or left to right, depending on the convention chosen) and the lines necessary

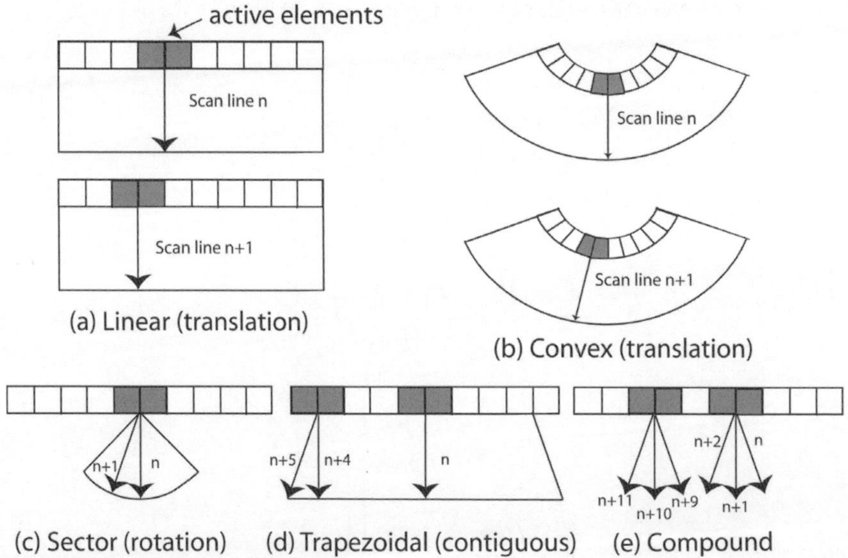


**Figure 6.28.** Time-sequenced image formats: (a) basic linear (translation), (b) convex or curved linear (translation), (c) basic sector (rotation), (d) trapezoidal (contiguous: rotation, translation, and rotation), and (e) compound (translation and rotation at each active aperture position).

for the frame are completed. The advantage of this arrangement is that wide coverage is achieved with a small aperture or "footprint." Transducers employing this scanning method are called phased arrays.

The last two scanning methods are combinations of the basic movements. In the trapezoidal or contiguous sweep of Figure 6.28(d), the ends are rotated with the center filled in with linear or translation scanning. Finally, in compound scanning, shown in Figure 6.28(e), scanning rotation or scanning over a small angular sector is performed at each active aperture position, then the active aperture is translated to a new sequential position.

## 6.9.2. TRANSDUCER TYPES

The types of transducers associated with various scan formats and clinical applications are shown in Figure 6.29. On the left is the positioning assembly, with the associated transesophageal transducer at the top. This phased array is a specialized unit that allows the transducer to be positioned on an articulated arm within the esophagus. Next is a convex array with the radiating surface pointing diagonally upward. This geometry is especially useful for abdominal imaging. To the right is a straight linear array. An image from a linear array can be seen in Figure 6.30, corresponding to the image format in Figure 6.28(a). The same type of array can produce the trapezoidal image of Figure 6.31, as explained in Figure 6.28(d). The T-shaped transducer is a stand-alone continuous wave Doppler transducer that consists of two single-element transducers as a transmitter–receiver pair. Next is a phased array. Compare its small size to the linear array. The small footprint is designed to fit in the intercostal spaces between ribs for cardiac imaging. An image generated by a phased array is shown in Figure 6.32 and corresponds to the image format of Figure 6.28(c). The next transducer is also specialized, a rotating phased array for 3-D image acquisition. Finally, the last transducer on the right is a small, high-frequency intraoperative linear array.

## 6.10. ADVANCED TOPICS

### 6.10.1. MULTIMODE OPERATION

As evident from Figure 6.29, ultrasound medical transducers appear in different forms suitable for various clinical applications. As transducer technology has evolved, especially with improvements in piezoelectric materials and in the manufacturing of high-frequency arrays, transducers have become more capable of performing different functions. In Figure 6.1, a transducer excited by an impulse added its own signature on both transmit and reception, as described by equations 6.30 and 6.31. As shown in Figure 6.16, the received output voltage pulse is dependent on the excitation used. In order to produce different modes, the excitation pulse is changed appropriately. Even though there is not space here to describe all the modes available in diagnostic ultrasound (see Szabo, 2004, for more details), three main modes will be discussed as examples. The first is B-mode, the pervasive gray-scale image that is used most often. In order to have excellent image quality, such as high resolution and subtle tissue texture differentiation, adequate bandwidth is necessary. The second mode is Doppler measurements and imaging, for which only a narrow bandwidth is needed. As the bandwidth of transducers increased, several modes, such as Doppler and B-mode imaging, could be performed with the same transducer by giving each mode a distinct excitation frequency.

With the recent development of domain-engineered single crystal materials, there is enough bandwidth for two or more imaging frequencies within the same overall transducer response. This

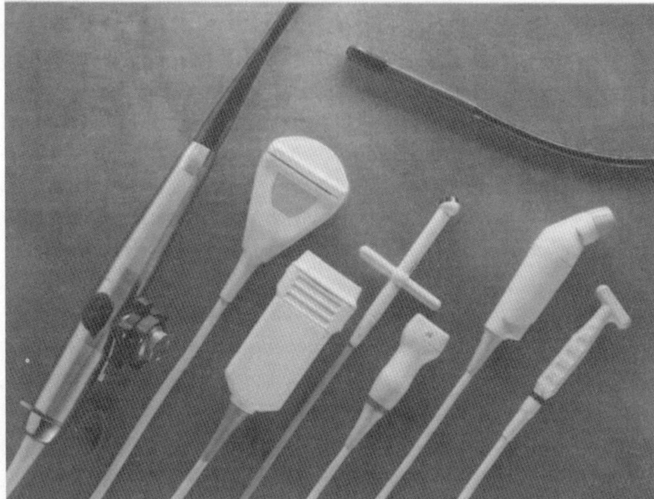

**Figure 6.29.** Transducer family portrait. Groups of array types (clockwise from top left corner): transesophageal phased array with positioning mechanism; convex array; linear array; stand-alone dual single-element continuous wave Doppler probe; phased array; rotating motorized phased array; and high-frequency intraoperative linear array. (Courtesy of Philips Medical Systems.)

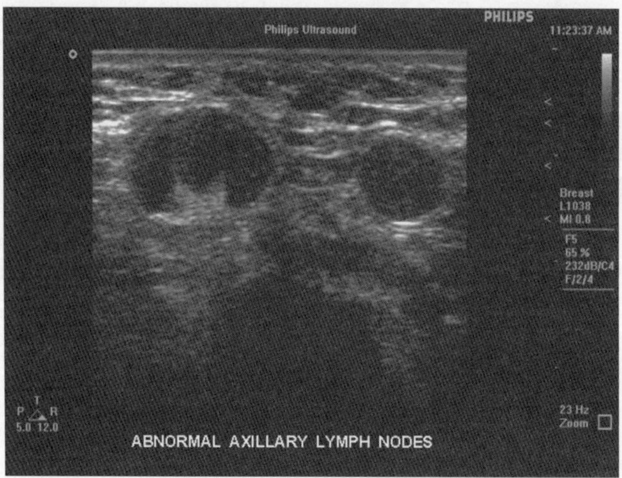


**Figure 6.30.** B-mode image of lymph nodes in the breast at 12 MHz; an example of a linear array format. (Courtesy of Philips Medical Systems.)

capability is shown in Figure 6.33(a) where several overlapping output voltage responses, $V_0/V_i(f_n)$ (see equation 6.30), distinguished by different center frequency pulse excitations, $P(f_n)$, are shown along with the overall transducer voltage transfer function, $V_f/V_g(f)$. What this development means is that a single multimode transducer can replace several narrower bandwidth transducers.

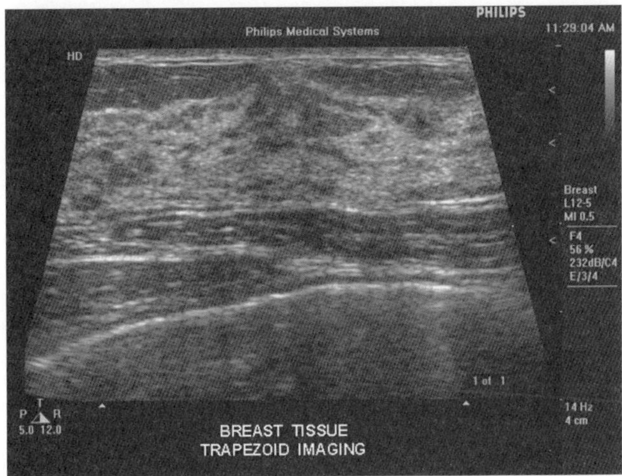



**Figure 6.31.** Trapezoidal format of a linear array with sector steering on either side of a straight rectangular imaging segment. (Courtesy of Philips Medical Systems.)

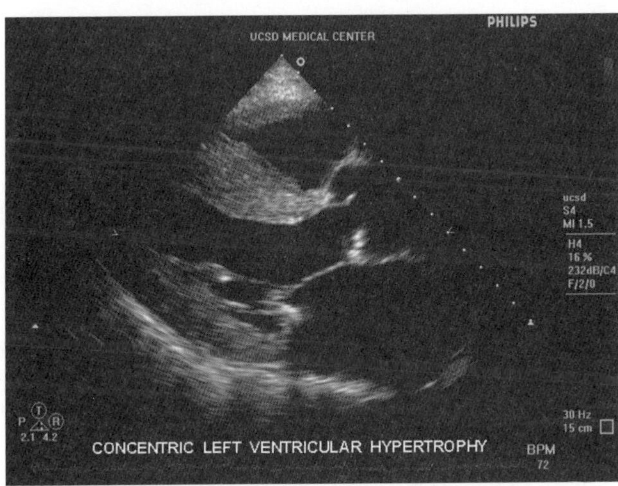



**Figure 6.32.** B-mode image of the heart at 4 MHz; an example of a sector array format. (Courtesy of Philips Medical Systems.)

The third mode, which is also the most demanding for bandwidth, is harmonic imaging. In this mode, the driving pulse is centered at a frequency $f_1$. Harmonic multiples of this frequency are generated by acoustic propagation in tissue, and the second harmonic, $2f_1$, is filtered out on reception for imaging, as illustrated in Figure 6.33(b). Earlier transducers with narrower bandwidths were not able to fully accommodate the full bandwidth of a second harmonic and lost substantial second harmonic signal strength in the high-frequency cutoff skirt of the transducer response.

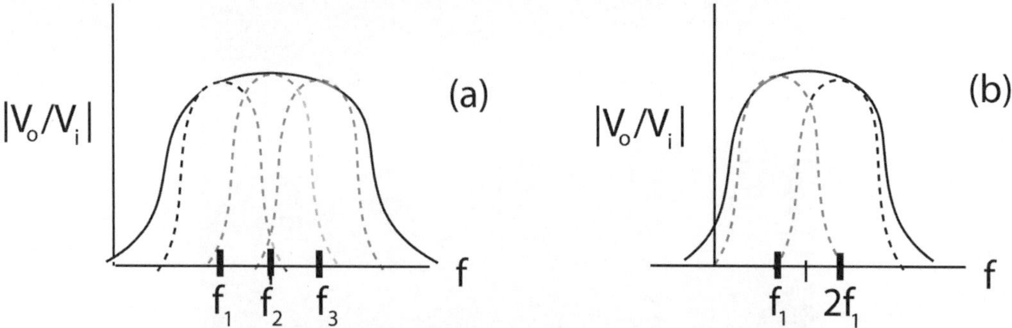

Figure 6.33. (a) Multiband operation depicted by the overall transducer transfer ratio compared to output responses to three different excitation frequencies, $f_n$. (b) Harmonic imaging transmit and receive bands compared to the overall transducer transfer ratio.

The range of transducer center frequencies is expanding. At the lower end, harmonic imaging uses fundamental frequencies of 1 MHz to 2 MHz and up. At the high end, 15 MHz is a typical upper limit, but this is being stretched, as 20 MHz transducer arrays are beginning to appear.

## 6.10.2. TWO-DIMENSIONAL ARRAYS

A major barrier to ultrasound imaging has been broken recently. Until this development, 1-D arrays were limited to $N = 128$ or 256 active channels. The main challenges are threefold. First, the manufacturing of a 2-D array with more than $N^2 > 2500$ individually addressable elements can be a wiring nightmare. Second, the standard method of connecting each element to the imaging system with an individual cable would be expensive and unwieldy (cables are the most costly part of an array). Third, in traditional architectures, an active receiving radio frequency channel is assigned to each element, so if this conventional approach is taken, the system could grow considerably, with corresponding amounts of needed electrical power. For example, a typical beam-forming board may have sixty-four channels, so the imaging system would jump from two boards to about forty.

Two alternatives for 2-D arrays have been realized. The first is a means of connecting to thousands of elements combined with low-power microbeam-forming electronics in the transducer handle. In this scheme, only the normal number of cables (128) are needed to connect to the system (Savord & Solomon, 2003). This approach to real-time 2-D imaging has been commercially implemented. The second type of 2-D array is a capacitive micromachined ultrasound transducer (CMUT), an alternative transduction technology based on existing silicon fabrication methods (Ladabaum et al., 1996). The CMUT is a tiny, sealed, air-filled capacitor. When a bias voltage is applied to this tiny membrane transducer, a stress is developed proportional to the voltage applied squared and the top electrode membrane deflects. The attractiveness of CMUT technology for imaging is their simpler and more flexible fabrication, integration with silicon electronics, high sensitivity, and broad bandwidth. Imaging with CMUT arrays has been demonstrated by Orlakan et al. (1997), Orlakan et al. (2002), and Panda, Daft, and Wagner (2003).

## ACKNOWLEDGMENTS

More in depth coverage of the topics in this chapter can be found in *Diagnostic Ultrasound Imaging: Inside Out*, by T. L. Szabo (Boston: Elsevier, 2004).

## REFERENCES

Berlincourt, D. A., Curran, D. R., & Jaffe, H. (1964). Piezoelectric and piezomagnetic materials and their function in transducers. In W. P. Mason (Ed.), *Physical Acoustics: Vol. 1A*. New York, NY: Academic Press.

Gururaja, T. R., Panda, R. K., Chen, J., & Beck, H. (1999). Single crystal transducers for medical imaging applications. *Proceedings of the IEEE Ultrasonics Symposium, 2*, 969–972.

Gururaja, T. R., Schulze, W. A., Cross, L. E., & Newnham, R. E. (1985). Piezoelectric composite materials for ultrasonic transducer applications. Part 11: Evaluation of ultrasonic medical applications. *IEEE Transactions on Sonics and Ultrasonics, SU-32*(4), 499–513.

Hosono, Y., & Yamashita, Y. (2005). Piezoelectric ceramics with high dielectric constants for ultrasonic medical transducers. *IEEE UFFC, 52*(10), 1823–1828.

IEEE. (2000). *Transactions on Ultrasonics, Ferroelectrics and Frequency Control, 47*(6), 1273–1624.

Kawai, H. (1969), The piezoelectricity of poly(vinylidene fluoride). *Japanese Journal of Applied Physics, 8*, 975–976.

Kino, G. S. (1987). *Acoustic waves: Devices, imaging, and analog signal processing*. Englewood Cliffs, NJ: Prentice-Hall.

Ladabaum, I., Jin, X., Soh, H. T., Pierre, F., Atalar, A., & Khuri-Yakub, B. T. (1996). Microfabricated ultrasonic transducers: Towards robust models and immersion devices. *Proceedings of the 1996 IEEE Ultrasonics Symposium, 1*, 335–338.

Leedom, D. A., Krimholtz, R., & Matthaei, G. L. (1978). Equivalent circuits for transducers having arbitrary even- or odd-symmetry piezoelectric excitation. *IEEE Transactions on Sonics and Ultrasonics, SU-25*, 115–125.

Newnham, R. E., Skinner, D. P., & Cross, L. E. (1978). Connectivity and piezoelectric-pyroelectric composites. *Materials Research Bulletin, 13*, 525–536.

Ohigashi, H., Koga, K., Suzuki, M., Nakanishi, T., Kimura, K., & Hashimoto, N. (1984). Piezoelectric and ferroelectric properties of P (VDF-TrFE) copolymers and their application to ultrasonic transducers. *Ferroelectrics, 60*, 264–276.

Oralkan, O., Jin, X. C., Degertekin, F. L., & Khuri-Yakub, B. T. (1997). Simulation and experimental characterization of a 2-D, 3 MHz capacitive micromachined ultrasonic transducer (CMUT) array element. *Proceedings of the 1997 IEEE Ultrasonics Symposium, 1*, 1141–1144.

Oralkan, O., Ergun, A. S., Johnson, J. A., Karaman, M., Demirci, U., Kaviani, K., . . . & Khuri-Yakub, B. T. (2002). Capacitive micromachined ultrasonic transducers: Next-generation arrays for acoustic imaging? *IEEE Transactions on Ultrasonics, Ferroelectrics, and Frequency Control, 49*, 1596–1610.

Panda, S., Daft, C., & Wagner, C. (2003). Microfabricated ultrasound transducer (CMUT) probes: Imaging advantages over piezoelectric probes. *Ultrasound in Medicine and Biology, 29*(5S), S69.

Park, S.-E., & Shrout, T. R. (1997). Characteristics of relaxor-based piezoelectric single crystals for ultrasonic transducers. *IEEE Transactions on Ultrasonics, Ferroelectrics, and Frequency Control, 44*, 1140–1147.

Redwood, M. (1963). A study of waveforms in the generation and detection of short ultrasonic pulses. *Applied Materials Research, 2*, 76–84.

Ritter, T., Geng, X., Shung, K. K., Lopath, P. D., Park, S.-E., & Shrout, T. R. (2000). Single crystal PZN/PT-polymer composites for ultrasound transducer applications. *IEEE Transactions on Ultrasonics, Ferroelectrics, and Frequency Control, 47*, 792–800.

Safari, A., Panda, R. K., & Janas, V. F. (1996). Ferroelectricity: Materials, characteristics, and applications. *Key Engineering Materials, 122–124*, 35–70.

Saitoh, S., Takeuchi, T., Kobayashi, T., Harada, K., Shimanuki, S., & Yamashita, Y. (1999). A 3.7 MHz phased array probe using $0.91Pb(Zn_{1/3}Nb_{2/3})O_3$–$0.09PbTiO_3$ single crystal. *IEEE Transactions on Ultrasonics, Ferroelectrics, and Frequency Control, 46*, 414–421.

Savord, B., & Solomon, R. (2003). Fully sampled matrix transducer for real time 3D ultrasonic imaging. *Proceedings of the 2003 IEEE Ultrasonics Symposium, 1*, 945–953.

Szabo, T. L. (2004). *Diagnostic ultrasound imaging: Inside out.* Boston, MA: Elsevier Academic.

## ABOUT THE AUTHOR

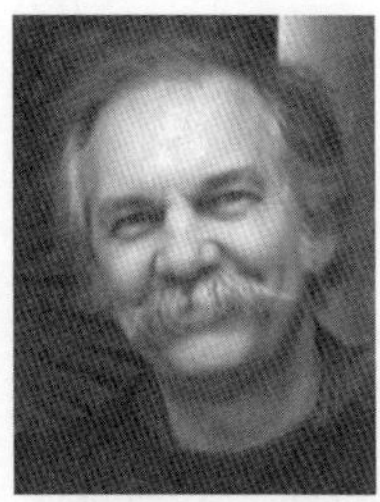

**Professor Thomas L. Szabo**, BS, MS, PhD has over forty years' acoustics research experience in government, industrial, and academic laboratories. From 1970 to 1981, he conducted research on signal processing acoustic devices at Air Force Cambridge Research Labs, later part of Rome Air Development Center. From 1979 through 1980, he was at Oxford University, United Kingdom, developing acoustic imaging for locating faults in coal seams. He joined Hewlett Packard in 1981 to develop ultrasonic imaging systems. Since 2001, he has been a research professor at Boston University in the Biomedical Engineering and Aerospace and Mechanical Engineering Departments exploring multimodal imaging and new applications of ultrasound. His publications include over eighty papers, four book chapters, and a book on ultrasound imaging. Among his awards are the 1973 Best Paper in IEEE Transactions on Sonics and Ultrasonics, a U.S. Meritorious Service Medal, and a Hewlett Packard Fellowship. He is a fellow of the Acoustical Society of America and the American Institute of Ultrasound in Medicine and a senior life member of the IEEE.

# CHAPTER 7

# CHEMICAL SENSORS FOR BIOMEDICAL APPLICATIONS

Gábor Harsányi

*Department of Electronics Technology*
*Budapest University of Technology and Economics*
*Budapest, Hungary*

## 7.1. INTRODUCTION

The largest group of chemical sensors for measuring concentrations of various analytes in biomedicine are applied for in vivo or ex vivo monitoring of blood components, such as the partial pressure of dissolved oxygen and carbon dioxide ($pO_2$ and $pCO_2$, respectively), pH, and the concentration of ionic compounds. The oxygen saturation of blood hemoglobin is monitored by physical sensors (photosensors) using the methods of oximetry, which is different from dissolved blood oxygen measurements. Although the majority of sensors are applied to blood analysis, their use in monitoring secretions (e.g., gastric acid, sweat, etc.) is becoming progressively more important. Gas sensors are also applied to the monitoring of inhaled and exhaled breath, in addition to their use in anesthesia. Humidity sensors may have very specialized applications, such as transepidermal water loss measurement. Beyond the following descriptions, further details about chemical sensors applied in biomedicine can be found in the literature (Diamond, 1998; Fraser, 1997; Göpel et al., 1991; Harsányi, 2000; Spichiger-Keller, 1998).

## 7.2. ELECTROCHEMICAL SENSORS FOR GASES AND IONS

### 7.2.1. ELECTROCHEMICAL SENSOR PRINCIPLES

Electrochemical cells are commonly used as sensors for the measurement of chemical quantities, typically ion or gas-molecule concentrations in different media. They also have wide applications in biomedical areas. In its simplest form, an electrochemical cell consists of a minimum of two electrodes with an ionic conductive material, called an electrolyte, situated between them. In practice, however, the sensor element itself is often only a part of a complete sensor unit. Accordingly, the following cases can be distinguished:

- The sensor element is the whole electrochemical cell and is isolated from the environment by, for example, a semipermeable membrane.
- The sensor consists of two electrodes, and the electrolyte between them is the actual analyte.
- The sensor element is a single electrode (the counterelectrode serves only for practical measurement purposes; see section 7.2.1.2).

Electrochemical cell sensors can be classified into three main categories according to the characteristics of the electrode reaction:

- Type A is characterized by direct participation of the mobile ions that are originally present in the electrolyte.
- Type B cells use the electrolytes as "solvents" for the charged products formed by reduction–oxidation (redox) reactions from neutral molecules that are present in the electrolyte or in the surrounding medium.
- Type C cells are characterized by competing or several-step electrode reactions.

Electrochemical sensors are based upon potentiometric, amperometric (more generally, voltammetric), or conductivity measurements. These different principles require specific designs for electrochemical cells. The operation of the sensors is based on reactions and their equilibria at the interfaces between electronic and ionic conductors on the electrode surfaces. Sometimes, transient behavior may also be applied for analytical purposes. These operating and measurement principles are summarized in the following sections according to the types listed previously.

### 7.2.1.1. Potentiometric Sensors for Ions

In potentiometric sensors, the potential difference between the reference electrode and the working electrode is measured without polarizing the electrochemical cell, which mandates only a very small allowed current. Thus the equilibrium electrode potential difference can be monitored, and this is given by the Nernst–Nicolsky–Eisenman equation (Sudhölter et al., 1989):

$$E = E_0 + \frac{R \cdot T}{z_i \cdot F} \cdot \ln\left[ a_i + \sum_j S_{ij} \cdot (a_j)^{z_i/z_j} \right], \tag{7.1}$$

where $E_0$ is the standard electrode potential of the sensor electrode; $a_i$ is the activity of the primary ion; $a_j$ is the activity of the interfering ions; $S_{ij}$ is the selectivity coefficient of the primary ion over the interfering ions; $R$ is the universal gas constant; $T$ is the absolute temperature; $F$ is the Faraday constant; $z_i$ is the valence of the primary ion; and $z_j$ is the valence for the interfering ion. The ion activity is generally approximated as a simple linear function of the concentration:

$$a_i = k_i c_i \ (k_i < 1), \tag{7.2}$$

where $k_i$ is the activity coefficient of the particular ion.

In the case of ideal ion selective electrodes (ISEs), the selectivity or cross-sensitivity constants ($S_{ij}$) can be neglected. In practice, however, they must be taken into consideration.

Conventional electrodes use generally metal, metal–salt, or metal–electrolyte–glass structures. Recently, for ISE purposes, another generation of electrodes—the membrane electrodes—is also used. These contain an internal reference electrode and an internal reference electrolyte in an isolation tube, which is closed by an ion-selective membrane that is generally a special polymer material. One side of the membrane is in contact with the analyte solution to be probed. The polymer–sample solution interactions can be divided into the following groups:

- The membrane contains active grains or ionic sites (called ionophores) that are the basis of ion exchange and complexion within the membrane. By reversible exchange of the ions between the analyte solution and the membrane phase or by a reversible penetration of the ions accompanied by the complexion process, a membrane charged double layer and a potential will be developed, which can be described by the Nernst equation. Recently sensor electrodes with nonionic grains, so-called neutral charge carriers, have been preferentially used for complexion processes with ions of the analyte.
- A surface charge and potential shift may also be developed by the sorption of ions onto the membrane surface. The process is typified by the adsorption of $H^+$ ions onto the surface of a glass electrode with a special composition that causes pH-dependent electrode potential variations. Glass electrodes are used as pH sensors.

In a conventional liquid junction ion-selective electrode, a reversible ion or electron transport mechanism is present not only at the membrane–analyte solution interface, but also at every phase boundary, resulting in well-defined interfacial potentials. Electrodes of this type usually exhibit little potentiometric drift, but the evaporation of water alters the electrolyte composition, causing problems with long-term stability.

Various other types of ion sensors have also been developed in which ion-selective polymeric membranes are deposited directly onto solid electrode surfaces with no internal electrolyte solution. This is called a solid-contact ISE, and is similar to a coated-wire electrode. Often, in this type of ISE, the membrane–solid interface is ill defined, leading to significant potentiometric drifts. A stable and reversible transition from electronic conductivity in the metal electrode to ionic conductivity in the polymeric membrane can be maintained by using double-membrane structures. Polymer electrolytes or hydrogel buffers are generally combined with permselective or ion-selective membranes. The mechanisms responsible for such improvements are still the subject of debate. Both adhesion and reaction mechanisms may influence the behavior of the electrodes.

In connection with potentiometric sensors, the role and nature of reference electrodes should also be clarified. These are so-called electrodes of the second class, that is, the metal electrode is covered by its solid salt and by a saturated solution of that salt. Their electrode potential is rather independent of the current density, thus it can be treated as a constant. Typical is the silver/silver chloride (Ag/AgCl) electrode, a silver wire coated by its chloride within a saturated potassium chloride (KCl) solution. Actually it is a chloride-sensitive electrode surrounded by a constant concentration solution.

### 7.2.1.2. Amperometric Sensors for Dissolved Gases

Amperometry is a method of electrochemical analysis in which the signal of interest is a current that is linearly dependent upon the concentration of an analyte. As the neutral chemical species (e.g., dissolved gas molecules) approach the working (or sensing) electrode, electrons are transferred from the analyte to the working electrode or to the analyte from the electrode. The direction of electron flow depends upon the properties of the analyte and can be controlled by the electric potential applied to the working electrode. To maintain charge neutrality within the sample, a counterreaction occurs at a second electrode, the counterelectrode. If a constant potential difference is maintained by the external circuit, a continuous current flow can be measured. Linear current versus ion concentration characteristics can be obtained by amperometry in diffusion-controlled processes via the so-called limiting current operating mode, where a plateau in the current–voltage characteristics is reached. Diffusion control can occur at several interfaces in the electrochemical cell:

- Diffusion of ions from the electrolyte to the surface of the electrode is used in the analytical method called polarography. Applying the Fick law of diffusion and the Faraday law for charge transfer, it can be easily shown that the current density, $i$, is proportional to the concentration, $c$, of the active component in the electrolyte:

$$i = \text{constant} \times c. \tag{7.3.a}$$

- Diffusion will also control the charge transfer process when particle flow limiting membranes are used on the surface of the electrolyte. This phenomenon is the basis of concentration measurements in the Clark-type oxygen sensors (Clark, 1956). The current density is proportional to the partial pressure of the dissolved gas analyte:

$$i = \text{constant} \times p. \tag{7.3.b}$$

- Particle flow limiting membranes can also be used on the surface of electrodes or within the electrolyte.

Setting the operating mode of the sensor in the limiting current region and keeping the voltage at a constant value, a current proportional to the concentration can be measured. To guarantee the constant potential difference between the working and counterelectrodes is independent from the current that polarizes the electrodes, the application of a potentiostat and a reference electrode is often necessary. The function of the potentiostat is to set the electrode potential of the working electrode always to a given value with respect to the reference electrode. The electrode potential of the reference electrode is independent of the current flowing through the cell, and it is also inert to the analyte to be examined.

### 7.2.1.3. Voltammetric Sensing Principle

The amperometric method is a special case of voltammetric measurement where the whole potential–current diagram is used for the analysis. Generally the potential of the working electrode, controlled by a potentiostat, is changed continuously with a constant scan rate. Any reaction at the electrode surface can usually be detected as a current superimposed on the base current due to double-layer charging. Thus, in these voltammograms, current peaks can be observed. The peak potential values can be used for qualitative analysis, and the height of the peaks is a function of analyte concentration. The structure of voltammetric sensors is generally the same as that of amperometric sensors and they are normally fabricated with reference, auxiliary, and working electrodes.

### 7.2.1.4. Conductimetric Sensors

These are based on the measurement of electrolyte conductivity, which varies when the cell is exposed to different environments. The sensing effect is based on the change in the number of mobile charge carriers in the electrolyte. If the electrodes are prevented from polarizing, the electrolyte shows ohmic behavior. Conductivity measurements are generally performed with an alternating current (AC) supply. As a first approximation, the conductivity ($\sigma$) can be expressed as

$$\sigma = \Sigma \mu_i z_i c_i e, \tag{7.4}$$

where $e$ is the elementary electric charge, $\mu_i$ is the mobility, $z_i$ is the valency, and $c_i$ is the volume number of ionic carriers in the electrolyte. Accordingly, the conductivity is a linear function of the ion concentration, thus it can be used for sensor applications. However, it is nonspecific for a given ion type, and both polarization and the limiting current operation mode must be avoided. For these reasons, small-amplitude alternating bias is used for the measurements with frequencies at which capacitive coupling is still not a factor in determining the impedance measurement.

All electrochemical sensor and measurement types discussed previously are based on equilibrium or stationary process stages. This is their main disadvantage: the response time is rather long and may be comparable to the time constants of the variations within the medium under observation. Another disturbing circumstance might be that long-lasting electrochemical processes at the electrode surfaces might alter the composition of an analyte present in small volumes. In such cases, techniques that are based on equilibrium stages cannot be applied because the equilibrium stage can never be reached.

Further details about electrochemical sensors can be found in the literature (Harsányi, 1995b, 2000).

### 7.2.1.5. Principles of pH, $pO_2$, and $pCO_2$ Sensors

The structures and operating principles of electrochemical pH, $pO_2$, and $pCO_2$ sensors suitable for biomedical use can be briefly summarized as follows:

For pH, ion-sensitive potentiometric glass and polymer-membrane electrodes are used. The basis of a pH-dependent Nernstian electrode potential measurable on these electrodes is selective and reversible $H^+$ ion adsorption onto special-composition glass surfaces, as well as a complex formation with ionophores within polymer membranes, respectively. Metal/metal oxide electrodes can also be used for pH measurements if the electrochemical oxidation of the metal is reversible.

Dissolved oxygen concentration (partial pressure) can be measured by means of a Clark-type amperometric sensor (Clark, 1958), in which the general structure (see Fig. 7.1) contains a reference Ag/AgCl electrode. The cathode is generally made of platinum or gold (but sometimes silver or graphite) and the electrolyte solution usually contains KCl with a buffering agent. The whole electrochemical cell is separated from the sample liquid by a diffusion membrane that is permeable to oxygen, but impermeable to water, ions, proteins, and blood cells. The most commonly used membrane materials are polytetrafluoroethylene (PTFE), polyethylene, and polypropylene. Its operation is based on the cathode reaction. The cathode is usually polarized at about 700 mV with respect to the reference electrode so that the sensor is operating in the diffusion-controlled limiting current region; thus the cell current is theoretically a linear function of the external oxygen concentration (see section 7.2.1.2). According to the reaction model currently accepted, the reduction of dissolved oxygen molecules proceeds via a two-electron pathway with the intermediate formation of hydrogen peroxide ($H_2O_2$):

$$O_2 + 2H_2O + 2e^- \Rightarrow H_2O_2 + 2OH^- \tag{7.5a}$$

$$H_2O_2 + 2e^- \Rightarrow 2OH^-. \tag{7.5b}$$

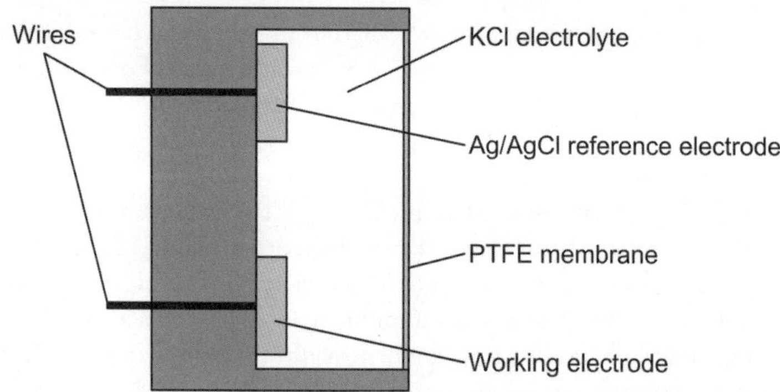


**Figure 7.1.** Schematic structure of the Clark-type oxygen sensor.

For the measurement of $pCO_2$, the Stow–Severinghaus-type potentiometric electrode can be used (Severinghaus & Bradley, 1958). This is a glass pH electrode covered by a membrane freely permeable to carbon dioxide molecules but impermeable to water, hydrogen ions ($H^+$), and bicarbonate ions ($HCO_3^-$). A sodium bicarbonate ($NaHCO_3$) layer is placed between the pH electrode and the membrane. Carbon dioxide molecules diffuse through the membrane to equilibrate with the electrolyte through the following reactions:

$$CO_2 + H_2O \Leftrightarrow H_2CO_3 \Leftrightarrow H^+ + HCO_3^-. \tag{7.6}$$

In equilibrium, the pH value is related to the $pCO_2$ by the equation

$$pH = constant - \log pCO_2. \tag{7.7}$$

Thus the glass electrode measures the external $pCO_2$ indirectly.

Another sensing principle has recently been proposed, based on the revealing of ion formation as described by equation 7.6 (Varlan & Sansen, 1997). This involves a conductimetric sensor in the closed cavity. The advantage is simplicity: only two electrodes are in the closed chamber.

### 7.2.2. SENSORS FOR MONITORING BLOOD GASES AND PH

Arterial blood gas analysis is one of the most frequently requested tests performed on critically ill patients both in the operating room and the intensive care unit. The $pO_2$ and $pCO_2$ in arterial blood, and also the pH, are determined to provide physicians with information about respiratory and metabolic imbalances as reflected by the adequacy of blood oxygenation and $CO_2$ elimination. With frequent measurement of blood gas parameters, the physician can correct these imbalances by adjusting mechanical ventilation, adjusting the ventilation gas composition, or administering pharmacological agents. Blood gas measurements are particularly important in premature (preterm) babies, who are vulnerable to respiratory illnesses because of immaturity of the lungs or inadequately developed mechanisms for the control of breathing. If the arterial $pO_2$ falls to a low level for only a short period of time, brain damage or even death may occur. If, on the other hand, the arterial $pO_2$ becomes too high as a result of the administration of oxygen, damage to the eyes can result and blindness may occur. Moreover, blood vessels in the brain may rupture as a consequence of fluctuations in cerebral blood flow caused partly by changes in $pCO_2$. The third parameter, pH, provides information about the general state of the patient's metabolism.

The technique of individual blood samples provides information at only one point in time, a snapshot of what is happening. However, it is known that large variations in blood gas levels can occur over the course of only a few minutes. Traditional and new-type small bedside analyzers suffer from several shortcomings: loss of patient blood each time a test is requested and both errors and loss of time during the transfer of the blood sample from the patient to the analyzer. Ideal blood analyzers should provide continuous and accurate measurements, and these can only be realized using appropriate sensors. Continuous in vivo blood monitoring can be performed either invasively or noninvasively and imply data collection directly from the body. Ex vivo sensors can be used to monitor blood samples that are continuously taken from the body by means of a catheter or cannula system.

Oxygen is carried in blood in two forms: oxygen chemically combined with hemoglobin (Hb) as oxyhemoglobin ($HbO_2$) and oxygen physically dissolved in the plasma. The degree to which it is chemically combined with Hb is most commonly expressed as blood oxygen saturation, which is defined according to equation 7.8:

$$SO_2 = (HbO_2)/(Hb + HbO_2). \qquad (7.8)$$

It is generally given as a percentage; normally arterial blood saturation ($SaO_2$) fluctuates around 98%, while venous blood saturation ($SvO_2$) is approximately 75%. These definitions assume that no other Hb species (e.g., combined with CO) are present in the blood.

Arterial $pO_2$ and $SaO_2$ are both good indicators of blood oxygenation. Their relationship is given by dissociation curves (Parker, 1987) that can be handled only by using exact measurements of blood pH. There are a number of other factors, however, any one of which can lead to a displacement of the dissociation relationships. In the saturation ranges, the derivation of real $SaO_2$ from the value calculated using $pO_2$ is likely to give large errors, thus the direct measurement of $SaO_2$ is preferred. On the other hand, patients breathing 100% oxygen will have a $pO_2$ greater than 66.6 kPa (500 mmHg), though in practice $pO_2$ values cannot be derived from $SaO_2$ measurements greater than 16 kPa (120 mmHg). Therefore the direct measurement of $pO_2$ values is desirable in anesthesia, in patients being artificially ventilated, and in babies in incubators. The conclusion is that, ideally, both parameters should be monitored directly. The necessary measurement range of $pO_2$ is 4 kPa to 80 kPa (30 mmHg to 600 mmHg) with a resolution of 0.133 kPa (1 mmHg) in the low concentration ranges and 1.33 kPa (10 mmHg) at high concentrations.

Carbon dioxide is carried by the blood both in a dissolved state and in combination with Hb and plasma proteins as carbamino compounds. The normal $pCO_2$ of arterial blood is approximately 5.3 kPa (40 mmHg), whereas that of venous blood is approximately 6 kPa (45 mmHg). Thus a measurement range of 2.7 kPa to 13.3 kPa (20 mmHg to 100 mmHg) with a resolution of 0.133 kPa (1 mmHg) is needed.

Normal physiological pH fluctuates between 7.0 and 7.4. The generally accepted measurement range is rather narrow (6.8 to 7.8), but high precision (0.01) is needed. It is considered that sensor-measured $pO_2$ and $pCO_2$ values that are within 5% to 10% of blood gas analyzer values and pH measurements that agree to within 0.02 to 0.04 pH units will lead to the same clinical treatment decisions.

Blood gas and pH measurements are a serious challenge for sensor technologies. The most important technical requirements are an operating temperature range of 20°C to 40°C; a response time of less than 3 minutes; minimal cross-sensitivity among $CO_2$, $O_2$, and pH; and insensitivity to anesthetic gases (Soller, 1994). The most important requirements are summarized in Table 7.1; others include ease of sterilization, rapid and easy calibration, low cost, disposability (especially for intravascular elements), biocompatibility (thromboresistant and nontoxic), and the capability of being inserted into 20-gauge (0.584 mm) catheters without compromising arterial pressure measurements.

### 7.2.2.1. Invasive Electrochemical Sensors

The invasive (intravascular) application of electrochemical sensors for blood gas and pH measurement would seem to be simple since only electrodes (coated wires) have to be placed into the vessels. In practice, however, not only a single electrode, but also electrode pairs or even whole electrochemical cells must be catheterized. There are three main approaches in the invasive application of sensors:

- Miniature membrane-covered cylindrical-shaped electrochemical cells on catheter tips for in vivo monitoring
- Electrochemical cells mounted into sample-taking cannula, catheter, or dome systems for ex vivo applications
- Miniaturized silicon sensors, made by microelectronic and micromachining processing methods, mounted either onto catheter tips or into cannula, catheter, or dome systems

The primary device for pH measurements is the glass electrode, and catheter-size versions have been produced using pH-sensitive soda-lime glass-covered platinum wires. Their main drawback is the possibility that the glass might break. For this reason, other solutions are being investigated. For example, an antimony/antimony oxide electrode can be employed (Buerk, 1993), its operation relying on the following anodic electrochemical reaction:

**Table 7.1.** Required specifications of blood gas and pH sensors

| | $pO_2$ | pH | $pCO_2$ |
|---|---|---|---|
| Measurement range | 4–80 kPa (30–600 mmHg) | 6.8–7.8 | 2.7–13.3 kPa (20–100 mmHg) |
| Resolution | 0.133 kPa (4–20) (1 mmHg) 0.667 kPa (20–40) (5 mmHg) 1.333 kPa (40–80) (10 mmHg) | 0.01 | 0.133 kPa (1 mmHg) |
| Temperature range | 20°C–40°C | 20°C–40°C | 20°C–40°C |
| Stability (per 72 hours) | <1.066 kPa | <0.03 | <0.8 kPa |
| Response time | <3 minutes | <3 minutes | <3 minutes |
| Insensitivity for | Anesthetic gases, pH, $pCO_2$ | Anesthetic gases, $pO_2$, $pCO_2$ | Anesthetic gases, pH, $pO_2$ |

Source: Reproduced with permission from Soller, B. R., 1994, "Design of Intravascular Fiber Optic Blood Gas Sensors," *IEEE Engineering in Medicine and Biology, 13*(3), pp. 327–335.

$$2Sb + 3H_2O \Leftrightarrow Sb_2O_3 + 6e^- + 6H^+. \qquad (7.9)$$

Thus the Ag/AgCl reference electrode has to be connected as a cathode, resulting in the following reaction:

$$O_2 + 4H^+ + 4e^- \Leftrightarrow 2H_2O. \qquad (7.10)$$

This is also the main shortcoming of the system, since the electromotive force of the cell depends on the dissolved oxygen concentration, which results in a disturbing cross-sensitivity in blood. However, with multisensor applications, this error can be compensated. Indium and palladium oxide electrodes can be operated without this problem, but their multiple valencies result in complicated pH-dependent characteristics.

Today, most potentiometric pH sensors are solid-state electrodes covered by ion-selective polymer membranes, mainly plasticized polyvinyl chloride (PVC) or silicone rubber with tri-n-dodecyl-amine ionophore additive, which is a neutral ion carrier, enabling selective and reversible complex formation with $H^+$ ions.

Silicon-based pH-sensitive ion-selective field effect transistors (ISFETs) can be fabricated employing either silicon dioxide/silicon nitride ($SiO_2/Si_3N_4$) or ion-selective PVC membrane gate-insulating layers. Also, by selecting an appropriate inert cover material, reference field effect transistors (REFETs) can be fabricated. Integrating them onto the same chip, the realizable small size makes possible their application on catheter tips.

Sensors for measuring blood $pO_2$ are almost exclusively based on the Clark principle. Figure 7.2 shows a typical catheter-tip sensor structure fabricated for practical applications (Rolfe, 1994). It contains the basis salt of the electrolyte in dry powder form between the surface of the electrodes and the plasticized PVC membrane. The membrane must allow water molecules to diffuse through it from blood into the electrolyte region, thereby dissolving the powder, forming a liquid electrolyte layer. The sensor uses a thimble silver cathode pushed over the tip of the catheter, with a hole at the anode Ag/AgCl reference electrode location. The illustrated type needs a water vapor permeable membrane, this being the reason for applying plasticized PVC.

The electrochemical cell demonstrated in Figure 7.2 employs a silver cathode for cost reduction. However, tests on various cathode materials have shown that the best results can be expected from gold.

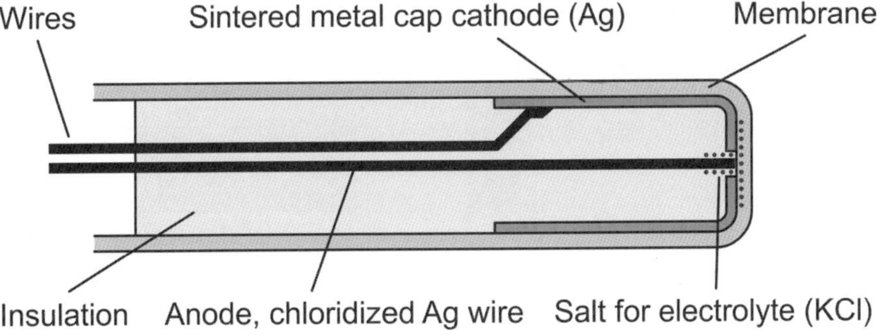


**Figure 7.2.** Conventional Clark-type blood oxygen sensor for catheter tip applications.

Platinum is less favorable, but its advantage is the possibility of preparing hermetic metal–glass bonding: thus platinum cathodes can be insulated well with good insulation glasses. A graphite cathode is inexpensive, but has a relatively high negative polarization voltage (less than –1 V) and considerable instability. The greatest disadvantage of silver cathodes is their instability due to electrochemical corrosion and migration of silver, which can cause a short-circuit formation or electrode consumption (Harsányi, 1995a). A saturated solution electrolyte can decrease the possibility of the latter effects, and generally a KCl solution is used as the electrolyte. Salt crystallization on electrode surfaces due to water evaporation may also result in disturbances. Water evaporation can be decreased by means of further sodium or potassium salt (phosphate, nitrate, or bicarbonate) additives.

Another promising approach for cost reduction is the application of thin- and thick-film processing instead of replacing gold or platinum with silver. The main problem with these solutions is the anodic reaction of the $H_2O_2$ that is developed at the cathode (see equation 7.5a), which leads to consumption of the Ag/AgCl electrode by its dissolution. This can be reduced by increasing the spacing between the electrodes, but this also implies a limit on scaling down (Harsányi, Péteri, & Deák, 1994).

Figure 7.3 shows the structure of a Clark-type sensor fabricated by means of silicon micromachining and thin-film processing that employs liquid electrolyte (Suzuki, Sugama, & Kokima, 1993). Its size (1 mm width, 15 mm length) enables catheter tip application. A glass substrate with a silver working electrode, gold counterelectrode, and Ag/AgCl reference electrode is bonded to a silicon substrate by field-assisted bonding. This is performed at 250°C in a nitrogen atmosphere by applying –1200 V to the glass substrate referred to the silicon substrate. This silicon substrate has anisotropically etched "V" grooves to provide small cavities to accommodate an electrolyte solution. Because the electrochemical reactions are localized in a very small amount of electrolyte, electrochemical cross talk between the electrodes must be eliminated. Therefore the container grooves are etched only over each electrode area and are connected by long narrow grooves. The oxygen-permeable membrane, made of

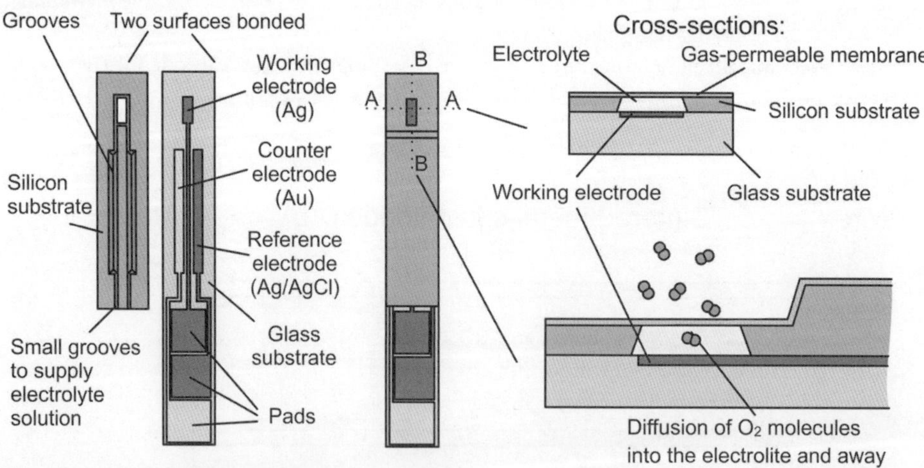


**Figure 7.3.** Structure of a micromachined Clark-type oxygen sensor. (left) The two parts of the sensor. (center) The complete structure. (right) Cross sections: A-A at the top, B-B below. Reprinted from Suzuki, H., Sugama, A., and Kokima, N., 1993, "Micromachined Clark Oxygen Electrode," *Sensors and Actuators B, 10*, pp. 91–98, with permission from Elsevier.

poly(fluoroethylene-propylene) (PFEP), is affixed thermally to the silicon substrate over an etched-through cavity above the working electrode. The electrolyte is incorporated by dipping the entire chip into the electrolyte solution within a centrifuge tube, placing it into a chamber, and evacuating. The channel system is closed by a droplet of silicone rubber that can easily be removed for electrolyte refreshing. The response of the resulting miniature amperometric sensor is about 30 nA/ppm $O_2$, with an average response time of 30 seconds and an almost zero residual current. The stable operation period of the sensor is 10 hours.

Figure 7.4 shows a silicon-based Clark-type sensor compatible with integrated circuit processing, thus the ISFETs and the circuitry components can be integrated onto the same silicon substrate (Gumbrecht et al., 1991). This sensor consists of a planar, thin-film, three-electrode system with two platinum electrodes and an Ag/AgCl reference electrode. Evaporated titanium layers were used to obtain good adhesion to the $SiO_2$. The silver was partly converted to chloride by chemical chloridization. A 30 μm thick photosensitive polyimide layer was deposited and patterned photolithographically to form a micropool above the electrode arrangement. Finally, the micropool was filled with a poly(hydroxyethyl methacrylate) (PHEMA) hydrogel. This is permeable to oxygen molecules and small ions, but protects the platinum working electrode from proteins that adhere to and poison the surface. The water content of the hydrophilic PHEMA membrane can vary within a wide range, thus it acts as both an electrolyte and membrane. Another construction was fabricated using a poly(vinyl alcohol) electrolyte buffer and a silicone rubber permselective membrane.

Very similar problems must be solved when fabricating $pCO_2$ sensors for blood gas measurements. The most important differences are the following:

- The cathode is a pH electrode.
- The electrolyte is generally $NaHCO_3$.
- Potentiometric or conductimetric measurement has to be applied.
- The applicable membrane material is PTFE or silicone rubber.

A novel sensing principle has also been proposed recently that is based on the revealing of ion formation, as described by equation 7.6 (Varlan & Sansen, 1997). This involves a conductimetric sensor in a closed cavity. The advantage of this is simplicity: there are only two electrodes in the closed chamber. This silicon micromachined sensor comprises two planar electrodes housed in a micromachined chamber formed between a silicon and a glass substrate. The cavity is filled with deionized water and

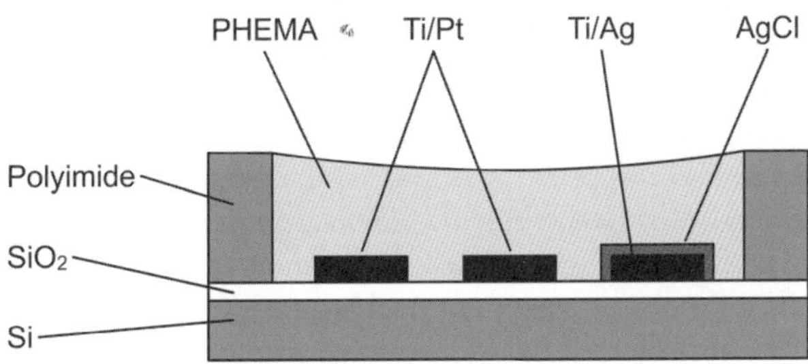


**Figure 7.4.** Schematic cross section of a thin-film Clark-type sensor. Reproduced with permission from Gumbrecht, W., Schelter, W., Montag, B., Bos, J. A. H., Eijking, E. P., and Lachmann, B., 1991, "Monitoring of Blood $pO_2$ with a Thin-Film Amperometric Sensor," *Proceedings of the 1991 International Conference on Solid State Sensors and Actuators [Transducers '91]*, San Francisco, CA, pp. 85–87.

is connected with the chemical environment via a sieve etched from the silicon and covered with a polymeric membrane.

### 7.2.2.2. Transcutaneous Electrochemical Sensors

Although intravascular monitoring remains an important part of intensive care, catheterization of arteries has some risks, especially in newborn babies. Such disadvantages have led to the advent and rapid growth of noninvasive blood gas monitoring methods. Of these, the transcutaneous technique has received considerable interest, as it enables blood gas measurements to be made through the skin.

Human skin is practically impermeable to gas molecules under normal conditions. However, Baumberger and Goodfriend (1951) revealed that if the skin temperature is increased, it may behave as a semipermeable membrane. Near 45°C, $pO_2$ measured at the surface can approach the arterial value quite closely. The estimation of arterial $pO_2$ and $pCO_2$ based on this noninvasive method is called the transcutaneous technique. In practice, the sensor elements used are Clark- and Stow–Severinghaus-type electrochemical cells equipped with heating elements and temperature sensors that enable operation within a well-controlled narrow temperature range.

A good estimation of arterial blood gas parameters depends on the correct choice of skin temperature (Huch, Huch, & Lübbers, 1972), but heating the skin causes several effects that must be considered in $pO_2$ measurements:

- Vasodilatation of dermal capillaries occurs, thereby "arterializing" the capillary blood.
- A rightward shift of the oxyhemoglobin dissociation curve takes place; that is, $pO_2$ increases at the sensor site.
- An increase of oxygen diffusion both through the stratum corneum of the skin and through the polymer membrane of the sensor will also occur.
- The increased rate of tissue metabolism increases the oxygen consumption, resulting in a decrease in $pO_2$.
- The overall operation of the electrochemical cell is strongly temperature dependent.

According to empirical results, phenomena that cause a virtual change in $pO_2$ at the sensor site may balance each other's effect at an appropriate choice of temperature. A sensor temperature of 43.5°C ± 0.5°C has been found to be optimum for reliable monitoring of arterial $pO_2$, ensuring good agreement between values measured by transcutaneous and invasive methods. However, temperature fluctuations in the sensor element must not exceed 0.1°C.

The structure of a conventional transcutaneous $pO_2$ sensor (Parker, 1987) is a specially designed Clark-type oxygen sensor in which a miniature heater coil is incorporated to maintain the skin at the necessary temperature. Temperature control is achieved using a thermistor, and a second thermistor acts as a safety cutout to prevent overheating of the sensor in the event of a primary thermistor malfunction. The cathode consists of several thin 20 μm platinum wires fused into glass and surrounded by a Ag/AgCl anode. The electrolyte is contained by a 25 μm thick PTFE membrane. Attachment of the sensor to the skin is performed by applying a double-sided adhesive tape to achieve a gas-tight seal around the circumference of the sensor. The typical current output of such a sensor is in the range of nanoamperes at a $pO_2$ of 20 kPa (150 mmHg).

The most important problem in conventional transcutaneous sensors is that they have a very complicated structure: a number of miniaturized elements must be integrated into a small device.

They are also generally expensive because of the difficult mounting process and the application of bulk precious metal electrodes.

Potential advantages are possible through the microfabrication of electrochemical biomedical sensors, including reduced size, reduced sample volume, fast response, and reduced cost because of the minimal precious metal consumption of the film electrodes. In addition, it should be possible to produce a highly uniform and well-defined microstructure of the electrode surface area using microelectronic technology. However, many special realization problems have to be solved, and complications may arise as the size of the electrodes and interelectrode distances are reduced.

A new type of transcutaneous $pO_2$ sensor structure is presented in Figure 7.5 (Harsányi, 1995b, 2000), which is based on the multilayer ceramic technology that is used in the fabrication of high-density electronic interconnection systems. The electrodes are made by thick-film technology using small amounts of precious metals. The heating element is an integrated thick-film resistor, and a pn-junction is used for temperature sensing. The disc-shaped ceramic sensor body has a groove at the edge for packaging purposes and a deep cavity in its center for the temperature sensor chip, which should be as close to the skin surface as possible for the necessary accuracy of temperature control. A diode chip is used for temperature-sensing purposes. The horseshoe-shaped heating resistor is screen-printed and fired on the top of the ceramic body using a common thick-film processing technique. It consists of several segments to give more freedom for heating.

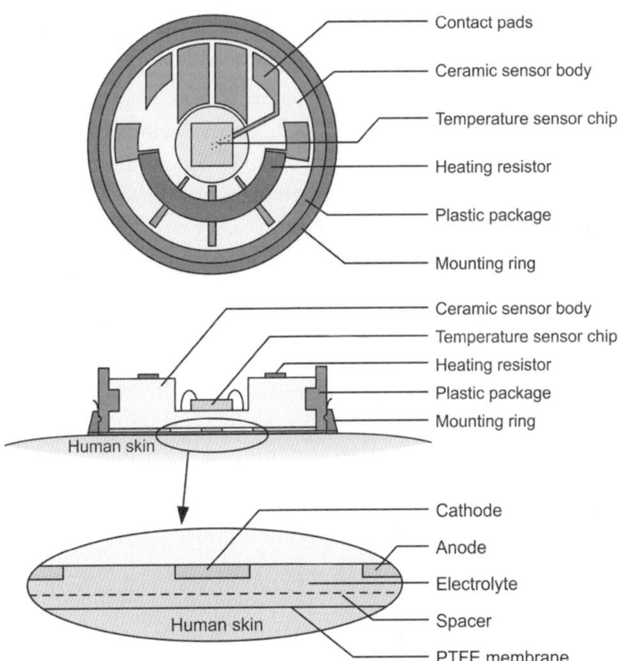


**Figure 7.5.** Structure of the ceramic transcutaneous blood $O_2$ sensor: (above) top view; (below) cross sections. Used with permission from Harsányi, G., 2000, "Sensors in Biomedical Applications," Technomic Publishing, Lancaster, PA, p. 184, with permission of CRC Press—a division of Taylor and Francis Books, Inc.

The sensing electrode (cathode) is fabricated using thick-film gold paste. The silver film for the Ag/AgCl reference electrode (anode) is also formed by thick-film techniques before being electrochemically chloridized in a 0.1M HCl solution. The total surface area of this Ag/AgCl electrode is 0.7 cm$^2$, while the area of the gold electrode is 1.77 mm$^2$. The ceramic body is molded into a plastic package. The 10 μm thick PTFE membrane is fastened with a mounting ring to the surface of the sensor, as shown in the cross section of Figure 7.5 (bottom). A conventional KCl solution with a buffering agent is used as the electrolyte. A thin, disc-shaped cellophane foil is placed between the electrodes and the membrane as a spacer. The application of multilayer wiring helps to produce an electrode separation that is appropriate for reducing the pickup of the $H_2O_2$ intermediate reaction product that causes electrochemical cross talk and electrode consumption. (This problem arises particularly in connection with film-type sensors, as the conventional types use bulk wire electrodes.)

Transcutaneous $pCO_2$ measurement relies on a similar technique. It is performed by means of heated Stowe–Severinghaus electrochemical sensors. Although the measurement technique is very similar, the transcutaneous estimation of blood $pCO_2$ differs in theory from that for $pO_2$ measurement because there is no balance-of-errors possibility: all the effects of heating (decreased solubility, increased rate of metabolism, increased diffusion) result in an increase of the measured transcutaneous $pCO_2$ compared to the real arterial $pCO_2$ value. Their relationship is expressed in equation 7.11:

$$(tc)pCO_2 = mpCO_2 + c, \tag{7.11}$$

where $m = 1.22$ and $c = 6.6$; these are empirical values that have gained general acceptance even though they might be somewhat dependent on the sensor size and shape.

A recent trend is to use a single sensor for both gases. This uses the same 0.6 mol L$^{-1}$ NaHCO$_3$/ ethylene glycol electrolyte for both the $pO_2$ and $pCO_2$ measurement and has a common reference electrode and a polymer diffusion membrane. The cathode is a 25 μm diameter platinum wire, and the pH-sensitive glass electrode for $CO_2$ measurement using the Stow–Severinghaus method is 2 mm to 3 mm in diameter. It also contains a heater coil and a temperature-controlling thermistor. The diffusion membrane is held in position by a PTFE ring, and the outer annulus is for attachment to the skin by means of a double-sided adhesive disc. The combined sensor is essentially a $pCO_2$ sensor with a cathode incorporated to measure $pO_2$. It is essential to limit the production of hydroxyl ions by the cathode so that the $pCO_2$ measurement is not affected by a change in the pH of the electrolyte. It can be shown that at a typical cathode current of 3 nA, the maximum average change in the electrolyte, will be less than $5 \times 10^5$ pH h$^{-1}$, which will not affect the $pCO_2$ readings.

A newer approach is the application of pH-ISFETs instead of electrodes. A novel miniature transcutaneous $pCO_2$ sensor was developed recently using a pH-ISFET, a conventional Ag/AgCl electrode, a hydrogel gate-membrane containing 0.1 mol L$^{-1}$ NaHCO$_3$ electrolyte, a heater coil, and a pn-junction temperature sensor (Jinghong et al., 1995). The whole structure is covered with a $CO_2$ gas permeable membrane. The sensor's measurement range is 0.53 kPa to 40 kPa (4 mmHg to 300 mmHg) with a response time of less than 2 minutes.

### 7.2.2.3. Combined Electrochemical Multisensors for Blood Gases and pH

Multisensors are capable of the simultaneous monitoring of several parameters from $pO_2$, $pCO_2$, pH, and temperature. This has great importance, especially in biomedical applications, for the following reasons:

- All four parameters are physiologically important.

- Blood gas sensors are sensitive to pH variations, hence the measurement of pH makes compensation for this effect possible.
- All sensors are temperature dependent, the compensation for which requires the application of temperature sensors.

Miniaturization is especially important when producing catheter-tip sensors. The following approaches are available:

- Building up compound electrochemical sensors using multielectrode systems
- Integrating multiple sensors onto silicon substrates

The example of Figure 7.6 demonstrates how three different sensor types can be integrated onto the same silicon substrate using compatible processing sequences (Tsukada, Miyahara, Shibata, &

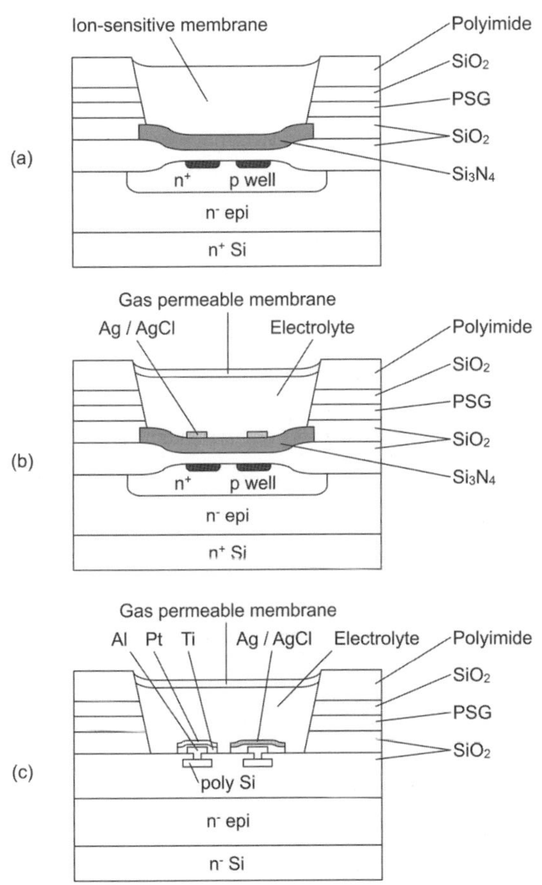


**Figure 7.6.** Cross-sectional structure of the elements in an integrated chemical sensor: (a) ISFET, (b) $pCO_2$ sensor, and (c) $pO_2$ sensor. Reproduced with permission from Tsukada, K., Miyahara, Y., Shibata, Y., and Miyagi, H., 1990, "An Integrated Chemical Sensor with Multiple Ion and Gas Sensors," *Sensors and Actuators B, 2*, pp. 291–295.

Miyagi, 1990). The combined sensor consists of a Clark-type $pO_2$ sensor with a platinum sensing electrode (Fig. 7.6[c]), a Stow–Severinghaus $pCO_2$ sensor with a $Si_3N_4$-gate pH-ISFET (Fig. 7.6[b]), and a pH sensor ISFET (Fig. 7.6[a]). Both gas sensors apply poly(vinyl alcohol) film for soaking the electrolyte: the KCl solution at the $pO_2$ sensor and the sodium chloride–sodium bicarbonate (NaCl-$NaHCO_3$) solution at the $pCO_2$ sensor, respectively. The gate membrane of the pH-ISFET is also $Si_3N_4$. Using plasticized PVC membranes with various ionophores, several ion-selective ISFETs can also be integrated onto the same chip.

## 7.2.3. ION-SELECTIVE SENSOR APPLICATIONS IN BLOOD AND OTHER SECRETIONS

Of great importance in blood compound monitoring are a number of ion concentrations (i.e., $Na^+$, $K^+$, $Ca^{2+}$, $Mg^{2+}$, $NH_4^+$, Cl), the monitoring of which can be accomplished by means of ion-selective sensors. Ion-selective electrodes for catheter-tip applications can be constructed using precious metal wires covered by plasticized PVC membranes with ion-selective neutral carriers. With a reference electrode, potentiometric measurement can be realized similar to pH electrodes (see section 7.2.1.1). A recent approach is the application of thin- and thick-film multilayer electrode systems and ISFETs integrated together for multisensors and also with signal processing circuitry on the same chip or substrate.

Figure 7.7 demonstrates the structure of a rather complicated thin-film ion-selective electrode for Na+/K+ (Keplinger et al., 1990). Metal layers were evaporated on glass substrates and shaped by photolithography. The internal reference electrode was established by the following metal multilayer sequence: titanium/gold/silver/silver chloride (Ti/Au/Ag/AgCl). The silver layer was chemically chloridized, and the insulating layer is a plasma enhanced chemical vapor deposition (PECVD) $Si_3N_4$ film. The salt layer was evaporated and structured by a liftoff technique and acts as an internal solid electrolyte. Finally, the structure was coated with the ion-selective membrane. For potassium electrodes

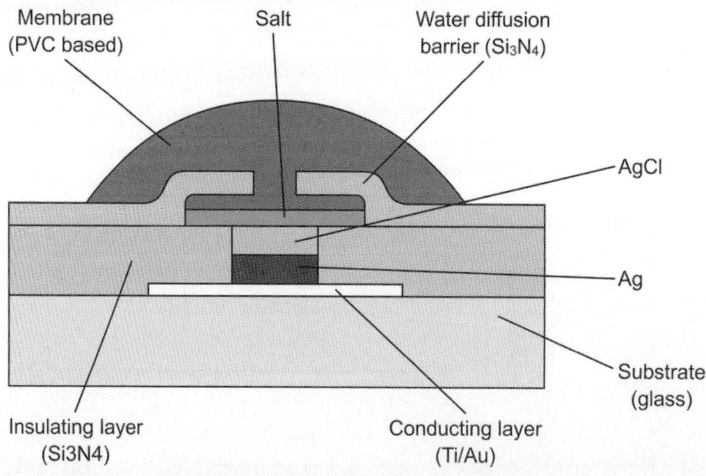


**Figure 7.7.** Cross section of a thin-film ion-selective device with water diffusion barrier. Reproduced with permission from Keplinger, F., Glatz, R., Jachimowicz, A., Urban, G., Kohl, F., Olcaytug, F., and Prohaska, O. J., 1990, "Thin-Film Ion-Selective Sensors Based on Neutral Carrier Membranes," *Sensors and Actuators B, 1*, pp. 272–274.

a composition of PVC-dioctyl-sebacate with valinomycin ionophore was chosen, and for sodium electrodes a PVC-nitrophenyl-octyl-ether with Na+-ionophore was chosen. To enhance long-term stability, an additional $Si_3N_4$ layer with a small aperture was introduced to limit the water transport across the membrane, thus achieving a lifetime of at least 3 days. The potential change is about 100 mV when the ion concentration is changed from 1 mmol $L^{-1}$ to 0.1 mol $L^{-1}$.

The cross section shown in Figure 7.8 is of an integrated micro multi-ion sensor using platinum gate ISFETs with several polymeric membranes (Tsukada et al., 1991). It consists of two kinds of ion sensors ($K^+$- and $Na^+$-ISFETs) and two complementary metal oxide semiconductor (CMOS) unity gain buffers. The ISFETs are buffered by high-impedance amplifiers. This configuration results in a linear dependence between the ion-selective membrane potential and the output voltage. In the chemically active area, the ion-selective membranes are formed on platinum/titanium/aluminum multilayer electrodes that are connected to n-channel metal oxide semiconductor (NMOS) gates. The platinum film is used as a protective layer against ion migration and hydration, and titanium is used as an adhesion layer. They were produced using a liftoff process. The $SiO_2$ and phosphosilicate-glass form passivation films. Finally, a polyimide layer is deposited and patterned photolithographically to form a well. The ion-selective membranes consist of PVC, ionophore, plasticizer, and additives. Almost-Nernstian sensitivities (49 mV per decade at 25°C; see equation 7.1) have been detected with good selectivity factors (log $S_{ij} < -2$).

Ion-selective sensors may have applications not only in monitoring blood compounds, but also in analyzing other secretions. As an example, an integrated probe for sweat analysis is considered here (Bezegh et al., 1987; Bezegh et al., 1988). Sweat, as a body fluid, can yield useful clinical information, and one of the few viable sweat tests is the determination of chloride concentration in the diagnosis of cystic fibrosis. Although the concentration in sweat may vary within a wide range, the local concentration measured in situ may provide useful information. A solid-state integrated differential-type probe based on $Na^+/Cl^-$ ISFETs was used to determine NaCl, the two silicon chips being attached to a flexible printed wiring substrate. Then, a blank membrane containing only the PVC polymer and

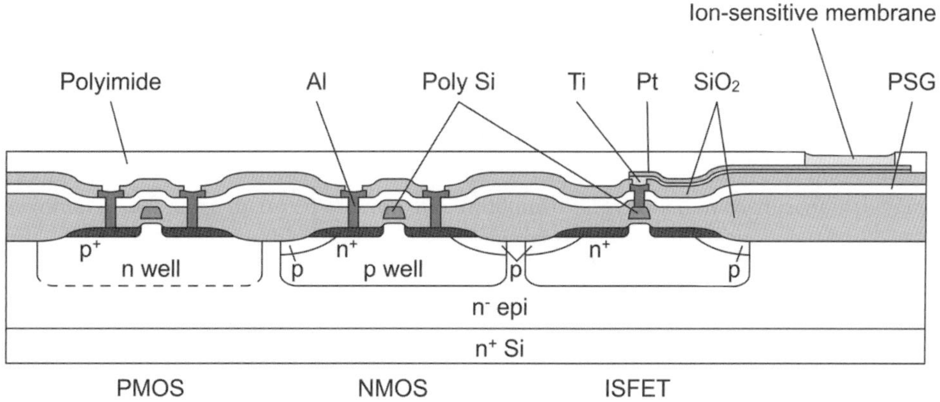



**Figure 7.8.** Cross-sectional structure of the integrated ISFET. Reproduced with permission from Tsukada, K., Miyahara, Y., Shibata, Y., and Miyagi, H., 1991, "An Integrated Micro Multi-Ion Sensor Using Platinum-Gate Field-Effect Transistors," *Proceedings of the 1991 International Conference on Solid State Sensors and Actuators (Transducers '91)*, San Francisco, CA, pp. 218–221.

plasticizer was applied as a continuous coating to the device surface. Electrochemical selectivity was introduced by doping this membrane with electroactive ingredients (ionophores). In practice, this was performed by dropping ionophores selectively onto the surface of the membrane. The device was attached to the surface of the skin in the same way as transcutaneous probes (see section 7.2.2.2). The difference in the two transistor currents was measured as a function of the NaCl concentration. The total amount of liquid required for the measurement is 0.3 µl, which is small compared to some 80 µl needed for conventional chloride titration.

A novel potentiometric sensor for potassium was developed by Schnakenberg et al. (1996) that provides several improvements and advantages resulting from the development of double-sided wafer processing (see Fig. 7.9). This sensor was fabricated in bulk silicon micromachining using double-sided wafer processing. A small channel was etched anisotropically in (100) silicon and the back side groove was metallized. To form an ion-selective electrode, an ion-selective membrane was deposited into the channel. In addition, the openings were shaped from the front side of the chip to provide microcontainments (channels) to improve the mechanical stability of the ion-selective membrane. For stable and reproducible potentiometric measurements, a reference electrode was deposited on the front side of the chip close to the openings. A novel evaporation process was developed for the deposition of a Ag/AgCl/Ag layer combination serving as a thin-film reference electrode. The small size of the sensor allows its localization in the tip of a three lumen catheter for medical applications. For the potentiometric measurement of potassium, different cocktails of ionophore-modified polymer membranes were prepared and deposited in the channel by a dispensing technique.

## 7.2.4. CHEMICAL PARAMETERS OF THE INNER EYELID

The eyelid sensor takes advantage of the unique function of the capillary bed in the palpebral conjunctiva, which is perfused by the internal carotid artery that supplies $O_2$ to the avascular cornea during sleep. The conjunctival oxygen sensor is essentially a miniaturized unheated version of a Clark-type $pO_2$ electrode mounted in an oval ophthalmic conformer ring (Mendelson, 1991). The conformer ring, which is made of a plastic biocompatible material, (poly[methyl methacrylate]; PMMA), is

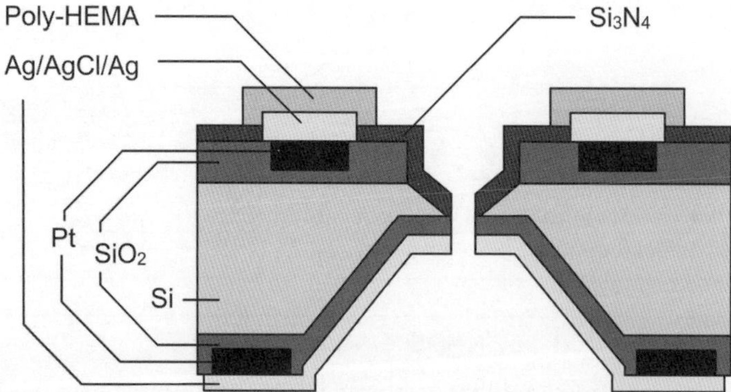


**Figure 7.9.** Structure of a miniature silicon-based potentiometric sensor. Used with permission from Schnakenberg, U., Lisec, T., Hintsche, R., Kuna, I., Uhlig, A., Wagner, B., 1996, "Novel Potentiometric Silicon Sensor for Medical Devices," *Sensors and Actuators B, 34*, pp. 476–480.

contoured to the shape of the sclera so that normal vision is not obstructed and free eye movement can be maintained. The inner eyelid is also a potential site for monitoring blood pH and oxygen saturation ($SaO_2$). A fiber-optic pH sensor and a pH-ISFET with a miniature reference electrode have demonstrated the possibility of pH monitoring, while the $SaO_2$ can be measured by a miniature reflectance oximeter sensor. The primary applications of these sensor types to date have been limited to emergency and critical care medicine.

## 7.2.5. MONITORING PH IN GASTRIC ACID

The ambulatory monitoring of pH in the upper gastrointestinal tract is also increasingly used for diagnostic and research purposes, and this involves a further application of inorganic component sensing beyond blood monitoring. Gastric acid measurements are currently performed with integrated glass and antimony electrodes; a severe drawback of these is encountered if several sensors must be installed in the gastroesophageal tract.

A new construction using ISFETs permits multiple mounting on a single catheter (Thybaud, Depeursinge, Rouiller, Mondin, & Grisel, 1990). This consists of several types of polymers, but the ISFET itself is not polymer-based. The gastric probe is composed of a supple PVC catheter in which the ISFETs are mounted on a floppy Kapton substrate, the passivating film being epoxy. The reference electrode is also installed at the catheter tip. The very small dimensions of the ISFET chips allow several ion-sensitive sensors to be mounted on a single catheter. Such multi-ISFET probes are expected to be very useful in the study of gastroesophageal reflux, which affects numerous people. The whole measuring system makes possible 24-hr ambulatory monitoring of pH and other ion concentrations in the gastrointestinal tract. The most recent, and obvious, approach is the application of telemetry, which enables the use of such probes without cabled catheters.

## 7.2.6. MEASURING AND MAPPING OF TISSUE PH AND PO$_2$

The direct measurement of tissue pH and $pO_2$ with minimal damage to the cells or to the microcirculation in the tissue produces a serious challenge for sensors. These micromeasurements are still a part of laboratory research and do not belong to everyday clinical practice. They can be applied in monitoring the brain, heart, muscle metabolism, and ischemia.

For practical measurements, microelectrodes have tip sizes in the range of living cell dimensions, which are much smaller than those utilized in conventional vessel catheters. Generally, compound glass–metal electrodes are fabricated using various special techniques of glass processing and metallurgy, such as glass pulling, mechanical and chemical polishing, grinding, chemical and electrochemical etch beveling, and so on. The structure of various pH and $pO_2$ microelectrodes are shown in Figure 7.10 (Buerk, 1993) without a detailed discussion about preparation methods. The first-generation microelectrodes employed open-tip glass or metal electrodes with the smallest possible tip sizes (typically in the range of 10 μm for glass and less than 1 μm for metal types) and a separate reference electrode (see Fig. 7.10[a] and 7.10[b]). Impurities can shift the characteristics of these type of electrodes after a few periods of use and the refreshing etch processes alter the tip geometry. Recessed-tip electrodes (see Fig. 7.10[c] and 7.10[d]) offer a significant improvement. Here, an open-tip microelectrode is prepared, then inserted into an insulating glass micropipette. However, one drawback of this design is a longer time response due to the increased diffusion distance from the tip to the transducer surface. The common shortcoming of all these types is that the measured electromotive force suffers interference

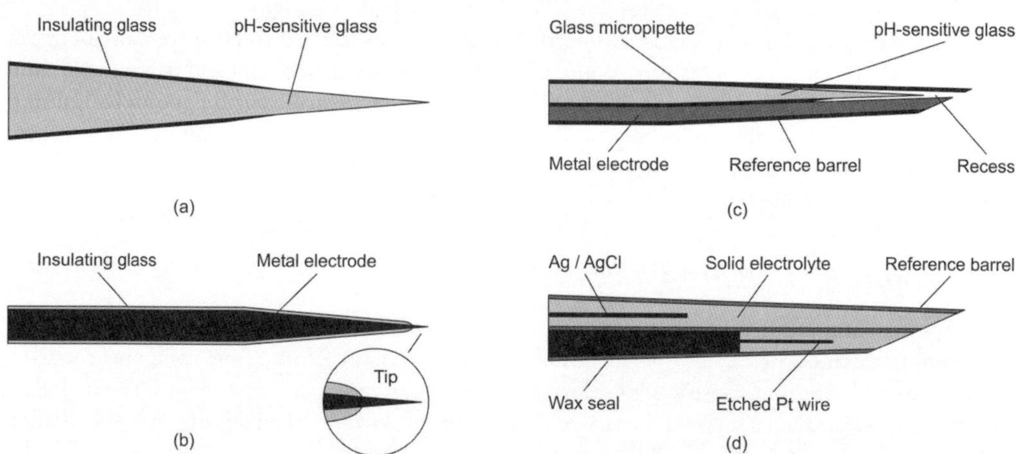



**Figure 7.10.** Typical structures for tissue pH and pO$_2$ microelectrodes: (a, b) open tip; (c, d) double-barrel recessed tip types. Used with permission from Buerk, D. G., *Biosensors, Theory and Applications*, 1993, Technomic Publishing Co., Inc., Lancaster, PA, pp. 98, 102.

by the cell membrane potential if an intracellular measurement is made with the reference electrode external to the cell. Double-barrel design (shown in Fig. 7.10[c] and 7.10[d]) combines the recessed type with a second barrel that is used as a reference electrode. Generally it contains a Ag/AgCl electrode and the barrel is filled with physiological saline. The two micropipette tips are fused together by local heating and pressure. Practical tip measurements are in the range of 10 μm to 35 μm.

Extremely fine probes have been developed that can be used to map out detailed surface features. In scanning electrochemical microscopy, a three-dimensional (3-D) representation of a region is made by systematically sweeping the probe across the sample. The fine tip of an electrochemical transducer is moved in small increments by a computer-controlled translation element. The resolution depends on the diameter of the scanning tip and the distance from the tip to the sample. (Of course, there are practical limitations on how close the probe can be placed to the surface, particularly if it is irregular or is moving.) Electrochemical mapping can be simplified by means of electrode arrays. Silicon micro-fabrication with electron-beam lithography and reactive ion etching (RIE) is a promising approach for preparing microelectrode arrays.

## 7.3. OPTICAL FIBER CHEMICAL SENSORS

Optical fiber sensors for blood gas and pH monitoring make possible invasive, generally intravascular, measurements and have optrode-type structures. There are both single-fiber and multiple-fiber types. In the case of a single-fiber optrode, the incident and emergent light have to be separated by means of a beam splitter. In indicator-mediated sensors, the absorbance is measured, therefore the reflection from the fiber tip should be increased by using reflecting surfaces. In fluorescent optrodes, secondary light emission is excited, thus reflection of the primary light has to be prevented. At present, low-cost appliances generally operate with light-emitting diode (LED) sources and photodiode detectors (Wolfbeis, 1991). Figure 7.11 shows the typical structure of a double-fiber, reflection-mode optrode catheter.

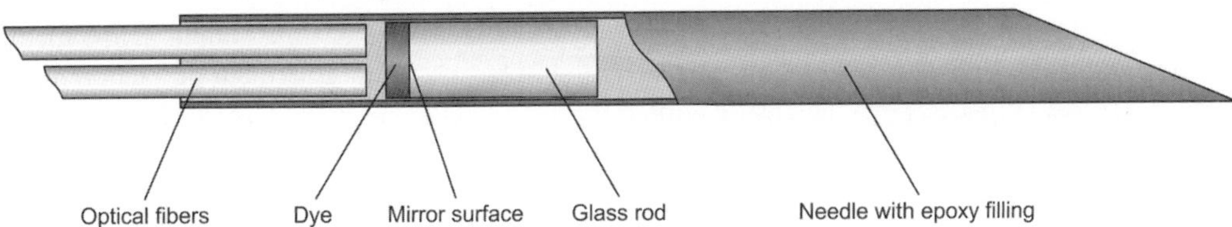


**Figure 7.11.** Typical structure of a double-fiber optrode for intravascular measurements.

## 7.3.1. OPTRODES FOR MEASURING BLOOD $PO_2$

Optrodes for measuring blood $pO_2$ are generally based on the fluorescent quenching of oxygen-sensitive fluorescent dyes such perylene-dibutyrate (Soller, 1994). The excited light intensity can be described by the Stern–Volmer equation. Neglecting the nonlinearity arising in the nonunit extension, the measurable intensity is

$$I = I_0/(1 + kpO_2),\qquad(7.12.a)$$

where $I_0$ is the fluorescent emission intensity in the absence of the quencher and $k$ is an empirical constant. This relationship results in a nonconstant sensitivity ($S$) for oxygen:

$$S = dI/dpO_2 = -kI_0/(1 + kpO_2)^2.\qquad(7.12.b)$$

Figure 7.12 is a plot of normalized absolute value sensitivity as a function of $pO_2$. The best sensitivity is achieved at less than 150 mmHg (20 kPa), and drops off considerably at higher levels, making it difficult to resolve small changes when the $pO_2$ is higher than 200 mmHg (26.6 kPa).

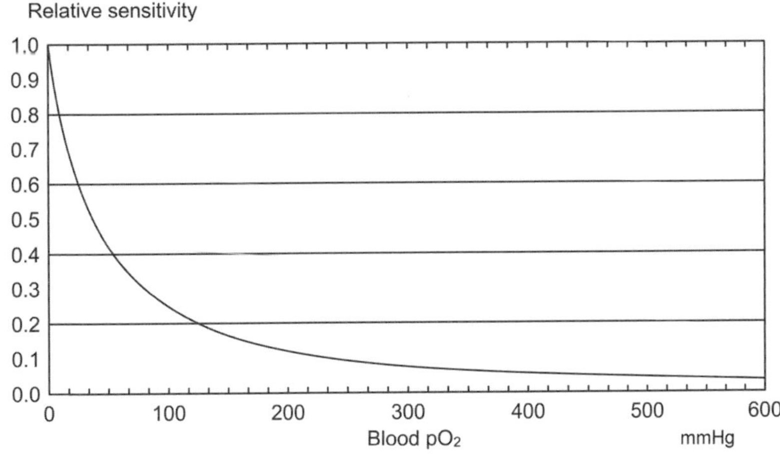


**Figure 7.12.** Relative sensitivity plot of a fluorescent blood oxygen optrode as a function of $pO_2$ (1 mmHg = 0.133 kPa). Reproduced with permission from Soller, B. R., 1994, "Design of Intravascular Fiber Optic Blood Gas Sensors," *IEEE Engineering in Medicine and Biology, 13*(3), pp. 327–335.

The fluorescent dye can be entrapped in a polystyrene membrane, for example, and kept in position at the fiber end with porous polyethylene tubing. The greatest measurement problem is interference due to anesthetic agents: narcotic halothane acts in the same manner as oxygen in fluorescent quenching. A method has been devised applying two sensors with different susceptibilities to quenching by oxygen and halothane, giving two independent signals that can be converted into oxygen and halothane partial pressures (Wolfbeis, 1991). Ruthenium-based fluorescent dye complexes have shown especially good lifetime and stability (Colvin et al., 1996). Further efforts have been reported about phosphorescence quenching of metalloporphyrins and terbium complexes used in blood oxygen optrodes (Papkovsky, 1993; Soller, 1994).

Recently membranes based on immobilized cobalt (II) porphyrins have been investigated for optical response to oxygen. It was found that in terms of chemical and optical stability, response, and lifetime, these types of oxygen-sensitive membranes exhibit better performance than earlier colorimetric sensor systems. The sensor response range was found to cover 1 hPa to 1000 hPa (mbar) of $pO_2$, that is, an oxygen content of 0.1% to 100% at atmospheric pressure. The peak performance of the sensor was observed with a membrane 20 μm thick, for which the 90% response time was reached in 5 seconds to 15 seconds and the operational lifetime was longer than 1 month (Röösli et al., 1997).

A new fiber-optic oxygen sensor has been developed by immobilizing tetraphenylporyphyrin (TTP) within the cross-linked silicone cladding of a conventional plastic-clad silica (PCS) optical fiber. The fluorophore was excited at 590 nm by an ultrabright yellow LED; the resulting fluorescence was collected at 650 nm (Mehrvar et al., 2000; Potyrailo & Hieftje, 1998).

A catheter-type optical oxygen sensor based on phosphorescence lifetime has been developed for medical and animal experimental use (Tsukada et al., 2003). Here, palladium-porphyrin was doped in a silicone-based polymer disc and was fixed at the edge of an optical fiber inserted in a catheter tube. The probe was 600 μm in diameter and 100 μm in thickness. In accuracy evaluations, excellent agreement was found between the $pO_2$ values measured through phosphorescence lifetime using the oxygen sensors and those measured as calibrating data using oxygen electrodes. The response time required to achieve 90% from reversible default values from 150 mmHg to 0 mmHg and from 0 mmHg to 150 mmHg was 15.43 seconds and 7.52 seconds, respectively. In animal experiments, the catheter-type oxygen sensor was inserted into a rat via the femoral artery and arterial oxygen pressure was monitored under asphyxiation. The sensor was valid in the range of oxygen concentration sufficient for biometry, and it is expected that it can be integrated with an indwelling needle.

## 7.3.2. OPTICAL FIBER BLOOD PH SENSORS

Optical fiber blood pH sensors are mostly reflection-type optrodes based on acid–base indicator dyes. The absorbance is generally measured at two wavelengths: one with maximal pH dependence, and the other, which is insensitive to pH, as a reference. The sensor signal ($I$) can be expressed as

$$I = I_0 \cdot e^{-bcl/(10^{(pK-pH)}+1)}, \tag{7.13}$$

where $I_0$ is the signal produced when no base form of the dye is present. This shows that the sensor properties depend on the inherent properties of the dye material ($b$ = extinction coefficient; pK = –logK; and K is the chemical equilibrium constant of the protonation–deprotonation process of the dye) and the manufacturing processes used to make the sensor ($c$ = the concentration of the dye material; $l$ = the optical path length). Blood pH measurements have to be performed in a narrow range with high accuracy (see Table 7.1). One of the most effective ways to achieve resolution goals is to optimize the pK of the dye material. Figure 7.13 shows the normalized response of a pH optrode for three different values of pK (Soller, 1994). When the pK of the dye is at the center of the range to be measured (7.4 in the case of blood pH), maximum sensitivity will be achieved.

The first blood pH optrodes employed phenol red indicator dye. Although phenol red has a pK of 7.9 in aqueous solutions, its value was lowered to 7.57 inside the polymer bed. Similar phenomena were found with various indicator types. Thus pH sensors can be designed with excellent resolution over the entire pH range by "tuning" the pK of the sensing material. This can be accomplished through proper choice of a functional group attached to the absorbing portion of the dye molecule or by immobilizing it into a polymer matrix with appropriate ionic characteristics. In this way, a pH sensor with phenol red was realized for the physiological detection range with an accuracy of 0.01 and with a temperature coefficient of 0.017 pH units °C$^{-1}$ (Peterson et al., 1980).

Fluorescence-based pH sensors have also been fabricated using the pH-dependent excitation spectra of hydroxypyrene-trisulfonic (HTPS) acid (Wolfbeis et al., 1983). The deprotonated form of HTPS bound to cellulose can be excited at 475 nm to give a fluorescence emission at 530 nm, the intensity of the latter being a function of the pH. The acid form of the dye can be excited at 410 nm to give fluorescence emission from the same band as the base form. When excited at the isoemissive wavelength of 428 nm (the excitation wavelength where the emission efficiency is the same both for acid and base forms), a pH-independent fluorescent signal is obtained that can be used for reference purposes. Other fluorescent indicator dyes are fluoresceinamine and dichlorofluorescein. pH sensors have also been fabricated using both colorimetric and fluorescent indicator dyes.

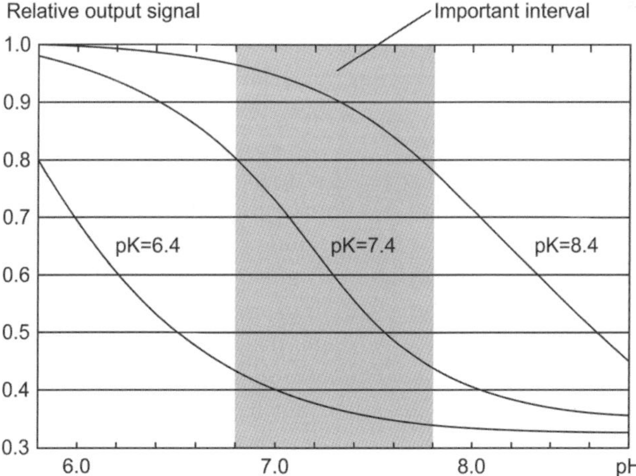


**Figure 7.13.** Characteristics of absorption-based pH sensors with various pK values. Reproduced with permission from Soller, B. R., 1994, "Design of Intravascular Fiber Optic Blood Gas Sensors," *IEEE Engineering in Medicine and Biology, 13*(3), pp. 327–335.

### 7.3.3. OPTICAL FIBER SENSORS FOR PCO$_2$

Most fiber-optic sensors for measuring pCO$_2$ use the same approach as the electrodes: a pH sensor is placed in contact with an internal solution of bicarbonate ion and is separated from the environment by a gas-permeable membrane such as silicone rubber or a copolymer of dimethylsiloxane. Both absorption-type optrodes with phenol red and fluorescence-based types applying dichlorofluorescein have been developed. The key for optimizing pCO$_2$ sensor design is to control the internal bicarbonate ion concentration. Figure 7.14 shows the pH–pCO$_2$ plot of the sensor for several bicarbonate ion concentrations (Soller, 1994). The graph shows that the resolution of the sensor does not change as a function of bicarbonate ion concentration. In order to achieve the desired pCO$_2$ resolution of 1 mmHg (0.133 kPa), the pH sensor must have a resolution of 0.009 pH units. However, the internal bicarbonate ion concentration determines the range of the pH response. To take advantage of the pH sensor designed to measure blood pH, the bicarbonate ion concentration should be chosen so that the internal pH varies between 6.8 and 7.8. As seen in Figure 7.14, a bicarbonate concentration of 0.035 mol L$^{-1}$ produces a pH response in the desired range. The bicarbonate may be soaked into the pH-dye layer or may be placed into a separate chamber resulting in multimembrane optrode structures. It is important to maintain a constant bicarbonate ion concentration, therefore water evaporation should be prevented. For this reason, sensors are stored in an aqueous buffer that can then also serve as one of the calibration solutions.

### 7.3.4. OPTICAL FIBER GASTRIC CATHETERS

Optical fiber sensors are also used as gastric pH catheters, their major disadvantages being their narrow pH range (maximum pH of 3) and their decreasing precision when the difference between the

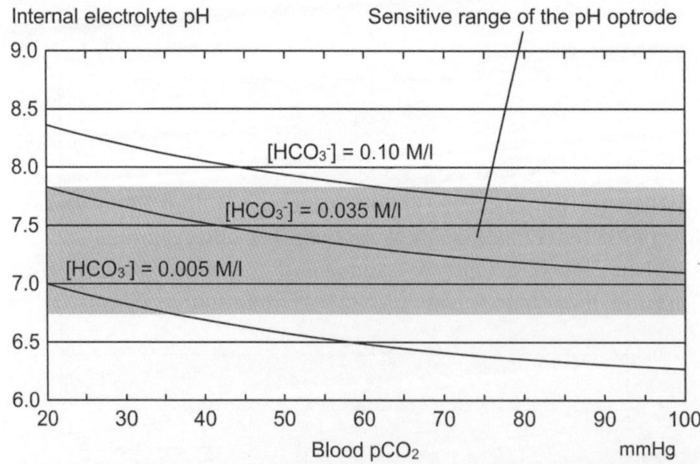


**Figure 7.14.** Internal pH characteristics of pCO$_2$ sensors with various internal bicarbonate ion concentrations (1 mmHg = 0.133 kPa). Reproduced with permission from Soller, B. R., 1994, "Design of Intravascular Fiber Optic Blood Gas Sensors," *IEEE Engineering in Medicine and Biology, 13*(3), pp. 327–335.

measured pH and the pK of the immobilized dye is increased. The determination of pH in blood is facilitated by this narrow range, but their medical application in gastric diagnostics calls for measurements over a large pH range from 0.9 to 7.7. There are two possibilities for mitigating these disadvantages: either use a dye having several pK values, as demonstrated with thymol blue for acid and basic media, or apply a more general solution—the coimmobilization of several dyes (Boisde, Blanc, & Machuron-Mandard, 1991). Here, a four-indicator-based pH optrode was developed and used successfully. The dye shows different behavior in solution and grafted into a poly(*N*-vinylimide-azole) (PVI) bed. Although the curve of output intensity against pH value consists of two almost linear zones with different sensitivities, it makes possible the determination of pH in the range of 0 to 12.

The fiber-optic approach is advantageous in intravascular measurements because it offers a means for sensor miniaturization so that even a fiber bundle can be introduced into the radial artery of a patient through a catheter. The working chemistries of the optrodes are placed at the tips of the fibers, while a thermocouple gives a direct reading of the sensor temperature at that tip. In one interesting solution, the sensors are incorporated onto an ophthalmoscope, thus providing sensor data as along with an image (Alcock & Turner, 1994). This device comprises an array of small fibers, each in contact with part of a chemically sensitive membrane covering the tip of the bundle—in effect resulting in an array of sensors interrogated via the pixels. Hybrid intravascular sensors have also been realized using the optical sensing of pH and $pCO_2$ combined with temperature measurement and electrochemical sensing of $pCO_2$.

## 7.4. OPTICAL SENSORS FOR INVASIVE AND NONINVASIVE OXIMETRY

Optical oximeter devices measure the $SaO_2$ of blood or tissue by exploiting the differences between the absorption spectra of organic compounds transporting oxygen, such as Hb and cytochrome $aa_3$. Oximetry is a technique for measuring a chemical-to-optical transduction effect without applying special indicator dyes, the latter being within the analyte itself. As a result, although the sensor elements are, in practice, physical sensors (e.g., photodiodes), the method is essentially chemical in nature.

### 7.4.1. THEORETICAL BASIS OF BLOOD OXIMETRY

Most oximeter sensors and appliances determine blood oxygen saturation (see equation 7.8 in section 7.2.2) based on the different absorption (extinction) spectra of Hb and $HbO_2$ (Parker, 1987). This is actually the cause of the different colors of arterial and venous blood. The measurement employs a minimum of two different wavelengths: one in the red range (generally around 660 nm) and another in the infrared (IR) range (between 805 nm and 1000 nm). The extinction coefficient is the same for Hb and $HbO_2$ at 805 nm, so this (isosbestic) wavelength can serve as a reference.

In reflection mode oximetry, backscattered light from the specimen is sampled at two different wavelengths ($\lambda_1$ and $\lambda_2$) and the oxygen saturation is estimated using the reflectance ratio, $R = \ln(I_0/I_r)$, where $I_0$ is the incident and $I_r$ is the reflected intensity, according to the following expression:

$$SO_2 = A - B[R(\lambda_1)/R(\lambda_2)], \qquad (7.14)$$

where $A$ and $B$ are empirical constants. Although scattering nonlinearity can be neglected in practice, the constants are of course dependent on the volume ratio of red blood cells, that is, the hematocrit. To compensate for this effect, the measurement is usually made at three wavelengths (Wolfbeis, 1991).

In transmission oximetry, the absorption of the light transmitted through the tissue is analyzed. According to the definition of optical density $(d)$,

$$d = \ln(I_0/I_t),  \tag{7.15.a}$$

where $I_0$ is the incident light intensity and $I_t$ is the transmitted light intensity. Applying the Lambert–Beer equation for a blood sample (see also equation 7.22, section 7.7.1.2.3):

$$d = l[h(\text{Hb})C(\text{Hb}) + h(\text{HbO}_2)C(\text{HbO}_2)],  \tag{7.15.b}$$

where $C$ is the concentration and $h$ is the extinction coefficient of the different compounds, and $l$ is the optical path length. This expression assumes linear contributions of the various compounds to the overall absorption. Performing optical density measurements at two different wavelengths ($\lambda_1$ and $\lambda_2$), the concentrations [$C(\text{Hb})$ and $C(\text{HbO}_2)$] can be determined from two linear equations, knowing the extinction coefficients [$h(\lambda_1,\text{HbO}_2)$, $h(\lambda_2,\text{HbO}_2)$, $h(\lambda_1,\text{Hb})$, $h(\lambda_2,\text{Hb})$] and the optical path length ($l$). However, the $\text{SaO}_2$ can be calculated without knowing $l$ exactly (Takatani & Ling, 1994):

$$\begin{aligned}
C(\text{Hb}) = {}& [h(\lambda_2,\text{Hb})d(\lambda_1) - h(\lambda_1,\text{Hb})d(\lambda_2)]/ \\
& l[h(\lambda_1,\text{HbO}_2)h(\lambda_2,\text{Hb}) - h(\lambda_2,\text{HbO}_2)h(\lambda_1,\text{Hb})],
\end{aligned}  \tag{7.16a}$$

$$\begin{aligned}
C(\text{HbO}_2) = {}& [h(\lambda_2,\text{HbO}_2)d(\lambda_1) - h(\lambda_1,\text{HbO}_2)d(\lambda_2)]/ \\
& l[h(\lambda_1,\text{Hb})h(\lambda_2,\text{HbO}_2) - h(\lambda_2,\text{Hb})h(\lambda_1,\text{HbO}_2)],
\end{aligned}  \tag{7.16b}$$

$$\text{SaO}_2 = C(\text{HbO}_2)/[C(\text{Hb}) + C(\text{HbO}_2)].  \tag{7.16c}$$

Because of the complicated absorption and scattering processes in blood, these results are often not accurate enough for practical applications. Measurements are then made at three or more different wavelengths and the $\text{SaO}_2$ is calculated from the measured densities according to equation 7.17, this being a more general form of equation 7.16 (Mendelson, 1991):

$$\text{SaO}_2 = \frac{a_0 + \sum\limits_i a_i \cdot d(\lambda_i)}{b_0 + \sum\limits_i b_i \cdot d(\lambda_i)},  \tag{7.17}$$

where $a_i$ and $b_i$ are constants that can be determined empirically by volunteers breathing varying $O_2$ concentrations.

In earlier times, the technique of oximetry was used for the analysis of in vitro blood samples. Nowadays, however, sensors and analyzer systems enabling continuous in vivo monitoring are the focus of interest.

### 7.4.2. INVASIVE OXIMETRY

For intravascular oximetry, plain optical fibers are used to guide the light signal inside the vessel and the light reflected from red blood cells back to the light detector. In estimating $\text{SaO}_2$, usually the reflectance values at two wavelengths, one in the red and the other in the near-IR range, are used with the empirical relation given by equation 7.14. According to the location of the measurement, both arterial and venous saturation can be measured separately.

The oximeter employs two different LEDs as light sources driven on alternate half cycles of the clock pulse (Wolfbeis, 1991). Light from the LEDs is tightly coupled into a branch of an optical fiber bundle. Reflected light is coupled to a photodiode, amplified, and delivered to a sample-and-hold circuit that reads the pulse heights, the ratio of which is computed and displayed. A typical operating frequency for the system is 200 Hz, and the empirical parameters can be set for the computations during in vitro calibration. Given an appropriate calibration, the accuracy of the system is about 1%.

One of the disadvantages of the fiber-optic oximeter is that any damage to the optical fibers results in large measurement errors. In order to circumvent this shortcoming, catheter-tip-type oximeters using hybrid-type miniature sensors have also been developed. The smart sensor elements, the red and IR LEDs, the photodiode, and the preamplifier chips are mounted in a planar arrangement onto the same substrate (Takatani & Ling, 1994).

### 7.4.3. NONINVASIVE EAR OXIMETRY

Because of the problems and risks of catheterization, methods of noninvasive oximetry have also been extensively developed. Noninvasive oximetry is essentially tissue oximetry. Tissue is a complicated medium in which blood vessels, both arteries and veins, are distributed nonhomogeneously. Since their distribution is unknown, the analysis of optical processes in tissue is rather complex. The ear oximeter, developed first by Hewlett Packard, has acquired some clinical success (Mendelson, 1991); the operating principle of the instrumentation is as follows. A high-intensity tungsten lamp generates a broad light spectrum. Eight narrowband interference filters are mounted on a rotating wheel that intercepts the light path sequentially to provide wavelength selection. These filtered light beam pulses enter a fiber-optic cable that carries them to the ear. A second fiber-optic cable guides the light pulses transmitted through the ear back to the instrument for detection and analysis. To measure arterial blood saturation ($SaO_2$), the ear probe is attached to the pinna of the ear after the ear has been rubbed briskly for about 20 seconds in order to increase local blood flow. A temperature-controlled heater within the probe maintains the temperature at 41°C, causing a local increase in blood flow and blood "arterialization" after the probe has been properly positioned on the ear. The computation circuits derive $SaO_2$ using equation 7.17. The accuracy of the measurement has been found to be better than 2.5% saturation regardless of skin color and ear thickness.

Another computational method subtracts the attenuation of bloodless tissue, and this measurement is made by compressing the ear using a transparent pressure capsule that is initially inflated to a pressure in excess of the arterial blood pressure, thus rendering the ear pinna practically bloodless. The main shortcomings of this method are discomfort for the patient caused by heat and pressure on the ear, and the relatively heavy weight of the optical cable, which is a particular disadvantage in monitoring neonates and premature infants.

In critical care and surgical settings, venous blood saturation ($SvO_2$) monitoring is especially valuable in patients with critical conditions, including hemodynamic instability, septic shock, high-risk cardiovascular conditions, severe burns, acute hypoxemic respiratory failure, and multisystem organ dysfunction.

### 7.4.4. PULSE OXIMETRY

Pulse oximetry is a noninvasive determination of blood $SaO_2$ that solves the problems inherent in ear oximetry. The basis of the technique is to measure the change in light transmitted through the skin that occurs as a result of arterial pulsation. The signal varies with pulsating changes in tissue blood volume, as shown by the plethysmographic diagram in Figure 7.15. It is assumed that the change in light transmitted through tissue during the inflow phase of the cardiac cycle (i.e., systole) is caused solely by the arterial blood, there is no pulse from the surrounding tissue, and the pulse of venous blood is normally insignificant. Consequently the pulsating component of the optical signal has to be measured. The optical signal is usually sampled at two wavelengths, one in the red (e.g., at 660 nm) and the other in the IR region (e.g., at the isosbestic wavelength 805 nm, or at 940 nm). A conventional linear regression according to equation 7.14 is applied to obtain arterial saturation. $SaO_2$ measured by pulse oximetry is often marked as $SpO_2$. Most pulse oximeters are of the transmission type, where forward-scattered light through the fingertip or the ear lobe is analyzed. Reflection-type pulse oximeters have also been developed, with more general applicability to any portion of the body, such as the forehead, cheek, calf, and thigh. However, in comparison to transmission, the reflection pulse oximeters have a poorer signal-to-noise ratio (SNR).

The breakthrough from oximetry to pulse oximetry came with new LED technology developed from 1982 to 1985. LED light sources are very small and easy to drive, and have the great advantage that they can be mounted within the sensor along with a photodiode receiver. For correct measurements, at least two LEDs emitting different wavelengths are necessary. A suitable combination consists of a red LED (650 nm) and an IR LED (940 nm). The red LED's wavelength has to occupy a narrow range, which is not normally possible with standard commercially available LEDs. One way to overcome this is to provide in each sensor a calibration resistor matched to the actual LED wavelength. Another way is to select only LEDs with a fixed wavelength. This method becomes practical if the LED wafer production yields a narrow wavelength distribution (Kästle et al., 1997).

Figure 7.16 shows a planar-structure reflection-type hybrid sensor (Mendelson, 1991). The hermetically sealed metal–glass package with a transparent cover lid contains an interconnection system on a ceramic substrate and four LEDs, with six large-area photodiodes around them, an arrangement

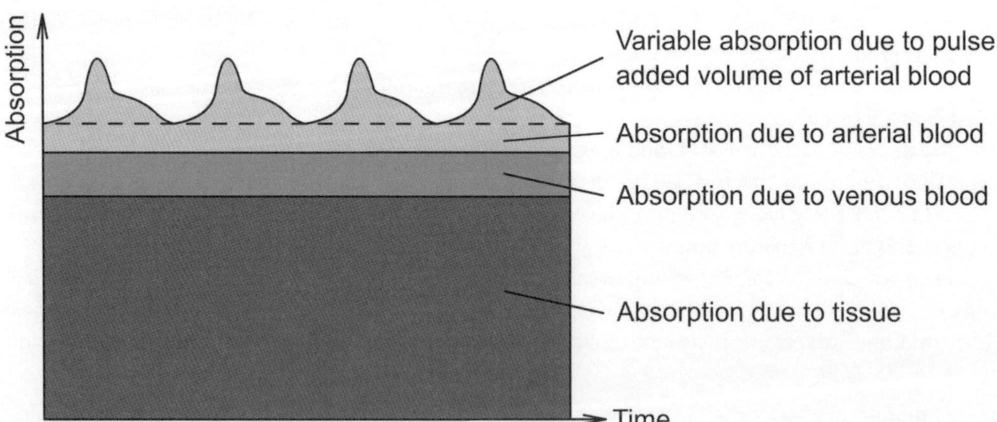


**Figure 7.15.** Variations in scattered or transmitted light attenuation by tissue, showing the rhythmic effect of arterial pulsation.

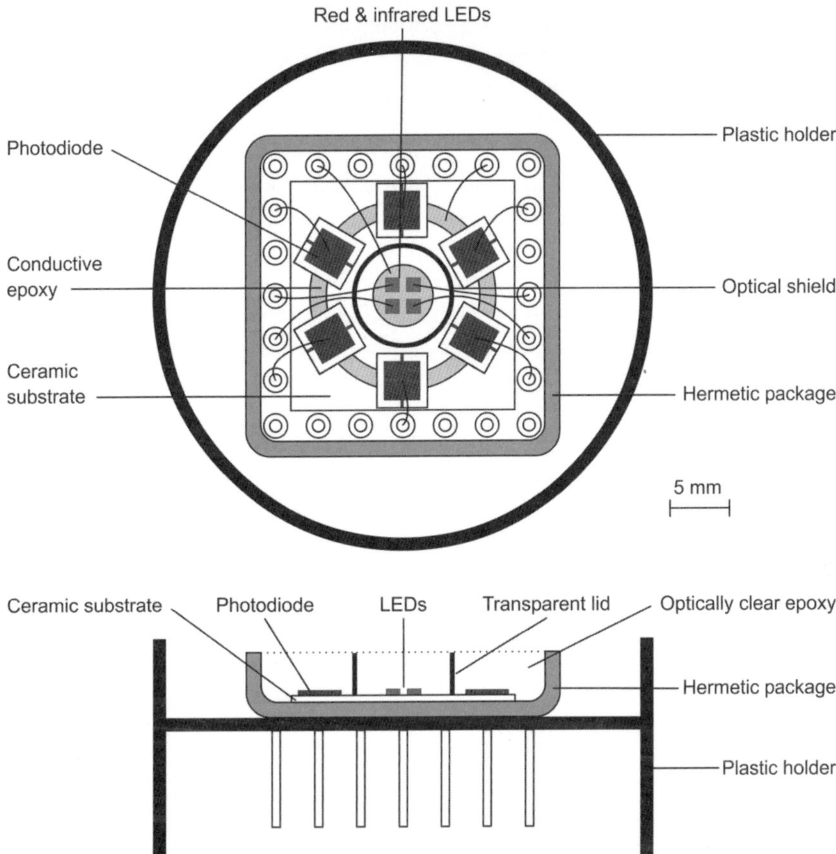


**Figure 7.16.** Noninvasive reflection oximeter sensor. Reprinted after Mendelson, 1991, "Invasive and Noninvasive Blood Gas Monitoring," in D. L. Wise (Ed.), *Bioinstrumentation and Biosensors*, Marcel Dekker, New York, NY, p. 271.

that makes possible the averaging of the spatial differences. The LEDs and photodiodes are optically shielded from each other and the metal package is molded into a plastic housing.

Newer $SpO_2$ measurement appliances employ only two LEDs and a single photodiode on ceramic substrates in a variety of sensor heads for several applications. These include the adult finger glove, pediatric finger glove, and neonatal foot strap, and earlobe clip, combined with a single measurement appliance (Kästle et al., 1997). Usually a time-multiplexed approach is applied in which the two LEDs are switched on and off alternately. The time periods usually consist of a minimum of three: active red, active IR, and a dark period in which the ambient light is measured. There can be more than three periods to allow more LEDs to be powered in one multiplexing time frame, or to allow additional dark periods; all these periods are similar in duration. The modulation frequency (the complete frame repetition rate) typically ranges from 200 Hz to 2 kHz. The frequency spectrum of such a time-multiplexed signal at the receiving photodiode consists of small bands (approximately 10 Hz) around the modulation frequency and its harmonics. Depending on the width of the individual LED pulses, the harmonic frequency content is of significant amplitude for several tens of harmonic orders.

Since pulse oximeters rely on adequate arterial pulsation, a significant reduction in peripheral vascular pulsation, such as in hypotension, vasoconstriction, or hypothermia, can produce a signal too small to be processed reliably by the oximeter. Furthermore, motion artifacts can cause erroneous readings. In practice, these artifacts are reduced by the digital processing of the analog signals and the averaging of the measured values over several seconds before they are displayed. The interference from electrosurgical units and high-intensity light sources, such as surgical lamps, can cause inaccurate readings, as can various compounds possibly present in the blood, such as intravenous dyes. Because interference could lead clinicians to apply incorrect care and therapy, possibly causing harm to patients, interference must be avoided at all costs. A major goal for sensor design is, therefore, optimum optical and electrical shielding. However, in spite of the various sources of error, the accuracy of pulse oximetry is sufficient for many clinical applications. Most manufacturers claim that their instruments are accurate to within 2% saturation in the range between 70% and 100%.

Despite the aforementioned limitations, pulse oximetry has become the most widespread and useful technique of blood oxygen measurement and monitoring. Recently it has been recommended as a standard of care for basic intraoperative as well as neonatal monitoring. All bedside patient monitoring systems (noninvasive and invasive) contain a pulse-oximeter module (e.g., Philips, HP, Ohmeda). Small appliances are also available for fingertip application, both as a single fingertip sensor with display and as sensor in contact with a wrist-wearable display system (e.g., Smith Medical PM Inc.; Nonin Medical Inc.).

This widespread application is due to several major advantages in comparison with all other methods used for measuring blood oxygenation:

- It is a noninvasive technique.
- It enables the direct determination of $SaO_2$ with good accuracy.
- It is not necessary to heat up the skin.
- There is no need for complicated computing and calibration processes.
- The sensors can be attached easily and quickly and the measurement also takes only a short time.
- The sensor elements do not contain any part that must be refreshed (such as electrolyte or a membrane), thus stable long-term operation is assured.

### 7.4.5. OTHER OXIMETRY METHODS

Cytochrome $aa_3$ (cytochrome oxidase) is the terminal enzyme of the mitochondrial respiratory chain and catalyzes approximately 90% of all $O_2$ utilization in the body. This enzyme is of particular importance in monitoring oxidative metabolism because it donates electrons to $O_2$. Therefore the redox state of cytochrome $aa_3$ is believed to be an indicator of intracellular $O_2$ sufficiency. In the oxidized state, this enzyme exhibits a distinctive absorption band in the 820 nm to 870 nm region of the spectrum. This band disappears upon reduction when $O_2$ delivery is compromised. Since Hb and $HbO_2$ also absorb in this spectral region, multiple wavelengths and the application of appropriate algorithms are required to eliminate this interference (Mendelson, 1991).

Noninvasive cerebral oxygenation monitoring can be performed by cytochrome $aa_3$ oximetry using three gallium-aluminum-arsenide (GaAlAs) laser diode light sources with peak emission wavelengths between 760 nm and 904 nm. The light is guided to the subject's forehead by an optical fiber, while the backscattered light from the brain is collected by another optical fiber located a few centimeters laterally from the incident entry beam. Using a third fiber close to the entry, and collecting backscattered light almost solely from bone, a differential measurement can be realized to minimize the effect of the skull. Deep-layer brain tissue information can be obtained in this way (Takatani & Ling, 1994).

Time-resolved spectroscopy can also be applied for obtaining information from deep-layer tissues. The basis of this technique is that very narrow duration (picosecond) excitation pulses are applied and the backscattered pulse waveforms are analyzed. The depth of the resultant information can be estimated in this way. Also, multiple detectors can be placed to focus at specific depths in the tissue, yielding 3-D mapping of oxygen in the tissue. Time-resolved spectroscopy is becoming important in neonatal cerebral monitoring.

Choroidal eye oximetry can be performed with special noninvasive tools by shining a multiple-wavelength light beam into the eye and measuring the amount of light that is backscattered from the ocular fundus using a special fundus camera. Blood oxygen saturation is computed, applying the usual methods of oximetry. Since choroidal blood is characteristic of the blood supply to the brain, this is an indirect method of brain oximetry.

## 7.5. MEDICAL GAS PHASE SENSORS

### 7.5.1. INHALED AND EXHALED $O_2$ AND $CO_2$ CONTROL

Fast, real-time measurements of $O_2$ and $CO_2$ in human breath are fundamental tasks in therapeutic and diagnostic medicine. For example, the shape of curves obtained by recording $O_2$ and $CO_2$ in expired gas is modified by airway obstruction, and the analysis of the deformation provides an indirect measurement of lung disorders. For several diagnostic methods, the determination of $CO_2$ alone is not sufficient. Distribution disorders of gaseous diffusion to or out of the blood system cannot be analyzed by $CO_2$ measurement alone because of the high diffusivity of $CO_2$ (about twenty times higher than for $O_2$). Thus the oxygen concentration in breath is an important additional parameter. Oxygen monitoring in pulmonary respiratory measurements involves a variety of clinical applications: adult and neonatal intensive care, anesthesia, pulmonary function diagnostics (breath-by-breath oximetry), and stress or exercise testing (sports medicine). While in clinical monitoring applications (anesthesia, intensive care) the measuring range covers 15 vol.% to 100 vol.% of $O_2$, the $O_2$ concentration range in diagnostic medicine (15 vol.% to 21 vol.%) is essentially limited to the breathing of ambient air.

Generally, mainstream measurements (gas mixture analysis in the primary flow directly at the patient's mouth) and sidestream measurements (a small stream of gas extracted from the primary flow) can be distinguished. Oxygen monitoring of gas mixtures in clinical applications is presently performed by instruments based on a variety of methods, and the conventional technical solutions may be classified as follows:

- Electrochemical sensors (polarographic or galvanic fuel cells) are commonly employed in slow-response applications and thus are restricted to the determination of the average oxygen concentration (Teledyne).
- Paramagnetic oxygen sensors are fast, but this technology is utilized successfully in sidestream configurations only.
- Zirconium oxide oxygen sensors show fast response times but cannot be used in the presence of anesthetic agents because of the high temperature (greater than 650°C) inside the measurement cell. Thus this principle in not frequently applied for medical purposes.

- Mass and Raman spectrometers are applied for sidestream measurements, with less suitability for widespread clinical applications because of their high price.
- Optical techniques for measuring oxygen in respiratory gas have also been suggested. For example, oxygen was measured based on its absorption band at 145 nm. However, various substances such as water vapor and $CO_2$ were found to interfere. Another instrument has been described that is based on the measurement of oxygen concentration using the very narrow absorption line at 760 nm.

An application of an optochemical oxygen sensor to respiratory gas monitoring was described by Kolle et al. (1997). This sensor was based on measurement of the quenching of the intensity of photoluminescence of the dye platinum (II) octaethylprophyrin ketone by molecular oxygen. The dye was immobilized in various polymers with and without plasticizer. The suitability of optochemical oxygen sensors for clinical use in respiratory gas-exchange measurements has been demonstrated in combination with a prototype instrument. These sensors require no moving parts, consequently they are more stable and cheaper to construct than paramagnetic instruments. It is possible to apply these sensors in vibrating and harsh environments.

Sidestream $CO_2$ modules work in conjunction with mainstream modules and are designed for use with intubated adult and pediatric patients to provide both waveforms and numeric values. The module samples an intubated patient's airway gases through a remote sample line that places less weight on the patient's airway adapter and reduces the risk of extubation. The remote sample cell is located on the front of the sidestream $CO_2$ module. From there, data are passed to the mainstream $CO_2$ module for analysis and display. The sidestream $CO_2$ module provides the following information: $CO_2$ waveform, end-tidal ($etCO_2$) numeric, and inspired minimum ($imCO_2$) numeric.

Bedside monitoring appliances all have the same role, the only differences being in the various application sites: hospital-based operating rooms, ambulatory surgical centers, and low-acuity procedural sedation (sedation procedures for developmentally disabled or incapacitated persons).

A complete metabolic monitor appliance is a special bedside unit (e.g., Philips). It is ideal for use with a ventilator or a canopy, and is equally suited to both spontaneously breathing and mechanically ventilated patients of all ages. The individual nutritional needs of critically ill patients vary widely; both overfeeding and negative energy balance are harmful. The only reliable method of designing and maintaining optimal nutrition in these patients is to measure their true energy expenditure. This is exactly what the metabolic monitor's indirect calorimeter is designed to do. It measures caloric needs and estimates substrate oxidation in patients by continuously monitoring $O_2$ consumption and $CO_2$ production. Measuring gas exchange makes it possible to study the complex interrelations between energy metabolism, nutrition, lung function, and ventilator dependency.

Currently successful electrochemical gas sensors are mostly steady type, or rather, the response of these sensors is measured with steady electrochemical methods under a steady operating state, such as Clark-type amperometric gas sensors and Nernst's potentiometric gas sensors. As a result, further improvement in sensor characteristics is restricted by this "steady-state" requirement, and usually this kind of steady electrochemical gas sensor is only able to detect a single gas component. In order to optimize the electrochemical sensor performance characteristics and develop sensor functions, new approaches for developing transient electrochemical multicomponent gas sensors have been proposed by Zhou et al. (2001)—porous thin-layer electrode coulometry (PTLEC) and modulated pulse potential amperometry (MPPA)—that work on thin-layer electrochemistry and transient electrochemistry principles, respectively. As compared with steady electrochemical methods for conventional electrochemical gas sensors, they represent breakthroughs in optimizing multicomponent gas-sensing performance characteristics in the detection of $O_2$ + $N_2O$ (nitrous oxide, an anesthetic gas) and $O_2$ + $CO_2$ (biorespiratory gases) gas mixtures.

The working electrode used in PTLEC was constructed using a hydrophobic porous thin-layer (less than 0.5 mm) gas electrode that consists of a hydrophobic porous layer made from a mixture of Teflon and acetylene black, a thin hydrophilic layer of catalyst, and a current collector between the layers. The PTLEC electrode is first exposed to the gas samples (1 to 2 seconds) and then immersed in the measurand liquid. The composition of the measurand liquid equilibrates with the help of a leveling bulb (the gas within the pores of the electrode) formed during the measurement, until the PTLEC electrode is fully immersed, and the electrochemical measurement is carried out. Voltammograms from the PTLEC electrode are recorded by the usual methods.

The modulated pulse potential amperometry (MPPA) approach was established by combining a computer-controlled fast modulated potential technique with a microelectrode method. The work was performed with an experimental setup controlled by a computer via an analog-to-digital (AD)/digital-to-analog (DA) converter. The controlling and measuring software programs provide a real-time and dynamic transduction technique integrated with the acquisition, treatment, and display of signals for rapid simultaneous detection of multicomponent gases, such as the biorespiratory gases $CO_2$ and $O_2$.

### 7.5.2. ANESTHETIC GAS MONITORING

Anesthetic gas monitoring (AGM; e.g., Philips) uses IR absorption technology to measure the five most commonly used anesthetic gases (halothane, isoflurane, enflurane, sevoflurane, and desflurane), plus $N_2O$ and $CO_2$. Oxygen is generally measured using paramagnetic or electrochemical techniques. The most important functions include the following:

- Automatic alert when anesthetic agent mixture is detected
- Inspiration and expiration values for all gases
- Individual alarm limits for each parameter
- Respiratory rate derived from $CO_2$ waveform
- Flow rate measurements
- Airway respiratory rate (awRR) monitoring

Phasein's IRMA mainstream probe, for example, is similar in size to a pulse oximeter finger sensor. It was designed using the latest advances in component and microprocessor technology to provide a complete mainstream monitoring system with unique versatility and design. The IRMA sensor head measures IR light absorption at ten different wavelengths in order to precisely determine gas concentrations in the mixture. An ultrarapid response time galvanic oxygen sensor cell integrated into the sensor head allows the proximal measurement of inspired/expired oxygen even for very small children.

A novel microdosage system consisting of a diaphragm pump and a piezoelectric nebulizer was developed by the Fraunhofer Institute for Integrated Systems and Device Technology (Fraunhofer IISB) in order to allow even the smallest quantities of anesthetics to be proportioned. This miniaturized multichannel gas measuring system is based on nondispersive IR spectroscopy and allows both anesthetic gases (such as fluorochlorinated hydrocarbons and $N_2O$) and expired $CO_2$ to be measured in the patient's main respiratory stream. To make possible a compact constructional design for the multichannel measuring equipment, a thermal radiator as the light source and the gas measuring cell itself are set up separately from each other. An IR light-guide fiber conducts the radiation to the gas-measuring cell where it is reflected through the patient's respiratory stream toward two multichannel detectors.

In order to develop a semiconductor-type gas sensor applicable to the monitoring of $N_2O$ in air, a search for semiconductor oxides sensitive to $N_2O$ was carried out by Kanazawa et al. (2001). Among the twenty-three kinds of single oxides tested, $SnO_2$ turned out to have the highest sensitivity to $N_2O$, although that sensitivity was not sufficiently high. However, it was found to be effectively improved when the $SnO_2$ was loaded with a small amount of a basic oxide such as SrO. A 0.5 wt.% SrO-loaded $SnO_2$ heated to 500°C exhibited an $N_2O$ sensitivity about three times that of pure $SnO_2$ and could detect $N_2O$ in air fairly well in the concentration range 10 ppm to 300 ppm.

## 7.5.3. EXHALATION GAS ANALYSIS FOR DIAGNOSTIC PURPOSES

Exhalation gas analysis is another potential application area for gas sensors, as it has been known since medieval times that the smell of human body odor or exhaled air can give an indication of the presence of disease. In modern times, the development of gas sensor systems has made possible the detection of disease marker gases in human exhaled air. These tests can be carried out at home or at the doctor's office.

One prerequisite for the realization of such applications is the existence of known and medically acknowledged marker gases that are detectable using appropriate gas sensor devices. The choice of the medical application is based on known clinical trials involving disease marker gases in breath. Some of the molecules investigated as markers include the following:

- Hydrogen ($H_2$): digestion $H_2$ as an indicator of the incomplete use of hydrocarbons
- Nitric oxide (NO): asthma, especially in children
- Ethanol: ethanol in the blood
- Carbon monoxide (CO): a marker for oxidative stress
- Ammonia ($NH_3$): protein digestion

The fact that an asthmatic person manifests a drastic increase in the concentration of NO in exhaled air is used for detection of the disease and for analyzing its severity. Having determined the NO concentration, it is possible to take timely measures aimed not only at preventing the onset of the disease, but also at terminating any respiratory tract inflammation. Together with NO, exhaled air may contain other gases such as acetone and CO in microconcentrations, and the level of oxygen in exhaled air may fall to 15 vol.%. For this reason the analysis of exhaled air should be comprehensive, and a multisensor approach was presented recently (Ivanova et al., 2004). Here, the level of NO in exhaled air was measured using a semiconductor sensor based on tungsten trioxide ($WO_3$), and the presence of acetone was determined using semiconductor sensors based on tin dioxide ($SnO_2$). The level of oxygen was determined using an electrochemical sensor of the amperometric type operating on a two-electrode measuring system. The concentration of CO was measured with the help of an electrochemical cell operating on a three-electrode measuring circuit. Because the characteristics of the sensors employed depend on such factors as temperature, humidity, and flow rate, there is a need to check these parameters in order to take them into account during measurements. For this reason, the multisensor complex was fitted with sensors for temperature (resistive type), humidity (a planar-type sorption-capacitance sensor), and flow rate (a thermoanemometer). The new multisensor complex is a multifunctional microprocessor-equipped measuring system intended for continuous measurements of the concentrations of NO, oxygen, acetone, and CO in exhaled air. In addition, real-time measurements of the temperature and humidity of the analyzed air are made, with further analysis and data saving by the computer.

The work presented by Fleischer and Simon (2005) was carried out in the course of the Low-Cost Gas Sensor System in Microsystems Technology for Medicine and Biotechnology (LOCMED) project. This joint university and industry research project targeted the development of innovative microelectromechanical system (MEMS) gas sensors for medical use and biological process control. Motivation for the selection of bronchial asthma as the medical target application was clear: besides the fact that it is a widespread disease with prevalence in the populations of industrialized countries of 5% to 15%, a well-defined and reasonably well-described marker gas exists. This is NO, which constitutes a general biomarker for pulmonary inflammation processes. Exhaled air is very humid, which strongly affects the signals from conventional low-cost gas sensors based on semiconducting oxides of the $SnO_2$ or $WO_3$ type, so this sensing technology was discarded for the selective detection of low NO levels.

An alternative and more modern type of gas sensor was selected and further developed, based on work function changes in a sensing material and read out via field effect transistors (FETs). This hybrid construction consists of two parts, a gateless FET and a suspended gate covered with a gas-sensitive layer, attached using an appropriate process. A construction based on flip-chip technology allows industrial use of this technology and low-cost production. In these devices, the gas to be detected adsorbs at the gas-sensitive layer and generates a small voltage (typically 100 mV) at the interface of the sensitive layer and the ambient gas (physically speaking, this is a change in the work function). This voltage then couples via the air gap capacitance to the transistor channel and modulates the source-drain current of the device. Advantages of this device type include its operability at temperatures from 120°C down to room temperature, as well as allowing a free choice of sensitive materials.

## 7.6. HUMIDITY SENSING

There are several special definitions relevant to humidity measurement techniques. Humidity is defined as the mass of vapor carried by a unit mass of vapor-free gas. The partial pressure of each species in the mixture is in direct proportion to its molar fraction. Thus

$$H = (M_A x_A)/(M_B(1 - x_A)), \qquad (7.18)$$

where $M$ is the molecular weight and $x$ is the molar fraction of the constituents; component $A$ is the water vapor and component $B$ is the air.

Relative humidity (RH) is defined as the ratio of the actual partial pressure of water vapor ($p$) to the saturated vapor pressure ($p_s$) of the water at the gas temperature:

$$RH = p/p_s. \qquad (7.19)$$

The dew point can also be used as a characteristic parameter for the water vapor content in the air. It is defined as the temperature ($T_d$) at which the gas becomes saturated during cooling:

$$p(T_d) = p_s(T), \text{ or } T_d = T_{p = ps}. \qquad (7.20)$$

The connections between the mentioned parameters are given by the laws of psychrometry (Norton, 1982), and a few examples are given in Table 7.2.

There are three major groups of humidity measuring methods: those that measure mechanical property changes; psychrometric measurements, which compare the latent heat of evaporation of a

**Table 7.2.** Connection between psychrometric properties

| Dew point, °C | Relative humidity at 20°C (%) | Water content (ppm) |
|---|---|---|
| −75 | 0.002 | ≈1 |
| −45 | 0.3 | 70 |
| −20 | 4.5 | $1 \times 10^3$ |
| 0 | 25 | $6.1 \times 10^3$ |
| 10 | 50 | $1.25 \times 10^4$ |
| 20 | 100 | $2.34 \times 10^4$ |

saturated environment to the environment in question; and those that respond to electrical or optical property changes such as resistance, capacitance, color, and so on and can be regarded as sensors. Because of the research efforts of the last few years, many different methods and types have been developed that can be categorized as follows:

- Temperature method
  - Dew point hygrometers
  - Psychrometers
- Sorption method
  - Impedance types (based on capacitance or resistance changes or on both, including dielectrics, electroconducting materials, and electrolytes)
  - Transistor structures based on material interactions
  - Mass sensitive devices (bulk or surface acoustic wave resonators)
  - Electrochemical cells
  - Fiber optic
- Propagation method
  - IR spectroscopy
  - Microwave propagation
  - Acoustic wave propagation

In practice, dew point sensors are physical sensors that detect water condensation on a cooled surface either optically or electronically by sensing changes in an interdigital impedance.

Many materials both adsorb and absorb moisture, and it is well known that water molecules undergo chemisorption and physisorption on solid surfaces. Chemisorption, which is the stronger process, causes dissociation of water molecules to form surface hydroxyls. Physisorption takes place on top of these. Water molecules in the first physisorbed layer are double hydrogen bonded to two surface hydroxyls, but are singly hydrogen bonded in the second and succeeding layers. In absorption, the adsorbed molecules penetrate the bulk material. If there are pores, capillary condensation of water takes place in addition to the absorption. Capillary condensation results in the presence of liquid water in all pores with radii up to the critical value according to Kelvin's law, which gives the relation between pore diameters and the saturated vapor pressure. A large number of empirical models exist to describe the absorption of water vapor into a solid, but there is a lack of accurate theoretical equivalents. Usually a porous humidity-sensitive polymer is composed of two phases, a solid polymer material, and water, absorbed and condensed (called quasi-liquid water). The relative permittivity values of polymers used in humidity sensors range from 3 to 10, whereas pure water has a far larger value of about 78 at 25°C. Therefore the capacitance of polymer layers changes with the absorption of water. Various types of polymer electrolytes have also been used for humidity sensors. When such polymer electrolytes sorb water vapor from the atmosphere their electrical resistivity decreases. Thus the easily measurable resistive impedance is a function of the humidity of the air surrounding the polymer. This has led to the well-known resistive-type humidity sensors.

Optical fiber systems are of interest partly as possible techniques for detecting gas species in the atmosphere. Several approaches have been reported for the realization of fiber-optic sensors for detecting environmental humidity. These operate using colorimetric, fluorescence, or luminescence effects in indicators that may be embedded into polymer materials, the latter acting simply as a host material. More about such materials and possible transducer types is discussed in the literature (Harsányi, 2000), while the remainder of this section will concentrate on the biomedical applications of humidity sensing.

## 7.6.1. MEASURING TRANSEPIDERMAL WATER LOSS

Human skin plays an important role in protecting the body from environmental influences and is responsible for many physiological functions. One of these is the water barrier function. Healthy skin optimally keeps water inside the body and has a so-called transepidermal water loss (TEWL) factor in a range specified for age, sex, and actual activity. Measurement of the TEWL factor (its units are grams per square meter per hour) is an important noninvasive method for assessing the efficiency of the skin as a protective barrier. The more perfect the skin protective barrier, the higher the water content of the body and the lower the TEWL.

Transepidermal water loss measurements permit the identification of disruptions in the skin protective function at an early stage, even before they are visible. Normal skin allows water loss only in amounts up to about 30 g m$^{-2}$ h$^{-1}$, measured in the crook of the left forearm. In the case of atopic skin, the TEWL is much higher. Determination of the TEWL is an important support in investigating the skin irritation that occurs due to various physical and chemical influences. Typical fields of application are allergy tests, occupational medicine, observation of newborns, supervising the healing process of skin damage and burns, and testing the effectiveness and biocompatibility of cosmetic products. Instruments for measuring the TEWL involve either surface skin impedance measurements or the application of open or closed chambers equipped with sorption humidity sensors. The former is strongly dependent on personal skin differences and sensor surface cleanliness. The latter is not a quick measurement due to a relatively long sensor time constant.

A new idea for measuring the moisture content in human skin using a fast dew point hygrometer sensor was presented recently (Jachowicz, Weremczuk, & Tarapata, 2004b). Here, the hygrometer construction was based on an integrated semiconductor sensor structure containing an interdigitated double-comb-shaped electrode arrangement for detecting condensation at the dew point, plus a thermoresistor and a heater. To speed up measurements, a fast silicon dew point hygrometer with a closed chamber can be applied. The semiconductor integrated sensor structure, located on a cooling Peltier couple module, was placed on an open side of the "closed chamber" measurement head. A flip-chip technology was used for the electrical structure input and output bonding to a flexible ribbon printed circuit board (PCB).

In operation, a special algorithm is used for very fast control of the detector surface temperature. When the open side of the measurement head is applied to the skin, the water molecules evaporating from the skin quickly increase the hygrometer readings. During the first 15 seconds to 20 seconds, a rapid increase in humidity in the air over the skin surface (in the closed chamber) can be observed. Full humidity stabilization is obtained after 100 seconds to 150 seconds. The measured values of saturated humidity as well as the analysis of humidity changes with time (e.g., the humidity derivative with respect to time) over a patient's skin can provide valuable information to physicians about the skin condition. It has been demonstrated that hygrometers can follow humidity changes with the relatively short delay times of 4 seconds for humidity increase and 10 seconds for humidity decrease.

## 7.6.2. HYGROMETERS FOR LARYNGOLOGY

One of the basic functions of the nose is the cleaning, heating, and humidifying of inhaled air. Thanks to rich vascularization, the presence of arteriovenous junctions, and numerous secretory cells, the nasal and sinusal mucosa produce from 800 mL to 1500 mL of fluid a day. This ensures that the nasal mucosa is moist and increases the humidity of the air passing through the nose. In some diseases the air reaching the larynx has too low a humidity, and this may become a cause of many respiratory tract disorders. Hygrometers on the market are too slow to follow and register precisely a breath humidity cycle. A new fast semiconductor dew point hygrometer for laryngology applications was presented by Jachowicz et al. (2004a). The semiconductor integrated sensor structure, located on a Peltier couple module, was placed in a gas flow chamber measurement head. The measured gas was sucked from the nasal sinus by a pipe connected to the hygrometer head. All operating and measuring functions were controlled by a microprocessor module. Preliminary tests of the whole measurement system were performed on a group of persons of different ages and genders.

## 7.7. SENSORS FOR METABOLITES IN BLOOD, TISSUE, AND SECRETIONS

### 7.7.1. BLOOD GLUCOSE SENSING AND MONITORING

One of the most important applications of biomedical sensors is the monitoring of blood glucose levels in diabetics by means of a glucose sensor. Normally, fasting blood glucose levels are in the range of 3.6 mmol $L^{-1}$ to 6.4 mmol $L^{-1}$ and the peak response to an oral glucose tolerance test should not exceed 11 mmol $L^{-1}$, falling below 7.8 mmol $L^{-1}$ 2 hours later. The diabetic will have a peak response exceeding 11 mmol $L^{-1}$, and the blood glucose will remain above this level after 2 hours. A person is diagnosed as diabetic when the fasting blood glucose level is greater than or equal to 7.8 mmol $L^{-1}$. The blood glucose level can even reach 30 mmol $L^{-1}$ in extreme conditions. One of the major medical advances of the twentieth century was the development of insulin to regulate glucose metabolism. The insulin dose for an individual must be adjusted to minimize hyperglycemia, while avoiding the serious condition of hypoglycemia. This requires frequent and accurate testing to monitor the diabetic's blood glucose level.

People with diabetes must check their blood sugar levels several times a day to help keep their diabetes under control. Most monitoring methods require a blood sample obtained by sticking a finger with a needle from an automatic device. Over the years, scientists have tried to find ways for people with diabetes to measure blood glucose without having to puncture the skin for a blood sample. Hundreds of research groups worldwide are currently attempting to develop a noninvasive glucose sensor.

The present solutions for glucose testing are the following:

- Traditional finger-prick measurements or alternate site testing
  - Invasive
  - Noncontinuous measurement
  - Painful
- Continuous monitoring for clinical use
  - Invasive
  - Uses interstitial fluid (ISF)
  - Must change the measurement site every few days
  - No real-time readings are available
- Continuous monitoring for home use, minimally invasive
  - Uses ISF
  - No real-time readings are available
  - Limited number of readings are available
  - Skin and tissue irritations may occur
- Continuous monitoring for home use, noninvasive
  - Uses optical or dielectric spectroscopy
  - Real-time readings are available
  - Continuous readings are available
  - Skin and tissue irritations do not occur

### 7.7.1.1. Reflectance Photometry

It is now possible for diabetics to determine their blood glucose levels at home using electronic home monitoring appliances. Usually the measurement should be done four times a day, before each meal and before bedtime. A drop of blood is obtained by pricking the finger. This sample is placed on a reagent strip that is analyzed by the instrument using reflectance photometry. This optical method is inherently nonlinear and requires somewhat more complicated signal analysis than other methods. Other disadvantages are the necessity for periodic recalibration and interference by various blood compounds such as erythrocytes and plasma proteins. In spite of these problems, the reagent strip method has been successfully implemented and a number of instrument types have been commercially available for many years.

### 7.7.1.2. Application of Glucose Biosensors

The goals of glucose biosensor research and development are to replace the reagent strip method with sensors and to produce portable instruments for in vivo or ex vivo blood glucose monitoring. Battery-operated portable appliances have employed electrochemical cells equipped with enzymatic membranes, first on $O_2$, and later on $H_2O_2$ transducer surfaces (Buerk, 1993). This form of instrument is simple to use, being operated by only one button, with instructions shown on a liquid crystal display. The instrument prompts the user to place either a calibration solution or a drop of blood into a small plastic well. The sample can be as small as 7 µl, and the plastic well holds it over an electrochemical sensor that is covered with the enzyme-activated membrane. This biosensor is linear with glucose concentration in the range from 0 mmol $L^{-1}$ to 30 mmol $L^{-1}$. Since the current required for the electrochemical biosensor is much less than that needed to operate the LEDs used in reagent strip photometric-type instruments, the appliance can be battery operated. Also, simpler electronics are required, thus allowing the instrument to be miniaturized to the size of a handheld calculator. It detects when the sample has been applied and automatically times the analysis, which is completed in 30 seconds. After making the measurement, the liquid crystal display prompts the user to wipe out the sample and place a drop of cleaning solution in the well. A tight plastic cover is then closed to prevent evaporation or spillage, keeping the membrane hydrated until the instrument is used again. Measurement tests have shown a good correlation with results using conventional analytical methods. Furthermore, interference by blood compounds is much less than for photometric instruments. The membrane has a lifetime of 500 to 1000 measurements or 6 weeks before there is a degradation in performance. The sensitivity of the instrument can be restored simply by replacing the enzyme-activated membrane. The only limitation of the glucose biosensor was found with measurements taken when the blood $pO_2$ was low, as anticipated from the rate-limited reaction. At the highest blood glucose levels, the instrument may underestimate the true level by approximately 10% when $pO_2$ is less than 5 kPa. When blood $pO_2$ is greater than 10 kPa, there is no practically detectable error due to $O_2$ limitation. Today, a number of pocket-portable instruments employ this measurement method.

Recent research and development has been directed toward the realization of implantable systems that are capable of either in vivo or ex vivo continuous monitoring of blood glucose. Ideally, a closed-loop system for regulating the delivery of insulin needs to be developed, using an implantable biosensor and an insulin pump actuator. A more tightly regulated control of insulin during the early stage of the disease may spare the diabetic more severe microcirculatory complications later in life. However, for widespread practical applications, a number of problems relevant to implantable glucose sensors must be solved, including the following:

- Miniaturization of the sensor elements and their integration with other sensors and circuitry components
- Improvement of biosensor lifetime and stability with sophisticated enzyme immobilization techniques
- Toxicology and stability problems due to mediator dissolution
- Biocompatible packaging and implantation methods
- Problems of enzyme refreshment, system recalibration, and sensor interchangeability

Glucose biosensors fabricated to date are based almost entirely on the catalytic effect of the glucose oxidase (GOD) enzyme according to the following net reaction scheme:

$$\text{glucose } (C_6H_{12}O_6) + O_2 \xrightarrow{\quad GOD \quad} \text{gluconolactone } (C_6H_{10}O_6) + H_2O_2. \quad (7.21a)$$

Glucose oxidase will return to its oxidized state in the presence of oxygen, resulting in $H_2O_2$ formation. The reaction product, $H_2O_2$, can also be used for amperometric transduction. Using a platinum or gold electrode polarized at a positive potential of 0.6 V to 0.7 V, $H_2O_2$ can be reduced electrochemically through the following reaction:

$$H_2O_2 \xrightarrow{\quad\quad} 2H^+ + O_2 + 2e^-. \quad\quad (7.21b)$$

Since $H_2O_2$ is generally absent from the external environment of the sensor, there is no necessity for dual-differential measurements, which is a great advantage over amperometric $O_2$ transducers. A detailed discussion of biosensor operation is beyond the scope of this section (see Chapter 8), but the most important applications of biosensors in the biomedical field include the following:

- Continuous monitoring in clinical practice
- Pharmacology: adjusting personal dosages and researching new medicines
- Portable and home monitors for patient self-control
- Implantable sensors for continuous monitoring in everyday life
- Implantable sensor-actuator systems that may replace the hormonal regulating function of one of the endocrine glands

The first two applications are still dominated by conventional analytical methods. The practical application of sensors in portable and home monitors is spreading, while implantable monitoring sensors are in the first stages of practical application. However, implantable regulating systems capable of long-term operation are still in the research and development stages. It is important to mention here that miniature, electronically controllable medicine pumps have already been realized for continuous medicine delivery using silicon micromachining, but there is a lack of reliable biosensors capable of long-term operation. Thus the realization of implantable regulating systems is hindered mainly by the instability and short lifetimes of the biosensor elements. An important recent research initiative is concentrating on body–sensor interface realization problems. Intravascular application, placing sensor elements into the bloodstream, is not an appropriate approach for long-term monitoring, and the taking of blood samples for analysis does not allow continuous operation of the system. Subcutaneous implantation seems to be the most promising approach, where the sample-taking dialysis cell or the sensor element itself is placed into the subcutaneous tissue, mainly in the abdominal fat. The analyte in this case is actually the tissue liquid, not the blood.

There are three main versions of the subcutaneous technique: microdialysis, ultrafiltration, and direct implantation. Based on the principles of diffusion, microdialysis is a method for removing chemical substances from extracellular body fluid without removing any liquid (Harsányi, 2000). The double-lumen microdialysis probe using hollow fibers (e.g., polysulfonic or cellulosic, generally with a molecular weight cutoff size of 15,000 to 20,000) functions as an artificial blood vessel: a physiological buffer solution is pumped at a constant flow rate (1 µl min$^{-1}$ to 100 µl min$^{-1}$) into the fiber placed subcutaneously and retrieves compounds of low molecular weight. The dialysate of the tissue is subjected to analytical methods. If, for example, GOD is contained in the dialysate, the resulting $pO_2$ may be taken as a measure of glucose concentration when determined by using appropriate sensors (Mascini, Moscone, & Bernardi, 1992). In other approaches, the enzyme is immobilized onto the transducer surface forming a real biosensor (Steinkuhl et al., 1996; Volpe et al., 1995). In both cases, however, the measurement is dependent on the flow rate, pressure, active membrane surface, and so on. In recent practical implementations, the probe is connected to a specially designed micromachined silicon-glass chip flow-through cell containing the integrated biosensor together with a system of capillaries and flow channels through which the dialysate is pumped (Steinkuhl et al., 1996). The electrodes of electrochemical-type biosensors are located in two pyramid-like microcontainments etched through the silicon by anisotropic etching. The amperometric current can be measured using miniaturized amplifier electronics with an LCD display that is contained in a handheld monitoring system with the overall size of a mobile phone. If an appropriately low pressure (vacuum) is applied through the subcutaneously inserted tubing of a sufficiently high molecular weight cutoff ultrafiltration membrane (Harsányi, 2000), the interstitial fluid may be sampled and analyzed directly. In the third version, the sensor element is directly implanted (Pickup, 1993). Nearly all these devices are laboratory designed and manufactured.

Considering time constants, microdialysis probes may provide an excellent description of glucose kinetics in subcutaneous tissue over relatively short intervals, but absolute glucose levels can be obtained only retrospectively. In contrast, the ultrafiltration technique may reveal the real glucose concentration in the subcutaneous interstitial fluid, but at relatively long intervals. All sample-taking methods suffer from a slow alteration of the real subcutaneous conditions. On the other hand, for the practical application of direct implantation of the sensor itself, a number of biocompatibility problems have to be overcome, including fibrosis, blood clotting, immunogenic effects, and the toxicity of enzyme or mediator leakage.

Sensors for Medicine and Science Inc. (SMSI) is developing a new approach to glucose monitoring. Here, an SMSI glucose sensor is implanted under the skin in a short outpatient procedure. This sensor is designed to automatically measure interstitial glucose every few minutes without any user intervention. It communicates wirelessly with a small external reader, thus allowing the user to monitor glucose levels continuously or on demand. The reader is designed to track the rate of change of glucose levels and warn the user of impending hypo- or hyperglycemia. The targeted operational life of the sensor implant is 6 to 12 months, after which it would be replaced.

Another innovation, GlucoWatch, by Cygnus, and is a small appliance that can be used as a watch on the wrist. This commercially available device operates with glucose biosensors. The measurement is based on reverse iontophoresis: the glucose molecules of the interstitial fluid are driven by a small current flowing through the intact skin. The glucose is gathered in two hydrogel collection discs in a single-use sensor that also contains the immobilized GOD enzyme. The enzymatic reaction produces $H_2O_2$ that is detected electrochemically (see Chapter 8). Glucose readings are provided as frequently as every 10 minutes for up to 13 hours of continuous monitoring time. Readings are stored in memory and can be viewed at the touch of a button. The second-generation GlucoWatch G2 Biographer is a glucose monitoring device for detecting trends and tracking patterns in glucose levels in adults (age 18 and older), and children and adolescents (age 7 to 17) with diabetes. This device is intended for use by patients at home and in health care facilities. It is indicated for use to supplement, not replace, information obtained with standard home glucose monitoring devices. It is also indicated for use in the detection and assessment of episodes of hypoglycemia and hyperglycemia, facilitating both acute and long-term therapy adjustments that may minimize these conditions. Interpretation of the results should be based on the trends and patterns seen with several sequential readings over time. It must be emphasized that there are circumstances in which patients should obtain a finger-prick test using a blood glucose meter. These situations include times when patients must calibrate the device, when patients' symptoms do not match the device readings, or when patients are considering making immediate changes in daily therapy or taking an insulin injection. In these instances, G2 Biographer results should not be the only source of information for making treatment decisions. The effectiveness of the device was assessed in different environments in multiple studies of similar design. These studies compared G2 Biographer readings with blood glucose test results. In all studies, the G2 Biographer readings closely matched the direction and speed of changes reflected in the blood glucose data. The median correlation coefficient was 0.87. There are some concerns, however, with the patient-oriented calibration process. The electrode surfaces may also cause skin irritation from the small direct current flowing through the skin, but such problems can be avoided by alternating the wearing of the device between both wrists.

### 7.7.1.3. Electrochemical Glucose Sensing

The detection of large molecular weight bioactive compounds is possible not only with biosensors, but also with conventional chemical sensors. The great advantage of these methods for biomedical applications is that they do not employ compounds of living things, which are the most critical lifetime limiting factors. Their common disadvantage is poor selectivity.

The use of direct electrochemical reactions for glucose sensing without the presence of an enzyme catalyst began more than 25 years ago. The first approaches almost all employed the concept of glucose oxidation. The perspective that glucose is an aldehyde that can not only be oxidized to an acid, but can also be reduced to an alcohol, and that this reduction and the redox couple can be utilized for a more selective sensing process, were exploited only much later. Amperometric and later voltammetric methods have been used in direct, three-electrode electrochemical techniques. Most sensors employ platinized platinum for the working and counterelectrodes, and sometimes carbon for the latter. The reference is usually a Ag/AgCl electrode. The physiologic buffer solution provides sufficient chloride ions for reference stability. In amperometry, the oxidation current of glucose is measured at a constant potential. The greatest disadvantages of this method are nonselectivity and a gradual loss in catalytic activity of the working electrode. Special techniques of cyclic voltammetry can ensure better selectivity (Yao, 1991):

- The overall voltammogram contains several peaks that are characteristic for glucose: by evaluating them together, some interference may be screened out.
- Using a suitable potential waveform, the interference of amino acids on glucose signals can be suppressed.
- By applying a technique of differential pulse voltammetry, interference by low molecular weight substances, such as urea, can be reduced in the linear response range of the glucose signal.
- The compensated net charge method involves the mathematical integration of the current of a cyclic voltammogram over one complete cycle: several sources of interference can be significantly diminished in this way.
- Low-potential cyclic voltammetry—an alternative approach for the enhancement of both the selectivity and sensitivity of the working electrode is to operate the voltammetry within a narrow potential range where the glucose signals are most pronounced and where the electrode is less susceptible to interference.

### 7.7.1.4. Application of Optical Polarimetry or Spectroscopic Methods for Noninvasive or Minimally Invasive Blood Glucose Monitoring

Noninvasive glucose monitoring is clearly the most attractive approach for patients with diabetes, allowing more frequent, and possibly even continuous, measurements without any pain or sensation. Such a system should also lead to a reduction in the number of undiscovered hypoglycemic events, as well as in the number of episodes and length of hyperglycemic periods. There are several categories of noninvasive glucose monitoring technologies involving electromagnetic waves: near-IR spectroscopy, mid-far-IR spectroscopy, optical rotation of polarized light, and impedance or dielectric spectroscopy.

Recent technological advances in the photonics industry have led to a resurgence of interest in optical glucose sensing and to realistic progress toward the development of an optical glucose sensor. Such a sensor has the potential to significantly improve the quality of life for the millions of diabetics worldwide by making routine glucose measurements more convenient. Currently more than 100 small companies and universities are working to develop noninvasive or minimally invasive glucose-sensing technologies, and optical methods play a large role in these efforts. Recent advances in optical glucose sensing have concentrated on optical absorption spectroscopy, polarimetry, Raman spectroscopy, and fluorescent glucose sensing.

### 7.7.1.4.1. Polarimetry

The measurement of glucose optical rotation activity on plane-polarized light has been used for the determination of D-glucose concentration in physiologic fluids because, assuming a constant optical path length, the rotation angle is a function of the concentration. Miniature optical integrated systems have been fabricated for such in vivo polarimetry measurements. Here, a (780 nm wavelength) laser diode/photodiode pair was mounted facing each other across a short (about 10 mm long) V-groove created by anisotropic etching into a silicon substrate. The V-groove, isolated with $Si_3N_4$ and covered with a semipermeable membrane, served as a reservoir for the glucose solution. Both diodes were covered with polarization films oriented perpendicularly to each other. The output signal is the photodiode current, which is simply the dark current if the reservoir does not contain glucose, and increases as a function of the glucose concentration. Amino acids and other blood or tissue fluid compounds having optical rotation effects may cause interference, so the efficiency of the permselective membrane has a significant effect on the operation (Burk, Arrieta, & Batich, 1987).

### 7.7.1.4.2. Raman Spectroscopy

Raman spectroscopy is a powerful analytical technique. It relies on the Raman effect, wherein inelastic collisions of photons of incident monochromatic light with molecules leads to some of the scattered light having wavelengths that differ from that of the source. The Raman technique is advantageous with respect to the specificity it can provide, making it a powerful technique for multicomponent blood analysis. However, the extremely weak signals cause it to be inappropriate for in vivo measurements; to achieve an acceptable SNR, the power of the light directed onto the tissue has to be unacceptably high.

### 7.7.1.4.3. Near-Infrared Glucometry

Infrared spectroscopy is a technique of organic analytical chemistry that employs IR absorption spectra of analytes for qualitative, quantitative, and structural analysis based on the phenomenon that various molecular groups and bond types give specific peak configurations in the spectra. The concentrations of particular molecules have linear relationships with the intensities of the relevant absorbance peaks (Beer's law), which can be used to predict the concentrations of those molecules in a substance. The intensity of an absorption peak is given by equation 7.22:

$$\ln(I_0/I) = e(\lambda)cl, \qquad (7.22)$$

where $I$ is the intensity, $I_0$ is the intensity of the incident light, $e$ is the absorptivity or extinction coefficient, $l$ is the path length, and $c$ is the concentration.

Glucose has many absorption peaks from the near-IR up to the mid-IR range (800 nm to 10 µm), although not all of them are specific for only this molecule. The peaks in the mid-IR range correspond to the fundamental vibrations, whereas in the near-IR range they correspond to overtone and combination vibrations. This results in weaker and broader peaks in the latter case. However, the near-IR range possesses some properties that make it more suitable than the mid-IR range for noninvasive in vivo diagnosis. In the mid-IR range, water, which is the dominant component of blood and tissue, absorbs light strongly, allowing only very shallow penetration depths. Therefore mid-IR spectroscopy has only been considered as basically an invasive technique. On the other hand, near-IR light can penetrate into the skin up to 1 cm. The great advantage of near-IR spectroscopy is the possibility of noninvasive blood glucose determination through the skin using the skin's "transmission window," which exists in the near-IR range from 0.7 μm to 2.5 μm. The concept for a near-IR glucometry device is simple: shine radiation through human tissue and analyze what emerges. In theory, the glucose in human tissue will provide a near-IR absorption or transmission fingerprint that can be used to calculate the glucose concentration. This process poses no threat to chemical bonds in the body. However, while working wonderfully for a glass of glucose and water, the approach encounters technical problems in reality because tissue components and other molecules that blur the glucose fingerprint attenuate the detectable signal. The resulting signal-to-noise problems demand complicated mathematical signal processing and amplification schemes.

Historically the mid-IR resonance peak at 9.676 μm characteristic for the C=O bond of glucose molecules was initially used for measuring glucose concentration by utilizing a tunable $CO_2$ laser light source. In vitro study of glucose in whole blood gave a resolution of 1.6 mmol $L^{-1}$. Since the interference of all blood-constituting molecules having C=O stretching vibration is the major problem, a multiple-wavelength approach is necessary (Mendelson et al., 1990).

Molecular transitions that occur within the near-IR spectrum are associated primarily with overtones and combinations of fundamental CH, NH, and OH vibration transitions (Arnold, 1996). The fundamental transitions are much stronger and appear in the mid-IR range. As mentioned, water strongly absorbs mid-IR radiation, which limits the depth of penetration into the human body to only a few hundred micrometers, making it impossible to perform noninvasive blood analysis. The fact that CH, NH, and OH stretches can be observed also in the near-IR spectrum, where the absorption of water is much less, potentially makes possible the noninvasive application of near-IR spectroscopy. Absorbance features directly associated with the glucose molecule are present in the long-wavelength portion of the near-IR spectrum. These features represent overtone and combination bands associated with CH vibrations within the glucose molecule and make this region preferred in terms of potential measurement selectivity and sensitivity. Since other organic molecules also show CH vibrations, their interference cannot be eliminated. The only solution could be multivariate calibration analysis using principal component regression with partial least squares methodology or neural network analysis. A description of these techniques is beyond the scope of this chapter; more about this topic can be found in the literature (Arnold, Burmeister, & Small, 1998; Burmeister, Arnold, & Small, 1998; Hazen, Arnold, & Small, 1998; Small & Arnold, 1998). Great research efforts have recently focused on multicomponent analysis systems for measuring glucose, cholesterol, urea, triglycerides, and lactate in vitro (Hazen et al., 1998). It must be stressed, however, that no one has ever successfully demonstrated the ability to measure in vivo glucose levels in a noninvasive manner (Arnold, 1996). On the other hand, the tremendous potential of this approach will continue to drive advancements in both spectroscopic and computer-based data analysis technologies.

In near-IR spectroscopy, photoacoustic interactions (excited by pulsed laser beams) also cause absorption peaks in the spectra that are more characteristic of the molecular weight and shape than the peaks characteristic for C-H bond resonance effects. Using laser photoacoustic near-IR spectroscopy at a wavelength of 1.7 μm, a relative absorption change of 20% was measurable within the glucose concentration range from 0 mmol $L^{-1}$ to 50 mmol $L^{-1}$. However, it is envisaged that any subsequent device will use multiple wavelengths for the analysis (Christison, 1993). Recently the evaluation method was combined with skin electrical impedance measurement to detect hypoglycemia (Pruna, 1995). Near-IR spectroscopy has also gained attention as a possible noninvasive method for monitoring blood oxygen (Liem, Hopman, & Oeseburg, 1992).

In spite of the obstacles, some groups (CME Telemetrix, InLight Solutions, and Sensys Medical [Instrumentation Metrics]) may have isolated, amplified, and analyzed in vivo and noninvasively a near-IR radiation signal from the forearm. Each group is either preparing for or entering clinical trials with a prototype. A near-IR glucometer would drastically reduce the consumables and discomfort associated with the best currently available monitoring methods, although infrequent drawing of blood samples may still be required for calibration of the device.

Table 7.3 provides a summary of the applied methods and the results published about near-IR glucometry appliances.

The investigational blood glucose monitor from Instrumentation Metrics seems to be one of the successful approaches. It utilizes near-IR diffuse reflectance spectroscopy to achieve a noninvasive measurement. Near-IR (750 nm to 2500 nm) spectroscopy in this application is the process of shining low-level radiation onto the forearm. A portion of the radiation, and the corresponding information within, is then reflected back to a detector. Analysis of the data derived from the first subjects to complete the study shows that the technology has been able to provide accurate measurements of blood glucose levels for at least 8 weeks after the device was personally calibrated for each user. The clinical trial demonstrated that Sensys Medical's noninvasive blood glucose device effectively measured blood glucose in 90% of people with diabetes. This multicenter national trial was the largest of its kind to evaluate a noninvasive testing method. The first commercial device, currently in early clinical testing, is the Sensys Glucose Tracking System (Sensys GTS). It is an upright console measuring 660 mm tall × 660 mm deep × 178 mm wide intended for use by consumers as well as in physician's offices, clinics, nursing homes, and hospitals. Users place their forearm on the device, like an armrest, to obtain a noninvasive blood glucose reading. The device is designed to provide people with diabetes an

**Table 7.3.** Comparison of available noninvasive glucose measurement methods applying near-IR spectroscopy

| Research group | Type of application | Estimated error, mmol L$^{-1}$ |
| --- | --- | --- |
| Rio Grande Medical Technology | Across fingertip | SEC[a] 1.1 |
| Heise et al. (1994); Marbach et al. (1993) | Diffuse reflectance on lip mucous membrane | SEP[b] 2.4 |
| Jagemann et al. (1995) | Across fingertip (applying artificial neural network analysis) | MRSE[c] 1–3 |
| Burmeister et al. (1998) | Transmittance across tongue | SEP[b] > 3 |
| Malin et al. (1999; Instrumentation Metrics) | Diffuse reflectance on forearm | SEP[b] 1.1 |

[a] SEC, standard error of calibration.

[b] SEP, standard error of prediction.

[c] MRSE, mean root square error.

easy and painless way to monitor blood glucose rather than relying on today's traditional blood-stick methods. The next-generation Sensys GTS is presently under development and will be a handheld monitor about the size of a personal digital assistant, such as a Palm Pilot. It is designed to provide portable self-testing.

### 7.7.1.4.4. Mid-Far-Infrared Glucometry

The near-IR method faces competition from mid-far-IR technology that could offer diabetics the same benefits. Mid-far-IR noninvasive systems use oscillating thermal gradient spectroscopy. The human body is a natural radiation source. Specific molecules, such as glucose, absorb, emit, and transmit radiation at particular wavelengths with signal intensities proportional to their concentrations. Glucose happens to absorb IR radiation strongly at 9.25 μm and weakly at 8.45 μm. For wavelengths between 6 μm and 12 μm, the water in our skin, which is approximately 65% of its composition, has a convenient transmittance window that permits analysis of the glucose absorption spectrum. By oscillating the temperature beneath the forearm between 25°C and 35°C once per second, modulated signals from glucose's absorption spectra can be detected and teased out of the body's natural IR emissions—all without an additional radiation source. Once these signals are isolated, computed differences between the 9.25 μm absorption maximum and the 8.45 μm absorption minimum reveal the glucose concentration. To improve this method's accuracy, multiple absorption spectra can be referenced against the base signal—not just those at the 8.45 μm and 9.25 μm wavelengths. OptiScan Biomedical Corporation is working intensively in this area.

### 7.7.1.4.5. Fourier Transform Infrared Spectroscopy

The classical ways of decomposing light into its spectrum are dispersive techniques. Dispersive spectrometers use gratings or prisms to disperse the light into a spectrum of its component wavelengths. A slit is then used to select which narrow "slice" is allowed to strike the detector. An alternative way to decompose light into its wavelength constituents is to use an interferometric technique utilizing Michelson interferometers. A collimated beam from a source enters the interferometer and strikes a beam splitter, at which half is reflected and half is transmitted. The beams reflected from a moving and fixed mirror are then recombined on the beam splitter and impinge on the detector. As one of the mirrors moves, the two recombined beams undergo amplitude interference due to the path difference. This produces an interferogram, which is seen by the detector and recorded by a computer. This interferogram is then Fourier transformed to give the spectrum of the light from the source; in this application, the light transmitted through the sample. In a dispersive system incorporating a grating and an exit slit, only one spectral element is sampled by the detector at a time. In contrast, in Fourier transform spectroscopy, all wavelengths arriving at the detector are examined simultaneously, resulting in higher throughputs. Another advantage of the interferometric technique is the superiority of its SNR. In theory, all spectrometers can show an improved SNR if spectra are averaged. However, this relies on the assumption that the spectra can be exactly superimposed. Any displacement error between spectra can cause band shapes to be distorted and, as a result, the SNR will fail to improve. Interferometric systems utilizing a helium–neon (He–Ne) laser for data acquisition, trigger, and motion control are very stable. Data can be acquired at very precise path differences, even if there are some jitters in the velocity of the moving mirror. However, it is clear that the method involves much more costly instrumentation than does the dispersive type. This is one significant limitation of applying it only for a single component (glucose) measurement.

Wide-range Fourier transform infrared (FTIR) spectrometry has proved to be a global, sensitive, and highly reproducible physicochemical analytical technique with which structural biomolecular moieties are characterized by their IR absorption. Since a biomolecule is defined by its unique structure, a unique FTIR spectrum will be exhibited by this biomolecule, representing its structural fingerprint. Furthermore, every biomolecular family present in the sample will exhibit almost similar and overlapping FTIR absorptions. FTIR analytical applications have allowed blood content determination using various materials and sample preparations. Concentrations of glucose, total proteins, creatinine, urea, triglycerides, and cholesterol in blood, plasma, and serum can be determined with clinical accuracy (Déléris & Petibois, 2003). However, important sample preparation, spectra manipulation, and mathematical treatment were necessary to obtain such results. Clinical analysis requires methods where sample manipulations are minimized because every one can be considered as a source of quantitative error affecting the predictive performance of the method used. Although wide-range FTIR spectrometry seems to be a very effective analytical method, it remains but a part of in vitro techniques using blood samples.

On the other hand, Tenhunen, Kopola, and Myllyla (1998) proposed the application of FTIR spectroscopy within the near-IR range for noninvasive glucose measurements. The wavelength range between 1500 nm and 1850 nm was selected in their study, and spectral measurements were performed using an FTIR spectrometer operating at 32 cm$^{-1}$ resolution. A halogen lamp was used as the light source and a fiber bundle was used as a transreflectance probe to achieve an appropriate penetration depth into the tissue. The fibers of this bundle were slightly pressed against the fingertip during measurement. A detector with a temperature-stabilized IR-sensitive InGaAs element was constructed for measuring the interferogram of the FTIR spectrometer. Wavelengths shorter than 1400 nm were filtered out to minimize the current noise and to guarantee maximal utilization of the dynamic range of the detector and the electronics. The partial least squares algorithm was used in calibration. The standard deviation of the error of prediction was 0.97 mmol L$^{-1}$ and 1.14 mmol L$^{-1}$ for measurements from water–glucose solutions and the test person, respectively.

Factors that have limited the acceptance of optical spectroscopy methods for noninvasive blood glucose sensing include signal variations due in part to changes in the skin tissue optics between patients, the lack of a repeatable path length inherent in using diffusely reflected photon approaches, temperature variations of the skin, and the pressure with which a probe is applied to the skin surface. Unfortunately most previous approaches to noninvasive glucose sensing have failed to address these important issues.

A unique property of IR multiple attenuated total reflectance (ATR) spectroscopy is that the spectra from an analyte are independent of the sample thickness. The basis of operation is that the reflectance spectrum of a large refractive index optical waveguide–sample analyte interface may be characteristic for the sample composition. The measurement could easily be realized in vitro, and by means of an optrode structure, also in vivo invasively. A system for in vitro spectral analysis of human blood serum was realized recently, based on ATR fiber-optic evanescent wave spectroscopy using a Fourier transform IR spectrometer. The blood serum samples were introduced into a special cell designed for the analysis, with an IR-transmitting silver halide fiber as the sensing element. The fiber was in direct contact with the sample. The transmission spectra were analyzed by models of neural networks, which is an effective tool for multicomponent analysis with undefined nonlinear cross-sensitivities. The concentrations of protein and cholesterol in uric acid in human blood serum were obtained, with good correlation with ordinary analytical methods. The method can be used for in situ real-time blood analysis (Gotshal et al., 1997).

McNichols and Gowda (2001) developed a novel skin port sensor that eliminates the effect of skin optics by using a stable, infection-free, dermal implant to provide a skinless "window into the body." The implant was designed to provide a fixed optical pathlength as well as features to minimize temperature and pressure variations. Preliminary experiments in a pig model demonstrated both a stable biological seal at the transcutaneous interface as well as ingrowth of vascular-containing granulation tissue within the sensing chamber. Furthermore, optical spectra acquired from the port demonstrated changes in glucose signatures related to concentration changes induced in the blood. The novel skin port sensor may provide the necessary platform for successful implementation of an optical approach to in vivo glucose sensing.

### 7.7.1.4.6. Glucose Sensing with Fluorescent Indicators

Another approach is the application of an implantable polymer "Smart Tattoo" based on fluorescent glucose sensing (McNichols & Coté, 2000). In the experimental process, two molecular compounds—dextran, a macromolecule composed of glucose subunits, and concanavalin A (conA), a protein that recognizes sugar—are encapsulated in polyethylene glycol (PEG) beads. PEG is a polymer commonly used for orthopedic implants because of its compatibility with human tissue. Dextran is tagged with one fluorescent dye color, or fluorophore, while conA is tagged with another. The experimental microgel beads, injected just under the skin, are too big to enter cells—unlike tattooing, in which cells absorb the pigment. Instead, the beads remain in the spaces between the cells—the interstitial spaces. Fluid in these spaces contains water and glucose molecules small enough to pass through the PEG and reach the fluorophore-tagged polymers. The level of glucose in interstitial fluid is related to the blood glucose level. The dextran molecules bind to the conA molecules, and together, under light from a laser or LED, they fluoresce, emitting a certain color. However, when glucose enters the picture, it competes with dextran, displacing the dextran molecules and binding to the conA. The fluorescent color changes according to the amount of glucose present. In preliminary studies, the researchers injected the microbeads under a rat's skin and found that the rat tolerated the implant. The beads did fluoresce under the rat's skin and indicated a change in glucose level.

GluMetrics Inc. (Irvine, CA, USA) has invented products that are based on a new type of glucose-sensing technology. GluGlow is a substance that glows in the presence of sugar. This boronic acid-based polymeric material is capable of detecting and measuring the blood sugar level of diabetics and other hospitalized patients in a way that will enable physicians to deliver higher quality care than before. Such a substance has long been sought as the "missing link" in the development of an artificial pancreas, which is likely to be the next major breakthrough in bionic physiology.

The benefits of GluGlow's remarkable chemistry are the following:

- It is stable and reversible with a high sensitivity and specificity for glucose.
- It is insensitive to its environment (particularly oxygen concentration).
- Its two-part system (dye and quencher) allows precise tailoring of fluorescence to optimize product performance.
- It has a low power requirement.

An invention by Medtronic Minimed Inc. (U.S. Patent 6766183) applies biosensor molecules that exhibit fluorescence emission at wavelengths greater than approximately 650 nm. Typical biosensor molecules include a fluorophore that incorporates an iminium ion, a linker moiety that includes a group that has an anilinic type of relationship to the fluorophore, and a boronate substrate recognition and binding moiety, which binds glucose. The fluorescence of molecules is modulated by the presence or absence of polyhydroxylated analytes such as glucose. This property, as well as their ability to emit fluorescent light at greater than approximately 650 nm, makes them particularly well suited for detecting and measuring in vivo glucose concentrations.

### 7.7.1.4.7. Infrared Emission Spectroscopy

A novel noninvasive blood glucose monitoring system was published by Malchoff et al. (2002). The human body emits strong electromagnetic radiation. The laws of physics state that all objects emit IR radiation and that the intensity of the radiation and spectral characteristics of the object are determined by its absolute temperature as well as by the properties and states of the object. Thus thermal radiation from the human body contains information about its spectral characteristics and is determined by absolute body temperature as well as by the properties and states of the emitting body tissues. It can therefore be concluded that blood spectral characteristics with different contents of glucose (or other analytes) will change the emissivity of the tympanic membrane, making it possible to measure the concentration of glucose in the blood. The tympanic membrane is known to be an excellent site for the measurement of body temperature because it shares its blood supply with the hypothalamus, the center of core body temperature regulation, and a tympanic thermometer measures the integral intensity (over all wavelengths) of IR thermal radiation. The radiation at the sensor has the spectral characteristics of the blood in the tympanic membrane. In this instrument, the spectral characteristics of various constituents of the blood were separated using analytical chemistry spectroscopic methods. The instrument relies on the use of IR filters placed in front of IR detector windows. One filter passes radiation corresponding to the thermal emission bands with glucose signatures and is placed in one of the IR detector windows, while the other IR detector window is covered by a filter capable of passing radiation that does not include emission bands characteristic of the analyte at wavelengths in the range of interest. A comparison of radiation intensity in the two detector windows provides a measurement that is proportional to the analyte concentration and can be correlated with the concentration of blood glucose.

### 7.7.1.5. Dielectric Spectroscopy

Dielectric spectroscopy (DS) has been tested over a period of time for noninvasive glucose monitoring. In complex biological systems, fast as well as ultraslow molecular rearrangements take place in the presence of microscopic, mesoscopic, and macroscopic organizations. DS is especially sensitive to intermolecular interactions and is able to monitor cooperative processes. It provides a link between the investigation, via molecular spectroscopy, of the properties of the individual constituents of complex biological material and the characterization of its bulk properties. It is well known that glucose does not affect the dielectric spectrum in the megahertz frequency band, and this is the reason its concentration cannot be measured directly. However, because of the specific reactions of blood and tissue cells to varying glucose concentrations, the electrolyte balance across the membranes of blood and underlying tissue is changed. Variations of glucose level and movement of glucose through the cell membrane, such as in erythrocytes, lead to a change in the electrolyte concentrations, and thus to an alteration in the interfacial polarization of the cell membrane—conductivity and permittivity variations. It has been shown that the sodium concentration is strongly correlated (oppositely) with the glucose concentration of the tissue. These effects cause changes in the electromagnetic properties of the human skin and underlying tissue, which are measured by the device. This is the reason why both AC and DC conductivity are sensitive to these subtle changes in electrolyte balance, which is related to the blood's glucose levels. The correct frequency has to be chosen in order to develop a glucose sensor based on DS that will be sensitive to the electrical changes in the body, particularly in blood.

As mentioned, glucose changes in blood are accompanied by significant conductivity variations that greatly influence the effect of electric polarization of cell membranes. This is the reason why the working frequency interval should not be too high, so as not to lose sensitivity to the dispersion (variations of impedance with frequency, resulting in nonlinear effects and huge signals) and ionic DC conductivity. At the same time, the frequency range should not be too low, so as to avoid problems with electrode polarization and huge signals from the dispersion in tissues. For this reason, a frequency in the 1 MHz to 200 MHz range should be chosen. The sensor uses electromagnetic waves in the selected frequency band that interact with the skin and underlying tissue in order to monitor their electrical properties. This is the reason why the sensor can be represented as a serial resonate contour terminated to the fringing working capacitance.

The impedance of the sensor at a given resonance frequency depends on impedance changes within the human skin and underlying tissue. The equivalent circuit of the sensor mounted on the skin is presented in Figure 7.17. The impedance of this resistor–inductor–capacitor (RLC) resonant circuit is measured over the specified frequency range by means of a vector network analyzer (VNA) or a resistive divider.

The typical impedance behavior of the sensor attached to the skin of a patient at different times when significant changes of blood glucose have been induced is shown in Figure 7.18. The data were obtained in the frequency range of 1 MHz to 200 MHz. The figure presents frequency changes of the modulus $|Z|$ and the phase of the impedance. It shows that the resonance frequency and the $|Z|$ minimum, in addition to the $Q$ factor of the resonant circuit, change with different blood glucose concentrations. In the defined frequency range, this sensor can thus provide sensitive measurements of the electrical properties of the skin and the underlying tissue. The sensitivity of the signal was between 20 mg dl$^{-1}$ glucose $^{-1}$ and 60 mg dl$^{-1}$ glucose $^{-1}$ (Caduff et al., 2003).

Based on these results, a commercial glucose-level monitoring device like a watch, called PEN-DRA, is available from Pendragon Medical Ltd. It does not extract any body fluids—it requires no

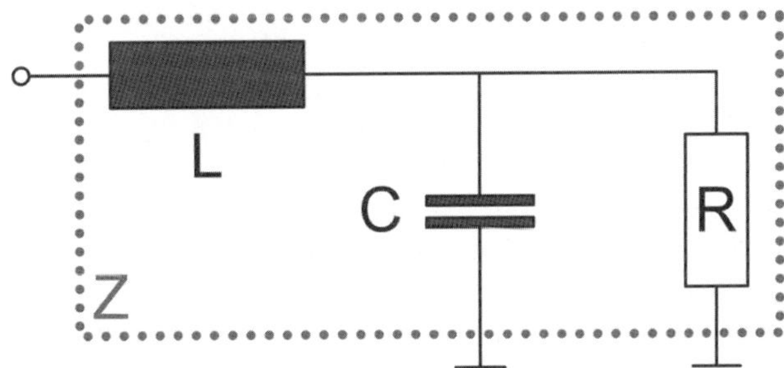


**Figure 7.17.** A simple electrical model of the sensor mounted on the skin. L is the inductance of the external coil, C is the fringing capacitance of the sensor attached to the skin, and R is the averaged resistance of the skin and underlying tissue. Reprinted from Caduff, A., Hirt, E., Feldman, Y., Ali, Z., & Heinemann, L., 2003, "First Human Experiments with a Novel Non-invasive, Non-optical Continuous Glucose Monitoring System," *Biosensors and Bioelectronics, 19*, pp. 209–217, with permission of Elsevier.

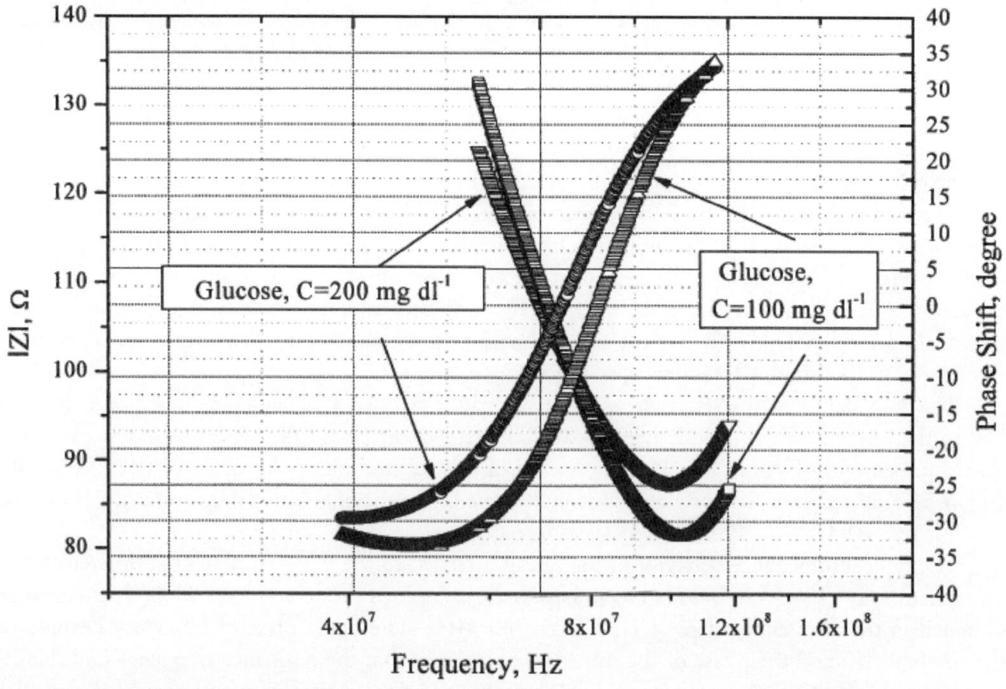



**Figure 7.18.** The modulus |*Z*| and the phase shift of the impedance of the sensor attached to the skin of a patient at different blood glucose concentrations measured by means of a vector network analyzer. Reprinted from Caduff, A., Hirt, E., Feldman, Y., Ali, Z., & Heinemann, L., 2003, "First Human Experiments with a Novel Non-invasive, Non-optical Continuous Glucose Monitoring System," *Biosensors and Bioelectronics, 19*, pp. 209–217, with permission of Elsevier.

blood or interstitial fluid samples. It is designed as an adjunctive device to supplement information obtained from standard blood glucose measuring devices. The device detects trends and patterns in glucose levels in patients with diabetes and can be used for real-time display at home as well as in health care facilities. It is a truly noninvasive method based on impedance spectroscopy that performs continuous measurement of glucose in real time, day and night, at one reading per minute and detects trends and patterns in glucose profiles. There is an adjustable alarm for signaling the onset of hypoglycemic conditions as well as hyperglycemic situations. Its benefits are as follows:

- Improves compliance for a tighter control of diabetes
- Helps to simplify the therapy management of diabetics—acute and long term
- Reduces diabetes complications by continuous monitoring and management of hypo- and hyperglycemic conditions
- Stores data of 1 month for glucose and alarm history
- Manages patient data with available user software

## 7.7.2. SENSORS FOR OTHER ANALYTES

Although the majority of studies and sensor developments in the field of blood and secretion analysis concentrate on glucose, analytes other than glucose are also important measurement targets. The accurate determination of biological parameters by means of rapid online measurements at low concentrations is an important task within the fields of pharmaceutical screening and medical diagnostics. However, in biological samples, the analytes of interest are present as minor components in complex mixtures and with interfering species.

Biosensors are the best candidates for these applications, providing direct solutions to this need for accuracy, but their intrinsic selectivity often excludes all the other components in a sample. A separation step introduced prior to the sensing component could allow for both an increase in selectivity with respect to the interfering species and the identification of a wide spectrum of molecular components in the sample. There has been an exponential increase in applications for biosensors in the fields of pharmaceutical screening and medical diagnosis, aimed at facilitating the real-time monitoring of biomolecular components (see Chapter 8). Researchers are also expanding the power and versatility of biosensors by using them together with other instruments, including mass spectroscopy (MS) and gas and liquid chromatography (GC, LC) systems (Jakeway, De Mello, & Russell, 2000; Weller, Schuetz, Winklmair, & Niessner, 1999). More and more technological methods are being developed that combine the advantages of both approaches in highly powerful analytical tools. Nevertheless, the application of such hybrid techniques is not yet very widespread, although additional approaches would be highly desirable.

Gas chromatography systems are important tools for analytical assays and have been proposed for biomedical, agricultural, environmental, and food industry applications. Gas chromatography is a separation process in which the substances to be separated are distributed between two immiscible phases. One of the two phases is stationary, while the other flows through the chromatographic separation path, making possible the transport of material in a mobile phase. The column and the detector are the main system components, although a gas injection system and electronics for data preprocessing play an important role from a system integration perspective.

Lorenzelli et al. (2005) discuss the development of a silicon-based integrated separation microsystem for gas chromatography aimed at biomedical applications, with particular emphasis on monitoring the homovanillic acid (HVA) and vanillylmandelic acid (VMA) ratios in mass population screening for neuroblastoma diagnosis and prognosis. The detection of neuroblastoma tumors can be accomplished by monitoring urinary levels of HVA and VMA as end products of the metabolism of the catecholamine-related molecules dopamine and norepinephrine, respectively. The miniaturized system consists of two main modules: a metal oxide semiconductor detector and a micromachined separation capillary column. As a first step, the metal oxide semiconductor's capability for detecting HVA and VMA has been demonstrated. Then, technology for a silicon separation capillary microcolumn, including an on-chip gas sensor housing, has been proposed and a first prototype has been developed. Traditionally flame ignition detectors and thermal conductivity detectors are commonly used in gas chromatography, but a semiconductor metal oxide gas sensor may be a suitable alternative to these detectors, as column separation can be improved by using selective layers, deposited on the membrane, to allow a better sensor response to a specific analyte. The proposed gas sensor consists of a microheater, a temperature sensor, and an interdigitated microelectrode covered by a $SnO_2$-based sensitive layer. The microheater is contained on a suspended membrane in order to provide better performance in terms of electrical power consumption and working condition monitoring. The capillary column is fabricated on a silicon wafer by means of deep reactive ion etching and anodic bonding techniques. Both the microchamber for the gas sensor housing and the inlets and outlets are produced by means of wet etching on the backside of the wafer. The gas sensor is packaged on the top of the column outlet by a flip-chip-like technique. Finally, a prototype of the gas sensor and the connected column system has been packaged to provide fluidic and electrical connections and to set the column temperature. The proposed microsystem is at an early stage of development, but represents a first step in the realization of a highly integrated, portable, and potentially low-cost miniaturized device for biomedical applications.

Fourier transform IR spectrometry was discussed in connection with glucose in section 7.7.1.4.5. Transmittance FTIR spectrometry was used in the study of Déléris and Petibois (2003) to analyze plasma microsamples (50 µl) using an iterative process. Results in accordance with clinical data were obtained from a single FTIR spectrum for the following biomolecules: amino acids, fatty acids, albumin, glucose, fibrinogen, lactate, triglycerides, glycerol, urea, a1-antitrypsin, a2-macroglobulin, transferin, Apo-A1, Apo-B, Apo-C3, IgA, IgD, IgG1, IgG2, IgG3, IgG4, IgM, haptoglobin, a1-acid glycoprotein, cholesterol, and cholesterol esters. Therefore, since only microsamples are necessary, frequent blood analysis becomes possible. A novel application of this method for the monitoring of inflammatory processes related to metabolic stresses in rugby players was also presented. It was shown that an FTIR spectrum constitutes a "metabolic photograph" of the subject, allowing classification between metabolic groups (pathologic or others). Difference spectra were used in order to improve the SNR by the elimination of the unvarying spectral contribution. In one study, it allowed the detection of overtraining in athletes several weeks before any physiologic or clinical symptoms occurred.

Alkaline phosphatase (ALP) is a well-known enzyme that exists in human blood. It is a nonspecific phosphomonoesterase that exhibits optimum activity at alkaline pH. The hydrolysis of phosphomonoesters in the presence of such an enzyme yields inorganic phosphate and corresponding alcohols, phenols, and so on. ALP in blood is mainly derived from liver and bone, and its activity increases if there is a problem in these organs. The rapid and convenient analysis of ALP in blood is important because the level of ALP activity is used as a preliminary diagnosis for many diseases, including hepatitis, cirrhosis, and tumors. A voltammetric measurement of ALP has been investigated to determine the feasibility of a health diagnosis sensor (Kim & Kwak, 2004). Simple photolithography with an office printer and transparency film was employed to construct an electrochemical sensor with an indium tin oxide (ITO) film on glass. ITO films can be easily patterned with a resolution of 50 µm, and an integrated sensor consisting of working, counter-, and reference electrodes on a single ITO plate was constructed by this method. P-nitrophenyl phosphate (PNPP) as the substrate for ALP was used. PNPP was hydrolyzed enzymatically and the product, p-nitrophenol, was detected by cyclic voltammetry and square-wave voltammetry at an oxidation potential of +1.1 V (versus a fabricated Ag/AgCl reference electrode) on a bare ITO electrode. According to this method, ALP can be detected in various media including fetal bovine serum, human serum, and untreated human blood. The linear dynamic range of ALP was 5 U L$^{-1}$ to 180 U L$^{-1}$. This method showed a performance that was acceptable for clinical applications and was sufficiently reproducible. Results were further examined via comparison with medical standard colorimetric analysis.

Early results from near-IR (see also section 7.7.1.4.3) spectroscopy-based systems that noninvasively measure total hemoglobin concentration and hematocrit levels for human subjects have recently been reported. Jeon et al. (2002) showed that hemoglobin can be measured using five LEDs with a wavelength of 569 nm to 975 nm, with an estimated accuracy of approximately 1 g dL$^{-1}$ in their initial study. Noninvasive hematocrit measurement has been demonstrated on surgical patients with large variations in blood hematocrit. These measurements were made with a full-spectrum fiber-optic sensor with a wavelength of 581 nm to 1000 nm (Zhang et al., 2000). Measurements were made by placing the sensor on the surface of the skin. Within single subjects, the measurement accuracy was excellent (1 hematocrit unit), but measurements between subjects were degraded because of variations in skin color, fat content, and instrument variability. Current research is focusing on developing methods to eliminate these factors and improve measurement accuracy for all near-IR spectroscopy-based chemical measurements. These noninvasive measurement techniques may have applications in assessing hematology during space flight, helping to ensure astronaut health and safety (Soller et al., 2002).

There is growing interest in the potential for using IR spectroscopy in health care, both for clinical analysis and for the detection of abnormalities in cells and biological fluids (Shaw et al., 1998). In the case of routine clinical analysis, one attraction is the promise of automated multianalyte determination using no reagents. Rather than reading the color and intensity produced by specific reagents, IR spectroscopic identification is based on the unique IR "color pattern" characteristics of the analyte itself (see also section 7.7.1.4.3). The simplicity of the measurement makes IR spectroscopy an attractive alternative to clinical methods that may be very labor intensive or imprecise, two such examples being fecal analysis and the determination of the lecithin:sphingomyelin ratio in amniotic fluid. As a diagnostic method, IR spectroscopy has shown promise as a nonsubjective adjunct to established tests for arthritis and cervical abnormalities.

Biological specimens present a challenge to the analytical IR spectroscopist. The spectrum of water is very intense. As a result, very short optical path lengths are required in order to provide usable mid-IR spectra ($400$ $cm^{-1}$ to $4000$ $cm^{-1}$) for native biological fluids. Several practical disadvantages conspire to limit the clinical applicability of transmission spectroscopy: while specialized cells can provide a path length of 10 μm, good path length reproducibility remains very difficult to achieve; cleaning between samples would likely require disassembly of the cell; small air bubbles are readily trapped; and automation of the sample preparation process would appear to be essentially impossible. Even if these issues could be addressed, there remains the concern that the extraordinarily intense absorptions of water may either degrade or completely mask certain solute absorptions, even at the shortest path lengths. One approach is to eliminate the water. Studies of serum, synovial fluid, and amniotic fluid have all yielded clinically relevant results from the spectra of films dried onto IR-transparent substrates (Shaw et al., 1998).

Progress in improving the quality of IR silver halide fibers has enabled the construction of several flexible fiber-optic probes of different geometries, which are particularly suitable for the measurement of small biosamples. Recent trends show that dry-film measurements by mid-IR spectroscopy could revolutionize analytical tools in the clinical chemistry laboratory (Heise, Kupper, & Butvina, 2002). IR diagnostic tools (ATR combined with FTIR) show promising potential for patients; minimally invasive blood glucose assays (see also sections 7.7.1.4.3 and 7.7.1.4.5) and skin tissue pathology investigations, in particular, can be accomplished using mid-IR fiber-based probes. Other applications (Heise et al., 2002; Kerslake & Wilson, 1996; Shaw & Mantsch, 1999) include the following:

- The measurement of skin samples, including penetration studies of vitamins and constituents of cosmetic cream formulations
- The microdomain analysis of biopsy samples from bog mummified corpses, and recent results on the chemistry of dermis and hair samples have been reported

- Investigations on pharmaceutical powder homogeneity
- Analysis of proteins and enzymes
- Analysis of lipids and biomembranes
- Analysis of nucleic acids, DNA, RNA, and their building blocks
- Analysis of sugars and complex carbohydrates
- Identification of malignant cervical tissue
- Detection of polydimethyl siloxane in lymph tissue (leakage monitoring of silicone implants)
- Online monitoring of dialyzed patients (urea in plasma)

Biomedical applications of novel spectroscopic methods have been increasing in the last few years. Matrix-assisted laser desorption and ionization time-of-flight (MALDI-TOF) and microscopic FTIR spectroscopy have been applied for the analysis of human blood samples in order to detect spectral peaks that might serve as biomarkers for the monitoring and identification of specific diseases (Huleihel et al., 2005). Samples of serum were obtained from healthy persons and patients suffering from diarrhea and analyzed by MALDI-TOF and advanced FTIR microscopy. The results showed consistent spectral peaks in all examined serums obtained from healthy persons when tested using MALDI-TOF and FTIR microscopy. In all tested patient samples, two unique and interesting peaks appeared in the MALDI-TOF spectra; however, when these samples were examined using FTIR microscopy, a peak completely disappeared in the FTIR spectra. These parameters could be used as a basis for developing a spectral method for the detection and identification of specific human diseases.

## 7.8. ACOUSTIC CHEMICAL SENSORS

Many important physical and chemical processes can be followed by observing the associated mass changes. The increased interest in using microbalances has resulted, in part, from rapid progress in scientific instrumentation. The quartz crystal microbalance (QCM) has found a wide range of applications in the areas of food, environmental, and clinical analyses since its discovery because of its inherent ability to monitor analytes in real time. The QCM depends on the well-known fact that the deposition of a small mass of material on the surface of a quartz microbalance lowers its resonance frequency. QCM sensors are commonly used for thin-film thickness monitoring in vacuum evaporation equipment. Similarly, the gravimetric sensor principle is based on changes in the fundamental oscillation frequency, $f_o$, upon adsorption or absorption of particles from a surrounding gas phase. For the first harmonic, the frequency shift ($\Delta f$) can be described by the Sauerbrey equation:

$$\Delta f / f_o = -\Delta m / m, \tag{7.23}$$

where $\Delta m$ is the mass change, $m$ is the mass, and $f_o$ is the operating frequency.

Many kinds of diseases are associated with the chemical composition of the patient's expiration; for example, the existence of acetone may be an indicator of diabetes, or the presence of dimethylamine suggests that liver function may be impaired. Sensors for disease detection have been intensively studied recently, not only for their ability to quickly detect diseases, but also for their noninvasive sensing properties. The acquisition of a highly sensitive, inexpensive, and convenient sensor is critical in this area. The QCM sensor modified with a proper molecule sifter is a possible answer, and research into QCM sensors coated with zeolite has recently begun. Mostly these sensors are employed to monitor harmful pollutants such as $SO_2$ and NO.

The application of a QCM modified with $Ag^+$-ZSM-5 zeolite for the diagnosis of diabetes was presented by Huang et al. (2004). Such a sensor is utilized in detecting acetone in nitrogen, and in this case, the concentration of acetone in a diabetic's breath. The zeolite type used here has nanometer cavities, the diameters of which approximate uniformly to 0.5 nm, which is very close to the molecular size of acetone (about 0.44 nm). When the zeolite is spin-coated on the QCM sensor, the nanometer cavities trap molecules smaller than their diameter and cause a mass change in the QCM sensor, resulting in a resonant frequency shift. The experimental results demonstrate high sensitivity and selectivity with good repeatability. A test to find the minimum detectable concentration of acetone vapor has obtained results of 1.2 ppm. The lower detection limit for acetone vapor is certain to be much lower; for example, 0.26 ppm has been identified in the diagnosis of diabetes. An average 90 seconds response time has been observed.

Recent advances in the design and construction of acoustic plate mode (APM) devices have allowed their use as sensors (Harsányi, 2000). This sensor consists of a piezoelectric plate, a receptor film, a fluid containment cell, and appropriate signal processing electronics. The piezoelectric plate supports APMs that are primarily horizontally polarized shear waves, thus the device is also called a shear horizontal acoustic plate mode (SH-APM) sensor. Typical plates are a few acoustic wavelengths thick. The waves are generated and detected by interdigitated electrodes on the lower surface and reflect between the upper and lower surface of the substrate. The beam interacts with the receptor polymer film and viscously coupled fluid sample as it reflects from the upper surface. Changes in the film due to mass loading or viscoelastic stiffening alter the phase of the reflected wave and result in a phase shift in the electrical signal. Similar to surface acoustic wave sensors, a dual delay line configuration can be used to compensate for nonspecific responses and undesired environmental effects. The advantage of the APM sensor is that electrical connections can be made on the surface of the device, which is not immersed in solution. Typical APM device frequencies are 25 MHz to 200 MHz.

A detailed understanding of the interactions of proteins with artificial surfaces is critical for many medical and biochemical applications. Such knowledge could, for example, improve the implementation of synthetic coatings for catheters and prostheses that come in contact with biological fluids. Other examples involve the nonspecific adsorption of pharmacological proteins at the walls of a container, which may reduce their activity, and the adhesion of pathogenic bacteria, which is determined by the affinity of the surface to proteins. What is needed to support technical progress is a rapid, online analytical tool capable of detecting proteins and determining their specific adsorption behavior for various surfaces. Contrary to traditional immunoassays, acoustic wave-based sensors allow the online and direct detection of label-free proteins, thus saving time and providing the opportunity to monitor the kinetics of the binding process. Chromium/gold-coated APM sensors have been used to investigate the interaction of immunoglobulin G (IgG) and fibrinogen with differently terminated self-assembled monolayers (SAMs) of thiols (Dahint et al., 1996). By this method, both the low affinity of hexa(ethylene glycol)-terminated alkanethiol SAMs and the high affinity of methyl-terminated surfaces toward protein adsorption were confirmed. It was found that the amount of bound proteins depends on the pH of the solution. At low pH values, protein binding to methyl-terminated surfaces is drastically reduced. The adsorption characteristics of fibrinogen at methyl-terminated surfaces are explained by a kinetic model that involves the initial binding of native proteins and a subsequent unfolding process. Complete regeneration of the sensor element is achieved by the use of sodium dodecylsulfate.

# REFERENCES

Alcock, S. J., & Turner, A. P. F. (1994). Continuous analyte monitoring to aid clinical practice. *IEEE Engineering in Medicine and Biology, 13*(3), 319–325.

Arnold, M. A. (1996), Non-invasive glucose monitoring. *Current Opinion in Biotechnology, 7*, 46–49.

Arnold, M. A., Burmeister, J. J., & Small, G. W. (1998). Phantom glucose calibration models from simulated noninvasive human near-infrared spectra. *Analytical Chemistry, 70*(9), 1773–1781.

Baumberger, I. P., & Goodfriend, R. B. (1951). Determination of arterial oxygen tension in man by equilibration through intact skin. *Federation Proceedings Federation of American Societies for Experimental Biology, 10*, 10–11.

Bezegh, K., Bezegh, A., Black, P. G., & Janata, J. (1988). Integrated probe for sweat analysis. *Journal of Clinical Laboratory Analysis, 2*, 16–18.

Bezegh, K., Bezegh, A., Janata, J., Oesch, V., Xu, A., & Simon, W. (1987). Multisensing ion-selective field-effect transistors prepared by ionophore doping technique. *Analytical Chemistry, 59*, 2846–2848.

Boisde, G., Blanc, F., & Machuron-Mandard, X. (1991). pH measurements with dyes co-immobilization on optrodes: Principles and associated instrumentation. *International Journal of Optoelectronics, 6*(5), 407–423.

Buerk, D. G. (1993). *Biosensors: Theory and applications.* Lancaster, PA: Technomic.

Burk, E. D., Arrieta, I. C., & Batich, D. C. (1987). The feasibility of an implantable opto-electronic glucose sensor. *Proceedings of the 9th Annual Conference of the IEEE Engineering in Medicine and Biology Society,* 788.

Burmeister, J. J., Arnold, M. A., & Small, G. W. (1998). Spectroscopic considerations for noninvasive blood glucose measurements with near infrared spectroscopy. IEEE Lasers and Electro-Optics Society *Newsletter, 12*(April), 6–9.

Caduff, A., Hirt, E., Feldman, Y., Ali, Z., & Heinemann, L. (2003). First human experiments with a novel non-invasive, non-optical continuous glucose monitoring system. *Biosensors and Bioelectronics, 19*, 209–217.

Christison, G. B. (1993). Summary of near infrared glucose sensing research towards a noninvasive measurement technique. *Chemical Sensors for In Vivo Monitoring, 11*(March), 8–10.

Clark, L. C. (1956). Monitoring and control of blood and tissue oxygen. *Transactions of the American Society for Artificial Internal Organs, 2*, 41–48.

Colvin, A. E., Phillips, T. E., Miragliotta, J. A., Givens, R. B., & Bargeron, C. B. (1996). A novel solid-state oxygen sensor. *John Hopkins APL Technical Digest, 17*(4), 377–385.

Dahint, R., Seigel, R. R., Harder, P., Grunze, M., & Josse, F. (1996). Detection of non-specific protein adsorption at artificial surfaces by the use of acoustic plate mode sensors. *Sensors and Actuators B, 35–36*, 497–505.

Déléris, G., & Petibois, C. (2003). Applications of FT-IR spectrometry to plasma contents analysis and monitoring. *Vibrational Spectroscopy, 32*, 129–136.

Diamond, D. (1998). *Principles of chemical and biological sensors.* New York, NY: John Wiley & Sons.

Fleischer, M., & Simon, E. (2005). Medical applications of gas sensors (LOCOMED). *Proceedings Sensor 2005, 12th International Conference,* Nuremberg, Germany, pp. 363–368.

Fraser, D. M. (1997). *Biosensors in the body: Continuous in vivo monitoring.* New York, NY: John Wiley & Sons.

Göpel, W., Jones, T. A., Kleitz, M., Lundström, I., & Seiyama, T. (1991). *Sensors: A comprehensive survey, Vol. 3, Part 2, Chemical and biochemical sensors.* New York, NY: John Wiley & Sons.

Gotshal, Y., Simhi, R., Ben-Ami, S., & Katzir, A. (1997). Blood diagnostics using fiberoptic evanescent wave spectroscopy and neural networks analysis. *Sensors and Actuators B, 42*, 157–161.

Gumbrecht, W., Schelter, W., Montag, B., Bos, J. A. H., Eijking, E. P., & Lachmann, B. (1991). Monitoring of blood $pO_2$ with a thin-film amperometric sensor. *Proceedings of the 1991 International Conference on Solid State Sensors and Actuators (Transducers '91),* San Francisco, CA, pp. 85–87.

Harsányi, G. (1995a). Electrochemical processes resulting in migrated short failures in microcircuits. *IEEE Transactions on Components, Packaging, and Manufacturing Technology, Part A, 18*(3), 602–610.

Harsányi, G. (1995b). *Polymer films in sensor applications.* Lancaster, PA: Technomic.

Harsányi, G. (2000). *Sensors in biomedical applications.* Lancaster, PA: Technomic.

Harsányi, G., Péteri, I., & Deák, I. (1994). Low cost ceramic sensors for biomedical use: A revolution in transcutaneous blood oxygen monitoring? *Sensors and Actuators B, 18–19*, 171–174.

Hazen, K. H., Arnold, M. A., & Small, G. W. (1998). Measurement of glucose and other analytes in undiluted human serum with near-infrared transmission spectroscopy. *Analytica Chimica Acta, 371*, 255–267.

Heise, H. M., Kupper, L., & Butvina, L. N. (2002). Bio-analytical applications of mid-infrared spectroscopy using silver halide fiber-optic probes. *Spectrochimica Acta B, 57*, 1649–1663.

Heise, H. M., Marbach, R., Koschinsky, T. H., & Gries, F. A. (1994) Non-invasive blood glucose sensors based on near-infrared spectroscopy. *Artificial Organs, 18*, 439–447.

Huang, H., Zhou, J., Chen, S., Zeng, L., & Huang, Y. (2004). A highly sensitive QCM sensor coated with $Ag^+$-ZSM-5 film for medical diagnosis. *Sensors and Actuators B, 101*, 316–321.

Huch, A., Huch, R., & Lübbers, D. W. (1972). Quantitative continuous measurement of partial pressure ($PO_2$ measurement) on the skin of adults and newborn babies. *Pflügers Archiv für die gesamte Physiologie, 337*, 185–198.

Huleihel, M., Karpasas, M., Talyshansky, M., Souprun, Y., Doubijanski, Y., & Erukhimovitch, V. (2005). Mass spectroscopic and IR spectroscopic evaluation of abnormal biological samples. *Vacuum, 78*, 557–562.

Ivanova, O., Chuprin, M., Krutovertsev, S., Pislyakov, A., Redina, O., Vdovichev, S., . . . & Konovalov, V. (2004). A multisensor system for detection of the composition of exhaled air. *Digest of Technical Papers Eurosensors XVIII*, Rome, Italy, P1.57.

Jachowicz, R., Weremczuk, J., Pczesny, D., & Rapiejko, P. (2004a). Fast dew-point hygrometer for laryngological applications. *Proceedings IEEE Sensors 2004*, Vienna, Austria, pp. 1488–1491.

Jachowicz, R., Weremczuk, J., & Tarapata, G. (2004b). Fast dew point hygrometer for measurements of human skin evaporation factor. *Digest of Technical Papers Eurosensors XVIII*, Rome, Italy, A2.4.

Jagemann, K. U., Fischbacher, C., Danzer, K., Muller, U. A., & Mertes, B. (1995). Application of near-infrared spectroscopy for non-invasive determination of blood/tissue glucose using neural network. *Zeitschrift für Physikalische Chemie-Leipzig, 191S*, 179–190.

Jakeway, S. C., De Mello, A., & Russell, E. L. (2000). Miniaturised total analysis systems for biological analysis. *Fresenius Journal of Analytical Chemistry, 366*, 525–539.

Jeon, K. J., Kim, S.-J., Kim, J.-W., & Yoon, G. (2002). Noninvasive total hemoglobin measurement. *Journal of Biomedical Optics, 7*, 45.

Jinghong, H., Dafu, C., Yating, L., Jine, C., Zheng, D., Hong, Z., & Chenglin, S. (1995). A new type of transcutaneous $pCO_2$ sensor. *Sensors and Actuators B, 24–25*, 156–158.

Kanazawa, E., Sakai, G., Shimanoe, K., Kanmura, Y., Teraoka, Y., Miura, N., & Yamazoe, N. (2001). Metal oxide semiconductor $N_2O$ sensor for medical use. *Sensors and Actuators B, 77*, 72–77.

Kästle, S., Noller, F., Falk, S., Bukta, A., Mayer, E., & Miller, D. (1997). A new family of sensors for pulse oximetry. *Hewlett-Packard Journal, 48*(2), 39–53.

Keplinger, F., Glatz, R., Jachimowicz, A., Urban, G., Kohl, F., Olcaytug, F., & Prohaska, O. J. (1990). Thin-film ion-selective sensors based on neutral carrier membranes. *Sensors and Actuators B, 1*, 272–274.

Kerslake, E. D. S., & Wilson, C. G. (1996). Pharmaceutical and biomedical applications of fiber optic biosensors based on infra red technology. *Advanced Drug Delivery Reviews, 21*, 205–213.

Kim, H.-J., & Kwak, J. (2004). Electrochemical determination of total alkaline phosphatase in human blood with a micropatterned ITO film. *Journal of Electroanalytical Chemistry, 577*, 243–248.

Kolle, C., Gruber, W., Trettnak, W., Biebernik, K., Dolezal, C., Reininger, F., & O'Leary, P. (1997). Fast optochemical sensor for continuous monitoring of oxygen in breath-gas analysis. *Sensors and Actuators B, 38–39*, 141–149.

Liem, K. D., Hopman, J. C. W., & Oeseburg, B. (1992). Method for the fixation of optrodes in near infrared spectrophotometry. *Medical & Biological Engineering & Computing, 30*, 120–121.

Lorenzelli, L., Benvenuto, A., Adami, A., Guarnieri, V., Margesin, B., Mulloni, V., & Vincenzi, D. (2005). Development of a gas chromatography silicon-based microsystem in clinical diagnostics. *Biosensors and Bioelectronics, 20*, 1968–1976.

Malchoff, C. D., Shoukri, K. A., Landau, J. I., & Buchert, J. M. (2002). Novel noninvasive blood glucose. *Diabetes Care, 25*, 2268–2275.

Malin, S. F., Ruchti, T. L., Blank, T. B., Thennadil, S. N., & Monfre, S. L. (1999). Noninvasive prediction of glucose by near-infrared diffuse reflectance spectroscopy. *Clinical Chemistry, 45*(9), 1651–1658.

Marbach, R., Koschinsky, T. H., Gries, F. A., & Heise, H. M. (1993). Non-invasive glucose assay by near-infrared diffuse reflectance spectroscopy of the human inner lip. *Applied Spectroscopy, 47*, 875–881.

Mascini, M., Moscone, D., & Bernardi, L. (1992). In vivo continuous monitoring of glucose by microdialysis and a glucose biosensor. *Sensors and Actuators B, 6,* 143–145.

McNichols, R. J., & Coté, G. L. (2000). Optical glucose sensing in biological fluids: An overview. *Journal of Biomedical Optics, 5*(1), 5–16.

McNichols, R. J., & Gowda, A. (2001). Development of an implantable skinport sensor for use as an in vivo optical glucose sensor. *Proceedings SPIE, 4263,* 11–19.

Mehrvar, M., Bis, C., Scharer, J. M., Moo-Young, M., & Luong, J. H. (2000). Fiber-optic biosensors: trends and advances. *Analytical Sciences, 16,* 677–692.

Mendelson, Y. (1991). Invasive and noninvasive blood gas monitoring (pp. 249–279). In: D. L. Wise (Ed.), *Bioinstrumentation and Biosensors.* New York, NY: Marcel Dekker.

Mendelson, Y., Clermont, A. C., Peura, R. A., & Lin, B.-C. (1990). Blood glucose measurement by multiple attenuated total reflection and infrared absorption spectroscopy. *IEEE Transactions in Biomedical Engineering, 37,* 458–465.

Norton, H. N. (1982). *Sensor and analyzer handbook.* Englewood Cliffs, NJ: Prentice Hall.

Papkovsky, D. P. (1993). Luminescent porphyrins as probes for optical (bio)sensors. *Sensors and Actuators B, 11,* 293–300.

Parker, D. (1987). Sensors for monitoring blood gases in intensive care. *Journal of Physics E: Scientific Instrumentation, 20*(9), 1103–1112.

Peterson, J. I., Goldstein, S. R., Fitzgerald, R. V., & Buckhold, D. K. (1980). Fiber optic pH probe for physiological use. *Analytical Chemistry, 52,* 864–869.

Pickup, J. C. (1993). Developing glucose sensors for in vivo use. *Trends in Biotechnology, 11,* 285–291.

Potyrailo, R. A., & Hieftje, G. M. (1998). Oxygen detection by fluorescence quenching of tetraphenylporphyrin immobilized in the original cladding of an optical fiber. *Analytica Chimica Acta, 37*(1), 1–8.

Pruna, S. (1995). Development of noninvasive method for in vivo sensing of glycaemia. *Chemical Sensors for In Vivo Monitoring, 19*(December), 30–33.

Rolfe, P. (1994). Intra-vascular oxygen sensors for neonatal monitoring. *IEEE Engineering in Medicine and Biology, 13*(3), 336–346.

Röösli, S. E., Pretsch, W., Morf, E., Tsuchida, E., & Nishide, H. (1997). Selective optical response to oxygen of membranes based on immobilized cobalt(II) porphyrins. *Analytica Chimica Acta, 338,* 119–125.

Schnakenberg, U., Lisec, T., Hintsche, R., Kuna, I., Uhlig, A., & Wagner, B. (1996). Novel potentiometric silicon sensor for medical devices. *Sensors and Actuators B, 34,* 476–480.

Severinghaus, I. W., & Bradley, A. F. (1958). Electrodes for blood $pO_2$ and $pCO_2$ determination. *Journal of Applied Physiology, 13,* 515–520.

Shaw, R. A., Eysel, H. H., Liu, K.-Z., & Mantsch, H. H. (1998). Infrared spectroscopic analysis of biomedical specimens using glass substrates. *Analytical Biochemistry, 259,* 181–186.

Shaw, R. A., & Mantsch, H. H. (1999). Vibrational biospectroscopy: From plants to animals to humans. A historical perspective. *Journal of Molecular Structure, 480–481,* 1–13.

Small, G. W., & Arnold, M. A. (1998). Data handling issues for near-infrared glucose measurements. Lasers and Electro-Optics Society *Newsletter, 12*(April), 16–17.

Soller, B. R. (1994). Design of intravascular fiber optic blood gas sensors. *IEEE Engineering in Medicine and Biology, 13*(3), 327–335.

Soller, B. R., Cabrera, M., Smith, S. M., & Sutton, J. P. (2002). Smart medical systems with application to nutrition and fitness in space. *Nutrition, 18,* 930–936.

Spichiger-Keller, U. E. (1998). *Chemical sensors and biosensors for medical and biological applications.* New York, NY: John Wiley & Sons.

Steinkuhl, R., Sundermeier, C., Hinkers, H., Dumschat, C., Cammann, K., & Knoll, M. (1996). Microdialysis system for continuous glucose monitoring. *Sensors and Actuators B, 33,* 19–24.

Sudhölter, E. J. R., Van der Wal, P. D., Skowronska-Patinska, M., Van den Berg, A., & Reinhoudt, D. N. (1989). Ion-sensing using chemically-modified ISFETs. *Sensors and Actuators, 17,* 189–194.

Suzuki, H., Sugama, A., & Kokima, N. (1993). Micromachined Clark oxygen electrode. *Sensors and Actuators B, 10,* 91–98.

Takatani, S., & Ling, J. (1994). Optical oximetry sensors for whole blood and tissue. *IEEE Engineering in Medicine and Biology, 13*(3), 347–357.

Tenhunen, J., Kopola, H., & Myllyla, R. (1998). Non-invasive glucose measurement based on selective near infrared absorption; requirements on instrumentation and spectral range. *Measurement, 24*, 173–177.

Thybaud, L., Depeursinge, C., Rouiller, D., Mondin, G., & Grisel, A. (1990). Use of ISFETs for 24h pH monitoring in the gastrooesophageal tract. *Sensors and Actuators B, 1*, 482–485.

Tsukada, K., Miyahara, Y., Shibata, Y., & Miyagi, H. (1990). An integrated chemical sensor with multiple ion and gas sensors. *Sensors and Actuators B, 2*, 291–295.

Tsukada, K., Miyahara, Y., Shibata, Y., & Miyagi, H. (1991). An integrated micro multi-ion sensor using platinum-gate field-effect transistors. *Proceedings of the Conference on Solid State Sensors and Actuators (Transducers '91)*, San Francisco, CA, pp. 218–221.

Tsukada, K., Sakai, S., Hase, K., & Minamitani, H. (2003). Development of catheter-type optical oxygen sensor and applications to bioinstrumentation. *Biosensors and Bioelectronics, 18*, 1439–1445.

Varlan, A. R., & Sansen, W. (1997). Micromachined conductometric p($CO_2$) sensor. *Sensors and Actuators B, 44*, 309–315.

Volpe, G., Moscone, D., Compagnone, D., & Palleschi, G. (1995). In vivo continuous monitoring of L-lactate coupling subcutaneous microdialysis and an electrochemical biocell. *Sensors and Actuators B, 24–25*, 138–141.

Weller, M. G., Schuetz, A. G., Winklmair, M., & Niessner, R. (1999). Highly parallel affinity sensor for the detection of environmental contaminants in water. *Analytica Chimica Acta, 393*, 29–44.

Wolfbeis, O. S. (1991). Biomedical application of fiber optic chemical sensors. *International Journal of Optoelectronics, 6*(5), 425–441.

Wolfbeis, O. S., Fürlinger, E., Kroneis, H., & Marsoner, A. (1983). A study on fluorescent indicators for measuring near neutral ("physiological") pH values. *Fresenius Journal of Analytical Chemistry, 314*, 119–124.

Yao, S. J. (1991). Chemistry and potential methods for in vivo glucose sensing (pp. 229–247). In: D. L. Wise (Ed.), *Bioinstrumentation and Biosensors*. New York, NY: Marcel Dekker.

Zhang, S., Soller, B. R., Kaur, S., Perras, K., & van der Salm, T. J. (2000). Investigation of noninvasive in vivo blood hematocrit measurement using NIR reflectance spectroscopy and partial least-squares regression. *Applied Spectroscopy, 54*, 294.

Zhou, Z. B., Feng, L. D., Liu, W. J., & Wu, Z. G. (2001). New approaches for developing transient electrochemical multi-component gas sensors. *Sensors and Actuators B, 76*, 605–609.

## ABOUT THE AUTHOR

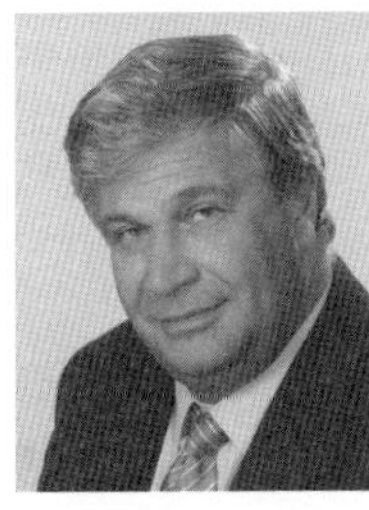

**Professor Gábor Harsányi** joined the Department of Electronics Technology, Budapest University of Technology and Economics (BME) in 1984 and is now head of the department. He graduated with a degree in electrical engineering from BME in 1981 and was awarded his PhD in electronics technology in 1992. In 2001 he received a DSc degree from the Hungarian Academy of Sciences. He has several years' industrial experience in sensor development. His main research interests are in electronic interconnection and packaging, MEMS, and sensors for industry and biomedicine. Publications include approximately two-hundred papers and two monographs. From 1993 to 1994, he was president of the Hungarian Chapter of the International Microelectronics and Packaging Society (IMAPS). Awards include Best Paper of Session at the 1991 International Symposium on Microelectronics in Orlando, Florida, and an IMAPS Fellowship in 1998.

# CHAPTER 8

# BIOSENSORS

J. Negandhi, A. Ray, and P. Vadgama

*Interdisciplinary Research Centre in Biomedical Materials*
*Queen Mary, University of London*
*London, UK*

## 8.1. INTRODUCTION

Biosensors (Arnold & Meyerhoff, 1988) are self-contained analytical devices that incorporate a biological recognition element combined with an artificial transducer. The latter may respond to a physical or chemical change resulting from the interaction of the biological element with the target molecule. In many cases, high selectivity is achieved with varying degrees of reversibility depending upon the exact bioaffinity system used. The activity of the (bio)chemical target species, typically in a biological sample, triggers the response cascade. Because biosensors depend for their activation on some form of initial binding, that is, an affinity reaction, then direct biofluid sample immersion or contact is usually unavoidable, and biosensor interfacial biocompatibility as well as integrated reactive chemistry can be issues of importance.

A convenient analytical target-based classification is drug, metabolite, protein, and nucleic acid biosensors with the last, based on complementary single-strand DNA or RNA binding, being a special form of affinity reaction. An alternative structure-based classification is often used for convenience, and of these, enzyme-based biosensors are by far the largest group, falling mainly within the category of metabolite biosensors. One of the first biosensors to be reported (Updike & Hicks, 1967) was such a device. It targeted glucose using an active enzyme membrane located over an oxygen probe. This demonstrated the core principle of biosensors, with close apposition of a biolayer and a sensing interface. The concentration of glucose was registered via a change in the response of the oxygen probe to a decrease in oxygen partial pressure over time, induced by the enzymatic reaction (discussed later).

In a biosensor, the biorecognition phase is designed to interact for a controlled period with the analyte, and the highly selective nature of this bioaffinity is typically exploited to produce a change in charge, optical property, oxidation state, mass, or some other specific interfacial change. The latter is now being increasingly explored in a more fundamental way in this expanding field. The description of different biosensors in this review uses a classification based partly on transducer type and partly on the biorecognition element, reflecting the differing ways in which particular devices are referred to in the literature, depending on the component being emphasized.

## 8.2. ENZYME-BASED BIOSENSORS

### 8.2.1. ENZYMES AS NATURAL CATALYSTS

Enzymes are proteins with catalytic properties that are highly selective. They are able to reduce the activation energy of complicated organic reaction sequences. In this way they permit reactive transformations to take place under mild, typically physiological, conditions and are used in nature as the universal catalyst, being able to facilitate and drive all key reactive conversions within a cell. They may, for example, convert high-energy compounds to those of lower energy, leading to the release of chemical potential energy and thereby underpinning the energy economy of the cell. The mild conditions involved (temperature, pH, ionic strength) are in fact prerequisites for an enzyme to work efficiently and for the enzyme structure to survive. For analytical purposes, this places a limit on how harsh any environmental assay conditions may be for enzyme-based conversions, whether in bulk solution or for an enzyme that is part of a biosensor.

### 8.2.2. SPECIFIC FUNCTIONAL PROPERTIES OF ENZYMES

Enzymes work by being able to coordinate the binding of one or more substrates in an optimal orientation as an initial step and as a prelude to making or breaking chemical structural bonds of the substrate. Their ability to catalyze the reaction is through stabilizing the transition state (the highest energy species in the reaction pathway) to augment the reaction rate. Notwithstanding the modified, immobilized state of the enzyme within a biosensor, this remains the basis of the resulting biosensing mechanism. Because a single, specific transition state is stabilized, a specific reaction pathway is promoted from a set of alternatives, and also a preset stoichiometry for the end product of transduction results. Enzymes in combination in natural systems can operate in a concerted manner, thus allowing the channeling of a unified network of catalytic activity and thereby transforming molecules along a pathway sequence of complex steps that inevitably involve the mutual gearing of multiple binding sites. This interenzyme combinatorial property could perhaps be a model for biocomputing, and for biosensing, and could extend the analytical repertoire beyond that achieved with just one or two enzymes.

Many enzymes require a nonprotein component to enable them to undertake their catalytic role. These nonprotein components—coenzymes or cofactors—require some form of interaction at the active site, and range from metal ions to large reduction–oxidation (redox) organic molecules such as nicotinamide adenine dinucleotide ($NAD^+$; Kress-Rogers, 1997). A redox compound is one that can be reversibly oxidized and reduced, and as such can alternately take and give up electrons. As a special example of activation, there are many enzymes in living organisms that are regulated by calmodulin, a 17 kD protein that has calcium affinity, and that could therefore serve as a reactive element for calcium sensing. When Ca²⁺ binds to calmodulin, it induces changes in structure that lead to calmodulin activation. As a result, the molecule has the potential to bind to other enzyme (and nonenzyme) target proteins (Stryer, 1995). So essentially this protein is a natural biological sensor (see Fig. 8.1) for calcium, and can in principle be harnessed in an artificial biosensor functionalized perhaps via an enzyme reaction.

An additional mechanism for natural enzyme regulation is covalent modification. This process involves controlled, reversible attachment to specific, functionally modifying peptide residues. Thus an enzyme may be synthesized in an inactive precursor form, but its activation can be switched on at a more appropriate moment required by the cell (e.g., by proteolytic degradation). Such a model system could be used to retain a dormant enzyme in a recognition system for later activation (e.g., to enhance storage lifetime or to report a proteolytic process).

## 8.2.3. ENZYMES WITHIN BIOSENSORS

In contrast to the use of soluble enzymes as reagents for bioanalytical methods, their incorporation into biosensors as solid-state elements allows them to be structural parts of such devices. The most important part of the enzyme molecule—the active site, the basis for molecular recognition—has to be protected in this phase conversion to the solid phase. There are a number of generalizations that can be made (Stryer, 1995) concerning the active site of an enzyme:

- It makes up a small part of total enzyme volume.
- It is three-dimensional (3-D).
- Substrate binding involves multiple, weak interactions.
- It takes the shape of a cleft or crevice in the enzyme molecule.
- Specificity of binding is determined by the 3-D organization of atoms presented at the active site.

This last concept was introduced by Emil Fisher using a lock-and-key analogy, but it is now evident that in some cases the active site of an enzyme may be modified by the act of binding of the substrate itself. Thus the active site can assume the shape of the substrate after the substrate has bound, a concept

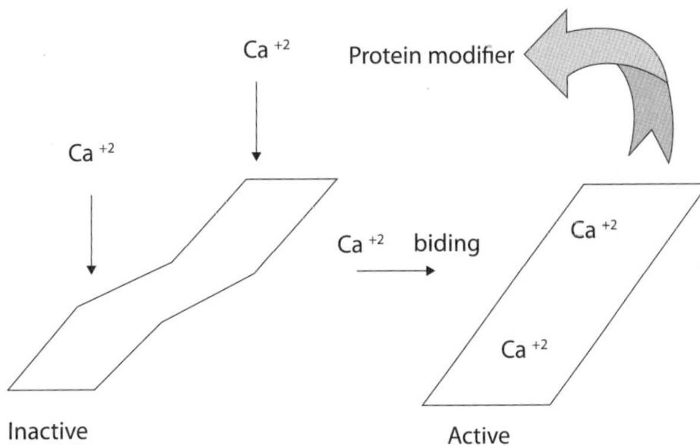


**Figure 8.1.** Schematic of a calcium-induced structural change in calmodulin allowing it to orchestrate the function of the other proteins.

referred to as induced fit. It is inevitable that immobilization of the enzyme protein distorts its active site, but with careful optimization and choice of method, not sufficiently to abolish catalysis.

## 8.2.4. GLUCOSE OXIDASE

Fortuitously for biosensors, one of the first enzymes to be used was glucose oxidase (GOD), which has turned out to have an exceptionally stable structure immune to a wide range of harsh treatments during immobilization. Figure 8.2 shows how GOD together with its cofactor flavin adenine dinucleotide (FAD) converts glucose to gluconic acid. This enzyme has been successfully used in many biosensing systems exploiting very many different approaches to immobilization to improve, for example, the sensitivity and catalytic efficiency of the resulting biosensor.

After successful immobilization, there is typically an improvement in performance in terms of thermal stability and retained enzyme activity across a broad pH range. In one example, Rauf et al. (2005) used a novel cellulose acetate–poly(methyl methacrylate) membrane to immobilize GOD and found that this improved resistance to the denaturation effects of pH, temperature, and urea, with maintained activity after repeated cycles of use and extended storage. Another recent study of interest used screen-printing via a cobalt phthalocyanine (CoPC) loaded in a water-based carbon ink to form the enzyme layer (Crouch et al., 2005). Optimization was achieved by varying the loading of the electrically active CoPC and GOD (CoPC acts as a mediator for hydrogen peroxide [$H_2O_2$] when incorporated into screen-printed carbon electrodes). Maximal linear range was observed when 20%(w/w) CoPC loading was used in relation to the weight of carbon, together with a GOD loading of 628 Ug$^{-1}$. The best potential for responses was found to be +0.5 V against a saturated calomel electrode reference with platinum as the counter. With a background supporting electrolyte of

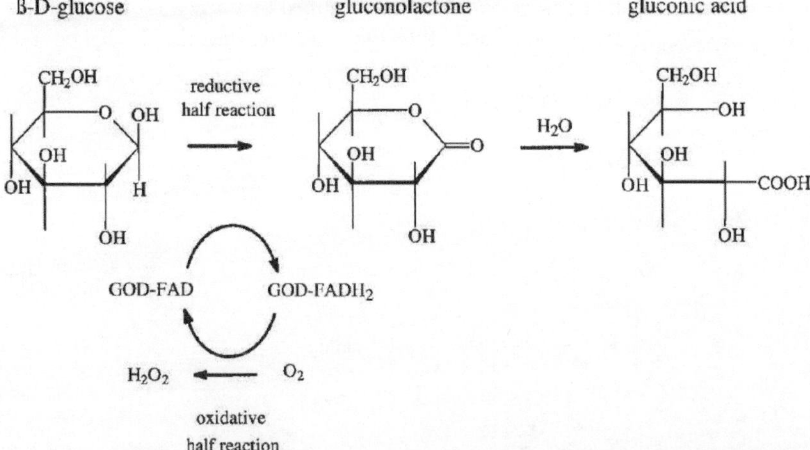


**Figure 8.2.** Diagrammatic representation of the conversion of glucose into gluconic acid by GOD. Adapted from Witt, S., et al., 2000, "Conserved arginine-516 of *Penicillium amagasakiense* glucose oxidase is essential for the efficient binding of b-D-glucose," *Biochemical Journal, 347,* pp. 553–559, with permission.

0.05 M phosphate buffer, pH 8.0, the glucose linear range was 0.2 mM to 5 mM with a response slope of 1.12 $\mu$A mM$^{-1}$. Such new immobilization strategies continue to hold promise for improved performance, even with a well-established enzyme. This is because the physical and chemical microenvironment has such a bearing upon the reaction and on the process for electron exchange, respectively, between substrate and enzyme and product and working electrode.

## 8.2.5. UREASE

Another common enzyme used in biosensors is urease. This enzyme catalyzes the conversion of urea into carbon dioxide ($CO_2$) and ammonia ($NH_3$) or to bicarbonate and ammonium ions, depending on the operational pH. Urea biosensors are important, as urea is invariably monitored in blood as an indicator of renal function. A variety of transducers have been used with urease. These typically include $CO_2$ and $NH_3/NH_4^+$ sensors (Arnold & Meyerhoff, 1988). One recent example is an interesting calorimetric biosensor with integrated microfluidic channels (Zhang & Tadigadapa, 2004). This device allowed the measurement of the enthalpy of an enzymic reaction on a real-time basis, and in more general terms could give an estimation of the thermal properties of a biological fluid. It was fabricated (see Fig. 8.3) as an independent microthermopile structure incorporated into a microfluidic

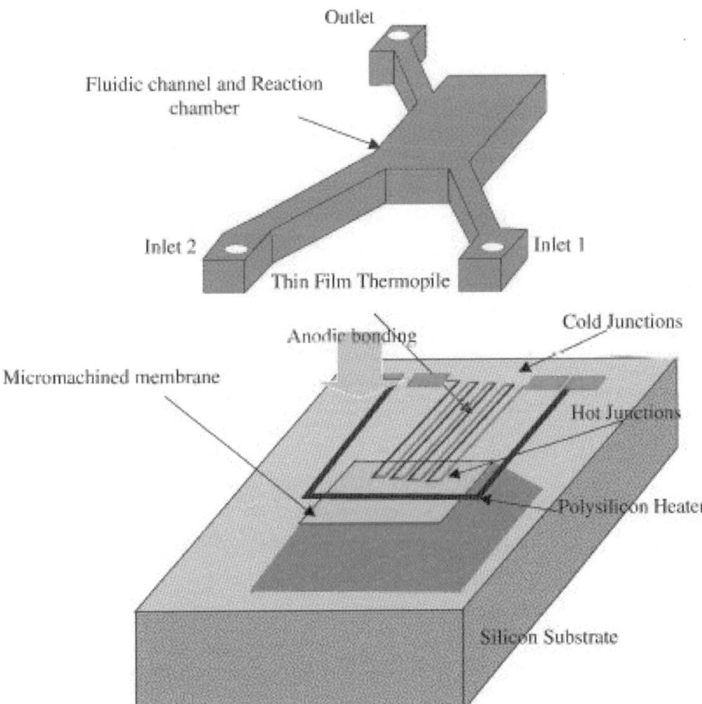


**Figure 8.3.** A 3-D schematic representation of the proposed microcalorimeter with integrated microfluidic channels. Adapted from Zhang, Y., & Tadigadapa, S., 2004, "Calorimetric biosensors with integrated microfluidic channels," *Biosensors and Bioelectronics, 19*(12), pp. 1733–1743, with permission.

measurement chamber. The thermopile, of gold and polysilicon, needed to be thermally isolated, and was fabricated on an insulating membrane. It showed high urea sensitivity and a short inherent time constant for thermal response.

Measurement of the heat of reaction from the catalytic action of urease was reported and GOD and catalase were also studied. Sensitivity was recorded by the conversion of thermal input into voltage. The thermocouple gave values of 17 $\mu V\ M^{-1}$ for urea. Glucose was also measured with a response of 53.5 $\mu V\ M^{-1}$, and $H_2O_2$ had a response of 26.5 $\mu V\ M^{-1}$. The system had the potential to measure more general enthalpic processes; as is frequently the case with broad-spectrum transducers, background effects needed to be corrected.

In the case of the $NH_4^+$ based device for urea, the measurement principle is that of a potentiometric ion-selective electrode. In one example, a $NH_4^+$-sensitive disposable electrode was produced using a double matrix membrane (Eggenstein et al., 1999). The electrode was prepared from filter paper silver-coated on one side and electrically insulated by means of a heat-sealing film. The polymeric ion-sensitive layer here was formed in combination with a filter paper matrix, which helped to improve reproducible fabrication. Urease was immobilized within poly(carbamoyl sulfonate) hydrogel, which served as an ion-sensitive membrane. The urea-sensitive electrode was combined with a disposable silver/silver chloride (Ag/AgCl) reference to achieve a fully disposable urea biosensor unit. The sensor provided reliable responses to urea in the range $7.2 \times 10^{-5}$ mM to $2.1 \times 10^{-2}$ mM.

## 8.3. ENZYME IMMOBILIZATION TECHNIQUES

### 8.3.1. GENERAL ISSUES

There are a number of techniques used to immobilize enzymes onto solid substrates, thus allowing them to be used repeatedly, notably for biosensing. The term immobilization simply indicates that the enzyme is placed in a fixed position with the active site accessible to the analyte. The advantages of immobilization are ease of use (and reuse), with an increase in enzyme stability along with more efficient, economical exploitation (Klibanov, 1979). With immobilization, an increase in molecular structural rigidity results that enhances stability, thus minimizing the impact of thermal and pH-induced factors leading to denaturation. The method of immobilization that is selected frequently influences parameters relevant to biosensors, such as detection limit, sensitivity, linear dynamic range, and reusability. Any tendency to nonspecific binding may also be affected (Schumacher, Mersal, & Bilitewski, 2005). Common methods used for enzyme immobilization include physical and chemical entrapment and adsorption onto support materials. While an initial choice of a suitable immobilization method may be based on the known physicochemical properties of the support and enzyme, the prediction of outcomes, such as activity stability, remains difficult.

### 8.3.2. PHYSICAL ENTRAPMENT

Physical entrapment involves an enzyme being held within an insoluble gel matrix, in a microcapsule, or retained at the matrix interface, although these may be difficult to distinguish (Fig. 8.4). Entrapment phases include polyacrylamide, alginate, and polyvinyl alcohol.

One current research method used in this area has involved stabilizing GOD in alginate microspheres with photoreactive diazoresin nanofilm coatings. By coating these microspheres, the stability

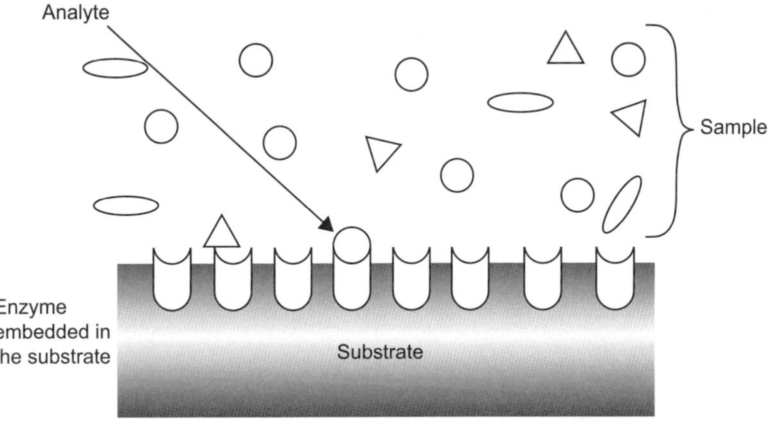



**Figure 8.4.** Physical entrapment of enzymes at a substrate used in biosensors.

and activity of the enzyme is retained for much longer than for spheres that are uncoated (Srivastava et al., 2005). Alginate fibers have also been used for physical entrapment (Hou et al., 2005) and subsequently used to allow cell attachment. In other research, more than one enzyme has been studied in a single type of matrix; for example, urease and glutamate dehydrogenase were retained in polypyrrole-polyvinyl sulfonate films by physical adsorption and also electrochemical entrapment (Gambhir et al., 2001). The mode of immobilization affects catalytic behavior. Entrapment avoids the need for covalent bond formation and thus is less distorting of the enzyme native structure. However, dense, high-level loading may be difficult, and loss through leaching from the matrix becomes a strong possibility.

### 8.3.3. CHEMICAL IMMOBILIZATION

Chemical immobilization involves attachment of the enzyme onto a support matrix by covalent bonding or by a multifunctional bridging reagent (see Fig. 8.5). An example of this is, again, the use of urease to detect urea.

Urease has been covalently attached, for example, onto conducting copolymer films, allowing high enzyme loading and stability due to the convoluted morphology of the polymeric phase. Unusually, an amperometric response was measured as a function of the concentration of urea with the redox film held at a fixed polarizing voltage (Rajesh, Takashima, & Kaneto, 2005). Other immobilization phases used include gelatin (Karacaoglu, Timur, & Telefoncu, 2003), polyvinyl chloride (PVC; Karakus, Pekyardimci, & Esma, 2005), polyethylenimine films (Lakard et al., 2004), and composite materials (Luo et al., 2004).

Covalent binding is commonly achieved through amino groups, accessible on the exposed surfaces of the protein. Typically these can react with aldehyde, epoxide, carboxylic, or amino groups once they have been activated (e.g., by an -imide derivative). Covalent binding of the enzyme directly to the surface of an electrode is generally the most robust approach to immobilization, and therefore potentially leads to the most stable structural integration. Such chemical bonding to a surface can be effected by nucleophilic amino acid side residues present on the protein (carboxylic acid, hydroxy,

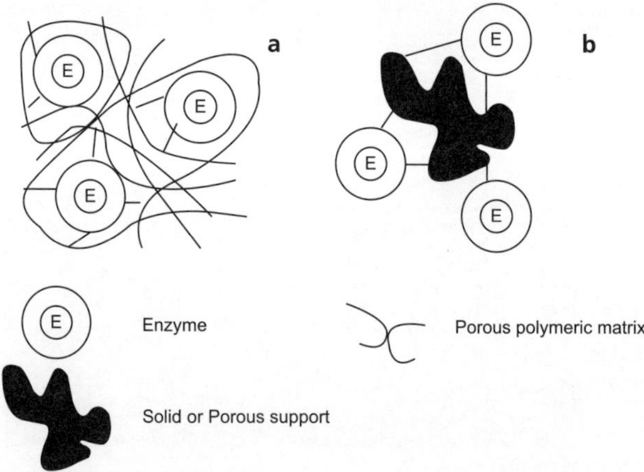



**Figure 8.5.** Schematic representation of chemical immobilization: (a) enzyme entrapped within an insoluble particle by a cross-linked polymer; (b) enzyme covalently attached to an insoluble particle.

thiol, imidazole, phenolic) but not directly involved in the biological function of the molecule. When immobilizing onto a working electrode, carboxyl groups may already be present or generated on the surface, for example, in the case of gold, by self-assembly of alkyl thiol compounds (Oh et al., 2004). These have to be further activated to allow covalent coupling of the protein, frequently achieved by incubation with a carbodiimide, such as 1-ethyl-3-(3-dimethyl-aminopropyl) carbodiimine hydrochloride (EDC) in the presence of N-hydroxysuccinimide (NHS). This latter functional group can also be generated in both polymers and gels. Active aldehyde groups have been generated by treatment with glutaraldehyde and by acidic hydrolysis of poly(3,3-diethoxypropyl methacrylate) in the presence of a photoactive generator (Christman & Maynard, 2005).

## 8.3.4. SURFACE ADSORPTION

Adsorption provides the simplest route to immobilization, but it leads to the least stable of all the outcomes. It relies on the tendency for protein macromolecules to form multiple noncovalent interactions at a surface. However, the enzyme is rather readily washed off the solid support surface, especially if it is used on a continuous basis within an aqueous sample (White & Turner, 1997). Successful immobilization should give initial high enzyme loading with high enzyme activity, leading to an efficient catalytic reaction in the device because little or no denaturation occurs. However, even here there may be a consequence of immobilization, manifested as a change in enzyme activity due to steric effects and other interactions of the enzyme with the solid support material. There may also be changes to the sample microenvironment near the enzyme due to the local charge properties of the support material. These latter can lead to altered partitioning and diffusion of solute into the biolayer phase or to conformational changes in the enzyme that could then lead to a shift in, for example, the optimal enzyme pH.

Typically adsorption is based on interactions between local dipoles existing at interacting functional groups. Alternating dipoles are induced in nonpolar regions of a molecule when two molecules approach each other, creating a distortion in electron density. While this is a common feature of all compounds, this is scaled up and, along with binding, is stronger for larger molecules. Common types of polar groups that are involved are –OH, –NH$_2$, =O, and =NH–, and these can form hydrogen bonds. Given the multiplicity of interactions, the technique is particularly appropriate for immobilizing macromolecules such as enzymes (Cao, 2005).

## 8.4. CLASSICAL AMPEROMETRIC DETECTION

This transduction mode frequently combines an enzyme with an electron acceptor or provider element, constituted from either a voltage-polarized electrode material or a mediator compound, near the electrode, that is able to create electron flow through an electrochemical circuit (Arnold & Meyerhoff, 1988). Typically a constant applied potential is used to drive the direction of electron flow to or from the redox phase with the current being monitored. The classical organization of the system utilizes a working, a reference, and a counterelectrode. The working electrode is the basis for the redox reaction, whereas the reference electrode is used to set the value of the applied potential at that working electrode. The counterelectrode is employed to divert current flow away from the reference electrode. If current flow is low and nominal voltage kept constant, it may be possible to rely on just the working and reference electrodes, with the latter being the source or drain of all the electrons (see Fig. 8.6).

### 8.4.1. OXIDASE-BASED ELECTRODES

Amperometric biosensors that use oxygen reduction and its subsequent monitoring, such as the one produced by Updike and Hicks (1967), are still used because they do not require a mediator and have been improved using functional membranes that are able to reduce biofouling. Therefore these types

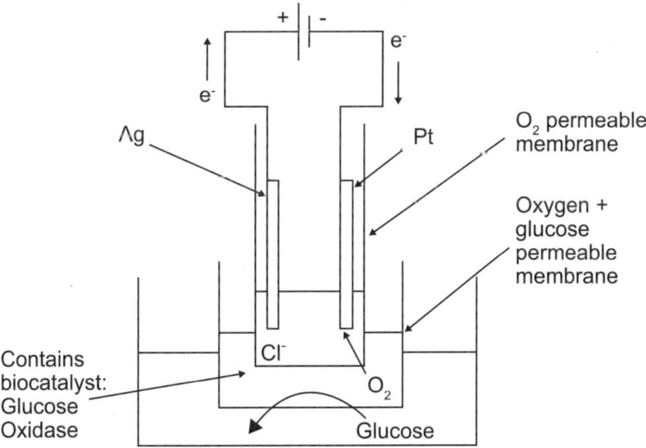


**Figure 8.6.** Schematic of a simple O$_2$ measurement-based amperometric biosensor. A potential is applied between the platinum cathode and a silver anode. This generates an O$_2$-dependent current that is carried between the electrodes by means of an electrolyte solution. This electrode compartment is separated from the biocatalyst (here, GOD) by a thin polymer membrane, permeable only to oxygen. The analyte solution is separated from the biocatalyst by another membrane, permeable to both the substrates and products.

of biosensors may be especially appropriate for in vivo applications. The biosensor that uses ampero-metric detection generally exploits an oxidoreductase enzyme. The advantage of using this or other types of biosensors for blood metabolite measurement is their insensitivity to chromogens and sample turbidity. Therefore the sample being assayed does not need to be modified, but rather can be used intact (e.g., whole blood). This approach to detection is highly applicable to blood enzyme–substrate systems, with utilization of a redox active product or cosubstrate.

For reactions such as those based on the oxidases, either detection of the enzymic consumption of oxygen or the production of $H_2O_2$ can be utilized (Atanasov et al., 1997; Liu, Hu, & Deng, 1997). By placing the enzyme in a sensor with a carefully engineered shape and structure, sensitivity and selectiv-ity can be improved, in addition to the biosensor being adapted with covering membranes to prevent electrode surface poisoning or contamination. In the pioneering concept for an enzyme electrode pro-posed by Clark and Lyons (1962), with GOD optionally immobilized onto an oxygen or other sensor surface, a local reactive change could be measured. If a gas permeable membrane (for $O_2$) is used, then the working electrode can be fully protected, whereby interference or passivation from low molecular weight polar species in the sample can be completely eliminated. The disadvantage of monitoring $O_2$ is that there is a need to derive the glucose-related signal from a decrease rather than an increase in the initial current, which makes the determination of glucose at low concentrations difficult. The system also requires an additional oxygen electrode, typically with inactive enzyme, to give ambient back-ground oxygen levels. Another problem is the need to ensure that there is excess oxygen in the catalytic layer so that the rate of enzymatic reaction is limited by glucose, not by $O_2$ (see Fig. 8.2).

One of the most successful in vivo glucose sensors based on oxygen consumption was developed as a catheter with a cylindrical gel containing immobilized GOD covered by an open-ended silicone rubber tube. This was essentially an amperometric oxygen sensor (Gough, Lucisano, & Tse, 1985), where oxygen could enter the immobilized enzyme region through both the exposed end and through the oxygen permeable silicone rubber layer, whereas glucose could only enter through the exposed end. This way, the relatively small surface access area for glucose versus oxygen entering the gel avoided oxy-gen limitation in the response. This potentiostatic sensor was one of many reported that used a gel or membrane to immobilize the enzyme for stable responses (Wang, Chen, Hocevar, & Ogorevc, 2000).

## 8.5. OPTICAL BIOSENSORS

Optical biosensors offer several advantages over other competing devices in terms of high speed, high precision, immunity to interference, and remote-sensing capabilities. With the introduction of new surfaces, the interactions of small molecules can now be studied reliably in real time, thus allowing kinetic parameters to be determined for the simultaneous testing of a wide range of analytes, including toxic agents and endocrine disruptors (Rodriguez-Mozaz et al., 2004). Optical biosensors are easy to miniaturize for the development of integrated, portable, and flexible devices.

### 8.5.1. OPTICAL ABSORPTION SPECTRA

Conventional spectrophotometric optical absorption measurements involve the recording of changes in the optical reflectivity or transmission of a surface due to absorption by the adsorbed molecular species as a function of wavelength. If incident light of intensity $I_{in}$ is reduced to $I_{out}$ after passing through a sample of thickness $d$, optical absorption is related to the properties of the material through an empirical relationship called the Beer–Lambert–Bouguer attenuation law (Schmid et al., 1997):

$$I_{out} = I_{in}\exp(-\alpha d), \qquad\qquad (8.1)$$

where $\alpha$ is the absorption coefficient or the molar absorptivity of the molecule. The value of the absorption coefficient $\alpha$ varies between different absorbing materials and also with wavelength for a particular material. A vast amount of information relevant to biosensor applications can be obtained from absorption spectra for the molecular species usually adsorbed on a surface (Hall, 1991). The technique becomes less sensitive if the surface coverage is one monolayer or less Wang, Ramirez, Wang, & Leblanc, 1999). In one example, diacetylene monomers were developed to be functionalized with biotin. When streptavidin in the molar ratio of 1:2 (streptavidin:biotin) was added to Langmuir–Blodgett films of polydiacetylene, visible optical absorption changes were seen due to the lower conjugation length of the $\pi$-electron system in the polymer backbone. Specific chemical species and the presence of surface-immobilized peptide were identified via time-of-flight secondary-ion mass spectrometry, which established surface species, and also by the use of X-ray photon spectroscopy (XPS; Geiger, Hug, & Keller, 2002). The measurement of redox active species as indicators of tissue oxidative damage, the quality of preservation in food stuffs, and of pollution levels was achieved by optically monitoring polyaniline films. With the use of GOD immobilized in such films, a combined capillary electrophoresis biosensor for monitoring physiological glucose was produced; the sensor showed excellent sensing stability, with most of the activity retained at 30 days (Bossi et al., 2003).

## 8.5.2. FIBER-OPTIC BIOSENSORS

Optical fiber waveguides are normally used for carrying optical pulses over long distances, but their application in monitoring optical changes in cells and tissues is an interesting development in biosensing. Fibers consist of a glass core with a refractive index of 1.5 surrounded by cladding with a slightly lower refractive index. For light entering the fiber face at an angle less than or equal to $\theta_A$ (acceptance angle), total internal reflection occurs (see Fig. 8.7), confining all the energy within the core if the angle of incidence at the core–cladding interface is greater than or equal to critical angle $\theta_C$. Fiber-optic cables are available as either single-mode (one acceptable ray-path per frequency) or multimode fibers. A variety of sensors have been produced, ranging from simple pH sensors to artificial olfaction sensors, high-density oligonucleotide arrays, and high-throughput cell-based arrays. A versatile sensing platform can be designed from high-density sensor packing ($2 \times 10^7$ cm$^{-2}$) of optical fiber bundles having diameters on the order of 3 µm to 10 µm. The individual fiber cores can be selectively etched to form high-density microwell arrays capable of housing complementary-sized microsensors (Epstein, Biran, & Walt, 2002). The miniature size can facilitate a faster response and a more-sensitive measurement capability, whether for monitoring single analytes or for more complex multiplexed assays.

For a sensor where an unmodified fiber core was inserted into a silica capillary tube, a charge-coupled device (CCD) was used as a multichannel detector, positioned alongside the capillary. This enabled mode-filtered light to be detected. By means of a sensor arrangement, acetic acid was assayed with a linear response to 90%(v/v) and a high correlation coefficient. The advantage of this arrangement was a rapid response and a relatively high signal-to-noise ratio (SNR), making the system appropriate for use in practical industrial analysis (Zhou et al., 2004).

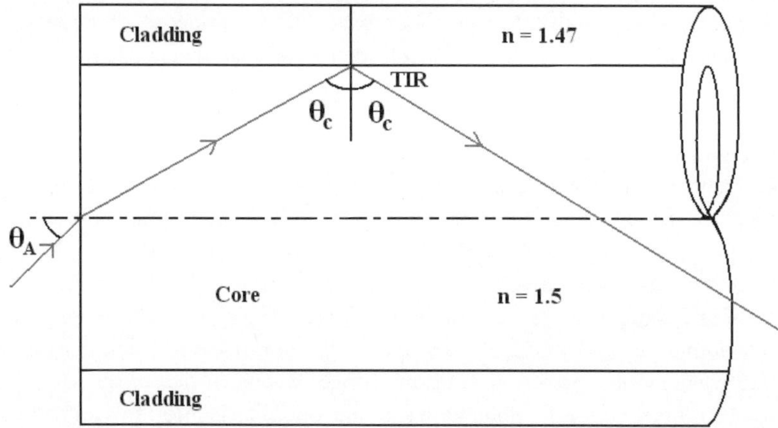


**Figure 8.7.** Schematic of an optical fiber.

## 8.5.3. SURFACE PLASMON RESONANCE

Surface plasmons are propagating electron density fluctuations in a thin metal layer confined to a metal–dielectric interface. They can be excited by plane-polarized light under total internal reflection. Resonance occurs when the momentum of the incoming light is equal to the momentum of the plasmons. For the wave vectors to match, light has to pass through a high refractive index (RI) material before striking the metal. By using a semicylindrical prism of high RI—$n_p$ in the Kretschmann configuration (see Fig. 8.8)—these waves can be excited by p-polarized light of wavelength $\lambda$ via an evanescent field (Kretschmann, 1971).

The wave vector of the incoming light is scanned, for example, by rotation of the prism or by a change in the wavelength, until a spectrum of wave vectors over reflected light intensity is obtained. The evanescent field is completely attenuated at a particular angle of incidence corresponding to resonance and thus there is no reflection. Of the metals that are usable, indium is expensive, sodium is reactive, copper and aluminum are broad in their surface plasmon resonance (SPR) response, and silver is too susceptible to oxidation. Gold is commonly chosen because it is highly resistant to oxidation and atmospheric contaminants, yet it is also compatible with many surface chemical modification systems. The thickness of the gold layer is required to be approximately 50 nm; thickness is of great importance for reliable sensing. In the Kretschmann arrangement (Fig. 8.8), the gold layer is coated directly onto the waveguide. A coating layer of an organic membrane can then be used to incorporate a biological affinity molecule for biosensing.

In the alternative Otto arrangement, there is a finite distance between the metal and the prism surface. This configuration is especially useful in the study of SPR in solid-phase media. However, since the distance between the metal and prism surface reduces SPR efficiency, it is less useful for applications with solutions. As an alternative, in one study a series of metallic nano-islands was formed on a glass surface using lithography, exploiting the morphology of glass monodisperse polystyrene nanospheres. The metal particles enhanced the local electromagnetic field through SPR and the particle size adjusted to optimize the local field for fluorophore absorption. The fluorophore used was Cy5

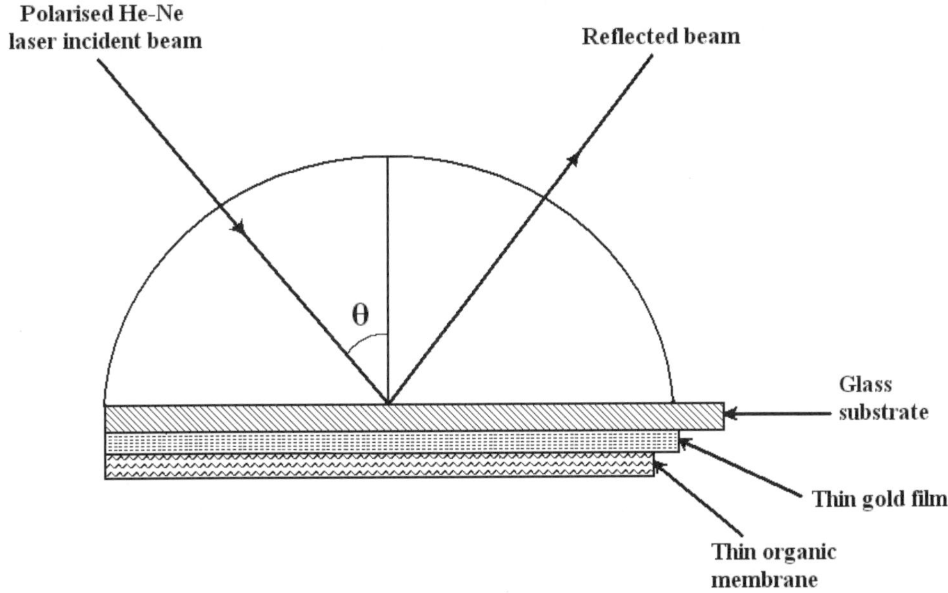


**Figure 8.8.** A Kretschmann-type configuration to measure surface plasmon resonance (SPR) data.

dye and the technique could enhance fluorescence and absorption by such plasmonic enhancement. A mean fluorescence enhancement by a factor of 8 was achieved in a simulated bioassay (Stranik, et al., 2005)—Cy5 dye is used as an indicator in optical immunoassay. In another study, binding of anti-bovine serum albumin (BSA) antibodies to a BSA layer was monitored by SPR as a model of immunoaffinity interaction to demonstrate the concept of additive assay, where surface accumulation of analyte can be related to concentration without surface regeneration (Chung et al., 2005). Polyethylene glycol-terminated monothiol and dithiol platforms on an SPR biosensor have been demonstrated to be very sensitive and specific for detection of microorganisms, notably *Staphylococcus aureus* (Naimushin et al., 2002). Detection of *S. aureus* using thiol self-assembled monolayers (SAMs) would appear to give added value to such sensing systems. The basic SPR protocol could be used to detect minute amounts of analytes such as pathogens, viruses, toxins, and proteins in a more complex sample (de Jong et al., 2005), and with dendritic SAMs, both direct and two-site (sandwich) immunoassays have been realized (Subramanian, Irudayaraj, & Ryan, 2006). Surface plasmon fluorescence spectroscopy can be applied simultaneously with SPR in order to increase the sensitivity and specificity of the binding assays (Xu et al., 2006). Here it was possible to register minor volume (i.e., depth) changes of a carboxymethyl dextran coating in relation to pH and in relation to film collapse, and was directly related to the number of available carboxyl groups and the extent of dextran cross-linking.

## 8.5.4. ATTENUATED TOTAL REFLECTION

Attenuated total reflection (ATR) at a silicon nitride ($Si_3N_4$) planar waveguide has been employed to monitor affinity activity. In one example, a 190 nm $Si_3N_4$ core layer sandwiched between two 1.5 μm silicon dioxide ($SiO_2$) cladding layers was used (see Fig. 8.9). The refractive indices are typically $n_1 \approx$ 1.46 and $n_2 \approx 2$ for the $SiO_2$ and $Si_3N_4$ layers, respectively, and the evanescent field volume attained is therefore reasonably high. Light is normally expected to propagate through the planar waveguide without significant attenuation, since both the $SiO_2$ and $Si_3N_4$ layers are transparent in the visible range. The input signal intensity $I_{in}$ becomes attenuated to $I_0$ after multiple reflections $N$ at the $Si_3N_4/$ thin-film interface, providing the sensing surface. The relationship between $I_i$ and $I_0$ is governed by the modified Beer's law (Plowman et al., 1994):

$$I_0 = I_{in}\exp(-\alpha_0 DN),$$
(8.2)

where $\alpha_0$ is the absorption coefficient of the sensing film prior to a biochemical or bioaffinity reaction (e.g., an enzymic reaction). The interaction length $D$ of the evanescent field depends upon the refractive index $n_J$ and thickness $d_J$ of the membrane in the following form (Nabok, Haron, & Ray, 2003):

$$D = \frac{5.5\, n_J\, d_J}{4 - d_J^2}\,.$$
(8.3)

The optical losses at each reflection are therefore dependent upon the absorption coefficient $\alpha_0$ and thickness $d_J$ of the sensing film. Changes in the film's properties parallel the attenuation of the transmitted light and provide a simple and effective tool for monitoring different biochemical reactions or protein deposition processes on the waveguide surface. Usually optical absorption spectroscopy involves a relatively short optical path through the membrane during a single step of light propagation, but the sensitivity of the waveguiding transducer becomes larger (Plowman et al., 1999) because of the number of multiple reflections (e.g., as many as 200).

Waveguides have also been produced using a silicon oxynitride (SiON) layer deposited onto a thermally grown $SiO_2$ layer. A multianalyte immunoassay has been developed, for example, utilizing multiple antibody-functionalized capture surfaces for detecting myocardial damage markers using a spatial arrangement, physical adsorption, and an integrated SiON optical waveguide (Plowman et al., 1999). A polyelectrolyte SAM layer bearing cyclo-tetra-chromotropylene as the indicator has allowed surface monitoring of GOD and urease layers (Haron & Ray, 2006).

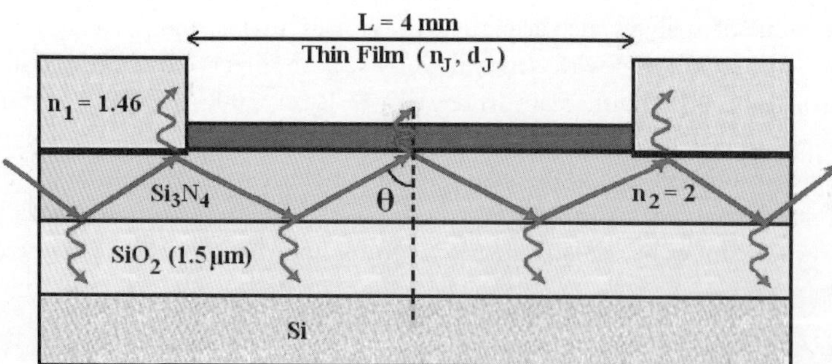


**Figure 8.9.** The structure of a $Si_3N_4$ planar waveguide, with useful dimensions and relevant optical parameters.

## 8.6. MODIFIED ELECTROCHEMICAL BIOSENSORS

### *8.6.1. MOLECULAR MEDIATORS*

Beyond the historically important classical systems discussed earlier, a new generation of modified electrodes offers an entirely different perspective on measurement. Most notably, the natural electron acceptor oxygen has been replaced in the oxidase reaction by a host of artificial electron acceptors. Figure 8.10 shows the prototypical setup of this so-called second-generation biosensor. Here the mediator is potentially in solution—an effective working example being ferricyanide—but the strategy has proved especially useful when the mediator has been in immobilized form. Essentially the enzyme catalyzes the oxidation of a substrate and, through this process, itself becomes reduced. The reduced state reverts to the original oxidized form by interaction with an electron mediator. The mediator can be continuously cycled into this oxidized state by the electrically polarized electrode surface. The net effect is a continuous shuttling of electrons from substrate to electrode, and thus a sustained current.

As previously summarized by Cardosi and Turner (1987), the artificial mediator must fulfill certain criteria:

- It should interact rapidly with the enzyme.
- It should exhibit reversible kinetics and be recyclable.
- The potential required for its electrochemical regeneration should be lower than that for oxidizing the enzyme active site.
- The oxidized and reduced forms need to be stable.
- In reduced form, the mediator should not react with ambient oxygen.

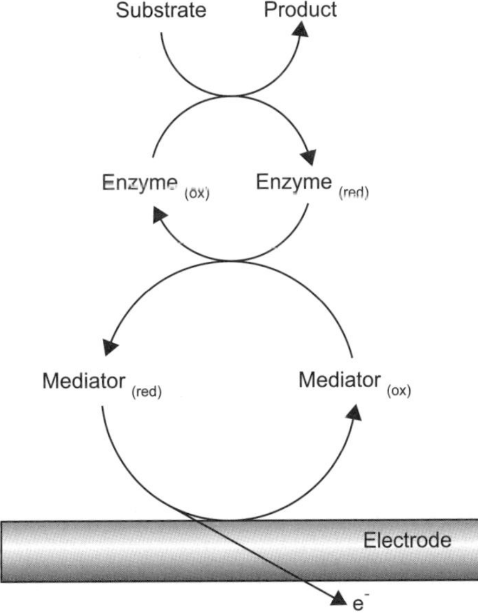


**Figure 8.10.** Reaction scheme for a mediated amperometric enzyme electrode: e = electron; ox = oxidized; red = reduced.

- The mediator must be nontoxic, although this may not be sufficient to allow for clinical in vivo use because of concerns about long-term effects.
- It is preferably insoluble in order to achieve reagentless measurement.

Efficient electron mediators establish electron rapid transfer between the enzyme active site and the electrode surface. The working potential employed with any given mediator species is usually significantly lower than that required to oxidize background interferents (e.g., ascorbate, urate, tyrosine, and acetaminophen), so selectivity is enhanced by being able to operate at low polarizing voltages.

One commercial biosensor, used for home glucose monitoring, uses ferrocene as an electrode-immobilized mediator. Ferrocene is an organometallic that is commonly used in amperometric sensors as a mediator molecule. One version of the amperometric ferrocene-modified glucose sensor was used for in vivo monitoring, reported by Claremont et al. (1986). They found that changes in sensor output were slower than blood glycemic changes and that the sensor configuration was difficult to construct. There have been many other mediators reported in the literature, such as quinone derivatives and organic conducting salts (Pandey, Upadhyay, & Upadhyay, 1997). Alfonso et al. (2004) immobilized GOD electrostatically onto carbon and platinum electrodes modified with mixed ferrocene-cobaltocenium dendrimers. Ferrocene remains the most common system used in biomedical analysis where there is a particular advantage to using biosensors able to operate in low-oxygen samples.

## 8.6.2. MEDIATOR CHAINS

Heller's group has carried out a significant body of work on mediated biosensors using polymer mediator chains. In the work of Zhang and Heller (2005), an amperometric sandwich immunoassay was reported for IgG that was able to register concentrations down to 7 pg mL$^{-1}$, with an extended measurement range to high concentrations. Here a hydrogel with redox properties was electrodeposited with avidin and two polyanions—poly(acrylic acid-co-maleic acid) and poly(acrylic acid)—used to quench cationic binding sites on the avidin. The polyanions variously bound by charge effects and by reacting with specific cysteine, lysine, and arginine residues on the avidin. Biotin-linked anti-rabbit IgG was retained by binding to the avidin phase, and served to capture target IgG. Subsequent binding by horseradish-peroxidase (HRP)-labeled anti-rabbit IgG led to HRP immobilization at the surface. The combined redox polymer and HRP unit was then able to effect electroreduction of $H_2O_2$. The two polyanions in the system proved effective in reducing adsorption effects and allowed for the broad analytical measurement range observed. In other work carried out by Heller's group (Barton et al., 2002), electroreduction of oxygen to water at pH 7 was achieved using another electron relay system, but with a laccase-activated cathode surface. Here, work using a *Pleurotus ostreatus* laccase was compared to results from previous work carried out involving electroreduction of oxygen to water with a *Coriolus hirsutus* laccase. The previous drawback of enzyme inhibition by chloride and loss of activity at neutral pH were overcome. The enzyme source can thus have a critical effect on enzyme performance, regardless of the inherent catalytic activity or nominal reaction chemistry.

## 8.6.3. ELECTROCHEMICAL IMMUNOASSAY

Many sensors use enzyme labels for amperometric detection of drugs (Holt et al., 1995), hormones (Athey, Ball, & McNeil, 1993a), and proteins (Della Ciana et al., 1996) as target analytes. Here, the enzyme label follows an immunoreaction and its activity is registered via an electrochemically active, soluble product (Treloar, Kane, & Vadgama, 1997). Enzymes used include GOD, horseradish peroxidase, β-galactosidase, alkaline phosphatase, and glucose-6-phosphate dehydrogenase (Gosling, 1990). Amperometric immunoassays for direct measurement (e.g., of theophylline) in whole blood have been reported (Athey et al., 1993b). To protect the electrode from biofouling by whole blood, a membrane overlay such as microporous polycarbonate has been used. Here, however, the enzyme product needs to be able to diffuse freely through the membrane, and if it is a soluble mediator, needs to shuttle unhindered as both a reduced and oxidized species. The mediator version of electrochemical immunoassay is thus analogous to the scheme shown in Figure 8.10, except that a permeable, low-fouling membrane needs to be placed directly on the electrode surface. Stable electrode-protecting membrane structures are particularly important for immunosensing because of the low current generated for the types of high-sensitivity assays undertaken, target molecules usually being at or below micromolar concentration.

Currently micromachined membranes are being developed that exhibit selective permeability and low biofouling; Desai et al. (2000) fabricated and characterized nanoporous silicon membranes based on microelectromechanical systems (MEMS) technology. When compared to polymeric membranes of similar pore size in protein-loaded samples, the silicon membranes allowed substantially greater glucose transport at 4 hr, while maintaining a complete barrier to albumin. In principle, such structures could function as low-barrier structures for mediator transport, thus creating a protected internal environment for stabilized electrochemistry. Moreover, such inorganic membranes were structurally stable with no evident degradation in protein-loaded solutions or biological samples at 37°C. One key advantage here was a uniform pore size and geometry (down to 10 nm), which could augment reproducibility and also design integration in future MEMS-based biosensors.

## 8.7. POTENTIOMETRIC DETECTION

### 8.7.1. GENERAL PRINCIPLES

The transducers in this type of biosensor system have the capacity to operate as pH probes and as ion-selective electrodes, mainly for inorganic ions. They are typically formulated as macroscopic potentiometric devices for routine analysis, or alternatively, as microelectronic sensors for specialist research use. Their stability is inevitably dependent upon the method of immobilization of the integral biological component, usually an enzyme. In the archetypal system, this consists of an immobilized enzyme film covering the probe, with the device connected to a high-impedance input meter such as that used for conventional pH measurement. In this instance, the catalyzed reaction generates or consumes hydrogen ions. There is a need for a retaining semipermeable membrane to surround the biocatalyst layer, the latter is often held in direct contact with the probe surface (e.g., the glass membrane of the pH electrode). The electrical potential generated between the internal Ag/AgCl electrode (in dilute hydrogen chloride [HCl] for pH) and an external reference electrode is measured.

Biosensors that involve enzyme-generated $H^+$ changes require the use of very weakly buffered solutions (e.g., less than 5 mM) for a significant change in pH to be registered. The relationship between pH change and substrate concentration is complex, including nonlinear effects due to pH-dependent enzyme activity variation, variable pH-dependent buffering, and the variable ionization of any weak acid or base produced by the enzyme. However, conditions can often be found where there is a linear relationship between measured pH change and substrate concentration. Provided there is sufficient enzyme loading, the change in potential approximates to the logarithm of the substrate concentration if the other cell potentials of the electrochemical cell, overall, remain constant (Pearson, Gill, & Vadgama, 2000). For a monovalent ion, this relationship is described by a simplified Nernst equation:

$$E = E^0 + (RT/F)\ln(a_m), \tag{8.4}$$

where $E$ is the electromotive force, $E^0$ is the electrode standard potential, $R$ is the gas constant, $T$ is the absolute temperature, $F$ is the Faraday constant, and $a_m$ is the activity of the measured ion m⁺. With high enzyme activity, an equivalent Nernstian relationship holds for the enzyme substrate. However, this equation cannot be applied precisely to biological samples due to the presence of multiple background ions and unknown overall ion activity and ion concentration in sample solutions.

Potentiometry is less sensitive than amperometry and its upper linear range is restricted compared with amperometric methods. Other disadvantages with potentiometric sensors are that they suffer from interference from other ions. In addition, there are fewer immediate enzymatic reactions that can be followed by potentiometric electrodes; those that are include the hydrolases (Pearson et al., 2000).

Ion-selective electrodes can be used for the analysis of urea, creatinine, and amino acids, achieved using immobilized enzymes and pH change as the detection mechanism (Kaun & Guilbault, 1997). In one potentiometric biosensor system for creatinine, creatinine iminohydrolase was immobilized on a chitosan membrane and coupled to a nonactin-based ammonium ion selective electrode (Magalhaes & Machado, 2002). In this study, response characteristics of three sensor variants with the enzyme immobilized by three different procedures were evaluated. Properties improved when chitosan coupling was via enzyme adsorption. The linear response was observed to be $10^{-4}$ to $10^{-2}$ M with response times of 30 s to 60 s and a lifetime of 44 days. The initial response to creatinine approached a theoretical monovalent ion slope (approximately 50 mV decade⁻¹).

A useful mode of application for potentiometric biosensors is incorporation into flow injection analysis (FIA). In one study (Koncki, Walcerz, & Leszczynska, 1999), the biosensor was formed by enzyme immobilization onto the active sensing surface of the electrode, and the FIA system allowed rapid urea and penicillin measurement. Automated analysis is possible with many devices and FIA has the ability to easily track calibration and baseline drift.

## 8.7.2. ENFETS

The microfabricated equivalent of the standard ion-selective electrode is the ion-selective field-effect transistor (ISFET), and in the present context, with an enzyme used as a biosensor, the enzyme-linked field-effect transistor (ENFET; Kauffmann & Guilbault, 1991). The active surface of an ENFET (see Fig. 8.11) is typically 500 μm × 50 μm with a depth of 300 μm. The main body comprises p-type silicon with two embedded n-type silicon areas: the negative source and the positive drain. The sensing interface is insulated by a thin layer of silica that serves as the gate of the FET. Above the gate region is a thin layer of H⁺-sensitive material that responds to a superimposed biocatalyst layer, typically a hydrolase. The sensitive elements of the FET require it to be protected by inert encapsulating material (e.g., polyimide photopolymer). When a potential is applied between the source and drain, current flows through the FET and is modulated by the potential generated at the ion-selective gate by its influence on electron density in the underlying silicon. Enzyme membranes retained on the ion-selective gates can alter pH, thereby altering the surface potential and current output of the device. The surface potential is measured against a reference electrode immersed in the same solution. The main advantage

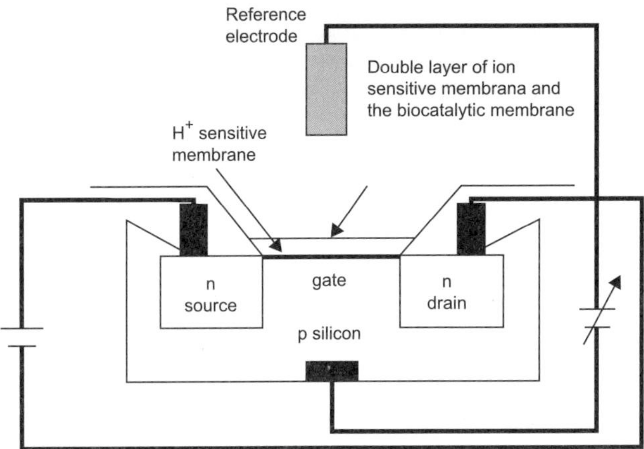


**Figure 8.11.** Schematic of the section across the width of an ISFET (the source is negative and the drain is at positive potential).

here is small size, mass production, and the general benefits of integrated circuit technology with the possibility of in situ signal processing. Urea-sensitive FETs (an ENFET containing bound urease with a separate reference electrode) are most commonly reported, especially because there are few nonpotentiometric routes to measuring urea by biosensor. Biosensor arrays of ISFETs and ENFETs offer a useful way of scale-up measurement, but as with other potentiometric devices, sensitivity may be affected by solution composition, ionic strength, and pH (Koncki et al., 1999).

Recent studies have shown some improvement in practical performance, making FETs more reliable. Work carried out by Luo et al. (2004) demonstrated a novel glucose ENFET based on the reactivity of manganese dioxide ($MnO_2$) nanoparticles. Generally, glucose-sensitive ENFETs are based on local pH change due to the formation of gluconic acid. However, with the ENFET fabricated by coimmobilizing GOD and $MnO_2$ nanoparticles on the ISFET gate, there was a significant local pH shift at the sensitive membrane with an increase in glucose concentration. The effect was achieved with the response of the ENFET being unaffected by pH or buffer concentration. The exact mechanism for this is unclear, but was possibly due to direct nanoparticle interaction with the $H_2O_2$ product of the enzyme reaction. This system gave a linear response to glucose over 0.025 mM to 1.90 mM, with an upper extension to 3.5 mM glucose (Luo et al., 2004). Other work has involved the application of the ENFET approach to penicillin (Wang, Li, Zhong, & Li, 1990) using penicillinase. A differential penicillin ENFET was constructed by modifying one of a dual set of ISFET gates with cross-linked BSA-penicillinase and the other with a blank membrane consisting of BSA alone. The linear range and sensitivity depended upon the buffer background: for 0.01 M and 0.02 M phosphate buffer, output was 6.5 mV mM$^{-1}$ to 7.0 mV mM$^{-1}$ and 3.2 mV mM$^{-1}$ to 3.6 mV mM$^{-1}$, respectively, over 0.5 mM to 14 mM and 0.5 mM to 25 mM penicillin concentrations, respectively. Storage in 0.01 M phosphate buffer at 4°C demonstrated a lifetime of more than 6 months.

Lakard et al. (2004) developed an electrochemical sensor consisting of a glass-sealed metal microelectrode coated by a polyethylenimine film. Enzyme was entrapped in a polymer matrix and four different protocols for immobilization were studied to determine the most reliable one. The greatest efficiency was obtained through physical adsorption of the enzyme coupled with surface reticulation using a dilute glutaraldehyde cross-linking solution. This sensor was advantageous, as it exhibited short response times (15 s to 30 s) and a response to urea over $1 \times 10^{-2.5}$ M to $1 \times 10^{-1.5}$ M with a viable response lasting 4 weeks.

## 8.8. PIEZOELECTRIC DETECTION

### 8.8.1. GENERAL PRINCIPLES

The interaction of antibodies with their corresponding antigens is an attractive basis for developing antibody-based chemical biosensors, that is, immunosensors. Theoretically, if an antibody can be raised against a particular analyte, an immunosensor can be developed to recognize it. Despite the high specificity and affinity of antibodies toward complementary ligand molecules, antibody–antigen interactions lead to only weak electronically measurable changes. However, the remarkable selectivity of antibodies has stimulated research in the field to overcome this problem (Luong & Guilbault, 1991; Muramatsu et al., 1987).

The piezoelectric effect in various crystalline substances is a useful property that allows the detection of analyte. Piezoelectric detection involves monitoring the change in mass at a sensor surface, either a piezoelectric crystal or an acoustic wave device. This type of biosensor has been used variously for environmental monitoring (Yokoyama et al., 1995), food microbial testing (Ye, Letcher, & Rand, 1997), and clinical analysis. The advantages of this type of sensor include solid-state construction, chemical inertness, durability, low cost, mass production, and the absence of any requirement to use a label to follow the mass reaction (Pearson et al., 2000). The types of piezoelectric crystals include lithium niobate, zinc oxide, gallium arsenide, and potassium sodium tartrate. However, the AT-cut quartz crystal is the most commonly used. This is because of its chemical stability and resistance to high temperature (Collings & Caruso, 1997). The piezoelectric immunosensor is thought to be one of the most sensitive analytical instruments developed to date, being capable of detecting antigens in the picogram range. Moreover, this type of device is believed to have the potential to detect antigens in the gas as well as the liquid phase (Kumar, 2000).

When a quartz plate is distorted in a defined direction, an electrical potential is generated between the two deformed surfaces due to charge separation. However, if a voltage is imposed, the crystal will distort, and with an oscillating voltage, it will vibrate. There is a natural vibration frequency for a crystal that is related to mass. Therefore if, for example, a protein is deposited on the surface of the crystal, a change in the natural or resonant frequency can be detected. This frequency shift is proportional to the mass change and can be represented by the Sauerbrey equation:

$$\Delta F = C_Q f^2 \Delta m / A, \qquad (8.5)$$

where $\Delta F$ is the change in fundamental frequency, $C_Q$ is sensitivity, and $f$ is the resonant frequency of the crystal. $A$ is the area of the crystal and $\Delta m$ is the mass change deposited (Sauerbrey, 1959). Admittedly this analysis is an oversimplification, since ionic, surface microviscosity, and dissipation, among other effects, are relevant to behavior in a liquid. However, correlation with deposited mass can nevertheless be made.

It can be seen from Figure 8.12 that such devices involve precoating the surface with the probe antibody (Skladal et al., 2005). This can be attached by many of the standard immobilization methods,

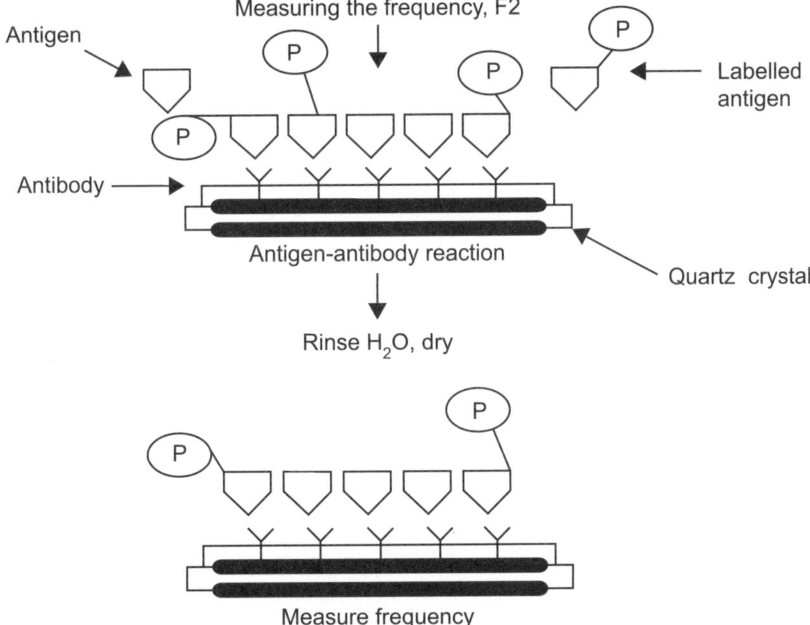



**Figure 8.12.** Use of a quartz crystal microbalance to detect a low molecular weight antigen. The presence of a heavy label (P) acts to increase the mass and hence the magnitude of the response upon binding. Here, the assay is in a dry format.

including cross-linking. When the analyte binds to the protein layer, the crystal mass increases, causing a decrease in resonant frequency. Disadvantages are that nonspecific adsorption is difficult to control and usually only high molecular weight analytes can be measured directly. For low molecular weight analytes, there is not a sufficient amount of molar mass to generate a change in frequency unless the molecule is prelinked to a high-mass structure (Fig. 8.12). It may also be necessary to compensate for background variables when performing analyses with piezoelectric sensors.

## 8.8.2. BIOSENSING OPPORTUNITIES

Some recent work with piezoelectric sensors has been aimed at microbial targets. Thus immunosensing to detect severe acute respiratory syndrome–associated coronavirus (SARS-CoV) from sputum in aerosol droplets has been attempted (Zuo et al., 2004). This was done by binding horse polyclonal antibody against SARS-CoV onto a piezoelectric crystal through protein A binding, facilitating orientation of the antibody binding sites toward the sample. Sample atomization using an aerosol increased the degree of antigen exposure to the antibody. A frequency-shift-based response was linearly related to antigen concentration in the range of 0.6 μg mL$^{-1}$ to 4 μg mL$^{-1}$. The sensor proved to be stable, and an analysis was possible in less than 2 minutes. In another study, Lin and Tsai (2003) used a piezoelectric immunosensor to detect staphylococcal enterotoxin B (SEB). Of the three methods for anti-SEB antibody immobilization on the gold surface of the piezoelectric driving electrodes, glutaraldehyde linkage to a polyethyleneimine precoating produced the best results. SEB was detected in the range 2.5 mg mL$^{-1}$ to 60 mg mL$^{-1}$ with a correlation coefficient of 0.997. The assay was relatively specific, with staphylococcal enterotoxin A providing a 6.44% response, while no response was seen for staphylococcal enterotoxin D. Storage under dry conditions stabilized the electrode over 3 days.

Skladal et al. (2005) reported the use of piezoelectric devices to investigate osteoprotegerin (OPG) interaction with ligands and antibodies. OPG is a secretory glycoprotein involved as a soluble factor in the regulation of bone mass with its ligand, RANKL, from the receptor activator of nuclear factor $\kappa$B (RANK) pathway. Its levels in serum indicate osteoclast formation activity. Any changes in the concentration ratio of the ligand and glycoprotein can result in bone loss, leading variously to osteoporosis, hypercalcemia, metastatic osteolytic lesions, and rheumatic bone degradation. Skladal et al. (2005) were able to immobilize monoclonal capture antibodies onto a piezoelectric quartz crystal and studied resonant frequency changes associated with OPG affinity reactions at the surface. This type of immunosensor appears promising for rapid diagnostics. Because of the microgravimetric principle of operation, other high-mass entities can be detected, and piezoelectric sensors are also suited to cell adhesion and deposition studies.

The thickness shear mode (TSM) quartz crystal resonator system has also been used, based on progress in the ability of oscillator circuits to deal with the solution dampening of shear displacement. Transduction exploits a propagated ultrasonic wave generated by imposing a sinusoidal field at the piezoelectric quartz resonator. Shear displacement alters at the solid–liquid interface due to adsorption, for example, and allows cell adhesion to surfaces to be monitored (Le Guillou-Buffello et al., 2005). The inhibiting properties of various bioactive polymers toward fibroblasts were followed by this technique. Thin films of various polymers bearing carboxylate or sulfonate functional groups were studied, and in contrast to traditional cell counting, dynamic cell adhesion activity could be followed.

Lee et al. (2005) used a monolithic piezoelectric structure, lead zirconate titanate [Pb(Zr$_{0.52}$Ti$_{0.48}$)O$_3$], as a cantilever, with SiN$_x$ as a support layer for following surface binding. Prostate-specific antigen (PSA) binding was measured via resonance frequency change due to interaction with antibody immobilized on the cantilever; the antibody was attached via calixcrown self-assembled monolayers on a gold coating. The resonant frequency shift depended on the cantilever size, but detection seemed possible down to 10 pg mL$^{-1}$.

### 8.8.3. NUCLEIC ACID DETECTION

There have been other more recent uses for piezoelectric sensors (e.g., as DNA probes). Skladal et al. (2004) coated a quartz crystal with oriented oligonucleotide probes used for the detection of hepatitis C virus (HCV) in serum. The gold electrode surfaces of the sensors were modified by self-assembly of cystamine, with glutaraldehyde bridging used to attach avidin or streptavidin. The latter allowed oriented binding of biotinylated DNA. When the devices were used in a flow cell, target DNA obtained through amplification by reverse transcriptase-polymerase chain reaction (RT-PCR) enabled identification of viral RNA. Piezoelectric assay here could be repeated on the same device; the assay time was 10 minutes. This type of approach could be valuable in extending its practical use into clinical, veterinary, medicolegal, and environmental sectors.

DNA sequence identification is, of course, central to molecular biology screening and genetic analysis. DNA techniques incorporating hybridization, amplification, and recombination all have complementary strand recognition as the starting point (Junhui, Hong, & Ruifu, 1997). For DNA biosensors especially, reliable sequence recognition is crucial. Tombelli, Minunni, and Mascini (2005) proposed focusing on the methodology for probe immobilization as a key step in any DNA biosensor development; analytical performance was likely to depend on a judicious choice of the immobilization phase. It was considered that the DNA needed to be attached to a solid support, yet retain its active conformation and binding ability through appropriate surface alignment. Any attachment also required that it be sustained over the period of an assay, with binding domains available to the solution phase DNA target.

## 8.9. ENZYME-BASED IMPEDIMETRIC BIOSENSORS

### 8.9.1. NUCLEIC ACID DETECTION

Impedance spectroscopy has been used as an effective method for observing the electrical changes on surface-modified electrodes. However, the approach can be time consuming for a full impedance spectrum taken over a broad range of frequencies.

In recent work by Lucarelli, Marrazza, and Mascini (2005), disposable oligonucleotide-modified screen-printed gold electrodes were used as genosensors. Thiol functionalized probe DNA was bound to a gold surface and impedance spectra obtained. From these, it was demonstrated that initial immobilization was determined by gold-thiol linkages. The technique allowed the use of a biocatalytically generated surface precipitate as the indicator parameter that changed impedance. In work by Davis, Nabok, and Higson (2005) with polymer-modified screen-printed carbon electrodes, impedance with single-strand DNA was characterized before and after target sequence binding. Complementary strand binding led to reduced impedance, not observed for DNA that remained unhybridized with unmatched target sequences.

### 8.9.2. IMMUNOSENSING

Impedimetric sensors have been developed for detecting immunobinding using antibodies. Cooreman et al. (2005) investigated the interaction between a semiconducting polymer and antibodies against the fluorescent dyes fluorescein isothiocyanate (FITC) and Cy5. The antibodies were physically adsorbed on polymer films and different surface loadings obtained based on the initial antibody concentration used. When differential impedance spectroscopy was used, the functionalized films showed a response to low (1 ppb) antigen concentration, with a time constant of 2 minutes to 3 minutes. Impedimetric immunosensors have also been fabricated by using electrodeposited biotin functionalized polypyrrole films to immobilize the antibody (Ouerghi et al., 2002). Attached biotinylated antibody to human IgG gave reproducible results with a detection limit of 10 pg mL$^{-1}$.

## 8.10. WHOLE CELL BIOSENSORS

### 8.10.1. BASIC STRATEGY

For the purposes of biosensing, whole cells provide a naturally prepackaged matrix of enzymes, enzyme cascades, and cofactors with a host of attendant high-affinity receptor systems. In contrast to isolated enzyme biosensors, such constructs, while usable as enzyme electrodes, inevitably respond to a rather broad range of analytes. However, there are important applications for such broad-spectrum devices, such as toxicity testing and environmental monitoring, where a broad response to a family of agents may be necessary, the nature of any included toxicant being unpredictable. The two main types of transducers used to monitor whole cell biocatalysts are electrochemical and optical. With electrochemistry, a naturally occurring species such as oxygen can be monitored through metabolic changes in cells, or an introduced chemical species can be monitored (e.g., a mediator interacting with the cell's electron transport chain; Bentley, Atkinson, Jezek, & Rawson, 2001).

## 8.10.2. SPECIFIC APPLICATIONS

The monitoring of aromatic hydrocarbons has been possible using bacterial cells with electrochemical detection (Paitan et al., 2004). The principle of operation was the fusion of a reporter gene to a promoter gene that was sensitive to the target analyte. A promoter region is generally utilized in gene coding for selective transcriptional regulation, and the constructs here led to a whole cell response to aromatic compounds but not to nonaromatics; the genes encoded enzymes able to generate electrochemically active products. Through this approach, micromolar concentrations of aromatic hydrocarbons such as xylene and toluene could be detected within minutes. The sensors were considered to be of possible use as early warning systems for environmental hazards. In another study (May et al., 2004), a whole cell potentiometric biosensor was developed based on a confluent layer of human umbilical vein endothelial cells (HUVECs). An ion-selective cellulose triacetate membrane was modified by covalent attachment of an arginine-glycine-aspartic acid (RGD) peptide sequence to enable cell adhesion. The cell-loaded biosensor was able to identify the presence of cell toxins by permeability effects at the stage when the cell monolayer was confluent; for such monolayers, increased ionic permeability correlated with higher levels of toxin, in this case histamine. This principle of operation could allow for measurement of a wide range of toxic agents for which there are no available bioaffinity molecules.

A microbial whole cell reporter has been demonstrated for the quantification of tetracycline using a green fluorescent protein reporter and a tetracycline-linked promoter gene (Bahl, Hansen, Licht, & Sorensen, 2004). The system could potentially be developed as a biosensor for this antibiotic (Chopra & Roberts, 2001). Another application has been to investigate the selectivity and sensitivity of immune cells in the body. Such cells in vivo undertake high-sensitivity immune recognition, and this capability in mast cells was exploited by detection of cell-released mediators (Page & Pizziconi, 1997).

## 8.11. NANOBIOSENSORS

### 8.11.1. HOLLOW CAPSULES

Nanosensing is an area of advanced research combining nanotechnology and biology. It opens up new areas and possibilities for detecting and manipulating atoms and molecules at the subcellular level. Measurements can be taken of intracellular environments as well as of molecular signaling processes in specific locations of the cell. Recent research has led, for example, to nanoscale spherical biosensors based on liposomes (Vamvakaki, Fournier, & Chaniotakis, 2005), in which an enzyme can be encapsulated in a stabilized microenvironment of the liposome, providing some defense against denaturation due to extreme conditions and to dilution effects. A coincorporated fluorescent pH indicator (see Fig. 8.13) was able to follow a hydrolytic internal enzyme reaction. Initially enzyme was introduced by repeatedly freezing and thawing liposomes. The liposome wall incorporated porin molecules to enable entry of low molecular weight substrate, while the large enzyme molecules remain entrapped. Small fluorescent indicator molecules were readily introduced for monitoring the reaction. The liposomal "package" has been extensively investigated for targeted drug therapy and controlled drug release, but

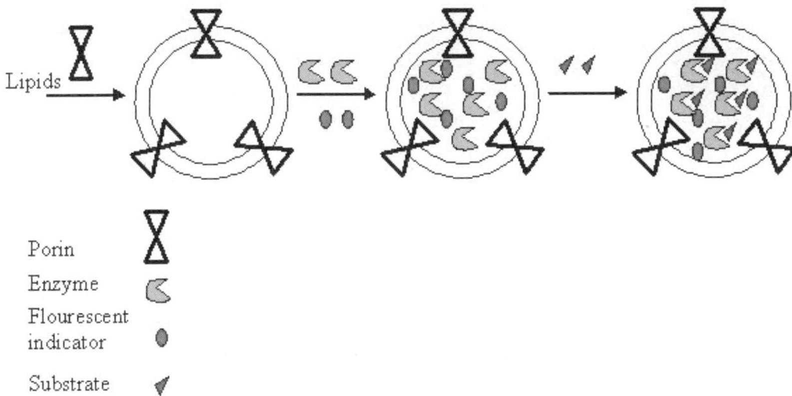



**Figure 8.13.** Schematic of the liposome biosensor design. Adapted from Vamvakaki, V., Fournier, D., & Chaniotakis, N. A., 2005, "Fluorescence Detection of Enzymatic Activity Within a Liposome-based Nano-biosensor," *Biosensors and Bioelectronics, 21*(2), pp. 384–388, with permission.

could also lead to new in vivo monitoring strategies. Other polymer encapsulants are also likely to emerge with advances in biocompatible film technology.

## 8.11.2. SOLID PARTICULATES

Zhou et al. (2005) enhanced the catalytic electrode surface of an amperometric glucose biosensor by dispersing platinum microparticles within a conducting nanofibrous polyaniline. The conducting property of the nanofibers allowed for effective $H_2O_2$ oxidation from the enzyme reaction by the platinum particles. Response to glucose was linear in the range $2 \times 10^{-6}$ M to $12 \times 10^{-3}$ M and was fast (7 s). In another study, Basu et al. (2004) developed a nanobiosensor for bacterial detection to diagnose human urinary tract infection. This condition is caused by *Escherichia coli* bacteria, with one aggressive variant being capable of producing a toxin-causing hemolytic uremic syndrome (HUS). Nanowires with gold surfaces were used to immobilize antibacterial antibody, and after target bacteria had been bound, alkaline phosphatase-conjugated second antibody was added, with the level of enzyme activity monitored by electrochemical and optical techniques. The work served to show how a nanosurface could increase biomolecule loading for more sensitive assays. Colloidal gold has been used to increase the surface area of a gold working electrode for electrochemical analysis (Cai et al., 2001). Here, an enhanced quantity of DNA was immobilized on the gold, lowering the detection limit for the target sequence. Solid spheres, based on polymeric materials, are being actively researched and may allow more versatile, distributed in vivo monitoring, or parallel processing if used in combination with dense detector arrays (Epstein et al., 2002).

## 8.12. BIOFOULING

### 8.12.1. EFFECT ON PERFORMANCE

Biosensors generally operate at a "macro" scale, and have been exploited for clinical use (Hall, 1991), particularly in point of care testing (POCT) and for continuous monitoring. As direct-contact devices, they need to be able to interface reliably with complex biological samples. While the bulk amounts of protein, colloid, and cells that transfer to a nearly exposed biosensor surface in a biomatrix are low in amount, the tissue masking and barrier effect on the device is the main cause of signal drift. In particular, where continued analyte flux is needed for a response, as is the case for enzyme electrodes, an immediate reduction in the response of the biosensor is evident (Gargiuli et al., 2005). Because of this, accuracy and precision in measurement are both lost. The transducer is not directly altered by these colloidal deposits, but there is a very strong influence from the external presence of nonspecific adherent elements. In the case of crystalloids that are surface active, however, diffusion to internal components is possible, and these can passivate the transducer functional elements. Thus free amino acids or thiol-containing molecules may be surface active and can modify a platinum or carbon working electrode of an electrochemical biosensor so that its surface activity is depressed and sensitivity distorted, notably when used with redox-dependent biosensors. Devices that are less affected are those where a true binding equilibrium is approached (e.g., antibodies, lectins, receptors, DNA/RNA). Here, response time may be extended, with less influence on the final equilibrium signal, unless there is masking of binding sites at the molecular scale.

## 8.12.2. BIOLOGICAL FACTORS

Biofouling occurs when the body reacts to a foreign object in contact with tissue or blood. This foreign body reaction is mediated by macrophages, fibroblasts, and capillaries to varying degrees, depending on the size, form, and topography of the foreign body. Eventually a fibrous capsule surrounds the biomaterial (fibrosis), isolating it from the local tissue environment (Gargiuli et al., 2005). For biosensors to function correctly, they need to be in intimate contact with the relevant sample compartment (e.g., blood). This makes them highly vulnerable to surface active agents, cells, and proteins designed to reject foreign material. As the sensor undergoes the biofouling process, there will be a reduction in both its steady-state and dynamic response. The various active redox components, polymeric packaging materials, metals, and conducting carbon of sensors all influence the precise characteristics of the reactive process in the body. If electrodes are implanted in tissue they cause a local inflammatory response, and if in contact with blood, thrombosis and embolism may result. Even when a biosensor material is "bio-inert" it will cause the same reaction as a foreign body. Essentially all materials are considered to provoke some response from the body, whether they have inherent reactive chemical properties or not. The overall effect on the performance of the sensor, however, is unpredictable, and herein lies the dilemma for successful deployment. In complex biosensors there may be leachable components, which can have significant local effects (Fischer et al., 1996). An example is the release of protein, which can act as an immunogenic trigger, especially if the biosensor is to be implanted repeatedly. A biosensor may present a biohazard, thus BSA, used in the past to cross link enzymes (Ahmed et al., 2004), is now no longer acceptable for in vivo use, given the dangers presented by possible contamination with bovine spongiform encephalitis (BSE) agent. Because of these problems, some current researchers are working on improving material properties in an attempt to produce new material compositions and new biological components that will pose fewer latent hazards.

In the case of biosensors for whole blood, stability has been improved by the inclusion of anticoagulant. In one study (Wang et al., 2000), electropolymerized films containing enzyme (GOD) and heparin on metal electrode transducers were used. Here, films from nonconducting poly(1,2-phenylenediamine) (PPD) were used to coentrap the enzyme. This method greatly improved the performance of the sensor after whole blood exposure, and platelet deposits and the formation of fibrin clots were avoided.

### *8.12.3. OPEN MICROFLOW*

Open microflow is a fluid injection system for tissue where a flowing liquid interface is formed between the sensor surface and the tissue sample matrix. This provides a continuously regenerating fluid filter and barrier that reduces cell or protein access to the sensor surface, thus reducing surface fouling (Rigby, Crump, & Vadgama, 1995). This type of liquid interface in tissue ensures reduced surface contamination and stabilizes biosensor interfacial contact. When used in vitro, there was retention of the electrode output to within 3% of the original glucose response and a tenfold reduction in baseline drift in the presence of blood over periods of 2 hours to 3 hours. When used in vivo, better tissue contact through tissue hydration eliminated any tissue versus blood differences; changes in glucose could also be registered more quickly. Whether improved performance through a liquid interface can have benefits during long-term implantation remains to be verified.

## 8.13. CONCLUSIONS

Although initiated as a basis for simplified measurement of complex parameters, biosensors have turned out to be a remarkable kaleidoscope of interfacial properties and challenges for practical utilization. The practical issues as yet defy ready transfer to widespread applied measurement. However, the armory of transducers, biomolecules, and formatting techniques, including MEMS, is continuing to expand, and it is likely that this will result in viable new systems. The concepts now being embodied extend well beyond the archetypal enzyme-based devices and demonstrate how target molecules might be tackled by a variety of new affinity systems. Cross-comparisons between systems now allow a further basis for optimization, promoting selection of the best combinations of biological and transducer elements. The field will need to address the more consumerist issues of robustness, lifetime, and operational stability, specifically for applied biological fluids. Thus it is likely that biocompatibility and questions concerning biosensor component materials will come to the fore in new research strategies.

## ACKNOWLEDGMENT

The authors are grateful to the EPSRC, DTI, and EU for generous funding during the preparation of this chapter.

## REFERENCES

Ahmed, S., Dack, C., Farace, G., Rigby, G., & Vadgama, P. (2004). Tissue implanted glucose needle electrodes: Early sensor stabilisation and achievement of tissue-blood correlation during the run-in period. *Analytica Chimica Acta, 537*(1–2), 153–161.

Alfonso, B., Armada, P. G., Losada, J., Cuadrado, I., Gonzalez, B., & Casado, C. M. (2004). Amperometric enzyme electrodes for aerobic and anaerobic glucose monitoring prepared by glucose oxidase immobilized in mixed ferrocene-cobaltocenium dendrimers. *Biosensors and Bioelectronics, 19*(12), 1617–1625.

Arnold, M. A., & Meyerhoff, M. E. (1988). Recent advances in the development and analytical applications of biosensing probes. *CRC Critical Reviews in Analytical Chemistry, 20*(3), 149.

Atanasov, P., Yang, S., Salehi, C., Ghindilis, A. L., Wilkins, E., & Schade, D. (1997). Implantation of a refillable glucose monitoring telemetry device. *Biosensors and Bioelectronics, 12*(7), 669–680.

Athey, D., Ball, M., & McNeil, C. J. (1993a). Avidin based electrochemical immunoassay for thyrotrophin. *Annals of Clinical Biochemistry, 30*(6), 570–577.

Athey, D., McNeil, C. J., Bailey, W. R., Hager, H. J., Mullen, W. H., & Russel, L. J. (1993b). Homogeneous ampero-metric immunoassay for theophylline in whole blood. *Biosensors and Bioelectronics, 8*(9–10), 415-419.

Bahl, M. I., Hansen, L. H., Licht, T. R., & Sorensen, S. J. (2004). In vivo detection and quantification of tetracycline by use of a whole-cell biosensor in the rat intestine. *Antimicrobial Agents and Chemotherapy, 48*(4), 1112–1117.

Barton, S. C., Pickard, M., Vazquez-Duhalt, R., & Heller, A. (2002). Electroreduction of $O_2$ to water at 0.6 V (SHE) at pH 7 on the "wired" *Pleurotus ostreatus* laccase cathode. *Biosensors and Bioelectronics, 17*(11–12), 1071–1074.

Basu, M., Seggerson, S., Henshaw, J., Jiang, J., del a Cordona, R., Lefave, C., . . . & Basu, S. (2004). Nano-biosensor development for bacterial detection during human kidney infection: Use of glycoconjugate-specific antibody-bound gold NanoWire arrays (GNWA). *Glycoconjugate Journal, 21*(8–9), 487–496.

Bentley, A., Atkinson, A., Jezek, J., & Rawson, D. M. (2001). Whole cell biosensors—electrochemical and optical approaches to ecotoxicity testing. *Toxicology In Vitro, 15*(4–5), 469–475.

Bossi, A., Castelletti, L., Piletsky, S. A., Turner, A. P. F., & Righetti, P. G. (2003). Towards the development of an inte-grated capillary electrophoresis optical biosensor. *Electrophoresis, 24*(19–20), 3356–3363.

Cai, H., Xu, C., He, P., & Fang, Y. (2001). Colloid Au-enhanced DNA immobilization for the electrochemical detection of sequence-specific DNA. *Journal of Electroanalytical Chemistry, 510*(1–2), 78–85.

Cao, L. (2005). Immobilised enzymes: Science or art? *Current Opinions in Chemical Biology, 9*, 217–226.

Cardosi, M. F., & Turner, A. P. F. (1987). The realisation of electron transfer from biological molecules to electrodes (pp. 257–275). In: A. P. F. Turner, I. Karube, and G. S. Wilson (Eds.), *Biosensors: Fundamentals and applications* Oxford, England: Oxford University Press.

Chopra, I., & Roberts, M. (2001). Tetracycline antibiotics: Mode of action, applications, molecular biology, and epide-miology of bacterial resistance. *Microbiology and Molecular Biology Reviews, 65*(2), 232–260.

Christman, K. L., & Maynard, H. D. (2005). Protein micropatterns using a pH-responsive polymer and light. *Lang-muir, 21*(18), 8389–8393.

Chung, J. W., Kim, S. D., Bernhardt, R., & Pyun, J. C. (2005). Application of SPR biosensor for medical diagnostics of human hepatitis B virus (hHBV). *Sensors and Actuators B:Chemical, 111*(S1), 416–422.

Claremont, D. J., Sambrook, I. E., Penton, C., & Pickup, J. C. (1986). Subcutaneous implantation of a ferrocene medi-ated glucose sensor in pigs. *Diabetologia, 29*(11), 817–821.

Clark, L. C., & Lyons, C. (1962). Electrode systems for continuous monitoring in cardiovascular. *Annals of the New York Academy of Sciences, 102*(1), 29–45.

Collings, A. F., & Caruso, F. (1997). Biosensors: Recent advances. *Reports on Progress in Physics, 60*(11), 1397–1445.

Cooreman, P., Thoelen, R., Manca, J., van de Ven, M., Vermeeren, V., Michiels, L., . . . & Wagner, P. (2005). Impedimet-ric immunosensors based on the conjugated polymer PPV. *Biosensors and Bioelectronics, 20*(10), 2151–2156.

Crouch, E., Cowell, D. C., Hoskins, S., Pittson, R. W., & Hart, J. P. (2005). Amperometric, screen-printed, glucose biosensor for analysis of human plasma samples using a biocomposite water-based carbon ink incorporating glucose oxidase. *Analytical Biochemistry, 347*(1), 17–23.

Davis, F., Nabok, A. V., & Higson, S. P. (2005). Species differentiation by DNA-modified carbon electrodes using an AC impedimetric approach. *Biosensors and Bioelectronics, 20*(8), 1531–1538.

de Jong, L. A. A., Uges, D. R. A., Franke, J. P., & Bischoff, R. (2005). Receptor-ligand binding assays: Technologies and applications. *Journal of Chromatography B: Analytical Technologies in the Biomedical and Life Sciences, 829*(1–2), 1–25.

Della Ciana, L., Bernacca, G., De Nitti, C., & Massaglia, A. (1996). Highly sensitive amperometric immunoassay for α-fetoprotein in human serum. *Journal of Immunological Methods, 193*(1), 51–62.

Desai, T. A., Hansford, D. J., Leoni, L., Essenpreis, M., & Ferrari, M. (2000). Nanoporous anti-fouling silicon mem-branes for biosensor applications. *Biosensors and Bioelectronics, 15*(9–10), 453–462.

Eggenstein, C., Borchardt, M., Diekmann, C., Grundig, B., Dumschat, C., Cammann, K., . . . & Spencer, F. (1999). A disposable biosensor for urea determination in blood based on an ammonium-sensitive transducer. *Biosensors and Bioelectronics, 14*(1), 33–41.

Epstein, J. R., Biran, I., & Walt, D. R. (2002). Fluorescence-based nucleic acid detection and microarrays. *Analytica Chimica Acta, 469*(1), 3–36.

Fischer, U., Bendtson, I., Bolinder, J., Reach, G., & Guy, R. H. (1996). Hypoglycaemia warning on the basis of intra-corporeal glucose monitoring. *Diabetes, Nutrition & Metabolism, 9*(1), 33–50.

Gambhir, A., Gerard, M., Mulchandani, A. K., & Malhotra, B. D. (2001). Coimmobilization of urease and glutamate dehydrogenase in electrochemically prepared polypyrrole-polyvinyl sulfonate films. *Applied Biochemistry and Biotechnology, 96*(1–3), 249–257.

Gargiuli, J., Gill, A., Schoenleber, M., Pearson, J., & Vadgama, P. (2005). Stable use of biosensors at the sample interface (Vol. 5, pp. 103–149). In: P. Vadgama (Ed.), *Surfaces and interfaces for biomaterials.* Cambridge, England: Woodhead.

Geiger, E., Hug, P., & Keller, B. A. (2002). Chromatic transitions in polydiacetylene Langmuir-Blodgett films due to molecular recognition at the film surface studied by spectroscopic methods and surface analysis. *Macromolecular Chemistry and Physics, 203*(17), 2422–2431.

Gosling, J. P. (1990). A decade of development in immunoassay methodology. *Clinical Chemistry, 36*(8), 1408–1425.

Gough, D. A., & Lucisano, J. Y., & Tse, P. H. S. (1985). Two dimensional enzyme electrode sensor for glucose. *Analytical Chemistry, 57*(12), 2351–2357.

Hall, E. A. H. (1991). *Biosensors* (North American ed.). Englewood Cliffs, NJ: Prentice-Hall.

Haron, S., & Ray, A. K. (2006). Optical biodetection of cadmium and lead ions in water. *Medical Engineering & Physics, 28*(10), 978–981.

Holt, P. J., Stephans, L. D. G., Bruce, N. C., & Lowe, C. R. (1995). An amperometric opiate assay. *Biosensors and Bioelectronics, 10*(6–7), 517–526.

Hou, Q., Freeman, R., Buttery, L. D., & Shakesheff, K. M. (2005). Novel surface entrapment process for the incorporation of bioactive molecules within preformed alginate fibers. *Biomacromolecules, 6*(2), 734–740.

Junhui, Z., Hong, C., & Ruifu, Y. (1997). DNA based biosensors. *Biotechnology Advances, 15*(1), 43–58.

Karacaoglu, S., Timur, S., & Telefoncu, A. (2003). Arginine selective biosensor based on arginase-urease immobilized in gelatin. *Artificial Cells, Blood Substitutes and Immobilization Biotechnology, 31*(3), 357–363.

Karakus, E., Pekyardimci, S., & Esma, K. (2005). Urea biosensors based on PVC membrane containing palmitic acid. *Artificial Cells, Blood Substitutes and Immobilizaton Biotechnology, 33*(3), 329–341.

Kauffmann, J. M., & Guilbault, G. G. (1991). Potentiometric enzyme electrodes. *Bioprocess Technology, 15*, 63–82.

Kaun, S. S., & Guilbault, G. G. (1987). Ion selective electrodes and biosensors based on ISEs (pp. 135–152). In: A. P. F. Turner, I. Karube, & G. S. Wilson (Eds.), *Biosensors: Fundamentals and applications.* Oxford, England: Oxford University Press.

Klibanov, A. M. (1979). Enzyme stabilisation by immobilisation. *Analytical Biochemistry, 93*(1), 1–25.

Koncki, R., Walcerz, I., & Leszczynska, E. (1999). Enzymatically modified ion-selective electrodes for flow injection analysis. *Journal of Pharmaceutical and Biomedical Analysis, 19*(3–4), 633–638.

Kress-Rogers, K. (1997). Biosensors and electronic noses for practical applications (pp. 3–39). In: K. Kress-Rogers (Ed.), *Handbook of biosensors and electronic noses.* Boca Raton, FL: CRC Press.

Kretschmann, E. (1971). Determination of optical constants of metals by excitation of surface plasmons. *Zeitschrift für Physik, 241*(4), 313–324.

Kumar, A. (2000). Biosensors based on piezoelectric crystal detectors: Theory and application. *Journal of the Minerals, Metals and Materials Society (Electronic Supplement), 52*(10). http://www.tms.org/pubs/journals/JOM/0010/Kumar/Kumar-0010.html

Lakard, B., Herlem, G., Lakard, S., Antoniou, A., & Fahys, B. (2004). Urea potentiometric biosensor based on modified electrodes with urease immobilized on polyethylenimine films. *Biosensors and Bioelectronics, 19*(12), 1641–1647.

Le Guillou-Buffello, D., Helary, G., Gindre, M., Pavon-Djavid, G., Laugier, P., & Migonney, V. (2005). Monitoring cell adhesion processes on bioactive polymers with the quartz crystal resonator technique. *Biomaterials, 26*(19), 4197–4205.

Lee, J. H., Hwang, K. S., Park, J., Yoon, K. H., Yoon, D. S., & Kim, T. S. (2005). Immunoassay of prostate-specific antigen (PSA) using resonant frequency shift of piezoelectric nanomechanical microcantilever. *Biosensors and Bioelectronics, 20*(10), 2157–2162.

Lin, H. C., & Tsai, W. C. (2003). Piezoelectric crystal immunosensor for the detection of staphylococcal enterotoxin B. *Biosensors and Bioelectronics, 18*(12), 1479–1483.

Liu, B. H., Hu, R. Q., & Deng, J. Q. (1997). Characterization of immobilisation of an enzyme in a modified Y zeolite matrix and its application to an amperometric glucose biosensor. *Analytical Chemistry, 69*(13), 2342–2348.

Lucarelli, F., Marrazza, G., & Mascini, M. (2005). Enzyme-based impedimetric detection of PCR products using oligonucleotide-modified screen-printed gold electrodes. *Biosensors and Bioelectronics, 20*(10), 2001–2009.

Luo, X. L., Xu, J. J., Zhao, W., & Chen, H. Y. (2004). A novel glucose ENFET based on the special reactivity of $MnO_2$ nanoparticles. *Biosensors and Bioelectronics, 19*(10), 1295–1300.

Luong, J. H. T., & Guilbault, G. G. (1991). Analytical applications of piezoelectric crystal biosensors (pp. 107–138). In: L. J. Blum & P. R. Coulet (Eds.), *Biosensor principles and applications.* New York, NY: Marcel Dekker.

Magalhaes, J. M., & Machado, A. A. (2002). Array of potentiometric sensors for the analysis of creatinine in urine samples. *Analyst, 127*(8), 1069–1075.

May, K. M., Wang, Y., Bachas, L. G., & Anderson, K. W. (2004). Development of a whole-cell-based biosensor for detecting histamine as a model toxin. *Analytical Chemistry, 76*(14), 4156–4161.

Muramatsu, H., Dicks, J. M., Tamiya, E., & Karube, I. (1987). Piezoelectric crystal biosensor modified with protein A for determination of immunoglobulins. *Analytical Chemistry, 59*(23), 2760–2763.

Nabok, A. V., Haron, S., & Ray, A. K. (2003). Planar silicon nitride waveguides for biosensing. *IEEE Proceedings Nanobiotechnology, 150*(1), 25–30.

Naimushin, A. N., Soelberg, S. D., Nguyen, D. K., Dunlap, L., Bartholomew, D., Elkind, J., . . . & Furlong, C. E. (2002). Detection of *Staphylococcus aureus* enterotoxin B at femtomolar levels with a miniature integrated two-channel surface plasmon resonance (SPR) sensor. *Biosensors and Bioelectronics, 17*(6–7), 573–584.

Oh, B. K., Kim, Y. K., Park, K. W., Lee, W. H., & Choi, J. W. (2004). Surface plasmon resonance immunosensor for the detection of *Salmonella typhimurium. Biosensors and Bioelectronics, 19*(11), 1497–1504.

Ouerghi, O., Touhami, A., Jaffrezic-Renault, N., Martelet, C., Ouada, H. B., & Cosnier, S. (2002). Impedimetric immunosensor using avidin-biotin for antibody immobilization. *Bioelectrochemistry, 56*(1–2), 131–133.

Page, D. L., & Pizziconi, V. B. (1997). A cell-based immunobiosensor with engineered molecular recognition. Part II: Enzyme amplification systems. *Biosensors and Bioelectronics, 12*(6), 457–466.

Paitan, Y., Biran, I., Shechter, N., Biran, D., Rishpon, J., & Ron, E. Z. (2004). Monitoring aromatic hydrocarbons by whole cell electrochemical biosensors. *Analytical Biochemistry, 335*(2), 175–183.

Pandey, P. C., Upadhyay, S., & Upadhyay, B. (1997). Peroxide biosensors and mediated electrochemical regeneration of redox enzymes. *Analytical Biochemistry, 252*(1), 136–142.

Pearson, J. E., Gill, A., & Vadgama, P. (2000). Analytical aspects of biosensors. *Annals of Clinical Biochemistry, 37*(2), 119–145.

Plowman, T. E., Durstchi, J. D., Wang, H. K., Christensen, D. A., Herron, J. N., & Reichert, W. M. (1999). Multiple-analyte fluoroimmunoassay using an integrated optical waveguide sensor. *Analytical Chemistry, 71*(19), 4344–4352.

Plowman, T. E., Garrison, M. D., Walker, D. S., & Reichert, W. M. (1994). Surface sensitivity of SION integrated optical wave-guides (IOWs) examined by IOW attenuated total-reflection spectrometry and IOW Raman-spectroscopy. *Thin Solid Films, 243*(1–2), 610–615.

Rajesh, B. V., Takashima, W., & Kaneto, K. (2005). An amperometric urea biosensor based on covalent immobilization of urease onto an electrochemically prepared copolymer poly (N-3-aminopropyl pyrrole-co-pyrrole) film. *Biomaterials, 26*(17), 3683–3690.

Rauf, S., Ihsan, A., Akhtar, K., Ghauri, M. A., Rahman, M., Anwar, M. A., & Khalid, A. M. (2005). Glucose oxidase immobilization on a novel cellulose acetate-polymethylmethacrylate membrane. *Journal of Biotechnology, 121*(3), 351–360.

Rigby, G. P., Crump, P., & Vadgama, P. (1995). Open flow microperfusion approach to in vivo glucose monitoring. *Medical & Biological Engineering & Computing, 33*(2), 231–234.

Rodriguez-Mozaz, S., Maria-Pilar Marco, M. P., Lopez de Alda, M. J., & Barceló, D. (2004). Biosensors for environmental monitoring of endocrine disruptors: A review article. *Analytical and Bioanalytical Chemistry, 378*(3), 588–598.

Sauerbrey, G. (1959). The use of quartz oscillators for weighing thin layers and for microweighing. *Zeitschrift fuer Physik, 155*(2), 206–222.

Schmid, B., Matzler, C., Heimo, A., & Kampfer, N. (1997). Retrieval of optical depth and particle size distribution of tropospheric and stratospheric aerosols by means of sun photometry. *IEEE Transactions in Geoscience and Remote Sensing, 35*(1), 172–182.

Schumacher, J. T., Mersal, G. A. M., & Bilitewski, U. (2005). Immobilisation of enzymes. In: A. Pandey, C. Webb, C. R. Soccol, & C. Larroche (Eds.), *Enzyme technology* (pp. 549–578). New Delhi, India: Asiatech.

Skladal, P., dos Santos Riccardi, C., Yamanaka, H., & da Costa, P. I. (2004). Piezoelectric biosensors for real-time monitoring of hybridization and detection of hepatitis C virus. *Journal of Virological Methods, 117*(2), 145–151.

Skladal, P., Jilkova, Z., Svoboda, I., & Kolar, V. (2005). Investigation of osteoprotegerin interactions with ligands and antibodies using piezoelectric biosensors. *Biosensors and Bioelectronics, 20*(10), 2027–2034.

Srivastava, R., Brown, J. Q., Zhu, H., & McShane, M. J. (2005). Stabilization of glucose oxidase in alginate microspheres with photoreactive diazoresin nanofilm coatings. *Biotechnology & Bioengineering, 91*(1), 124–131.

Stranik, O., McEvoy, H. M., McDonagh, C., & MacCraith, B. D. (2005). Plasmonic enhancement of fluorescence for sensor applications. *Sensors and Actuators B: Chemical, 107*(1), 148–153.

Stryer, L. (1995). *Biochemistry* (vol. 8, 4th ed., pp. 181–233). New York, NY: W H Freeman.

Subramanian, A., Irudayaraj, J., & Ryan, T. (2006). Mono and dithiol surfaces on surface plasmon resonance biosensors for detection of *Staphylococcus aureus*. *Sensors and Actuators B: Chemical, 114*(1), 192–198.

Tombelli, S., Minunni, M., & Mascini, M. (2005). Piezoelectric biosensors: Strategies for coupling nucleic acids to piezoelectric devices. *Methods, 37*(1), 48–56.

Treloar, P. H., Kane, J. W., & Vadgama, P. M. (1997). Electrochemical immunoassays (pp. 481–509). In: C. P. Price & D. J. Newman (Eds.), *Principles and practice of immunoassays* (2nd ed.). New York, NY: Stockton Press.

Updike, S. J., & Hicks, G. P. (1967). The enzyme electrode. *Nature, 214*(5092), 986.

Vamvakaki, V., Fournier, D., & Chaniotakis, N. A. (2005). Fluorescence detection of enzymatic activity within a liposome based nano-biosensor. *Biosensors and Bioelectronics, 21*(2), 384–388.

Wang, J., Chen, L., Hocevar, S. B., & Ogorevc, B. (2000). One-step electropolymeric co-immobilization of glucose oxidase and heparin for amperometric biosensing of glucose. *Analyst, 125*(8), 1431–1434.

Wang, S., Ramirez, J., Wang, P. G., & Leblanc, R. M. (1999). Surface chemistry, topography, and spectroscopy of a mixed monolayer of 10,12-pentacosadiynoic acid and its mannoside derivative at the air-water interface. *Langmuir, 15*(17), 5623–5629.

Wang, Z. X., Li, S. Y., Zhong, L. C., & Li, G. X. (1990). Research and application of enzyme FET sensitive to penicillin. *Chinese Journal of Biotechnology, 6*(2), 149–156.

White, S. F., & Turner, A. P. F. (1997). Enzymes cofactors and mediators (pp. 43–58). In: K. Kress-Rogers (Ed.), *Handbook of biosensors and electronic noses*. Boca Raton, FL: CRC Press.

Witt, S., Wohlfahrt, G., Schomburg, D., Hecht, H.-J., & Kalisz, H. M. (2000). Conserved arginine-516 of *Penicillium amagasakiense* glucose oxidase is essential for the efficient binding of b-D-glucose. *Biochemical Journal, 347*(2), 553–559.

Xu, F., Persson, B., Lofas, S., & Knoll, W. (2006). Surface plasmon optical studies of carboxymethyl dextran brushes versus networks. *Langmuir, 22*(7), 3352–3357.

Ye, J. M., Letcher, S. V., & Rand, A. G. (1997). Piezoelectric biosensor for detection of *Salmonella typhimurium*. *Journal of Food Science, 62*(5), 1067–1073.

Yokoyama, K., Ikebukuro, K., Tamiya, E., Karube, I., Ichiki, N., & Arikawa, Y. (1995). Highly sensitive quartz crystal immunosensors for multisampling detection of herbicides. *Analytica Chimica Acta, 304*(2), 139–145.

Zhang, Y., & Heller, A. (2005). Reduction of the nonspecific binding of a target antibody and of its enzyme-labeled detection probe enabling electrochemical immunoassay of an antibody through the 7 pg/mL–100 ng/mL (40 fM–400 pM) range. *Analytical Chemistry, 77*(23), 7758–7762.

Zhang, Y., & Tadigadapa, S. (2004). Calorimetric biosensors with integrated microfluidic channels. *Biosensors and Bioelectronics, 19*(12), 1733–1743.

Zhou, H., Chen, H., Luo, S., Chen, J., Wei, W., & Kuang, Y. (2005). Glucose biosensor based on platinum microparticles dispersed in nano-fibrous polyaniline. *Biosensors and Bioelectronics, 20*(7), 1305–1311.

Zhou, L., Wang, K., Choi, M. F., Xiao, D., Yang, X., Chen, R., & Tan, W. (2004). A fibre-optic mode-filtered light sensor for general and fast chemical assay. *Measurement Science and Technology, 15*(1), 137–142.

Zuo, B., Li, S., Guo, Z., Zhang, J., & Chen, C. (2004). Piezoelectric immunosensor for SARS-associated coronavirus in sputum. *Analytical Chemistry, 76*(13), 3536–3540.

## ABOUT THE AUTHORS

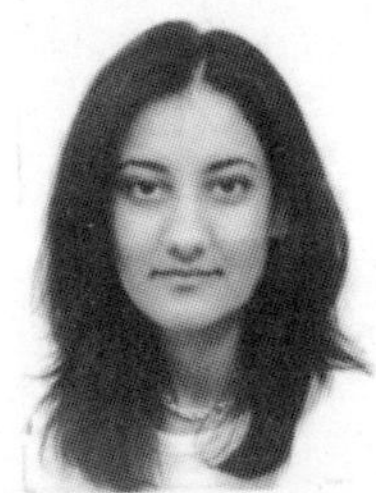

**Jaina Negandhi** graduated with a BSc in biomedical materials science from the University of Manchester, United Kingdom, with First Class Honors. She has been working on the development of permselective and biocompatible membranes for microbioreactors and in microfluidic systems for polymer membrane fabrication. Her goal has been to establish viable reactor systems for nerve cell lines incorporating controlled, dual flow circuits with continuous monitoring of lactate output.

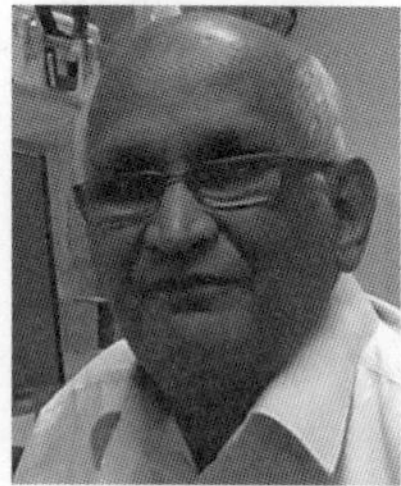

**Professor Asim K. Ray**, BSc, MSc, PhD, DSc is a chartered engineer and chartered physicist. He is a Fellow of the Institution of Engineering and Technology (UK) and the Institute of Physics (UK). He leads a research group of three postdoctoral fellows, two visiting fellows, and two PhD students. He holds the Chair of Functional Materials at Queen Mary University of London. His specific research interests lie in thin-film technologies for the fabrication of nanostructures and chemical and biosensors. He is a college member of the Engineering and Physical Science Research Council (UK). He is editor-in-chief of the journal *IET–Circuits, Devices & Systems*.

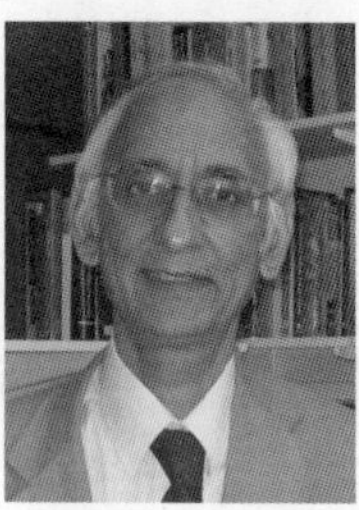

**Professor Pankaj Vadgama** is currently director of the Interdisciplinary Research Centre (IRC) in Biomedical Materials, Queen Mary University of London, and professor of clinical biochemistry at Queen Mary's School of Medicine and Dentistry at the University of London. He has developed permselective, biocompatible, and biomimetic polymeric membranes for stable transduction in whole blood and tissue. Both in vivo and in vitro work has been undertaken, including the use of miniaturized devices for glucose and lactate monitoring.

# CHAPTER 9

# Sensors for Medical Thermography and Infrared Radiation Measurements

E. F. J. Ring,* R. A. Thomas,[†] and K. J. Howell[‡]

*Medical Imaging Research Unit, Faculty of Advanced Technology
University of Glamorgan, Pontypridd, UK

[†]Faculty of Applied Design and Engineering
Swansea Metropolitan University, Swansea, UK

[‡]Centre for Rheumatology
Royal Free & University College Medical School, Hampstead Campus, London, UK

## 9.1. BACKGROUND

The living human body is warm, usually warmer than the environment, and techniques for imaging body temperature now play a useful role in modern science. Convection currents of heat emitted by the human body have been imaged by a technique called Schlieren photography, in which the change in refractive index with density in the air around the body is made visible by special illumination (Ring, 1995). This method has been used to monitor heat loss in experimental subjects, especially in the design of protective clothing for people working in extreme physical environments.

Heat transfer by radiation is of greater value in medicine. The human body surface requires variable degrees of heat exchange with the environment as part of the normal thermoregulatory process (Houdas & Ring, 1982). Most of this heat transfer occurs in the infrared (IR) spectrum, which can be imaged by electronic thermal imaging. IR radiation was undefined before 1800, when Sir William Herschel performed his famous experiment to measure heat beyond the visible spectrum. Nearly 200 years before, Italian observers noted the presence of reflected heat. John Della Porta, in 1698, observed that when a candle was lit and placed before a large silver bowl in church, he could sense the heat on his face. When he altered the positions of the candle, bowl, or his face, the heat was no longer experienced.

William Herschel, in a series of careful experiments, showed that not only was there a "dark heat" present, but that heat itself behaved like light—it could be reflected and refracted under the right conditions. William's only son John Herschel repeated some experiments after his father's death and successfully made an image using solar radiation. This he called a thermogram, a term still in use today to describe an image made by thermal radiation (Fig. 9.1). John Herschel's thermogram was made by focusing solar radiation with a lens onto a suspension of carbon particles in alcohol. This process is known as evaporography (Ring, 2000).

A major development came in the early 1940s with the first electronic sensor for IR radiation. This was made from indium antimonide (InSb), and was mounted at the base of a small dewar (vacuum) vessel to allow cooling with liquid nitrogen. The first medical images taken with a British prototype system, the "Pyroscan," were made at Middlesex Hospital in London and the Royal National Hospital for Rheumatic Diseases in Bath in 1959 to 1961. By modern standards these thermograms were very crude. A mark II Pyroscan was made for medical use in 1962, with improved images. However, the mechanical scanning was slow and each image needed from 2 minutes to 5 minutes to record. The final picture was written line by line on electrosensitive paper. During this time, the potential for thermal imaging in medicine was being explored by an increasing number of researchers. Earlier work by the American physiologist J. Hardy (1934) had shown that human skin, regardless of color, is a highly efficient radiator, with an emissivity of 0.98, close to that of a perfect blackbody (1.0). Cancer detection was a high-priority subject. With hopes that this new technique would be a screening tool for breast cancer, many centers across Europe, the United States, and Japan became involved. A British surgeon, K. Lloyd Williams (1969), showed that many tumors are hot, and the hotter the tumor, the poorer the prognosis. By this time, images were displayed on a cathode ray screen in black and white. Image processing by computer had not arrived, so there was much discussion about schemes to subjectively score the images and to look for hot spots and asymmetry of temperature in the breast. This

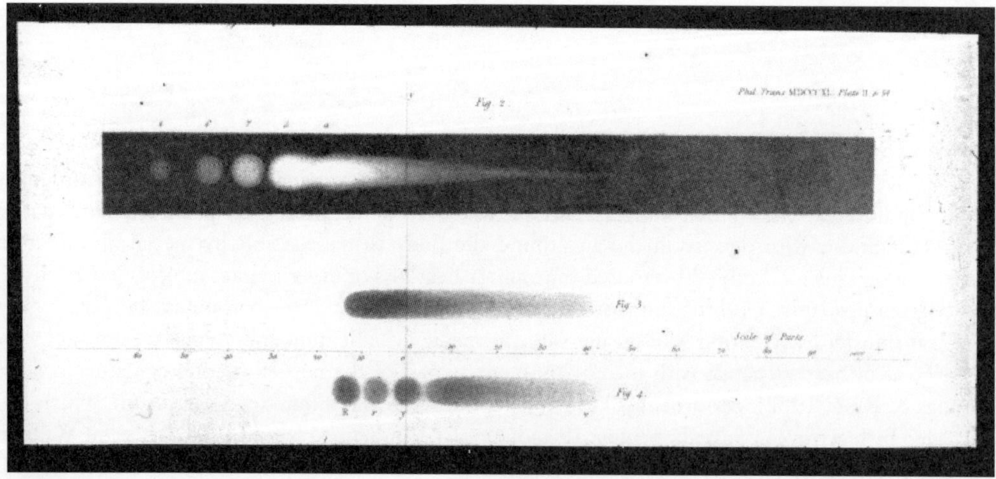

**Figure 9.1.** A solar evaporagram, called a thermogram by Sir John Herschel in 1840.

was confounded by changes in the breast during the menstrual cycle in younger women. The use of false-color thermograms was only possible with photography at this time. A series of bright isotherms were manually ranged across the temperature span of the image, each being exposed through a different color filter, and superimposed on a single frame of film.

By the mid-1970s the first computer systems offered basic image processing. With computerization, many problems associated with thermal imaging of the human body began to be resolved. The images could be archived in digital form, standard regions of interest could be selected, and temperature measurements could be obtained from the images. Manufacturers of thermal imaging equipment slowly adapted to the call for quantification, and some supplied thermal radiation calibration sources to aid in the standardization of techniques. Medical workshops on thermal imaging, which started in the late 1960s, became a regular feature, and in Europe, a major conference was held in Amsterdam in 1974 on the physiological and medical applications of IR imaging. Standardization groups were also formed to determine guidelines for good practice. These included requirements for patient preparation, conditions for thermal imaging, and criteria for the use of thermal imaging in medicine and pharmacology (Engel, Cosh, Ring, Page-Thomas, & Van Waes, 1979; Ring, Engel, & Page-Thomas, 1984).

Infrared imaging has many useful applications in medicine. In rheumatic diseases it can be used as an objective measure of inflammation and as a means of determining the effectiveness of anti-inflammatory treatments (Bacon, Ring, & Collins, 1977). Changes in blood perfusion, especially in the hands and feet, often result in an increase or decrease in skin temperature. One example is Raynaud's phenomenon, where fingers undergo color changes and cold extremities can occur regardless of the surrounding temperature. Tests based on a thermal challenge with cold water immersion are used as a means of quantifying the severity of this condition (see Fig. 9.2). Skin diseases (Fig. 9.3), nerve injuries where circulation is affected, and injuries from industry and sport have all been investigated with the help of IR imaging. Recently, following the severe acute respiratory syndrome (SARS) outbreak in

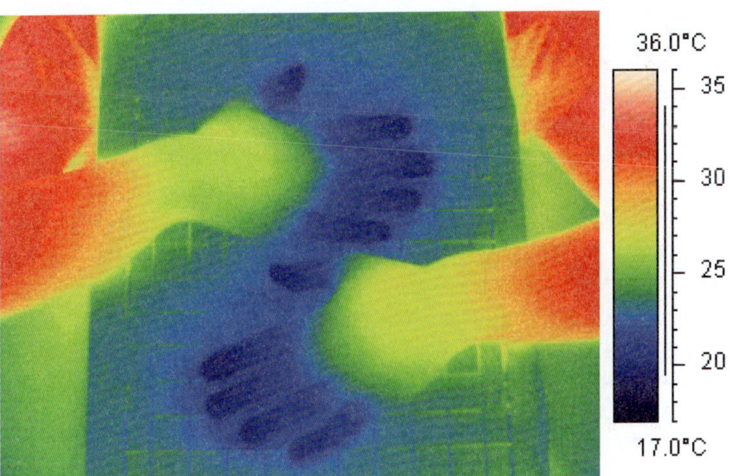


**Figure 9.2.** Hands of a Raynaud's phenomenon patient 10 minutes after cold challenge in water at 15°C for 1 minute, demonstrating delayed rewarming of the fingers (FLIR SC500, 320 pixel × 240 pixel FPA microbolometer detector, 7.5 μm to 13 μm).

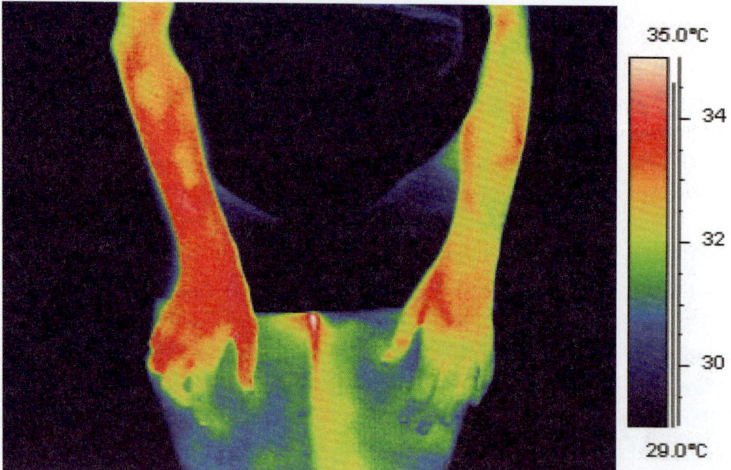



**Figure 9.3.** The inflammatory skin condition morphea, extending along the right forearm and hand (FLIR SC500; from Sampaio et al., 2006).

Southeast Asia, there has been fresh interest in its potential for screening traveling passengers for fever now that high-resolution systems at lower cost are available. Continuous imaging with uncooled detector systems is now providing better stability and accuracy than has been previously available.

Improvements in thermal imaging cameras have had a major impact, both on image quality and speed of image capture. Early single-element detectors were dependent on optical mechanical scanning. Image resolution, both spatial and thermal, was inversely dependent on scanning speed. Some earlier single-element systems in the 1960s, such as the Bofors and some American imagers, operated at a scanning rate of 1 frames $s^{-1}$ to 4 frames $s^{-1}$. AGA cameras were introduced at that time, scanning at 16 frames $s^{-1}$ and using interlacing to smooth the image. Multielement arrays were developed in the United Kingdom and were tested in thermal cameras in the 1970s (e.g., EMI and the Rank Organization). Alignment of the elements was critical, and a poorly aligned array produced characteristic banding in the image. The first significant detector for faster high-resolution images was produced by Elliott (1981), subsequently becoming known as the "signal processing in the element" ("Sprite") detector. This detector was used in the Rank Taylor Hobson high-resolution system called "Talytherm." This camera also had a high-specification IR zoom lens with a macro attachment. Superb images of sweat pore function, eyes with contact lenses, and skin pathology were recorded with this system (see Fig. 9.4). Only a few of these systems were produced.

From the multielement arrays came the first focal plane array (FPA) detectors, with increased numbers of pixels and elements yielding high resolution at video frame rates. Uncooled bolometer arrays have also been shown to be adequate for many medical applications. Without the need for electronic cooling systems, these cameras are almost maintenance free.

Good software with enhancement and analysis is now expected in thermal imagers. Many commercial systems use general imaging software, which is primarily designed for industrial users of the technique. A few dedicated medical software packages have been produced, many of which can enhance the images from older cameras (http://www.medimaging.org). As standardization of image capture and analysis becomes more widely accepted, the ability to manage images and, if necessary,

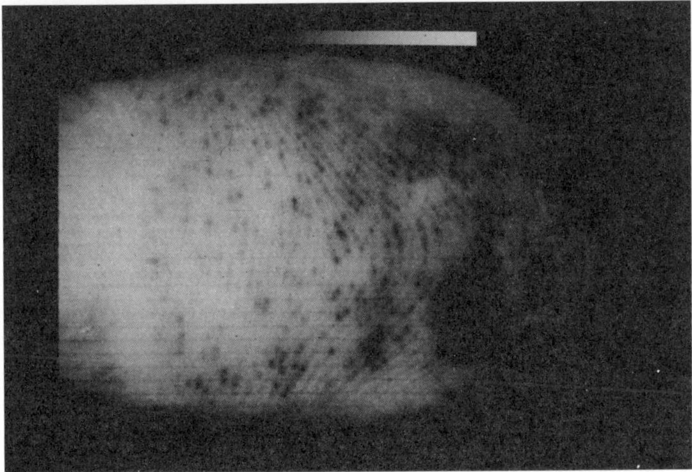

**Figure 9.4.** High-resolution thermogram showing sweat distribution on a finger.

transmit them over an intranet or the Internet has become possible. Future developments will enable the operator of thermal imaging systems to use reference images and reference data as a diagnostic aid. However, this will depend on the level of standardization that can be provided by the manufacturers, and by the operators themselves (Ammer & Ring, 2008; Ring & Ammer, 2000). Modern thermal imaging is already digital and quantifiable, and ready for integration into hospital and clinical computer networks.

## 9.2. INTRODUCTION

Medical interest in the detection of fever can be traced to the earliest records of medical observation. Physicians recognized the importance of a raised temperature in humans long before the arrival of any objective instruments of measurement. For centuries this remained a subjective skill, and the concept of measuring temperature was not developed until the sixteenth century with the advent of Galileo's thermoscope. This used a glass tube filled with a liquid and functioned as an unsealed thermometer, but was subject to influence by atmospheric pressure as a result. Further developments in thermometry led to the nineteenth century pioneering work of Carl Wunderlich (1871), who established the value of monitoring human temperature over time with the clinical thermometer (see Chapter 1 for more details). As has already been described, the ability to image the temperature distribution over an object or the human body is a relatively modern concept that has now become an established tool in medicine, science, and industry.

Since 2008 there has been an increased use of thermal imaging as a means of screening airline passengers for fever, and the International Standards Organization has published a standard and operational guidelines for fever screening: ISO/IEC 80601-2-59, *Medical electrical equipment: Particular requirements for the basic safety and essential performance of screening thermographs for human febrile temperature screening*. There is also a second document: ISO/IEC TR80600, *Medical electronic equipment: Deployment, implementation and operational guidelines for identifying febrile humans using a screening thermograph*. These documents specify the use of radiometric thermal imaging and the appropriate implementation methods required in order to discriminate correctly between passengers or personnel with and without clinical fever.

## 9.3. INFRARED RADIATION

### 9.3.1. THE IR SPECTRUM

In objects at a temperature above absolute zero, –273.16°C (or 0 K), every atom and every molecule vibrates kinetically. According to the laws of electrodynamics, an oscillating electric charge is associated with a variable electric field and an alternating magnetic field. These vibrations produce electromagnetic waves that radiate from the object at the speed of light. The transfer of radiant energy by electromagnetic waves in the thermal range occurs between 0.1 μm and 100 μm, as shown in Figure 9.5.

The optimum wavelength of an IR radiometer is determined by the wavelength distribution of the emitted radiation and the type of detector. Another consideration is the transparency of the atmosphere for the transmission of IR radiation between the object and the radiometer. At particular wavelengths there is a "lack of radiative transparency" within segments of the IR spectrum. There are, for example, high levels of IR transparency between 3.5 μm and 4.1 μm (with poor transmission at 4.2 μm due to carbon dioxide absorption) and between 8 μm and 14 μm (although there is a marked reduction above 12.5 μm), as seen in Figure 9.6.

The IR segment of the electromagnetic spectrum is at wavelengths just beyond the visible spectrum, as shown in Figure 9.7, and can be divided into three more segments by wavelength. These, measured in micrometers, are

- 0.8 μm to 2.0 μm: near IR;
- 2.0 μm to 5.6 μm: middle IR;
- 7.5 μm to 15 μm: far or long-wave IR.

### 9.3.2. NEAR IR

"Near IR" refers to a narrow wavelength range from 0.8 μm to 2.0 μm. Examples of near-IR measurement instruments include spot radiometers, line scanners, and radiometric imagers. Typical

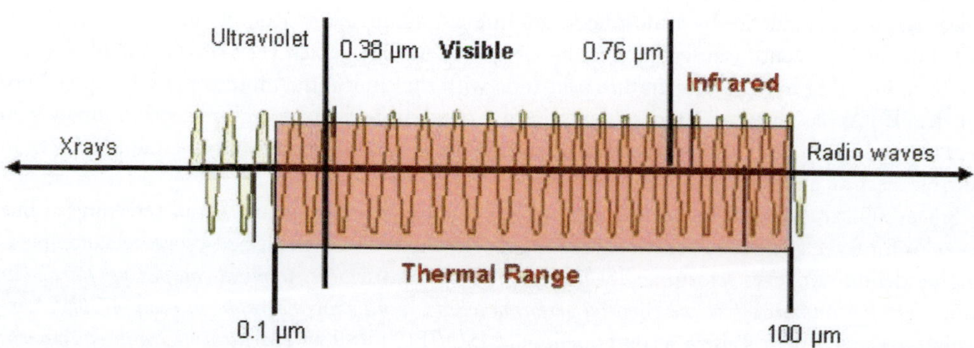


**Figure 9.5.** Thermal range of electromagnetic radiation.

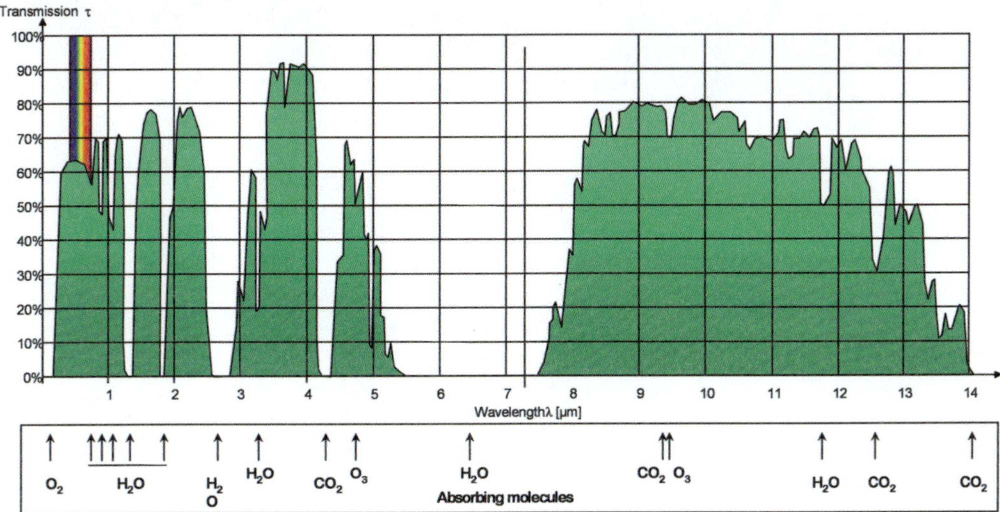



**Figure 9.6.** Propagation of electromagnetic radiation through the atmosphere. Courtesy of FLIR Systems with permission.

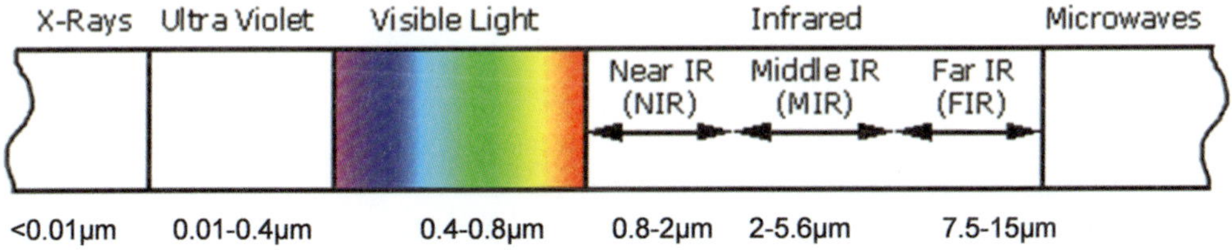



**Figure 9.7.** Infrared segments of the electromagnetic spectrum (average values of wavelength).

applications include night vision surveillance and industrial process monitoring, usually at high temperatures greater than 350°C.

### 9.3.3. MID IR

"Mid IR" refers to a wavelength range from 2 μm to 5.6 μm. The mid IR range is utilized by instruments that are usually cooled, including radiometric imagers in medicine, and line scanners and imagers used in fire and rescue. There is good thermal contrast in the mid wave (image on the right in Fig. 9.8) as compared to an identical object in the long wave (image on the left in Fig. 9.8), especially when measuring human tissue.

Most common detector materials such as InSb, platinum silicide (PtSi), and mercury cadmium telluride (MCT) can be used for these wavelengths.

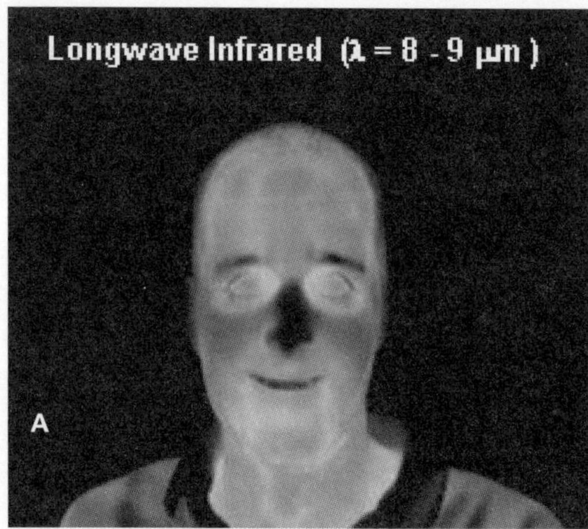


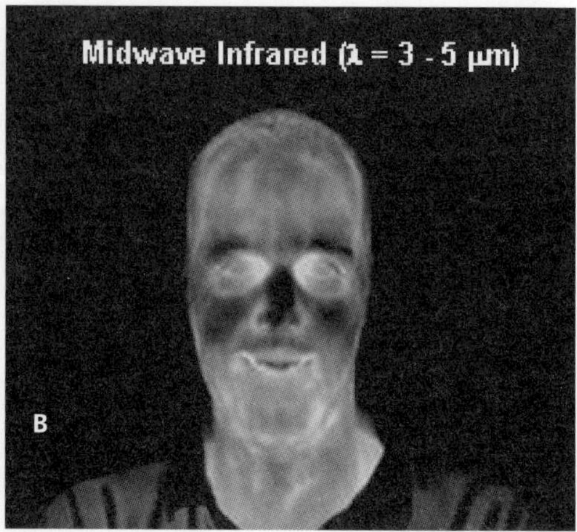


**Figure 9.8.** Infrared camera thermal contrast and wavelength (courtesy of FLIR Systems with permission).

### 9.3.4. FAR IR

"Far IR" refers to a wavelength range from 7.5 µm to 15 µm and represents wavelengths used by a larger group of IR radiometers, usually uncooled, and applied in both biomedical and industrial applications. In contrast with the mid-IR technology used in medicine, far-IR instruments work extremely well at ambient temperatures and when measuring low temperatures up to 100°C. However, these instruments can be more sensitive to emissivity changes and have a wide dynamic range, but with lower thermal contrast. Germanium is typically the lens material.

### 9.3.5. BLACKBODIES AND THE STEFAN–BOLTZMANN LAW

Any object whose temperature is above absolute zero emits radiant energy according to the Stefan–Boltzmann law:

$$\text{Total radiated power, } Q = \sigma \varepsilon A T^4 \text{ [W].} \tag{9.1}$$

This equation gives the radiated power from a real object sometimes known as a gray body (not a blackbody, where the emissivity $\varepsilon$ would be unity and theoretically would have no effect on the radiated value). It is a relationship between the radiated energy (electromagnetic radiation) emission rate $Q$ and the absolute temperature of the body $T$, which is affected by the emissivity (where $\varepsilon$ is less than 1) at the surface of area $A$. The constant $\sigma$ is the Stefan–Boltzmann constant, whose value is $5.67 \times 10^{-8}$ W m$^{-2}$ K$^{-4}$ (see Chapter 5 for the definitions of radiometric quantities). The equation was discovered experimentally by Jožef Stefan (1835–1893) in 1879 and derived theoretically, using thermodynamics, by Ludwig Boltzmann (1844–1906) in 1884.

A blackbody is defined as an object that absorbs all radiation that impinges on it at any wavelength. Kirchoff's law states that any body that is capable of absorbing all radiation is equally capable of the emission of radiation. An example of a blackbody radiator is a lightproof box with a small hole and with the following characteristics:

- Any radiation that enters the hole is scattered and absorbed by continued reflection within the box, resulting in almost no energy escaping.
- The box, when heated, becomes a cavity radiator that radiates energy, the characteristics of which are determined only by the temperature.

## 9.3.6. EMISSION OF RADIATION

The radiant energy absorbed by an object is converted to internal energy $(U)$, which is equivalent to heat flow having taken place, and thus the temperature of the object rises (if no change of state takes place). If there is no conduction or convection or any other energy input, the temperature of the body rises until the rate of radiant emission becomes equal to the rate of absorption. If this does not happen, then the object will continue to absorb radiation and the temperature will rise indefinitely until destruction occurs.

The emissivity $\varepsilon$ quantifies the rate of emission or absorption for different surfaces and is a correction factor that indicates how well an object emits or absorbs radiant energy. This correction factor has values between zero and one. The emissivity of a surface depends on the wavelength of the radiation being emitted (or absorbed). The following equation is an example of the need to consider the background conditions. The power $Q$ is the detected power, and the last term now accounts for the contribution from the reflection of background radiation from an opaque object, where it can be shown that the reflectivity $\rho = (1 - \varepsilon)$:

$$Q = \sigma\varepsilon AT^4_{abs} + \sigma(1 - \varepsilon)AT^4_{Bgrd\text{-}abs}. \tag{9.2}$$

In this equation $T_{abs}$ and $T_{Bgrd\text{-}abs}$ are the absolute temperatures of the body and the background, respectively. A surface whose emissivity is 0.9 at 10 μm may have an emissivity of 0.1 at 100 μm. This is known as a selective surface.

## 9.4. INFRARED CAMERA CHARACTERISTICS

### 9.4.1. DEFINITIONS RELATING TO IR CAMERA PERFORMANCE

*Radiometric accuracy* for an IR camera is defined as the accuracy of the temperature measurement obtained by the radiometric device compared to that of the true undisturbed surface temperature (McIntosh & Thomas, 2009).

*Repeatability* defines the consistency of this accuracy from measurement to measurement.

*Uniformity* is the deviation of a single measurement when measured from different points over the entire field of view (FOV).

*Sensitivity* is the lowest detectable temperature difference on a surface.

When manufacturers state a figure for accuracy, they will often confuse these issues, or at least not define them in a manner that makes it easy to compare instruments. Furthermore, all figures of merit produced by manufacturers are usually defined only for blackbody surfaces, and are usually best-case numbers at a specific absolute temperature (typically 303 K, 30°C, 86°F).

Originally conversion of the camera output signal to a temperature value was not performed within the camera, but externally, using manual calculations involving calibration curves and a calculator. Today the process is the same, but the calibration curve has been programmed into the camera's memory, and calculations to convert the electrical signal to temperature are performed internally by a microprocessor. It is important to understand the conversion process, especially if there is a need to recalculate the temperatures because incorrect values of emissivity, background, or optical transmission were initially used. If new universal analytical software techniques are to be developed independently of specific camera models, then emulation of this process will be essential.

## 9.4.2. INFRARED CAMERAS AND THE STEFAN–BOLTZMANN RELATIONSHIP

There is a widespread belief that IR camera response is a direct function of the Stefan–Boltzmann relationship. This assumption would be correct only if the camera were a 100% efficient energy detector over an extremely wide band of wavelengths, and no spectral modification of the signal by the atmosphere and optics occurred. The realities for most IR cameras are the following:

- They only detect a very small percentage of the overall energy emitted.
- Many detectors and optics do not have a combined flat response over their bandwidth.
- As the temperature of the object changes, the percentage of energy falling in the particular camera bandwidth changes.

The net result is that as the temperature of the surface of an object increases the resultant detector signal response may be a function of that temperature, ranging from a linear to a power function. Table 9.1 shows the band radiance (in units of watts per square meter per steradian) for a blackbody at temperatures of 0°C, 20°C, and 40°C for three different wavelength ranges. It is clear that as the temperature of the body increases, the radiance emitted over each wave band also increases, but with deviations from linearity. Note that the power emitted in the near waveband is extremely low at these near-ambient temperatures.

The larger percentage increase in signal in the mid-wave band versus the long-wave is one of the reasons that there are many reports that mid-wave cameras produce images having "more contrast" than those taken of an identical object with a long-wave camera (see Fig. 9.8). The reason for this is that the temperature difference is the same, but the image appears to have more contrast because the signal is increasing at a faster rate in the mid-wave case. This occurs because mid-wave (2 μm to 5.6 μm) cameras (looking at objects at temperatures of less than about 250°C, 523 K) are concentrated on the left side (the steep slope) of the peak of the Planck curves, while long-wave (7.5 μm to 15 μm) cameras are concentrated on the right side (the gentle slope) of the peak of Planck curves (see Fig. 9.9).

**Table 9.1.** Radiance across three wave bands for a blackbody at temperatures of 0°C, 20°C, and 40°C, with the percentage increases in radiated power

| Temperature | Near wave (0.8 μm–2 μm) | | Mid wave (2 μm–5.6 μm) | | Long wave (7.5 μm–15 μm) | |
|---|---|---|---|---|---|---|
| | *Band radiance, W m$^{-2}$ sr$^{-1}$* | *% Increase* | *Band radiance, W m$^{-2}$ sr$^{-1}$* | *% Increase* | *Band radiance, W m$^{-2}$ sr$^{-1}$* | *% Increase* |
| 0°C (273 K) | $1.1 \times 10^{-6}$ | | 1.5 | | 42.5 | |
| 20°C (293 K) | $7.5 \times 10^{-6}$ | 581% | 3.1 | 107% | 59.5 | 40% |
| 40°C (313 K) | $3.9 \times 10^{-5}$ | 420% | 5.9 | 90% | 80.3 | 35% |

Note: Data calculated at http://www.spectralcalc.com.

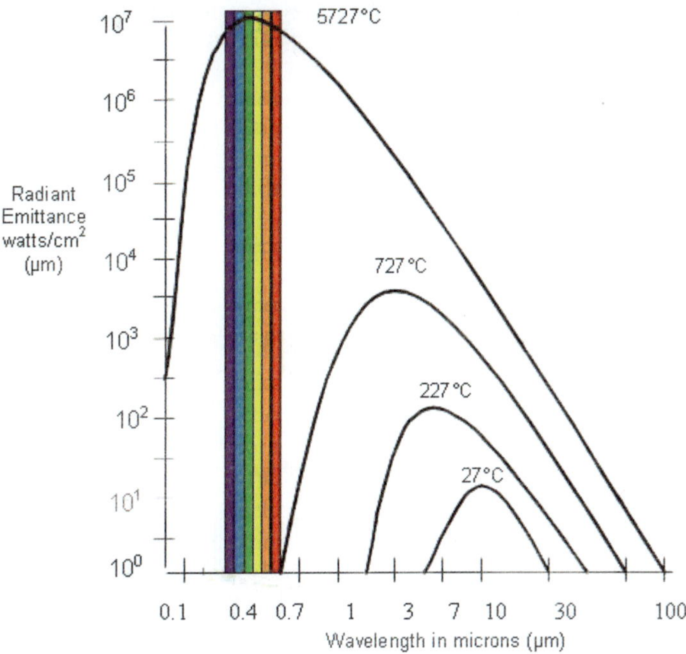


**Figure 9.9.** Planck radiation curves of a perfect emitter (blackbody).

Unfortunately it is not as straightforward as curve-fitting the response in Figure 9.9. Generally the mathematical model used is of the form blackbody signal equals some function of the object temperature, $f(T)$, as shown in equation 9.3. Since camera manufacturers calibrate IR instruments against blackbody simulators, and temperature must be measured on real bodies, taking emissivity and reflected background into account, the basic formula to correct for temperature becomes

$$Signal = \varepsilon f(T_{object}) + (1 - \varepsilon)f(T_{background}). \tag{9.3}$$

But what mathematical function best describes the $f(T)$ relationship? Should it be linear, exponential, a polynomial, or something else? Depending on how wide a temperature range is required, any of these functions could provide a good curve fit. To cover the entire temperature range of a detector, however, a complex equation has to be used. As an example, the following curve-fit equation was published by AGEMA (now FLIR Systems) in its Thermovision® 900 Series operating manuals:

$$Camera\ Signal = R/(e^{[B/T]} - F), \tag{9.4}$$

where $T$ is the absolute blackbody temperature in kelvin, $R$ is a response factor, $B$ is a spectral factor, and $F$ is a shape factor.

Typically a camera manufacturer will measure the camera signal against a series of blackbody temperatures and a best fit of their specific mathematical model will be used. In the previous case, a unique value for $R$ and $F$ is calculated since the spectral factor will be determined by the midpoint of the spectral response for that model of camera. While best-fit formulas like this have evolved and been perfected over the years by various manufacturers, it is illustrative of the empirical, rather than theoretical, nature of instrument calibration.

### 9.4.3. CURRENT CHALLENGES

As indicated previously, details of the methods for conversion from signal to temperature remain in the realm of the manufacturers' proprietary information. As they strive to produce instruments of higher measurement accuracy (currently evolving to values better than ±2°C or ±2%), they are maintaining proprietary control of their signal data conversion algorithms, and hence their software. For example, one manufacturer has sold more than fifteen different software programs, most of which had data formats not directly compatible with each other, and some that could not even be converted with a utility. Some view this as positive marketing, maintaining control over the customer base and increasing profit margins on camera sales by selling high-priced software. Yet this philosophy is inhibiting the development and growth of generic specialty analysis software, especially for medical, electrical apparatus, machine, and building diagnostics.

The need for a certain degree of proprietary control of signal conversion is recognized, and probably essential. But if the industry is to mature, a universal standard 14-bit image format needs to be developed, allowing users to have generic software analysis capability in order to change values of emissivity, background, and optical transmission. Only then will powerful industry-wide software analysis tools emerge.

## 9.5. INSTRUMENTS FOR IR RADIATION

There are essentially two types of IR instruments: spot thermometers (sometimes known as "single-point" devices) and portable IR thermal imaging cameras (IR radiometers).

### 9.5.1. INFRARED THERMOMETERS

Infrared spot radiometers measure the energy radiated from a small area of the object using a sensor, such as a micromachined thermopile, and convert this energy into temperature. For example, the ear is an easily accessible site for temperature measurement because the eardrum shares the same blood supply as the temperature control center in the brain, the hypothalamus. Thus it can reflect changes in core body temperature without a significant time lag. However, the accuracy of the measurement can be affected by instrument drift or errors, spot size, emissivity, and ambient changes such as temperature and convection. The typical accuracy of an ear (tympanic membrane) thermometer is ±0.2°C (see Chapter 1 for further details). A spot radiometer aimed at a moving object will create a temperature profile (in time) along the object. The measurement resolution for spot radiometers is almost always given as a ratio of distance to spot size. Typically 30:1 or 60:1 work well for general use. Radiometers without a sighting device, or only a single projected laser spot to define the measurement region, are less reliable.

The advantages of spot radiometers are the following:

- Small size
- Single output, making emissivity compensation easier

- Low data rates, which are easy to process
- Controls that are easy to interface
- Stable, proven, rugged technology with tens of thousands of installed units
- Narrow FOV, making it easy to install into sight tubes
- Low cost

The limitations of such devices are the following:

- The measurement only covers one spot.
- Response times are slow.
- There are no overall indications of temperature variances on an object.

## 9.5.2. INFRARED RADIOMETERS

Infrared radiometers, commonly known as IR thermal imagers, are instruments for detecting and measuring spectral radiance from a surface and displaying the results as a two-dimensional temperature distribution. IR radiometers measure the spectral radiance that leaves a surface and passes through the atmosphere and the camera optics to eventually impinge on the radiation detector.

As outlined in section 9.4.2, to transform the signal from the detector to an accurate surface temperature reading requires a mathematical model involving four fundamental considerations:

- Calibration against known radiant sources (blackbodies) over the entire detector temperature range
- Empirical modeling of detector/optics/atmosphere response within a specific spectral range
- Subtraction of the signal due to background irradiance
- Correction of the signal to that equivalent to a blackbody (see Fig. 9.10)

A number of IR radiometers exist, some offering similar performance characteristics. The design of thermal imaging cameras has moved away from earlier mechanical scanning technology to fixed focal plane arrays (FPAs), as outlined in section 9.5.3. More recently the uncooled microbolometer detector has become a popular option (and is also described later). Table 9.2 lists some of the advantages and disadvantages of cooled and uncooled IR radiometers.

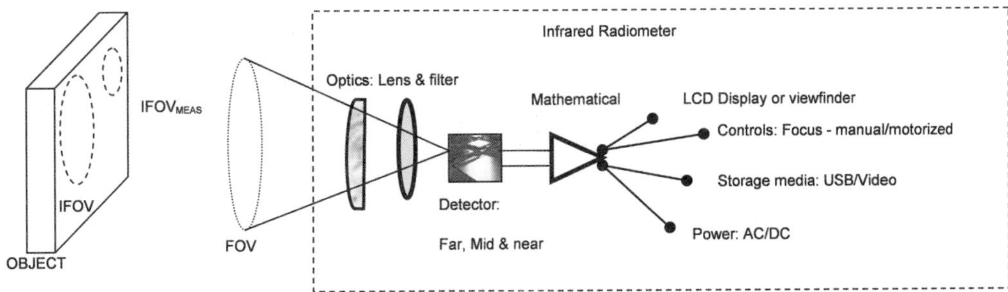


**Figure 9.10.** Propagation of electromagnetic radiation from object to detector and subsequent signal processing in an IR radiometer (FOV, field of view).

**Table 9.2.** Radiometer types with cooled and uncooled detectors

| | Cooled detector | Uncooled detector |
|---|---|---|
| Advantages | Less weight because of a reduction in mechanical parts (no mechanical scanner): more portable, lighter, reliable, and with improved battery life; Excellent resolution (dependent on the number of pixels); Generally have fast frame rates of 30 Hz to 60 Hz. | Mechanical simplicity; Improved reliability of camera: no cooling required. |
| Disadvantages | Complex, expensive detector arrays with multiplexing electronics; Detector needs cooling; Startup time—cooler has to work hard to attain low temperatures because of the larger mass of detector material. | Internal temperature stability; Compensation required for internal thermal noise; Fill factors can be as low as 40%. |

The selection and purchase of an IR radiometer for medical applications requires consideration of the capability and suitability of the instrument to perform the desired task, which is to accurately measure (and with high levels of thermal and spatial sensitivity) temperature differences across the skin surface. To accomplish this, a number of technical specifications need to be understood:

- The *noise equivalent temperature difference* (NETD) is defined as the temperature difference that will produce a signal-to-noise ratio (SNR) of unity. It describes the system's electronic noise, which for a given signal will vary depending on the temperature of the object.
- The *instantaneous field of view* (IFOV), also known as spatial resolution, can be expressed as the angle given by the ratio of the projected size of a pixel, or the smallest detectable target, divided by the distance to the target (usually described as parts of a degree or milliradians).

There are many others, such as minimum detectable temperature (MDT), thermal resolution, accuracy, frame rate and nonuniformity correction.

### 9.5.3. FOCAL PLANE ARRAYS IN IR RADIOMETERS

As mentioned previously, in thermal imaging cameras the multielement electronically scanned FPA has replaced systems using a very small number of detector elements and mechanical image scanning. Sometimes called a "staring array," this term refers specifically to the use of array detectors, each detector element of which looks at one point of the total image projected onto the FPA by the optical train, as illustrated in Figure 9.11.

#### 9.5.3.1. The Development of Detector Arrays for Thermal Imaging Cameras

Historically detector arrays evolved as follows:

- First generation (during the 1960s)—scan-to-image scanning systems
- Second generation (during the 1970s)—electronically scanned "staring" systems with FPAs
- Third generation (currently)—multicolor detectors sensing IR radiation in more than one spectral band (Anbar, 1995) and on-chip functionality in the 1990s

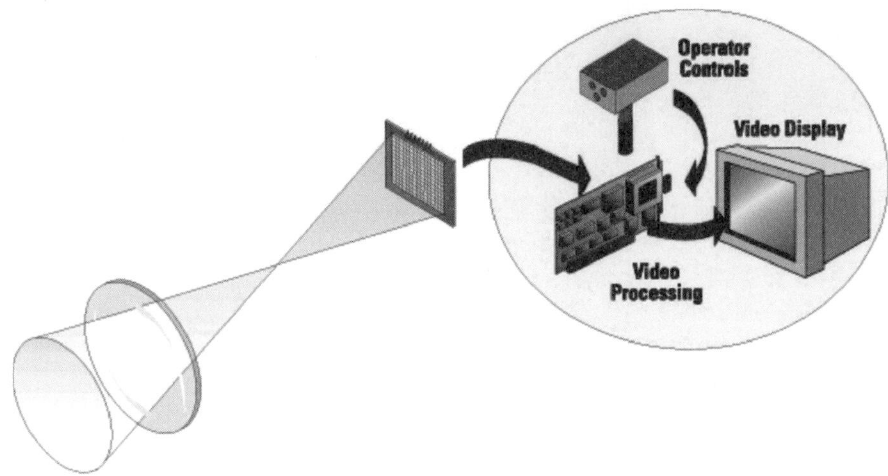


**Figure 9.11.** Principle of the FPA.

Figure 9.12, as described by Rogalski (2009), is a useful guide to these stages and illustrates key developments in the adoption of various IR detector materials.

The spatial resolution, and ultimately the picture quality, is determined not only by the number of pixels within the detector array, but more importantly, by the physical size of each detector. The ratio of active IR sensing surface area to inactive area surrounding each detector in an FPA is known as the fill factor. Higher fill factor detectors typically exhibit better sensitivity and lower power consumption. There are a number of FPA formats currently available:

- Low resolution—160 pixels × 120 pixels (19,200 pixels)
- Medium resolution—320 pixels × 240 pixels (76,800 pixels) uncooled or 256 pixels × 256 pixels (65,536 pixels) cooled
- High resolution—640 pixels × 480 pixels (307,200 pixels) uncooled or 640 pixels × 512 pixels (327,680 pixels) cooled

Larger formats are now appearing. A 512 pixel × 512 pixel PtSi FPA has been fabricated using charge-coupled device and complementary metal oxide semiconductor (CCD/CMOS) technology that has high performance and good pixel-to-pixel uniformity. Typical pitches between pixels are in the range of 20 μm to 50 μm. Lack of uniformity of the detector elements across the array can affect performance, and individual pixel response characteristics can differ considerably across the array. Therefore pixel correction is required prior to forming the final camera image. This involves calibrating each individual pixel by exposing the array to calibrated surfaces of known temperature.

## 9.6. THERMOGRAPHIC CAMERA SENSORS

### 9.6.1. DETECTOR TYPES AND FIGURES OF MERIT

Thermal sensitivity/resolution, or NETD, is considered to be one of the most useful measurement parameters in medical thermography, particularly with reference to measuring small temperature

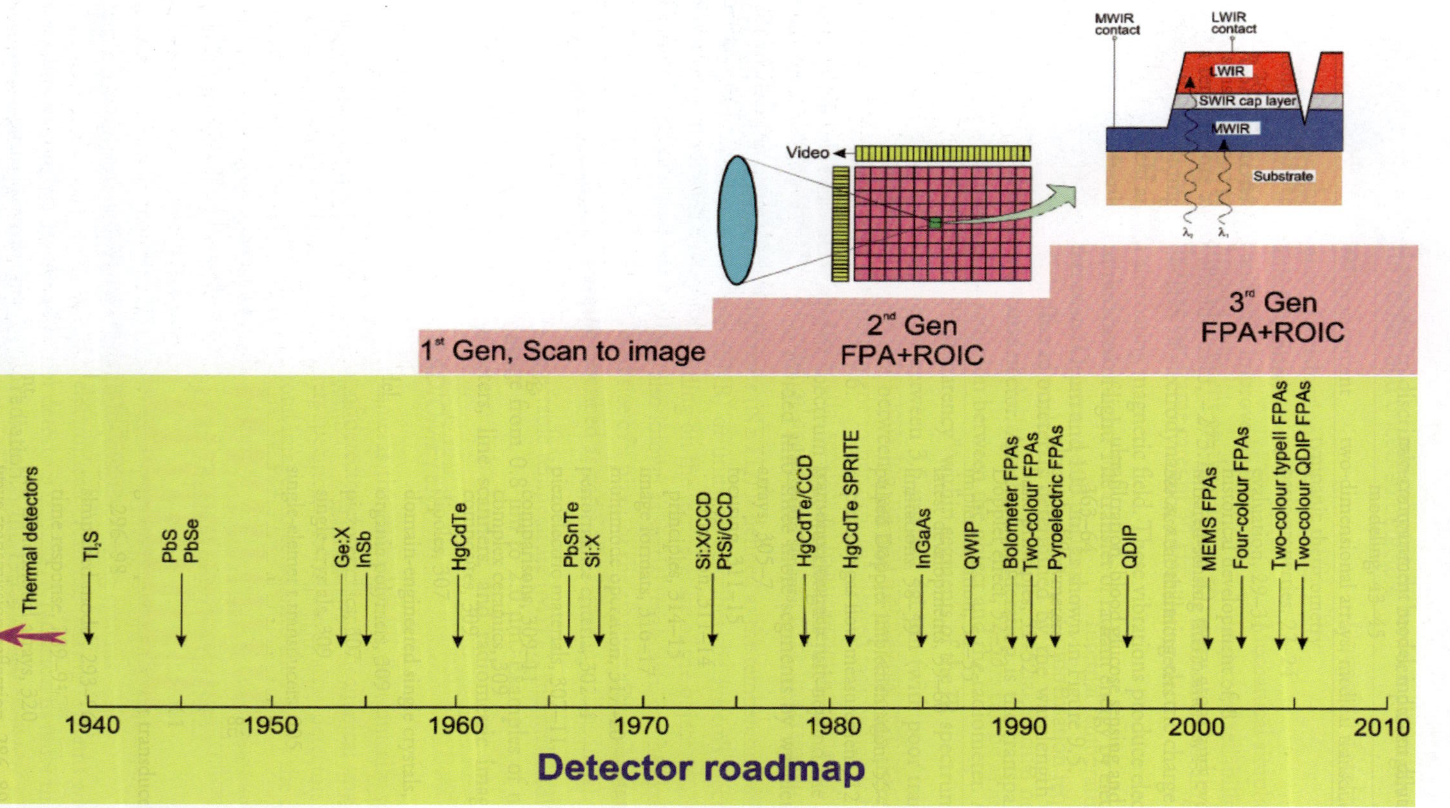


**Figure 9.12.** The evolution of the FPA and a time line for developments in the adoption of detector materials (ROIC, readout integrated circuit; from Rogalski, 2009).

differences on the skin surface. It is a measure of the performance of the detector and processing electronics. Grenn (1996) measured the NETD for first- and second-generation IR cameras (mechanical scanners and FPAs) from the analog video outputs with wide FOV optics and found that the new detectors reveal a tenfold increase in sensitivity. There is no single figure of merit that measures the quality of an IR image, but NETD has been widely adopted.

Most IR detectors operate using quantum mechanical interactions between incident photons and electrons in the detector material. They can take several different forms depending on the particular mechanisms involved. However, in all thermographic systems, the type of detector used to convert the incident radiation into a meaningful signal ultimately shapes the functionality of the IR camera. The actual detector used depends on the wavelengths to be detected.

Infrared detectors can be divided into two groups: thermal detectors and photon (quantum) detectors.

## 9.6.2. THERMAL DETECTORS

The operation of thermal detectors relies on a two-step process. The absorption of IR radiation in these detectors raises the temperature of the device, which in turn changes some temperature-dependent parameter, for example, electrical conductivity. The major advantage of thermal detectors is that they can operate at room temperature, but their sensitivity is lower and response time longer (several milliseconds) than for photon detectors. Nevertheless, this makes thermal detectors suitable for FPA operation, where the latter two properties are less critical.

The most important of the thermal detectors is the microbolometer, which absorbs thermal energy over a range of wavelengths and does not require cryogenic cooling, even when operating in the far IR. The uncooled microbolometer array has a tiny absorptive, temperature-sensitive element that is thermally linked to a temperature reference in vacuum. Each pixel detector element is free standing "in the air," supported only by two thin legs at each side, as shown in Figure 9.13. As IR radiation is absorbed,

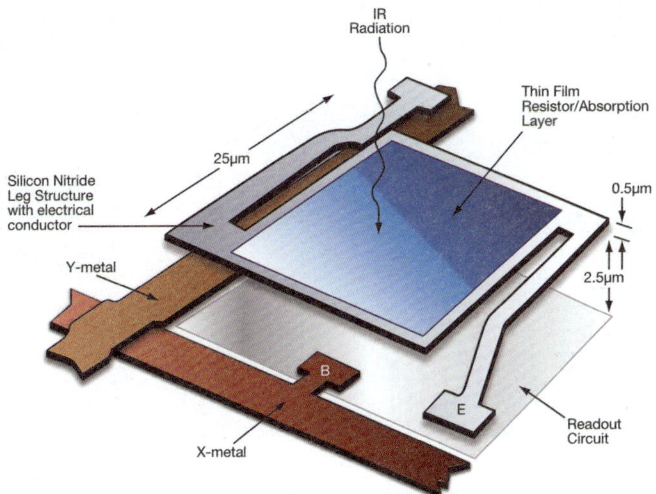


**Figure 9.13.** Basic structure of an uncooled microbolometer camera pixel. Courtesy of Electrophysics, with permission.

the temperature of the element increases. Sensing this temperature change provides a measure of the incident IR power level. The microbolometer output is the change in conductivity (which is relatively easy to measure) for each pixel in the array, and these data are transferred out for processing using the integrated readout circuit. The system is very gain stable, direct current (DC) coupled, and radiometric.

Although microbolometers provide very good linearity and gain stability, the radiation from internal parts can be as much as ten times higher than the object radiation. However, any effects arising from this can be minimized by the use of advanced automatic temperature compensation systems based on accurate internal temperature sensors, a temperature reference, and a neural network algorithm in the signal-processing electronics.

The general trend seems to be that microbolometers are being increasingly utilized, particularly for low-cost industrial applications.

There are other, less important classes of thermal detectors. Ferroelectric and pyroelectric sensors sense changes in capacitor charge, and being alternating current (AC) coupled, need chopper systems in the radiation path. Since it is difficult to get a flat radiometric response across the detector waveband, these detectors are not commonly used today in biomedicine, although there was some use of low-resolution pyroelectric systems in the 1990s prior to the widespread availability of uncooled microbolometer devices (Darton & Black, 1991; see Fig. 9.14).

## 9.6.3. PHOTON DETECTORS

In contrast to thermal detectors, all photon detectors (or quantum detectors) convert radiation directly to an electrical signal. For example, the absorption of far-IR radiation results directly in some specific quantum events, such as the photoelectric emission of electrons from a surface or electronic interband transitions in semiconductor materials. In the latter case, when IR photons impinge on the photon detector, electrons are excited from the valence band across an energy gap into the conduction band,

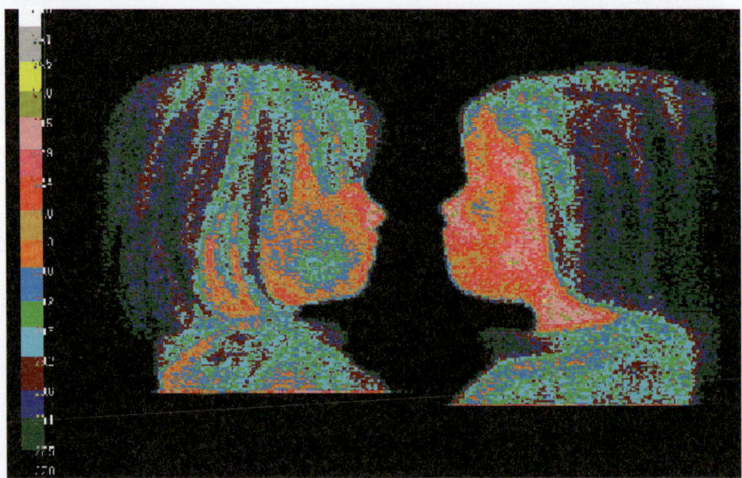

**Figure 9.14.** Skin inflammation at the left side of the face (STARSIGHT pyroelectric imager, Insight Vision Systems, Great Malvern, UK; deuterated triglycerine sulfate detector, 8 µm to 14 µm; from Martini et al., 2002).

provided the photon energy exceeds that of the gap. The output of photon detectors is governed by the rate of absorption of photons, not directly by the photon energy.

At room temperature, all electrons possess significant thermal energy, and some are excited into the conduction band where they contribute to the signal as a noise current. Also, as the temperature increases, progressively more electrons have sufficient energy to make the transition from the valence to the conduction band, giving a larger noise current. This is called the dark current. When its magnitude is comparable to that of the signal current, it defines the lower limit of usefulness of the sensor. If the detector is cooled down to cryogenic temperatures, few electrons have sufficient thermal energy to jump the gap to the conduction band. The result is a very significant reduction in the unwanted noise current. For this reason it is usual to cool the detector down to cryogenic temperatures (77 K with liquid nitrogen, or 4 K with liquid helium) to reduce any excessive dark current. The result is improved performance with smaller response times, but at the expense of larger detector assemblies. Photon detectors are very sensitive and stable, but they need cooling.

There are two types of photon detector, characterized by the response of the semiconductor material to interactions with photons of the radiation: photoconductive (generates free carriers in a semiconductor that in turn increase the conductivity), and photovoltaic (generates a potential difference across a p-n junction or a small current through it, depending on the load applied). However, in some materials (e.g., PtSi), the junction is a Schottky barrier type.

### 9.6.3.1. Photoconductive Detectors

The operation of photoconductive detectors is based on the direct generation of electron-hole pairs of charge carriers by incident photons in a semiconductor. The photons must be sufficiently energetic to excite an electron across the energy gap. These free charge carriers increase the conductivity of the device material and provide a means of measuring the rate of photon absorption. The current–voltage characteristics of photoconductive devices are symmetric with respect to the polarity of the applied voltage. Typical photoconductive detector materials include MCT, InSb, lead sulfide (PbS), and lead selenide (PbSe).

In most cases photoconductive detectors are cooled to cryogenic temperatures, although there are some exceptions where thermoelectric cooling to 200 K seems to be sufficient, as in 3 μm to 5 μm MCT detectors.

### 9.6.3.2. Photovoltaic Detectors

In a photovoltaic detector, IR radiation is incident on a semiconductor diode with a p-n or Schottky junction. The latter is a metal–semiconductor junction with rectifying characteristics similar to those of a p-n junction, but with a lower junction voltage. If the photons have sufficient energy, an electron is excited from the valence band into the conduction band, leaving behind a hole that can also contribute to conduction. Photovoltaic detectors absorb photons to create electron-hole pairs across the p-n junction, where an internal potential barrier with a built-in electric field separates them. The presence of this electron-hole pair can be monitored as an electrical signal to provide IR detection.

Because of the diode junction, the current–voltage characteristics of photovoltaic devices exhibit rectifying behavior to the polarity of any applied voltage, in contrast to the symmetric behavior of photoconductive devices. However, these detectors are operated in the photovoltaic electrical mode in which zero external voltage bias is applied to the p-n junction and there is a parallel load resistor. The resistance of the load may vary from zero, when the output photocurrent is directly proportional to the irradiance incident on the detector, to infinity, when the voltage generated is logarithmically related to the irradiance.

Such photovoltaic devices can be manufactured as part of an array that includes a capacitor that stores a charge proportional to the incident radiation in a manner similar to that of a CCD. Typical photovoltaic detector materials include PtSi, MCT (or HgCdTe), and InSb.

### 9.6.3.2.1. Mid-IR and Far-IR Photon Detectors

Mid-wave photons have higher energies than far-IR photons and are more likely to excite electrons over the gap. Therefore the gap can be made wider; this means that the detector does not need to be cooled down as much as for far-IR photons. A common detector material used in the mid wave is PtSi, while quantum well-type detectors are used in the far IR (see section 9.8).

A PtSi photon detector with a Stirling cycle engine cooler from a mid-wave IR radiometer (Inframetrics SC1000) is shown in Figure 9.15.

Detectors with band gap energies small enough to respond to longer wave IR radiation (8 µm to 12 µm region) must be cooled to cryogenic temperatures between 77 K and 25 K to eliminate thermally generated carriers. To maintain these temperatures, the detector must be enclosed in a vacuum housing called a dewar, with a suitable window transparent at the required IR wavelengths.

## 9.7. WAVELENGTH DEPENDENCE OF DETECTOR RESPONSES

Almost all IR detectors are wavelength sensitive. Figure 9.16 shows the variation with wavelength of the responses of three detectors, two photon types—PtSi and gallium arsenide (GaAs) quantum well IR photodetector (QWIP; see section 9.8)—along with a thermal type, a microbolometer. The detectors have different response profiles, with maximum responses at differing wavelengths. Interestingly, in the far-IR range, both the GaAs and microbolometer peak at 8.5 µm, while the mid-IR PtSi detector peaks at 3.5 µm.

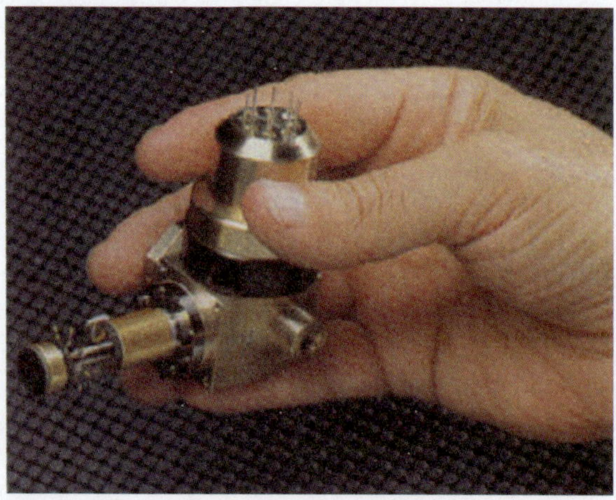

**Figure 9.15.** Platinum silicide photon detector with Stirling cooler. Courtesy of Inframetrics with permission.

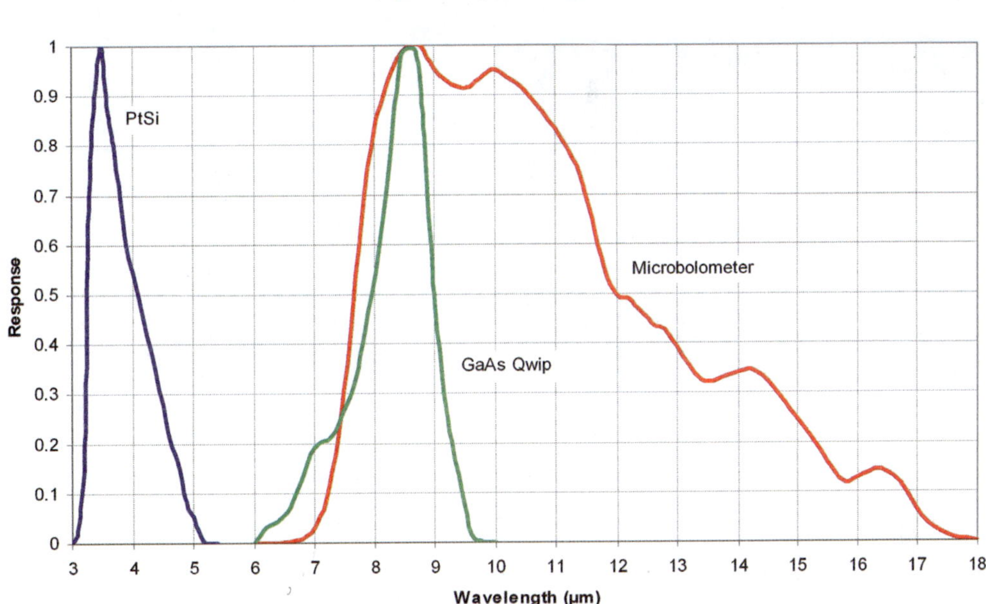


**Figure 9.16.** Detector response curves. Courtesy of FLIR Systems, with permission.

## 9.8. QUANTUM WELL IR PHOTODETECTORS

The QWIP is a more recent and particularly useful type of detector. These devices consist of quantum wells in semiconductor material where the resultant electronic levels can be tailored to absorb radiation in the 3 μm to 20 μm wavelength region. Given special grating structures, they can achieve a high quantum efficiency. Figure 9.17 illustrates the grating structure and the increase in responsivity with the grating.

Some typical characteristics associated with QWIPs are a thermal sensitivity of 20 mK at 30°C, a spatial resolution of 1.1 mrad, real-time 14-bit digital output, and data acquisition rates up to 900 Hz (via reduction in spot size area), often with a minimum 320 pixels × 240 pixels (76,800 detectors) FPA.

The FPAs of QWIPs require cooling using miniature Stirling coolers, normally operating between 70 K and 75 K.

Table 9.3 compares the characteristics of a QWIP with those of detectors made with two other materials, MCT and InSb.

## 9.9. CONTACT THERMOGRAPHY

Liquid crystal sensors for temperature became available in usable form in the 1960s (see Chapter 1). Originally they were painted on the skin, which had previously been coated with black paint. Three or four colors became visible if the paint was at the critical temperature range for the subject. Microencapsulation of these substances, primarily cholesteric esters, resulted in plastic sheet detectors. Later these sheets

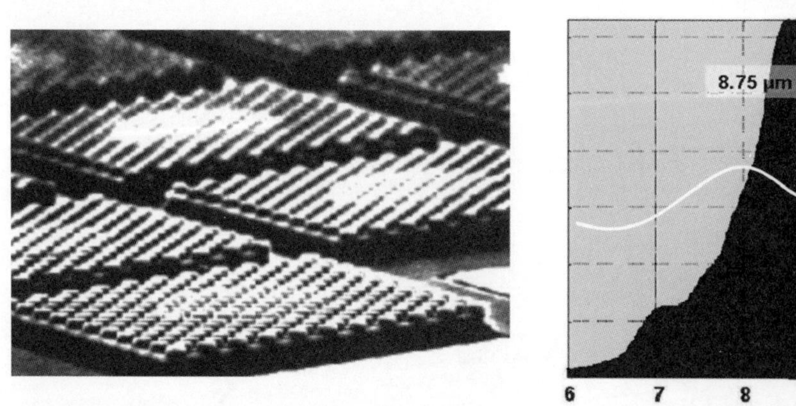


**Figure 9.17.** Photomicrograph of a QWIP detector array with grating (SC 3000) and its spectral response curves. Courtesy of FLIR Systems, with permission.

**Table 9.3.** Characteristics of three different detector materials

|  | QWIP (AlGaAs/GaAs/InGaAs) | MCT | InSb |
|---|---|---|---|
| Wavelength | Mid IR/far IR | Mid IR/far IR | Mid IR |
| NETD | <20 mK | 20 mK | 20 mK |
| Uniformity | Good | Bad | Good |
| Optics | Si/Ge | Si/Ge | Si |
| Cooling | 70 K | 77 K | 77 K |
| Operability | High | Good | Good |

were mounted on a soft latex base to mold to the skin under air pressure using a cushion with a rigid, clear window. Polaroid photography was then used to record the color pattern while the sensor remained in contact with the skin. The system was reusable and inexpensive. However, sensitivity declined over 1 to 2 years from manufacture, and many different pictures were required to obtain a subjective pattern of skin temperature (Flesch, 1984). This technique is no longer in common use because it cannot compete with the highly efficient modern IR imaging systems that are available today.

## 9.10. MEDICAL THERMOGRAMS ILLUSTRATING ADVANCES IN IMAGE QUALITY

Examples of medical thermal images are shown in Figure 9.18: an early single-detector, mechanically scanned AGA camera image and a modern image taken with a microbolometer FPA camera. It is evident that the quality of the modern image is very much improved compared with the image obtained in 1984.

## 9.11. THE FUTURE

Advances in IR detector technology continue. Overall, modern imaging systems offer great improvements in image quality and stable performance. Computing and image processing power continues

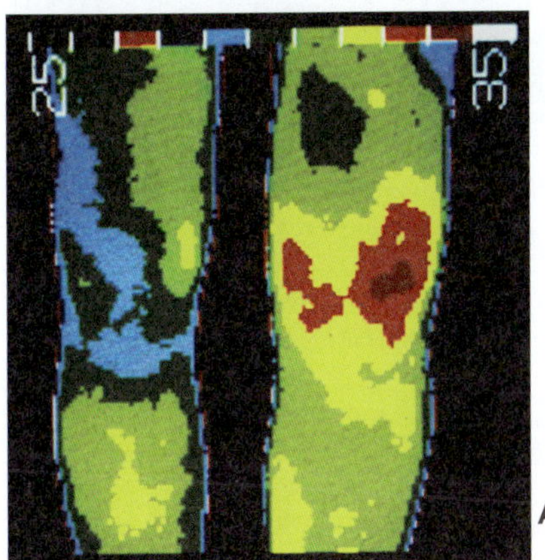
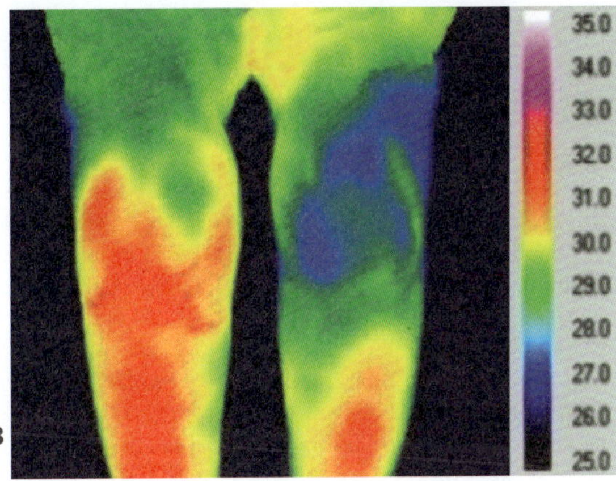

**Figure 9.18.** (a) A knee thermogram (hot area showing inflammatory arthritis) recorded with an AGEMA 782 (1984), mechanically scanned, single-element, InSb detector cooled by liquid nitrogen (3 μm to 5 μm). (b) Inflammatory arthritis affecting one knee, recorded by a FLIR SC500 (2002), 320 pixel × 240 pixel FPA uncooled microbolometer (7 μm to 13 μm). It has a spatial resolution (IFOV) of 1.3 mrad and a thermal sensitivity at 50 Hz to 60 Hz of 0.08°C at 30°C.

to develop, with major advantages for thermal imaging and its many applications. It is envisaged that future IR detectors will have higher spatial and thermal resolution, a reduced need for cooling, and lower cost.

The move to increased array sizes with higher pixel densities will achieve some of these goals, particularly with reference to higher spatial resolution. Higher thermal resolution will allow identification of the smallest of temperature differences required in medicine (Abedin et al., 2004; Norton et al., 2006; Thomas, 1999).

## REFERENCES


Abedin, M. N., Refaat, T. F., Bhat, I., Xiao, Y., Bandara, S., & Gunapala, S. D. (2004). Progress of multicolor single detector array development for remote sensing. *Proceedings SPIE, 5543*, 239–247.

Ammer, K., & Ring, E. F. J. (2008). Standard procedures for infrared imaging in medicine (pp. 22-1–22-14). In: N. A. Diakides & J. D. Bronzino (Eds.), *Medical infrared imaging*. Boca Raton, FL: CRC Press.

Anbar, M. (1995). Uses of infrared multiple wavelength cameras in clinical thermology (pp. 50–55). In: K. Ammer & E. F. J. Ring (Eds.), *The thermal image in medicine and biology*. Vienna, Austria: Uhlen-Verlag.

Bacon, P. A., Ring, E. F. J., & Collins, A. J. (1977). Thermography in the assessment of anti-rheumatic agents (pp. 105–110). In: *Rheumatoid arthritis: Assessment.* J. L. Gordon & B. L. Hazleman (Eds.). Amsterdam, Netherlands: Elsevier Biochemical.

Darton, K., & Black, C. M. (1991). Pyroelectric vidicon thermography and cold challenge quantify the severity of Raynaud's phenomenon. *British Journal of Rheumatology, 30*, 190–195.

Elliott, C. T. (1981). New detector for thermal imaging systems. *Electronics Letters, 17*, 312.

Engel, J. M., Cosh, J. A., Ring, E. F. J., Page-Thomas, D. P., & Van Waes, P. (1979). Thermography in locomotor diseases: Recommended procedure. *European Journal of Rheumatology and Inflammation, 2*, 299–306.

Flesch, U. (1984). Thermographic techniques with liquid crystals in medicine (pp. 283–299). In: E. F. J. Ring & B. Phillips (Eds.), *Recent advances in medical thermology*. New York, NY: Plenum.

Grenn, M. W. (1996). Recent advances in portable infrared imaging systems. *Proceedings of the 18th International Conference of the IEEE Engineering in Medicine and Biology Society, 5*, 2083–2084.

Hardy, J. D. (1934). The radiation of heat from the human body. III. The human skin as a black-body radiator. *Journal of Clinical Investigation, 13*(4), 615–620.

Houdas, Y., & Ring, E. F. J. (1982). *Human body temperature, its measurement and regulation.* New York, NY: Plenum.

Lloyd Williams, K. (1969). Thermography in the prognosis of cancer. *Bibliotheca Radiologica, 5*, 62–67.

Martini, G., Murray, K. J., Howell, K. J., Harper, J., Atherton, D., Woo, P., . . . & Black, C. M. (2002). Juvenile-onset localized scleroderma activity detection by infrared thermography. *Rheumatology (Oxford), 41*, 1178–1182.

McIntosh, G. B., & Thomas, R. A. (2009). Infrared camera signal conversion to temperature. *Thermology International, 19*(3), 70–72.

Norton, P. R., Horn, S. B., Pellegrino, J. G., & Perconti, P. (2006). Infrared detectors and detector arrays (pp. 37-1–37-25. In: J. D. Bronzino (Ed.), *The biomedical engineering handbook (3rd ed.): Medical devices and systems.* Boca Raton, FL: CRC Press.

Ring, E. F. J. (1995). The history of thermal imaging (pp. 13–20). In: K. Ammer & E. F. J. Ring (Eds.), *The thermal image in medicine & biology.* Vienna, Austria: Uhlen-Verlag.

Ring, E. F. J. (2000). The discovery of infrared radiation in 1800. *Imaging Science Journal, 48*, 1–8.

Ring, E. F. J., & Ammer, K. (2000). The technique of infrared imaging in medicine. *Thermology International, 10*(1), 7–14.

Ring, E. F. J., Engel, J. M., & Page-Thomas, D. P. (1984). Thermological methods in clinical pharmacology. *International Journal of Clinical Pharmacology, 22*(1), 20–24.

Rogalski, A. (2009). Multispectral infrared detector arrays. *Proceedings of the 8th Conference on Thermography and Thermometry in Practice*, Ustron, Poland, Politechnic University Lodz, Poland.

Sampaio, C., Visentin, M. T., Howell, K., Woo, P., & Harper, J. (2006). Morphoea (synonym: localized scleroderma) (pp. 2020–2029). In: J. Harper, A. Oranje, & N. Prose (Eds.), *Textbook of pediatric dermatology.* Oxford, England: Blackwell Publishing.

Thomas, R. A. (1999). *Thermography monitoring handbook.* Oxford, England: Coxmoor.

Wunderlich, C. A. (1871). *On the temperature in diseases. A manual of medical thermometry* (translation from German by W. Bathurst Woodman). London, England: New Sydenham Society.

## ABOUT THE AUTHORS

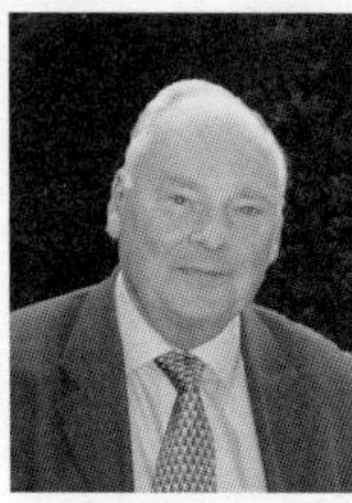

**Professor E. F. J. Ring** has been involved with infrared thermal imaging since 1959 and developed a system of quantification for the clinical research trials of new drugs used for the treatment of rheumatic diseases. He was awarded a Doctor of Science degree for this work by Bath University, United Kingdom, in 1995. As an author of over three-hundred papers and books and organizer of conferences in the United Kingdom and overseas, he was awarded a medal from the combined colleges of The Royal College of Medicine, The Royal College of Surgeons, and The Royal College of Obstetricians and Gynaecology in 2008. After retirement from the health service as head of medical imaging at the Royal National Hospital for Rheumatic Diseases in Bath, he has been head of the Medical Imaging Research Unit at The University of Glamorgan, United Kingdom, since 2001.

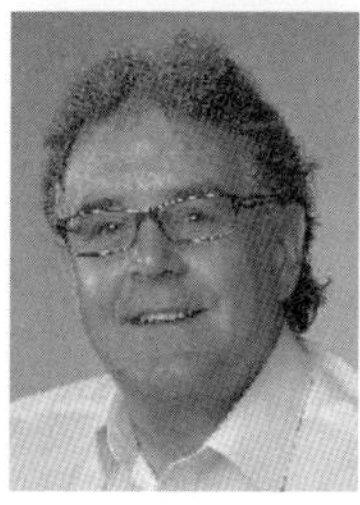

**Professor R. A. Thomas** has a PhD in infrared thermography and over twenty years' experience as an academic in the area of condition monitoring, including research fellowships in thermography at UK and South African universities. He is chairman and organizer of QRM, an International Biennial Nondestructive Testing Conference in Condition Monitoring, author of the *Thermography Monitoring Handbook*, and has contributed to *The Biomedical Engineering Handbook (3rd Edition)* and *Handbook of Non-Invasive Methods and the Skin (2nd Edition)*. He is technical editor of the journal *Thermology International* and guest editor of the journal *Quality and Reliability Engineering International*. Professor Thomas is a member of IEC/SC/65B/WG5 charged with the task of implementing the specification of infrared thermal imagers within medicine. He is a chartered engineer and fellow of the IET (formerly Institution of Electrical Engineers).

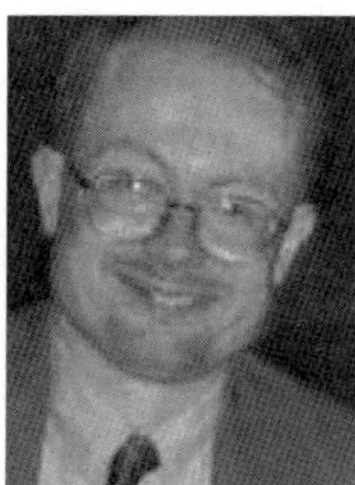

**Dr. Kevin Howell** is a clinical scientist at the Rheumatology Department of the Royal Free Hospital, London. He gained a BSc in physics from the University of Birmingham, United Kingdom, in 1991 and an MSc in medical electronics and physics from the University of London in 1995. In 2009 he completed a PhD at the University of Glamorgan on infrared thermography in rheumatology. Infrared research at the Royal Free is focussed on the detection of Raynaud's phenomenon from studying hand rewarming rates after cold challenges and the assessment of skin inflammation in childhood connective tissue disease. In his spare time Kevin is a tennis official who has worked as an umpire at numerous Davis Cup ties, the U.S. Open, and every Wimbledon Championship since 1991.

# Index